NEW PESTICIDES AND SOIL SENSORS

NEW PESTICIDES AND SOIL SENSORS

Nanotechnology in the Agri-Food Industry, Volume 10

Edited by

ALEXANDRU MIHAI GRUMEZESCU

Department of Science and Engineering of Oxide Materials and Nanomaterials, Faculty of Applied Chemistry and Materials Science, University Politehnica of Bucharest, Bucharest, Romania

ELSEVIER

ACADEMIC PRESS

An imprint of Elsevier

elsevier.com

Academic Press is an imprint of Elsevier
125 London Wall, London EC2Y 5AS, United Kingdom
525 B Street, Suite 1800, San Diego, CA 92101-4495, United States
50 Hampshire Street, 5th Floor, Cambridge, MA 02139, United States
The Boulevard, Langford Lane, Kidlington, Oxford OX5 1GB, United Kingdom

Library of Congress Cataloging-in-Publication Data
A catalog record for this book is available from the Library of Congress

British Library Cataloguing-in-Publication Data
A catalogue record for this book is available from the British Library

ISBN: 978-0-12-804299-1

Publisher: Nikki Levy
Acquisition Editor: Patricia Osborn
Editorial Project Manager: Jaclyn Truesdell
Production Project Manager: Caroline Johnson
Designer: Mark Rogers

Typeset by Thomson Digital

CONTENTS

LIST OF CONTRIBUTORS

Semra Akgönüllü
Hacettepe University, Department of Chemistry, Ankara, Turkey

Saad Alkahtani
King Faisal University, College of Agriculture and Food Sciences, Arid Land Agriculture Department, Al-Ahsa, Kingdom of Saudi Arabia

José Luis Alonso-Prados
National Institute for Agricultural and Food Research and Technology (INIA), DTEVPF, Plant Protection Products Unit, Madrid, Spain

Laxmi P. Bagri
Government Model Science College, Bose Memorial Research Laboratory, Department of Chemistry, Jabalpur, Madhya Pradesh, India

Anil Kumar Bajpai
Government Model Science College, Bose Memorial Research Laboratory, Department of Chemistry, Jabalpur, Madhya Pradesh, India

Paul Cătălin Balaure
University "Politehnica" of Bucharest, Faculty of Applied Chemistry and Materials Science, "Costin Nenitzescu" Department of Organic Chemistry, Bucharest, Romania

Nilay Bereli
Hacettepe University, Department of Chemistry, Ankara, Turkey

Ana R.J. Cabrita
REQUIMTE, LAQV, ICBAS, Institute of Biomedical Sciences Abel Salazar, University of Porto, Rua Jorge Viterbo Ferreira, Porto, Portugal

Mariana Carmen Chifiriuc
Faculty of Biology and Research Institute of the University of Bucharest - ICUB, University of Bucharest, Bucharest, Romania

Duygu Çimen
Hacettepe University, Department of Chemistry, Ankara, Turkey

Carmen Curutiu
Faculty of Biology and Research Institute of the University of Bucharest - ICUB, University of Bucharest, Bucharest, Romania

Ilda Czobor
Faculty of Biology and Research Institute of the University of Bucharest - ICUB, University of Bucharest, Bucharest, Romania

Adil Denizli
Hacettepe University, Department of Chemistry, Ankara, Turkey

Ali Derazshamshir
Hacettepe University, Department of Chemistry, Ankara, Turkey

Alka Dwevedi
University of Delhi, Sri Aurobindo College, South Campus, New Delhi, India

António J.M. Fonseca
REQUIMTE, LAQV, ICBAS, Institute of Biomedical Sciences Abel Salazar, University of Porto, Rua Jorge Viterbo Ferreira, Porto, Portugal

Nawal Gaafar
National Research Centre, Pests and Plant Protection Department, Dokki, Cairo, Egypt

Irina Gheorghe
Faculty of Biology and Research Institute of the University of Bucharest - ICUB, University of Bucharest, Bucharest, Romania

Jyotirmoy Ghosh
Banwarilal Bhalotia College, Chemistry Department, Asansol, West Bengal, India

Adriana Marcia Graboski
Department of Food Engineering, URI, Erechim, Erechim, Brazil

Dragoş Gudovan
University "Politehnica" of Bucharest, Faculty of Applied Chemistry and Materials Science, "Costin Nenitzescu" Department of Organic Chemistry, Bucharest, Romania

Iulia Gudovan
University "Politehnica" of Bucharest, Faculty of Applied Chemistry and Materials Science, "Costin Nenitzescu" Department of Organic Chemistry, Bucharest, Romania

John Hayles
The University of Adelaide, School of Chemical Engineering, Adelaide, SA, Australia

Josef Jampílek
Comenius University, Department of Pharmaceutical Chemistry, Faculty of Pharmacy, Bratislava, Slovakia

Lucas Johnson
The University of Adelaide, School of Chemical Engineering, Adelaide, SA, Australia

Arvind M. Kayastha
Banaras Hindu University, School of Biotechnology, Institute of Science, Varanasi, India

Ozcan Konur
Yildirim Beyazit University, Faculty of Engineering and Natural Sciences, Department of Materials Engineering, Keçiören Ankara, Turkey

Katarína Kráľová
Comenius University, Institute of Chemistry, Faculty of Natural Sciences, Bratislava, Slovakia

Pravita Kumar
University of Delhi, Sri Aurobindo College, South Campus, New Delhi, India

Promod Kumar
University of Delhi, Sri Aurobindo College, South Campus, New Delhi, India

Yogendra Kumar
University of Delhi, Sri Aurobindo College, South Campus, New Delhi, India

Veronica Lazar
Faculty of Biology and Research Institute of the University of Bucharest - ICUB, University of Bucharest, Bucharest, Romania

Fabio Lima Leite
Department of Physics Mathematics and Chemistry (DFMQ), Nanoneurobiophysics Research Group, Federal University of São Carlos (UFSCar), Sorocaba, Brazil

Carmen López-Goti
National Institute for Agricultural and Food Research and Technology (INIA), DTEVPF, Plant Protection Products Unit, Madrid, Spain

Dusan Losic
The University of Adelaide, School of Chemical Engineering, Adelaide, SA, Australia

Larisa Lvova
University "Tor Vergata," Department of Chemical Science and Technologies, Rome, Italy

Alexandra Manzoli
Department of Food Engineering, URI, Erechim, Erechim, Brazil

Luminita Marutescu
Faculty of Biology and Research Institute of the University of Bucharest - ICUB, University of Bucharest, Bucharest, Romania

Marina Nadporozhskaya
St. Petersburg State University, Faculty of Biology, St. Petersburg, Russia

Hugo M. Oliveira
REQUIMTE, LAQV, ICBAS, Institute of Biomedical Sciences Abel Salazar, University of Porto, Rua Jorge Viterbo Ferreira, Porto, Portugal

Marcela Popa
Research Institute of the University of Bucharest-ICUB, Bucharest, Romania

Prabhakaran Rajkumar
Madurai Kamaraj University, Department of Biochemistry, School of Biological Sciences, Madurai, Tamil Nadu, India

Tharmarajan Ramprasath
Madurai Kamaraj University, Department of Biochemistry, School of Biological Sciences, Madurai, Tamil Nadu, India; Georgia State University, Center for Molecular and Translational Medicine, Atlanta, GA, United States

Rajesh Kumar Saini
Government Model Science College, Bose Memorial Research Laboratory, Department of Chemistry, Jabalpur, Madhya Pradesh, India

Pilar Sandín-España
National Institute for Agricultural and Food Research and Technology (INIA), DTEVPF, Plant Protection Products Unit, Madrid, Spain

Crina Saviuc
Research Institute of the University of Bucharest-ICUB, Bucharest, Romania

Yeşeren Saylan
Hacettepe University, Department of Chemistry, Ankara, Turkey

Govindan Sadasivam Selvam
Madurai Kamaraj University, Department of Biochemistry, School of Biological Sciences, Madurai, Tamil Nadu, India

Beatriz Sevilla-Morán
National Institute for Agricultural and Food Research and Technology (INIA), DTEVPF, Plant Protection Products Unit, Madrid, Spain

Yogesh K. Sharma
University of Delhi, Swami Shraddhanand College, North Campus, New Delhi, India

Parames C. Sil
Bose Institute, Division of Molecular Medicine, Kolkata, West Bengal, India

Krishnendu Sinha
Bose Institute, Division of Molecular Medicine, Kolkata, West Bengal; Jhargram Raj College, Department of Zoology, Jhargram, West Bengal, India

Clarice Steffens
Department of Food Engineering, URI, Erechim, Erechim, Brazil

Juliana Steffens
Department of Food Engineering, URI, Erechim, Erechim, Brazil

Juan José Villaverde
National Institute for Agricultural and Food Research and Technology (INIA), DTEVPF, Plant Protection Products Unit, Madrid, Spain

Nabil El Wakeil
King Faisal University, College of Agriculture and Food Sciences, Arid Land Agriculture Department, Al-Ahsa, Kingdom of Saudi Arabia; National Research Centre, Pests and Plant Protection Department, Dokki, Cairo, Egypt

Clare Worthley
The University of Adelaide, School of Chemical Engineering, Adelaide, SA, Australia

Fatma Yılmaz
Abant İzzet Baysal University, Department of Chemistry Technology, Bolu, Turkey

SERIES FOREWORD

The emergence of nanotechnology has reached impressive heights in recent years and the development of special nanodevices and nanomaterials has found intriguing applications in agriculture and food sector. Most of the investigated nanotechnological approaches initially aimed to solve evolving problems in the agri-food industry in order to impact on the economic potential. Soon after the implementation of new technologies and approaches that were using nanostructured materials, the worldwide concern was rapidly extended to numerous applications that could be developed by using the science of nanosized materials. Smart materials, biosensors, packaging materials, nutraceuticals, and nanodevices have been designed to address numerous agri-food related issues with direct impact in health, economy, ecology, and industry. As the engineering of nanostructures has constantly progressed and extended its applications, there is virtually unlimited potential in this sector. However, the widely differing opinions on the applicability and usefulness of nanotechnology between both specialists and the general public has hampered progress. The main concern manifested by people is related to the potential risk for health and the environmental impact of the recently developed nanoengineered materials and devices. Therefore, current approaches are strictly considering these concerns when designing nanotechnological solutions for agriculture and food sectors.

This multivolume series was developed by the constant need to discover current inquiries and approaches on the field of agri-food science and also to learn about the most recent progress, approaches, and applications that have emerged through nanotechnology.

As agriculture is the backbone of most developing countries, nanotechnology has the potential to revolutionize the agriculture and food sector by promoting productivity through genetic improvement of plant and animal foods. It can also ensure the delivery of drugs, genes, and pesticides to specific sites at cellular levels in targeted plants and animals, by limiting side effects. Nanotechnology can be used to evaluate gene expression under different stress condition for both plant and animal foods through the development of nanoarray-based gene-technologies. Additionally, this technology can detect fertilizers, pesticides with high precision by smart nanosenors for an adequate management of the natural resources. Moreover, numerous industrial-related applications with direct impact on economy have emerged. For example, nano- and micro-structured arrays can detect the early presence of pathogens, contaminants, and food spoilage factors. Other applications for this technology are smart integration systems for food processing and packaging, as well as nanoemulsion-based decontaminants for food equipment and storage compartments, and nanoparticles that facilitate the bioavailability and delivery of nutrients directly to cells.

The potential benefits of nanotechnology for agriculture, food, fisheries, and aquaculture were identified and supported by many countries, which invested a significant amount of money in the development of applications. Also, numerous campaigns are currently trying to increase awareness on the developing process and recent technologies in order to influence the acceptance of customers. Although nanoagri-food industrialized concept could help to find a sustainable solution for the current global food crisis, the offered advantages should balance the concerns regarding soil, water, environment, and health related issues that such approach could bring.

The series entitled *Nanotechnology in the Agri-Food Industry* brings comprehensive and recent knowledge regarding the impact of the science of nanometer-sized materials on the field of agriculture and food industry, but also discuss the current inquiries regarding risks of these applications in all relevant fields such as environment and health, aiming to increase awareness to a wider amount of readers.

Dr Alina Maria Holban

Department of Microbiology and Immunology, Faculty of Biology, University of Bucharest, Romania

Dr Monica Cartelle Gestal

Harvill Lab, University Of Georgia, Athens, GA, United States

SERIES PREFACE

About the Series (Volumes I–X)

In a permanently changing society, health and well being remain the key drivers for the food industry. Despite the technological progress made in the agri-food industry, a true food crisis emerges in several areas of the globe. This can be explained by insufficient food but mostly by inadequate food for a very distinct range of consumers. In this context, innovative technologies represent the core throughout the whole food chain from raw materials/ingredient sourcing, food processing, quality control of finished products, and packaging. Nanotechnology, coupled with novel interdisciplinary approaches and processing methods, has enabled some important advances recently flourishing in many of these areas. The science of nanosized materials can improve and even resolve the huge challenges faced by the food and bioprocessing industries for developing and implementing systems that can produce qualitative and quantitative foods that are safe, sustainable, environment friendly, and efficient. This emerging tool finds its applications in various fields and represents an endless approach for the development of innovative strategies in food development, processing, and packaging.

This multivolume set aims to bring together the most recent and innovative applications of nanotechnology in the agri-food industry, but also to present the future perspectives in the design of new or alternative foods.

The series contains 200 chapters organized in 10 volumes, prepared by outstanding research groups that made significant impacts on the field of nanotechnology and food-related research sectors. This comprehensive set represents an updated and highly structured material for undergraduate and postgraduate students in food science, biotechnological, engineering fields, but also a valuable resource of recent scientific progress, along with most known applications of nanomaterials on the food industry to be used by researchers, engineers, and academia. Moreover, novel opportunities and ideas for developing or improving technologies in the agri-food industry by innovative companies, biotechnological industries, and other economical structures are highlighted and their potential is widely dissected. This series may be also valuable for the wide audience interested in recent nanotechnological progress in the agri-food field worldwide.

These 10 volumes cover almost all aspects related to the applications of *Nanotechnology in the Agri-Food Industry* and are named as:

Volume I Novel Approaches
Volume II Encapsulations
Volume III Emulsions
Volume IV Nutraceuticals
Volume V Nutrient Delivery
Volume VI Food Preservation
Volume VII Food Packaging
Volume VIII NanoBioSensors
Volume IX Water Purification
Volume X New Pesticides and Soil Sensors

Each volume contains 20 chapters, which were carefully composed and illustrated to highlight the most innovative and intensively investigated applications of nanotechnology on particular wide interest domains of the agri-food industry field.

Alexandru Mihai Grumezescu
*University Politehnica of Bucharest,
Department of Science and Engineering
of Oxide Materials and Nanomaterials,
Faculty of Applied Chemistry and
Materials Science, Bucharest, Romania
http://grumezescu.com/*

VOLUME PREFACE

Nanotechnology has the potential to make a huge impact on the agri-food sector, minimizing issues of current agricultural practices on environment and human health, improving food security and productivity, while promoting social and economic equity. The development of intelligent nanosystems has allowed for the immobilization of nutrients and their controlled release in soils, improved the uptake of nutrients by plants, mitigate eutrophication, improved the structure and function of pesticides by increasing solubility, enhanced resistance against hydrolysis and photodecomposition, provided a more specific and controlled-release toward target organisms, enhanced the water-holding capacity of soil, enabled sensitive biosensing, and may be used to absorb environmental contaminants.

Nanopesticides are intensively investigated for the potential benefits they could bring, which include the potential to increase efficacy and durability of a pesticide while at the same time reducing the amount of active ingredients and minimize or eliminate any potential hazards. In agriculture and soil science, nanosensors may be used to diagnose various soil diseases, contaminants, physicochemical quality, composition, but may be used in the same time as nanofertilizers able to deliver nutritive substances on the required areas or as decontaminating nanoagents, since they contain encapsulated suitable agents.

This book offers a wide and up-to-date perspective regarding the scientific and applicative progress that has been made in recent years in the design of pesticides, soil sensors, nanodetectors, and how the science of nanostructured materials impacted on the progress of agricultural practices in the last 20 years. Environmental, clinical, and economical related aspects of nanopesticides and new sensors are revealed and debated within the volume.

Volume X contains 19 chapters, prepared by outstanding international researchers from Brazil, Australia, Portugal, Spain, Italy, Slovakia, Czech Republic, Romania, Russia, Egypt, Saudi Arabia, India, and Turkey.

Irina Gheorghe et al., in Chapter 1, entitled *Lessons From Inter-Regn Communication for the Development of Novel, Ecofriendly Pesticides,* review the progress made in biopesticides development, focusing on microbial- and plant-derived products and in the field of chemical pesticides biodecontamination by using microbial enzymes.

Chapter 2, prepared by Krishnendu Sinha et al., entitled *New Pesticides: A Cutting-Edge View of Contributions From*

Nanotechnology for the Development of Sustainable Agricultural Pest Control, focus on how nanotechnology promises a breakthrough in refining our present understanding regarding the expansion of new-generation nanocides and safe carriers, nanotechnology-based biocides, and chemical pesticides. New ideas about nanotechnology-based surveillance and control of pests, diseases as well as insect pest management are also discussed.

In Chapter 3, entitled *Nanopesticides: Preparation, Targeting, and Controlled Release,* written by Josef Jampílek et al., the focus is on the methods of preparation of nanoengineered active ingredients, their formulation to nanocarriers for targeted biodistribution/controlled release and their biological effectiveness. Benefits and environmental risks of nanopesticides are also dissected.

Paul Cătălin Balaure et al., in Chapter 4, entitled *Nanopesticides: A New Paradigm in Crop Protection* describes how to overcome main drawbacks in crop production by using nanopesticide delivery systems. The most significant achievements in the field are illustrated by carefully selected up-to-date examples, in each case highlighting the superior performances of nanopesticides relative to their bulk counterparts in terms of selectivity, efficiency, and reduction of the harmful environmental impact.

Chapter 5, entitled *Nanopesticides: A Review of Current Research and Perspectives,* prepared by J. Hayles et al., gives an overview regarding the improvement of the water solubility of poorly soluble pesticide active ingredients to improve bioavailability, which involves formulation of the active ingredients into nanoemulsions and dispersions. Also, encapsulation of pesticide active ingredients within permeable nanoparticles are reviewed and discussed.

Juan José Villaverde, in Chapter 6, entitled *An Overview of Nanopesticides in the Framework of European Legislation* reviews the recent state of knowledge on nanopesticides, highlighting their physicochemical properties and analytical challenges that should be optimized or overcomed to allow their authorization in Europe.

Nabil El Wakeil et al., in Chapter 7, entitled *Is Nanotechnology a Promising Field for Insect Pest Control in IM Programs?,* provide impressive information about the effects of nanoparticles on insects and their impact in insect management, along with revealing potential effects on humans health and environment.

Luminita Marutescu et al., in Chapter 8, entitled *Botanical Pesticides With Virucidal, Bactericidal, and Fugicidal Activity,* review the main biopesticides of vegetal origin (plant extracts and essential oils) with virucidal, bactericidal, and fungicidal activity, while discussing their potential advantages and applications over classical pesticides.

Irina Gheorghe et al., in Chapter 9, entitled *Present and Perspectives in Pesticides Biosensors Development and Contribution of Nanotechnology*, present the current state and perspectives in the development of novel pesticides biosensors and the contribution of nanotechnology to the design of more sensitive and versatile sensors.

Carmen Curutiu et al., in Chapter 10, entitled *Pesticides and Antimicrobial Resistance: From Environmental Compartments to Animal and Human Infections*, summarize the aspects regarding bacterial resistance to pesticides and the impact of these substances in the emergence of antibiotic resistance in clinical strains.

Luminita Marutescu et al., in Chapter 11, entitled *Molecular Mechanisms of Pesticides Toxicity* summarize the molecular targets and mechanisms of pesticides toxicity, highlighting the main experimental models (cell cultures, invertebrates, nonmammalian or mammalian models) and methodological approaches currently utilized to investigate toxicity of pesticides.

Chapter 12, entitled *A Simple Whole Cell Microbial Biosensor to Monitor Soil Pollution*, prepared by Prabhakaran Rajkumar et al., explore the recent advances in bacterial biosensor and their implications in soil pollution management.

In Chapter 13, entitled *Flow Analysis as an Analytical Tool for Soil Monitoring: From Wet Chemistry Assays to Nanomaterials-Based Sample Preparation*, Hugo M. Oliveira et al., present the most recent contributions of flow analysis for the analysis of soils as follows: fundamentals of flow analysis and their major evolutions; the recent advances in the flow analysis-based methodologies for the analysis of nutrients and contaminants in soils, with a particular emphasis in the methodologies that incorporated the use of nanomaterials and the challenges and opportunities in the soil analysis field that result from the combination between flow analysis and nanomaterials.

Chapter 14, prepared by Rajesh Kumar Saini, entitled *Smart Nanosensors for Pesticides Detection*, presents state-of-the-art updates in the technology of pesticide biosensors and provide a critical evaluation of recent advances in this area and newer trends in biosensors such as tailor-designed biomolecules that include aptamers and molecularly imprinted polymers, optical, electrochemical, and piezoelectric materials.

Alka Dwevedi et al., in Chapter 15, entitled *Soil Sensors: Detailed Insight Into its Research Updates, Significance and Future Prospects*, entails all the recent development on soil sensors, obtained data analysis, and their applications in fields as well as their shortcomings.

Clarice Steffens et al., in Chapter 16, entitled *Nanosensors for Detection of Pesticides in Water*, highlight the structure, operation, and applicability of cantilevers nanossensors for pollutants in water. Also, this chapter presents the surface functionalization methods, the limits of detection and mechanism of pesticide recognition.

Chapter 17, entitled *Chemical Sensors for Soil Analysis: Principles and Applications*, prepared by Larisa Lvova et al., offer an up-to-date overview about the principles and selected application of chemical sensors and multisensory systems for the assessment of soils and main soil nutrition components detection performed over the last two decades.

Fatma Yılmaz et al., in Chapter 18, entitled *Surface Plasmon Resonance Based Nanosensors for Detection of Triazinic Pesticides in Agricultural Foods*, focused on the production of triazine pesticide imprinted surface plasmon resonance nanosensors and their impact in agriculture and food industry.

Chapter 19, entitled *Scientometric Overview in Nanopesticides*, prepared by Ozcan Konur, highlights important papers influencing the development of the research field of the newly emergent domain of nanopesticides and also determines the key research areas in the field of pesticides. The research in this field has strong public policy implications providing strong incentives for the key stakeholders involved in this field.

Alexandru Mihai Grumezescu
*University Politehnica of Bucharest,
Department of Science and Engineering
of Oxide Materials and Nanomaterials,
Faculty of Applied Chemistry and
Materials Science, Bucharest, Romania
http://grumezescu.com/*

1

LESSONS FROM INTER-REGN COMMUNICATION FOR THE DEVELOPMENT OF NOVEL, ECOFRIENDLY PESTICIDES

Irina Gheorghe*, Marcela Popa, Luminita Marutescu*, Crina Saviuc**, Veronica Lazar*, Mariana Carmen Chifiriuc***

**Faculty of Biology and Research Institute of the University of Bucharest - ICUB, University of Bucharest, Bucharest, Romania; **Research Institute of the University of Bucharest-ICUB, Bucharest, Romania*

1 Introduction

A pesticide is represented by any substance or mixture of substances used for preventing, destroying, or controlling any pest including vectors of human or animal diseases, undesired species of plants or animals causing either harmful effects or otherwise interfering with the production, processing, storage, or marketing of food, agricultural commodities, wood and wood products, or animal feedstuffs, or which may be administered to animals for the control of insects, arachnids, or other pests. The term includes chemicals used as growth regulators, defoliants, desiccants, fruit thinning agents, or agents for preventing the premature fall of fruits, and substances applied to crops either before or after harvest to prevent deterioration during storage or transport. Despite their beneficial effects exhibited by the inhibitory effects against pests harmful for plants and animals, the chemical pesticides could also be toxic for harmful effects on other organisms that must not be effected and tend to pollute the environment. If used in high quantities they can be evenly lethal. Biopesticides are used instead of chemical pesticides as the negative effects are low compared to chemical pesticides.

New Pesticides and Soil Sensors. http://dx.doi.org/10.1016/B978-0-12-804299-1.00002-3

2 Classification of Pesticides

Pesticides are classified depending on their origin and chemical structure (organic, natural rotenone, pyrethrumor synthetic, e.g., DDT, permethrin, malathion, 2,4-D, glyphosphate, or inorganic molecules), mode of action (Tables 1.1 and 1.2), spectrum of activity (broad spectrum pesticides with unselective harmful effects against reptiles, fish, pets, and birds, e.g., chlorpyrifos, chlordane/selective pesticides which are active only against a specific or group of pests, e.g., 2,4-D which affects broad-leaved plants), target pest (insecticides, algaecides, herbicides, bactericides, fungicides, rodenticides, larvicides, repellents by taste or smell, desiccants acting drying plant tissues, ovicides which inhibit the growth of insects and mites egg, virucides, molluscicides, acaricides, nematicides, avicides, moth balls, lampricides, piscicides), formulations (stable, emulsifiable, oil in water suspensions concentrates; wettable powders or granules obtained by mixing the active ingredient with clay; baits obtained by mixing the active ingredient with a food base; dusts which are applied dry in carriers as clay, talc, silica gel, or diatomacious earth; fumigants, which are gaseous insecticides usually packaged under pressure and stored as liquids, tablets, or pellets), route of entrance in the target pest (Table 1.3) (Drum, 1980; Zacharia, 2011; Pesticide Application Safety, 2016).

Table 1.1 Classifications of Pesticides Depending on Their Mode of Action

Type	Characteristics	Examples
Contact (nonsystemic)	They are not penetrating the plant tissues and do not reach plant vascular system They need direct cotnact with pest	Paraquat Diquat dibromide
Systemic	They penetrate efficiently the plant tissues and are transported thorough the vascular system The exhibit toxicity after ingestion (Buchel, 1983)	2,4-D and glyphosate

Table 1.2 Classifications of Pesticides Depending on Their Chemical Composition (Buchel, 1983; Zacharia, 2011)

	Group of Pesticides			
Characteristics	**Organochlorines**	**Organophosphorous**	**Carbamates**	**Pyrethroids**
	Organic compounds with five or more chlorine atoms; the first synthetic organic pesticides; widely used as insecticides; have a long-term residual effect in the environment since they are resistant to most chemical and microbial degradations	Chemical substances produced by the reaction between phosphoric acid and alcohols	Esters of carbamic acids	Synthetic analogs of the naturally occurring pyrethrins extracted from pyrethrum plant (*Chrysanthemum cinerariaefolium*) flowers The synthetic derivatives of ketoalcoholic esters of chrysanthemic and pyrethroic acids are more stable in sunlight than natural pyrethrins.
Mechanisms of action	Nervous system disruptors leading to convulsions and paralysis of the insect and its eventual death	Nervous system disruptors by inhibiting the action of acetyl cholinesterase (AChE) enzyme, causing irreversible blockage, accumulation of the enzyme andmuscular overstimulation	AchE inhibitors	Neuro-endocrine poisons causing paralysis
Examples	DDT, lindane, endosulfan, aldrin, dieldrin, chlordane	Insecticides, nerve gases, herbicides	Insecticides	Deltamethrin, cypermethrin

3 Pesticides Toxicity and Carcinogenicity

Pesticides are classified in four classes by the World Health Organization (WHO), and respectively by the International Agency for Research on Cancer (IARC), according to the potential toxicity and carcinogenicity risks to human health caused by the accidental contact to human being, i.e.,class Ia = extremely hazardous; class Ib = highly hazardous; class II = moderately hazardous; class

Table 1.3 Classifications of Pesticides Depending on the Route of Entry and Type of Exposure

Route of Entry	
Stomach	• Acquired during feeding • Represented by bacteria/bacterial toxins applied to water (for combating mosquito or black fly larva) or incorporated in baits (for combatingants, cockroaches, and other pest insects with chewing mouthparts) Examples: ingested anticoagulants with delayed action, to prevent the occurrence of bait shyness and to allow the administration of antidote (vitamin K)
Contact	• Supplied by water or aerosols or surfaces • Induce lesions at the level of nerve and respiratory centers of arthropods
Fumigants	• Volatile compounds that enter the bodies of insects in a gaseous phase • Rarely used in present to combat rodents
Systemic	• Absorbed by plants, pets, or livestock and are disseminated throughout the organism via the vascular system • Quickly lethal action or interference with normal development-typically used for tick and flea control on pets, and for dog heartworm prevention
Chemical repellents	• Used to prevent bloodsucking insects (mosquitoes, black flies, ticks) from biting humans, livestock, or pets • Examples (dimethyl toluamide) (Pesticide Application Safety, 2016)

III = slightly hazardous; class IV = products unlikely to present acute hazard in normal use (Zacharia, 2011). However, this classification can be versatile, due to the cummulative and chronic effects (Table 1.4), reasons for which there is a strong need for novel criteria of pesticides (re)classification (Líska and Kolesár, 1982). Regarding carcinogenicity, class 2 (hazardous agents) is subdivided into three subclasses (2A, 2B, and 2C) (Turusov and Rakitskiĭ, 1997). The pesticide toxicity is affected by the state of the chemical, that is, solid, liquid, or gas. Liquids or gasses can penetrate the body via skin, the mouth, the lungs, and the eye, while solid particles are entering through the skin or mouth (Table 1.4).

4 Biopesticides

Biopesticides are naturally occurring or derived materials from living organisms or their metabolites, which depending on their origin can be classified in: (1) microbial pesticides (often derived from *Bacillus thuringenesis*) which are active against bacteria,

Table 1.4 Classification of Pesticides Toxicity to Humans

Number of exposures to a poison and the time it takes for toxic symptoms to develop	
Acute toxicity	A person is exposed to a single dose of a pesticide (e.g., acute dermal exposure, acute inhalation)
Chronic exposure	Repeated or continuous exposure to a pesticide by a person (e.g., chronic dermal, oral, inhalation toxicity)
Subchronic exposure	Repeated or continuous exposure to a pesticide, but without any measurable toxic effects
Delayed toxicity	Exposure to a chemical (fipronil, asbestos) is most often only discovered in retrospective epidemiological studies
Body system affected and route of entry	
Dermal exposure Absorption through the skin as a result of a splash, spill, or drift when mixing, loading, or disposing of pesticides, exposure to large amounts of residue	Cutaneous Toxicity Most often associated with petroleum based products, pyrethroids, and some herbicides 1/3 of all pesticide-related occupational illnesses Symptoms: dermatitis (skin rash associated with inflammation and redness): • *Primary irritant dermatitis*: caused by chemical substances (herbicides, pesticides used in vector control—pyrethroids) that directly irritates the skin (such as acids or bases) with minor irritation or severe, with blisters or ulcerations • *Allergic contact dermatitis*: caused by chemical substances that stimulate development of an allergic reaction The degree of dermal absorption hazard depends on the dermal toxicity of the pesticide (highly irritant, irritant, moderately irritant, slightly irritant, and nonirritant), the extent of the exposure, the way the pesticide is formulated (emulsifiable concentrates are better absorbed than wettable powders, dusts, and granular pesticides) (very good resorption, good resorption, and low resorption), and the part of the body contaminated (male scrotum is very susceptible).
Oral exposure Accidental or intended oral exposure High risks are associated with pesticides transfer from their original labeled container to an unlabeled bottle or food container	In high doses, ingested pesticides may cause serious illness, severe injury, or even death
Respiratory exposure Vapors and extremely fine particles have the greatest potential for poisoning via respiratory exposure Respirators and gas masks can provide protection	Damages to nose, throat, and lung tissues
Eye exposure Eye protection with shields or goggles is always needed when measuring or mixing concentrated and highly toxic pesticides or when there is a risk of exposure to dilute spray or dusts that may drift into the eyes. Granular pesticides present a special hazard to eyes because of the size and weight of the individual particles	Immediate threat of blindness, illness, or even death

fungi, or viruses, exhibiting their inhibitory effect by binding to the larval gut receptor causing starvation; (2) biochemical pesticides, which are nontoxic pest controllers that include pheromones, natural plant, and insect regulators, enzymes, biorepellents, or attractants and (3) plant incorporated protectants, which are produced by genetically modified plants. Currently, there is much interest in the development of new biocontrol agents aiming to extend the area of application and the spectrum of target pests (Chin-A-Woeng et al., 2003; Diallo et al., 2011; Hynes et al., 2008). Food security (a pressing issue for all nations) faces a threat due to population growth, land availability for growing crops, climate change leading to increases in both a biotic and biotic stresses, increasing consumer awareness of the risks related to the use of agrichemicals, and also the reliance on depleting fossil fuel reserves for their production. Legislative changes in Europe mean that fewer agrichemicals will be available in the future for the control of crop pests and pathogens. In this context, the need for the implementation of a more sustainable agricultural system globally, incorporating an integrated approach to disease management, has become a top priority. Biological control has been shown to be an environmentally friendly alternative. There were developed research projects, such as VALORAM (Valorizing Andean Microbial Diversity) (http://valoram.ucc.ie) aiming to examine the role of microbial communities in crop production and protection to improve the productivity, but also sustainability, food security, and environmental protection.

4.1 Microbial Pesticides

The rhizosphere is the soil-plant root interface, consisting of the soil adhering to the root besides the loose soil surrounding it. Plant growth-promoting rhizobacteria (PGPR) are potential agents for the biological control of plant pathogens. PGPR are the rhizosphere bacteria that can enhance plant growth by a wide variety of mechanisms, like phosphate solubilization, siderophore production, biological nitrogen fixation, rhizosphere engineering, production of 1-Aminocyclopropane-1-carboxylate deaminase (ACC) and other enzymes, quorum sensing (QS) signal interference and inhibition of biofilm formation, phytohormones production, HCN, phenazines, pyrrolnitrin, and pyoluteorin, antibiotics, and antifungals, production of volatile organic compounds (VOCs), induction of systemic resistance, promoting beneficial plant–microbe symbioses, interference with pathogen toxin production (Bhattacharyya and Jha, 2012). A biocontrol strain should be able to protect the host plant from pathogens and have the ability of strong colonization.

The presence of root exudates has a pronounced effect on the rhizosphere where they serve as an energy source, promoting growth and influencing the root system for the rhizobacteria. In certain instances, they have products that inhibit the growth of soilborne pathogens to the advantage of the plant root. In exchange, plant growth promoting substances are likely to be produced in large quantities by the rhizosphere microorganisms. Recent progress in the understanding on the diversity of PGPR in the rhizosphere along with their colonization ability and mechanism of action should facilitate their application as a reliable component in the management of sustainable agricultural system (Bhattacharyya and Jha, 2012). Various rhizosphere bacteria are potential (micro)biological pesticides which are able to protect plants against diseases and improve productivity. They offer an alternative to the use of chemical fertilizers, pesticides, and other supplements.

A major source of concern is reproducibility in the field due to the complex interaction between the plant (plant species), microorganisms, and the environment (soil fertility and moisture, day length, light intensity, length of growing season, and temperature).

The PGPR, which are used as biocontrol agents are represented by rhizospheric and endophytic microorganisms that can survive and compete favourably well with soilborne fungal pathogens, such as *Fusarium* sp. which pose serious constraints on agroproductivity (Saraf et al., 2014). By multiple mechanisms, such as indole acetic acid production, siderophore production, phosphate solublilization, systemic resistance induction and antifungal volatile production among others (Ajilogba and Babalola, 2013). They include species from *Bacillus* and *Pseudomonas* genera.

Pseudomonas spp. are particularly suitable for application as agricultural biocontrol agents since they: (1) can use many exudate compounds as a nutrient source (Lugtenberg et al., 1999a); (2) are abundantly present in natural soils, in particular on plant root systems, which is indicative for their adaptive potential; (3) have a high growth rate relative to many other rhizosphere bacteria; (4) possess diverse mechanisms by which they can exert inhibitory activity toward phytopathogens and thereby mediate crop protection (Dunlap et al., 1996; Lugtenberg et al., 1999b), including the production of a wide range of antagonistic metabolites (Gutterson, 1990); (5) are easy to grow in vitro; (6) can subsequently be reintroduced into the rhizosphere by seed bacterization (Lugtenberg et al., 1994); and (7) are susceptible to mutation and modification using state of the art genetic tools (Galli et al., 1992). Several strains have already been marketed as commercial biocontrol products, such as Cedomon (BioAgri

AB, Uppsala, Sweden), a seed treatment based on a phenazine-producing *Pseudomonas chlororaphis* strain providing protection against seedborne diseases in barley and oats.

The strategies through which biocontrol agents can antagonize soilborne pathogens are generally divided into four categories: (1) competition for niches and nutrients (niche exclusion), (2) predation, (3) antibiosis, and (4) induction of a plant defence response (ISR) (Chin-A-Woeng et al., 2003).

Microscopy analysis of a root surface colonized by *Pseudomonas* sp. bacteria, including the phenazine-producing strain PCL1391, shows that they mainly colonize the root in microcolonies at the junctions of epidermal cells (Chin-A-Woeng et al., 1997). The fungal pathogen *Fusarium oxysporum* f. sp. *radicis-lycopersici* colonizes the tomato root surface at the same locations, as was observed using an autofluorescent protein-marked fungus (Lugtenberg et al., 1999b).

An example of competition for nutrients is limitation of iron. Iron is an essential cofactor for growth in all organisms, but the availability of solubilized Fe^{3+} in soils is limited at neutral and alkaline pH. Most organisms, including fluorescent *Pseudomonas* spp., take up ferric iron ions through high-affinity iron chelators, designated as siderophores, which are released from bacterial cells under Fe^{3+} limiting conditions. The complexed iron is taken up via specialized cell surface-located uptake systems and thus provides a route for the iron uptake. The ability to produce efficient siderophores is sometimes combined with the ability to take up related siderophores from other organisms (Koster et al., 1993, 1995). The ability to scavenge iron under Fe^{3+} limitation provides the biocontrol organism with a selective advantage over pathogens or deleterious organisms that possess less efficient iron binding and uptake systems. Siderophore-deficient mutants were found to be less suppressive to pathogens than the isogenic parental strain.

Fluorescent *Pseudomonas* spp., isolated from tomato and pepper plants rhizosphere soil, was evaluated in vitro against the causal agents of tomatoes damping-off (*Sclerotinia sclerotiorum*), root rot (*Fusarium solani*), and causal agents of stemcanker and leaf blight (*Alternaria alternata*). For this purpose, dual culture antagonism assays were carried out to determine the effect of the strains on mycelial growth of the pathogens. In addition, strains were screened for their ability to produce exoenzymes and siderophores. All the strains significantly inhibited *A. alternata*, protease was produced by 30% of the strains, but no strain produced cellulase or chitinase. The selected *Pseudomonas* Psf5 strain was evaluated on tomato seedling development and as a potential candidate for controlling tomato damping-off. In vivo studies resulted in significant increases in plant stand, as well as in root dry weight. Psf5 was able to establish and survive in tomato plants rhizosphere after 40 days following the planting of bacterized seeds (Hammami et al., 2013).

Some important biocontrol traits, such as chemotaxis and motility and antibiotics production have been established using the *P. chlororaphis* PCL1391 strain. It has been shown that a nonmotile mutant of the *P. chlororaphis* PCL1391, producing phenazine-1-carboxamide (or chlororaphin) as the active metabolite, were at least 1000-fold impaired in competitive tomato root tip colonization compared with the wild type. Consequently, the colonization-impaired mutant lost its ability to suppress disease, while still being able to produce the same amounts of antifungal activity as the wild type (Chin-A-Woeng et al., 2003). A *cheA*– chemotaxis mutant of *Pseudomonas fluorescens* WCS365 was also strongly reduced in competitive potato and tomato root colonization under gnotobiotic conditions, as well as in potting soil (Weert de et al., 2002; Simons et al., 1996).

Foliar spray and microinjection of PGPR rhizobacterial species, such as *P. fluorescens* and *Pseudomonas aeruginosa* on chickpea infected with *S. sclerotiorum* induced synthesis of phenylalanine ammonia-lyase (PAL). Induction of PAL was also associated with increased synthesis of phenolic compounds, such as tannic, gallic, caffeic, chlorogenic, and cinnamic acids. Treatment with *P. fluorescens* was found to be more effective in inducing phenolic compounds as compared to *P. aeruginosa,* but the last one induced a more persistent response. Foliar application was found to be superior to microinjection in terms of rapid PAL activity (Basha et al., 2006).

The effectiveness of PGPR, especially *P. fluorescens* isolates were tested against charcoal rot of chickpea both in green house, as well as in field conditions. Most of the isolates reduced charcoal rot disease and promoted plant growth in green house (Kumar et al., 2007). A marked increase in shoot and root length was observed in *P. fluorescens* treated plants. The *P. fluorescens* Pf4-99 isolate effectively promoted plant growth (significantly increasing the biomass of the chickpea plants, shoot length, root length, the total number, and weight of seeds, seeds protein content, seed germination associated with a high vigor index of seedlings, while decreasing seeds microflora), produced indole acetic acid, inhibited the mycelial growth of the *Macrophomina phaseolina* under in vitro conditions and reduced the disease severity (Kumar et al., 2007).

The combined used of PGPR with conventional pesticides may increase their efficacy and broaden the disease control spectrum. The effect of four different *Bacillus* sp. PGPR strains (*Bacillus subtilis* GB03 and FZB24, *Bacillus amyloliquefaciens* IN937a, and *Bacillus pumilus* SE34) applied individually and in mixtures, as well as in combined use with acibezolar-S-methyl (ASM) and hymexazol, on plant growth promotion and on the control of *Fusarium* crown and root rot (FCRR) of tomato was evaluated. All PGPR strains, and particularly SE34, promoted the tested plant growth characteristics significantly. After 28 days of incubation, SE34 strain populations remained stable. The GB03 and FZB24 strains provided a higher disease suppression when applied individually. However, application of IN937a in a mixture with GB03 provided a higher control efficacy of *F. oxysporum* f. sp. *radicis-lycopersici* (Forl). Treatment of tomato plants with ASM resulted in a small reduction in disease index, while application of hymexazol provided significantly higher control efficacy. Combined applications of the four PGPR strains with either ASM or hymexazol were significantly more effective. The results of the study indicate that, when PGPR strains were combined with pesticides, there was an increased suppression of Forl on tomato plants (Myresiotis et al., 2012).

Another study investigated the effect of seven *Bacillus*-species PGPR seed treatments on the induction of disease resistance in cowpea against mosaic disease caused by the blackeye cowpea mosaic strain of bean common mosaic virus (BCMV). Initially, although all PGPR strains recorded significant enhancement of seed germination and seedling vigor, GBO3 and T4 strains were very promising. In general, all strains gave reduced BCMV incidence compared with the nonbacterised control, both under screen-house and under field conditions. Cowpea seeds treated with *Bacillus pumilus* (T4) and *Bacillus subtilis* (GBO3) strains offered protection of 42 and 41% against BCMV under screen-house conditions. Under field conditions, strain GBO3 offered 34% protection against BCMV. The protection offered by PGPR strains against BCMV was evaluated by indirect enzyme-linked immunosorbent assay (ELISA), with lowest immunoreactive values recorded in cowpea seeds treated with strains GBO3 and T4 in comparison with the nonbacterised control. In addition, it was observed that strain combination worked better in inducing resistance than individual strains. Cowpea seeds treated with a combination of strains GBO3 + T4 registered the highest protection against BCMV. PGPR strains were effective in protecting cowpea plants against BCMV under both screen-house and field conditions by inducing resistance against the virus. Thus, it is proposed that PGPR strains, particularly GBO3, could be potential inducers against BCMV and growth enhancers in cowpea (Udaya et al., 2009).

Phenazines and phloroglucinols are major determinants of biological control of soilborne plant pathogens by various strains of fluorescent *Pseudomonas* spp. (Chin-A-Woeng et al., 2003). Phenazine derivatives kill fungi but the phenazine derivative pyocyanin, produced by certain *P. aeruginosa* strains, which are also animal and human pathogens (Mahajan et al., 1999).

Phenazines encompass a large family of heterocyclic nitrogen-containing brightly colored pigments with broad-spectrum antibiotic activity. They are synthesized almost exclusively by bacteria. Their production has been reported for *Pseudomonas, Streptomyces, Nocardia, Sorangium, Brevibacterium,* and *Burkholderia* species (Turner and Messenger, 1986). Although phenazines have been known for their antifungal properties, the interest in phenazines increased with the resurgence of research in biocontrol in the 1980s, driven in part by trends in agriculture toward greater sustainability and an increased concern about the use of chemical pesticides. Phenazine derivatives produced by Pseudomonads can be easily extracted from spent growth supernatant of cultures and analyzed using high performance liquid chromatography and detected with a diode array detector (Fernandez and Pizarro, 1997). The most commonly identified derivatives produced by *Pseudomonas* spp. are *pyocyanin, PCA, PCN,* and a number of *hydroxy-phenazines* (Turner and Messenger, 1986). They play a pivotal role in biological control (Chin-A-Woeng et al., 1998). In addition, PCA was shown to play a role in ecological fitness (Mazzola et al., 1992). The mechanisms for the action of phenazines in antifungal interactions are poorly understood (Chin-A-Woeng et al., 2003). Phenazines are toxic to a wide range of organisms including bacteria, fungi, and algae (Toohey et al., 1965). The conditions at which phenazine derivatives are active can be diverse (Turner and Messenger, 1986). The PCA-producing strain *P. fluorescens* strains 2–79 (Thomashow and Weller, 1988) and *P. aureofaciens* strain 30–84 (Pierson et al., 1995) showed no significant biocontrol activity in a *F. oxysporum* f. sp. *radicis-lycopersici* assay, whereas strain PCL1391, which produces the closely related PCN, inhibits this pathogen under identical conditions.

Microbial volatile organic compounds (mVOCs) of 27 rhizobacterial isolates were identified using gaschromatography/mass spectrometry (GC/MS), and their antifungal activity against *Rhizoctonia solani* was determined in vitro and compared to the activity of as election of pure volatile compounds. Five of these isolates, *Pseudomonas palleroniana* R43631, *Bacillus* sp. R47065, R47131, *Paenibacillus* sp. B3a R49541, and *Bacillus simplex* M3-4 R49538 trialled in the field in their respective countries of origin, that is, Bolivia, Peru, and Ecuador, showed significant increase in the yield of potato. This screening strategy may offer a template for the future isolation and determination of putative biocontrol and plant growth-promoting agents, useful as part of a low-input integrated pest management system (Velivelli et al., 2015).

4.2 Plant-Derived Biopesticides

Essential oils (EOs) are widely used as biopesticides and to control bacterial infections (Table 1.5). EOs from *Aloysia triphylla*, *Cymbopogon nardus*, *Lippia origanoides*, *Hyptis suaveolens*, *Swinglea glutinosa*, and *Eucalyptus globulus* were classified as repellents of Class IV, IV, IV, III, II, and II, respectively, whereas the commercial repellent IR3535 in Class II after 2 h exposure. All EOs presented small, but significant inhibitory properties against the QS system in *Escherichia coli* (pJBA132) at 25 μg/mL after 4 h exposure. Morerover, alcoholic or water extracts, as well as EOs majoritary compounds, such as acetophenone, (E)-anethole, (+)-aromadendrene, *cis*-asarone, benzyl alcohol, bisabolene, L(−)-borneol, bornyl acetate, 7-hydroxycalamenene, α-cadinol, camphene, camphor, carvacrol,1-butyl-3,4-methylenedioxybenzene, β-caryophyllene, caryophyllene oxide, (−)-α-cedrene, 1,8-cineole, citral, (S)-(−)-β-citronellol, *p*-cymene, ethyl cinnamate, ethyl rho-methoxycinnamate, *trans*-cinnamaldehyde, *trans*-cinnamyl alcohol, confertifolin, curcuminoids, dimethyl trisulfide, methyl propyl disulfide, 1-dodecanol, β-elemol, eugenol, β-eudesmol, (e)-β-farnesene, (+)-fenchone, (1R)-(−)-fenchone, geraniol, germacrene D, guaiol, A-humulene, Isoeugenol, (−)-isolongifolene, isopimpinellin, hydrocinnamyl alcohol, limonene, linalool, linalool oxide, 13-epi-manool, menthol, menthone, (E)-*p*-methhoxycinnamaldehyde, 2-isopropyl-5-methylcyclohexanone, methyl chavicol, methyl eugenol, myrcene, myristicin, 4aα,7α,7aβ-nepetalactone, (+)-terpinen-4-ol, Nerol, Nerolidol, α-pinene, β-pinene, 1-phenyl-1-ethanol, l-perillaldehyde, *p*-cresyl methyl ether, pogostone, rotundifolone, safrole, spathulenol, styrene,γ-terpinene, α-terpineol, terpinyl acetate, (−)-α-thujone, thymol, 1-tridecanol, ar-turmerone, and zerumbone alone or in different combinations have been proved efficient against different pests, exhibiting postingestion, contact or systemic toxicity and acting as repellents, fumingants, antiQS agents, and so on (Table 1.1). These data suggest that the plant-derived compounds and formulations are sustainable, promising new sources of natural pesticides with diverse mechanisms of action and routes of entry (Cervantes-Ceballos et al., 2015).

Table 1.5 EOs with Pesticidial Activity

Compound/Extract	Plant Species	Pest Species	Activity	References
Alcohols, aldehydes, and monoterpenes of citronella oil		*Triatoma rubida* (Uhler), *Triatoma protracta* (Uhler), *Triatoma recurva* (Stal)	Repellence	Zamora et al. (2015)
Three plant oils	*Achillea*	*Khapra beetle, Trogoderma granarium* (Everts) (Coleoptera: Dermestidae)	Fumingation	Alamir et al. (2015)
Monoterpenes: • Menthyl acetate • Geraniol		*Rhodnius prolixus* Ståhl (Hemiptera: Reduviidae)	Repellence	Lutz et al. (2014)
Thymol isoeugenol		*Lucilia sericata Fannia* sp. *Musca domestica Muscina stabulans Ophyra aenenscens Coproica* spp. *Leptocera* spp.	Influence of the production of flies	Lynch Ianniello et al. (2014)
• Thymol • Carvacrol • l-Perillaldehyde		*Culex pipiens pallens*	Fumigant	Ma et al. (2014)
Terpenes: • Eugenol • Geraniol • Citral		*Dermanyssus gallinae*		Sparagano et al. (2013)
Monoterpenes: menthone, menthol, menthyl acetate, limonene, citral, 1,8-cineole		*Musca domestica* L.	Repellent, pupicidal toxicity	Kumar et al. (2014)
Poly(ethylene glycol) (PEG) nanoparticles containing EOs		*Tribolium castaneum Rhizopertha dominica*	Lethal and sublethal activity	Werdin González et al. (2014)
Microemulsions (ME): oil in water (o/w) geranium EO and geraniol MEs and emulsions		*Culex pipiens pipiens*: larvae	Larvicidal	Montefuscoli et al. (2014)

(*Continued*)

Table 1.5 EOs with Pesticidial Activity (*cont.*)

Compound/Extract	Plant Species	Pest Species	Activity	References
β-Pinene		*Phalaris minor, Echinochloa crus-galli, Cassia occidentalis*	Affects germination, root length, and shoot length	Chowhan et al. (2013)
Thymol		*Helicoverpa armigera*	Larvicidal, egg development and oviposition impairment	Bovornnanthadej et al. (2013)
EOs	12 species of *Zingiberaceae* plants	*Aedes aegypti Culex quinquefasciatus*—fourth in star larvae and pupae	Larvicidal and pupicidal activity	Phukerd and Soonwera (2013)
EO	*Adenocalymma alliaceum, Piper callosum*	*Bemisia tabaci* (Genn.) biotype B (Hemiptera: Aleyrodidae)	Inhibition of the settlement and oviposition of *B. tabaci* biotype B adults	
EOs	*Ageratum conyzoides* L., *Coleus aromaticus* Benth. *H. suaveolens* (L.) Poit	*Tribolium castaneum* Herbst	Fumigant	Jaya et al. (2014)
EO and its components: • Dimethyl trisulfide • Methyl propyl disulfide	*Allium macrostemon* Bunge (Liliaceae)	*Aedes albopictus*	Larvicidal	Liu et al. (2014b)
Extract	*Allium sativum*	*Dermanyssus gallinae* (Acari: Mesostigmata)	Field efficacy	Faghihzadeh Gorji et al. (2014)
EO	*Allium tuberosum* Rottler ex Sprengle roots and its constituents	*Aedes albopictus* Skuse—larval mosquitoes	Larvicidal	Liu et al. (2015b)
EO and methanolic extract and 1,8-cineole	*Alpinia galanga (L.)*	*Coptotermes gestroi* (Wasmann) and *Coptotermes curvignathus* (Holmgren) (Isoptera: Rhinotermitidae)	Antifeedant and repellent	Abdullah et al. (2015)
EO and its constituents: • Limonene • Eucalyptol	*Amomum tsaoko* Crevost et Lemarie fruits	*Tribolium castaneum* (Herbst) *Lasioderma serricorne* (Fabricius)		Wang et al. (2014b)

EOs and its constituents: • 1-Dodecanol • 1-Tridecanol	*Angelica dahurica* and *Angelica pubescentis* root	*Colletotrichum acutatum, Colletotrichum fragariae, and Colletotrichum gloeosporioides, Aedes aegypti, Stephanitis pyrioides*	Antifungal, biting deterrent and insecticidal	Tabanca et al. (2014)
EOs	*Araucaria columnaris, Agathis moorei, Agathis ovata, Callitris sulcata, Neocallitropsis pancheri*	*Rhipicephalus (Boophilus) microplus*	Acaricidal	Lebouvier et al. (2013)
Chloroform extract	*Artemisia absinthium*	*Rhipicephalus sanguineus*	Adult immersion test, egg hatchability test and larval packet test	Godara et al. (2014)
EO and its constituents: • D-Camphor • Linalool • Cineole • α-Terpineol • L(−)-borneol	*Artemisia annua* L.	*Solenopsis invicta* Buren	Fumigants, contact, insecticides, repellents	Zhang et al. (2014a)
EO and its components: eucalyptol β-pinene β-caryophyllene camphor	*Artemisia argyi* Lévl. et Van	*Lasioderma serricorne* adults		Zhang et al. (2014b)
EO and its major components: • Camphor • Eucalyptol • Terpine-4-ol • Germacrene D • Caryophyllene oxide-caryophyllene	*Artemisia gilvescens*	*Anopheles anthropophagus*	Larvicidal	Zhu and Tian (2013)
EOs	*Artemisia herba alba, Rutachalepensis Satureja calamintha*	*Tribolium castaneum Tribolium confusum*	Toxicity	Abbad et al. (2014)

(*Continued*)

Table 1.5 EOs with Pesticidial Activity (*cont.*)

Compound/Extract	Plant Species	Pest Species	Activity	References
EOs	*Artemisia herba-alba, Lippia citriodora, Mentha pulegium, M. spicata, Myrtus communis, Rosmarinus officinalis, Thymus satureioides*	*Spodoptera littoralis, Myzus persicae, and Rhopalosiphum padi* *Meloydogine javanica*	Antifeedant and nematicidal	Santana et al. (2014)
EOs	aerial parts of *Artemisia nilagirica* and *Artemisia maritima*	*Colletotrichum acutatum, Colletotrichum fragariae, Colletotrichum gloeosporioides* *Aedes aegypti*	Antifungal, mosquito biting deterrent, larvicidal activities	Stappen et al. (2014)
EO and its constituents: • α-Terpinyl acetate • α-Terpineol • 4-Terpineol • Linalool	*Artemisia rupestris* L. aerial parts	*Liposcelis bostrychophila* Badonnel	Insecticidal, repellent activity	Liu et al. (2013a)
EO and its constituents: • Eucalyptol • β-Pinene • Camphor • Terpinen-4-ol	*Artemisia stolonifera* (Maxim.) Komar.	*Tribolium castaneum, Lasioderma serricorne*	Toxicity, repellent	Zhang et al. (2015)
EOs	*Azadirachta indica, Piper nigrum, Mentha spicata, Cammiphora myrrha, Elettaria cardamomum, Zingiber officinale, Curcuma longa, Schinus molle, Rosmarinus officinalis*	*Rhynchophorus ferrugineus*—cell line	Cell proliferation inhibition	Rizwan-ul-Haq and Aljabr (2015)

EOs and its constituents: • Nerolidol • Limonene	*Baccharis dracunculifolia* DC	unengorged larvae and engorged females of *Rhipicephalus microplus* (Acari: Ixodidae)	Acaricidal	de Assis Lage et al. (2015)
EOs mixed with either sunflower oil or ethul alcohol	Basil, geranium, balsam fir, lavender, lemongrass, peppermint, pine and tea tree	Horn flies	Repellent	Lachance and Grange (2014)
EOs	*Boesenbergia rotunda Zingiber zerumbet, Litsea petiolata, Curcuma zedoaria Zingiber cassumunar*	*Aedes aegypti Culex quinquefasciatus*	Repellent	Phukerd and Soonwera (2014)
EO	*Brassica nigra*	*Aspergillus niger, Aspergillus ochraceus, Penicillium citrinum*	Fungicidal	Mejía-Garibay et al. (2015)
EO	*Callistemon citrinus* (Curtis)	*Callosobruchus macullatus* (F.)	Insecticidal, repellent	Zandi-Sohani et al. (2013)
EO	*Carum copticum* seeds	*Aspergillus flavus* *Aspergillus niger*	Antiaflatoxin B1 activity	Kazemi (2015)
EO	*Cinnamomum glaucescens*	Callosobruchus chinensis Aspergillus flavus LHP-10	Insecticidal, antifungal, antiaflatoxin, antioxidant	Prakash et al. (2013)
EO and polyvinyl alcohol strips	*Cinnamomum zeylanicum*	*Plodia interpunctella*	Repellent	Jo et al. (2013)
EO	Cinnamon	*Pyrus pyrifolia*	Decay incidence	Wang et al. (2014c)
EO	Citronella	*Alternaria alternata*	Antifungal	Chen et al. (2014)
EOs	Citronella, hairy basil, catnip, and vetiver	*Aedes aegypti, Aedes albopictus, Culex quinquefasciatus, Anopheles minimus*	Behavioral responses of colony populations	Sathantriphop et al. (2014)
EOs and its constituents: • Limonene • Citral	Citrus limon [L.] Burm. *C. paradisi* Macfadyen	*Anastrepha fraterculus* (Wiedemann) and *Ceratitis capitata* (Wiedemann) immature stages	Insecticidal	Ruiz et al. (2014)

(*Continued*)

Table 1.5 EOs with Pesticidial Activity (*cont.*)

Compound/Extract	Plant Species	Pest Species	Activity	References
EOs	*Citrus limonum* (Sapindales: Rutaceae), *Litsea cubeba* (Laurales: Lauraceae), *Cinnamomum cassia*, *Allium sativum* L. (Asparagales: Alliaceae)	6th instars and adults of *Alphitobius diaperinus* (Panzer) (Coleoptera: Tenebrionidae)	Fumigant, contact, and repellent activities	Wang et al. (2014a)
EO	*Citrus paradisi*	*Aedes aegypti*	Toxicity, ovicidal and larvicidal activity	Ivoke et al. (2013)
EOs	*Citrus sinensis*, *Cymbopogon citratus*, *Eucalyptus glubulus*, *Illicium verum*, *Lavandula angustifolia*, *Mentha piperita*, *Zingiber cussumunar*	*Musca domestica* L.	Oviposition deterrent, ovicidal activities	Sinthusiri and Soonwera (2014)
Acetone, chloroform, ethyl acetate, methanol, and petroleum benzine leaf extracts	*Clausena dentata* (Wild) (Rutaceae)	*Anopheles stephensi*, *Culex quinquefasciatus*, and *Aedes aegypti* (Diptera: Culicidae)	Larvicidal	Manjari et al. (2014)
EO and thymol	*Coleus aromaticus*	*Culex tritaeniorhynchus*, *Aedes albopictus*, *Anopheles subpictus*	Larvicidal	Govindarajan et al. (2013a)
EO	*Conyza newii* (Asterale: Asteracea, Oliv. & Hiern)	*Anopheles gambiae* s.s.	Repellent	Mayeku et al. (2014)
EO	*Coriandrum sativum* L. (Apiaceae)	*Aedes albopictus* Skuse (Diptera: Culicidae)	Larvicidal, repellent	Benelli et al. (2013)
EO	*Cotinus coggyria* Scop.' leaves	*Acanthoscelides obtectus* *Tribolium castaneum*		Ulukanli et al. (2014a)

EO constituent-7-hydroxycalamenene	*Croton cajucara*	*Absidia cylindrospora, Cunninghamella elegans, Mucor circinelloides, Mucor circinelloides* f. *circinelloides, Mucor mucedo, Mucor plumbeus, Mucor ramosissimus, Rhizopus microsporus, Rhizopus oryzae, Syncephalastrum racemosum* *Rhizopus oryzae*		Azevedo et al. (2014)
EO and α-terpineol	*Cryptomeria fortunei* Hooibrenk	*Reticulitermnes chinensis*	Antitermitic	Xie et al. (2013, 2014)
EO	*Cryptomeria japonica* leaf	*Anopheles gambiae sensu stricto*	Larvicidal	Mdoe et al. (2014)
EOs	*Cucurbita maxima* *Lupinus luteus* *Allium sativum* *Mentha piperita*	*Cephalopina titillator*	Larval immersion tests	Khater (2014)
EO	*Cuminum cyminum*	1230 fungal isolates—*Aspergillus flavus* LHP(C)-D6	Antifungal, antiaflatoxigenic and fumigant	Kedia et al. (2014)
EO	*Cunila angustifolia* (Benth)	*Alphitobius diaperinus* (Panzer)	Larvicidal, insecticidal	Do Prado et al. (2013)
EO and ethanolic extracts and hexane-soluble fraction: • β-Elemol • α-Cadinol	*Cunninghamia konishii* Hayata	*Coptotermes formosanus* Shiraki (Isoptera: Rhinotermitidae)	Insecticidal activity	
EO	*Cupressus arizonica* var glabra (Sudw.) Little—female cones, male cones, needle-twings, wood-bark	*Colletotrichum acutatum, C. fragariae, C. gloeosporioides* *Aedes aegypti*	Larvicidal, biting deterrent and antifungal activity	Ali et al. (2013c)
EOs	*Cupressus arizonica, Cupressus benthamii, Cupressus macrocarpa, Cupressus sempervirens, Cupressus torulosa, Chamaecyparis lawsoniana, Juniperus phoenicea, Tetraclinis articulata*	*Aedes albopictus*	Larvicidal, repellent	Giatropoulos et al. (2013)

(*Continued*)

Table 1.5 EOs with Pesticidial Activity (*cont.*)

Compound/Extract	Plant Species	Pest Species	Activity	References
EOs and extract of ar-turmerone and curcuminoids	*Curcuma longa*	*Aedes aegypti* (L.) and *Anopheles quadrimaculatus* (Diptera: Culicidae)	Larvicidal, deterrent activity	Ali et al. (2015b)
EOs	*Cymbopogon citratus, Cymbopogon giganteus, Cymbopogon schoenanthus, Eucalyptus citriodora, Eucalyptus tereticornis, Cochlospermum tinctorium, Cochlospermum planchonii, Securidaca longepedunculata, Chenopodium ambrosioides*	*Anopheles gambiae*	Insecticidal	Bossou et al. (2013)
EOs and major constituents: -Citral -1,8-Cineole	*Cymbopogon citratus*	*Musca domestica* L. (Diptera: Muscidae)	Contact toxicity, fumigation, pupicidal	Kumar et al. (2013)
EO and mixture of citral, myrcene and oil.	*C. nardus* *Cymbopogon citratus*	*Aedes aegypti*	Insecticidal, repellent	Hsu et al. (2013)
Chemically modified EOEOs	*Cymbopogon* spp. *Corymbia citriodora*	*Rhipicephalus (Boophilus) microplus*	Acaricidal	Chagas et al. (2014)
EO	*Cymbopogon winterianus* *Syzygium aromaticum*	*Rhipicephalus (Boophilus) microplus*	Influence on the development stages	de Mello et al. (2014)
EOEOs and its constituents: 4-terpineol D-limonene	*Dahlia pinnata*	*Sitophilus zeamais Sitophilus oryzae*	Contact toxicity, fumigant	Wang et al. (2015b)
Crude methanolic extracts	*Datura stramonium, Azadirachta indica, Calotropis procera leaves, Allium sativum* cloves, and *Carica papaya* seeds	*Rhipicephalus (Boophilus) microplus*	Acaricidal	Shyma et al. (2014)

EO and its major constituents: • Carvone • Limonene	Dill seads	*Zymoseptoria tritici* (teleomorph: *Mycosphaerella graminicola*)	Antifungal	Deweer et al. (2013)
EOs	*Echinophora lamondiana* B.Yildiz et Z.Bahcecioglu—flower, leaf, and stem	*Aedes aegypti* (L.) and *Anopheles quadrimaculatus* Say (Diptera: Culicidae)	Biting deterrent, larvicidal	Ali et al. (2015a)
EO	*Elionurus muticus*	*Artemia salina*	Cytotoxic effect	Füller et al. (2014)
EO nanoemulsion	Eucalyptus	*Culex quinquefasciatus*	Larvicidal	Sugumar et al. (2014)
Monoterpens from the EO: oxygenated monoterpenes (α-terpineol, 4-terpineol, and 1,8-cineole) and terpene hydrocarbons (γ-terpinene, *p*-cymene, α-pinene)	Eucalyptus	*Aedes aegypti* (L.) (Diptera: Culicidae)	Larvicidal activity, knockdown effect	Lucia et al. (2013)
EOs	*Eucalyptus camaldulensis* Dehnh. (Myrtales: Myrtaceae) *Heracleum persicum* Desf. (Apiales: Apiaceae)	*Callosobruchus maculatus F.* (Coleoptera: Bruchidae)	Lethal and sublethal activities	Izakmehri et al. (2013)
EO	*E. globulus* *E. lehmannii*	*Orgyia trigotephras* third and fourth larval stages	Insecticidal	Slimane et al. (2014)
EO	*Eucalyptus urograndis* (Myrtaceae)	*Rhodnius neglectus* Lent (Hemiptera: Reduviidae)	Insecticidal	Gomes and Favero (2013)
EO	*Eugenia caryophyllus*	*Dermatophagoides pteronyssinus*	Acaricidal	Mahakittikun et al. (2014)
EOs	*Evodia calcicola* and *Evodia trichotoma* leaves	*Tribolium castaneum* adults *Lasioderma serricorne* adults *Liposcelis bostrychophila.*	Repellent	Yang et al. (2014)
EO	*Feronia limonia*-leaves	*Anopheles stephensi, Aedes aegypti, Culex quinquefasciatus*	Larvicidal	Senthilkumar et al. (2013)

(*Continued*)

Table 1.5 EOs with Pesticidial Activity (*cont.*)

Compound/Extract	Plant Species	Pest Species	Activity	References
EO	*Foenicultm vulgare*—aerian parts	*Aedes aegypti*	Larvicidal activity against third instar larvae	Rocha et al. (2015)
EO and its major constituents	*Geranium maculatum* L.	*Musca domestica* L.	Insecticisdal	Gallardo et al. (2015)
EO	*Hoslundia opposita* Vahl (Lamiaceae)-leaves	*Tribolium castaneum*	Contact toxicity and repellent	Babarinde et al. (2014)
EO and constituents: • Myristicin • Safrole • 1,8-Cineole	*Illicium henryi* (Illiciaceae) root bark	*Liposcelis bostrychophila*	Fumigant	Liu and Liu (2015)
Silica gel enhanced with EO	*Juniperus oxycedrus* L. *ssp. oxycedrus* (Pinales: Cupressaceae)	*Sitophilus oryzae* (L.) (Coleoptera: Curculionidae) *Tribolium confusum* Jacquelin du Val (Coleoptera: Tenebrionidae)	Insecticidal	Athanassiou et al. (2013)
EO and its constituents: 1,8-cineole, ethyl cinnamate, ethyl rho-methoxycinnamate, *trans*-cinnamaldehyde	*Kaempferia galanga* L. rhizomes	*Liposcelis bostrychophila* Badonnel	Repellent and insecticidal	Liu et al. (2014a)
EO	*Laurus nobilis* leaves	*Alternaria alternata*	Antifungal	Xu et al. (2014)
EO	*Lippia alba* (Miller) N.E. Brown	*Trichophyton rubrum, Epidermophyton floccosum, Microsporum gypseum*	Antidermatophytic potential, inhibits peptidase and keratinase activities	Costa et al. (2014)
EO and maijor components: • Carvacrol • Thymol	*Lippia gracilis* Schauer	*Rhipicephalus (Boophilus) microplus*	Acaricidal	Cruz et al. (2013)
EO	*Lippia sidoide*	Unengorged larvae and nymphs of *Rhipicephalus sanguineus* and *Amblyomma cajennense*	Acaricidal	Gomes et al. (2014)

LPP1 with the EO	*Lippia sidoides*	*Rhipicephalus microplus* - females Entomopathogenic nematodes *Heterorhabditis bacteriophora* HP88 and *Heterorhabditis indica*	Hatching percentage of larvae	Monteiro et al. (2014)
EOs	*Lippia sidoides, Croton zehntneri, Croton nepetaefolius, Croton argyrophylloides, Croton sonderianus*	*Aedes aegypti*	Insecticidal	de Lima et al. (2013)
EO	*Lippia triplinervis*—aerial parts	*Rhipicephalus microplus* - unengorged larvae and engorged females	Acaricidal	Lage et al. (2013)
EOs and its components: benzyl alcohol, acetophenone, 1-phenyl-1-ethanol, hydrocinnamyl alcohol, *trans*-cinnamyl aldehyde, *trans*-cinnamyl alcohol, *cis*-asarone, styrene, *cis*-ocimene	*Liquidambar orientalis* *Valeriana wallichii*	*Japanese termite* (Reticulitermes speratus)	Fumigant	Park (2014)
EO	*Liriope muscari*—aerial parts	*Tribolium castaneum, Lasioderma serricorne and Liposcelis bostrychophila* adults	Contact toxicity and repellent	Wu et al. (2015)
EOs	*Litsea cubeba (LC), Litsea salicifolia (LS), Melaleuca leucadendron* (ML)	*Aedes aegypti*	Behavioral responses	Noosidum et al. (2014)
EOs	*Melaleuca alternifolia* (Myrtales: Myrtaceae), *Carapa guianensis* (Sapindales: Meliaceae)	*Haematobia irritans* (L.) and *Musca domestica* L. (both: Diptera: Muscidae)	Insecticidal and repellent	Klauck et al. (2014)
EOs	*Melaleuca alternifolia* *Lavandula angustifolia*	*Bovicola ocellatus* (Piaget) (Phthiraptera: Trichodectidae)	Contact and vapour toxicity	Ellse et al. (2013)
EO	*Melaleuca alternifolia, Carapa guianensis*	*Haemotobia irritans* *Chrysomya megacephala*	Repellent	Klauck et al. (2015)

(*Continued*)

Table 1.5 EOs with Pesticidial Activity (*cont.*)

Compound/Extract	Plant Species	Pest Species	Activity	References
EOs and extract	*Melaleuca alternifolia, Syzygium aromaticum, Mimosa tenuiflora*	*Alternaria alternata, Botrytis cinerea* and *F. oxysporum f. sp. lycopersici* (races 1 and 2)	Antifungal	La Torre et al. (2014)
EOs	*Mentha piperita* L. (Lamiales: Lamiaceae), *Satureja thymbra L.,Lavandula angustifolia Mill, Ocimum basilicum* L., *Citrus limon* L. (Sapindales: Rutaceae), *C. sinensis* L.	*Planococcus ficus* (Signoret) (Hemiptera: Pseudococcidae)	Insecticidal	Karamaouna et al. (2013)
EO, rotundifolone and 15 analogues of the rotundifolone	*Mentha x villosa*	*Aedes aegypti*	Larvicidal	Lima et al. (2014)
EO	*Monarda bradburiana* Beck *Monarda fistulosa* L.	*Aedes aegypti* larvae	Repellent	Tabanca et al. (2013b)
EO	*Morinda lucida*	*Callosobruchus maculatus*	Insecticidal	Owolabi et al. (2014)
EO	*Murraya microphylla* branches and leaves	*Lasioderma serricorne* adults	Contact toxicity, and repellent	You et al. (2015)
EO/methanolic extract	*Myrtus communis* L.	*Leishmania tropica Cryptococcus neoformans Epidermophyton floccosum, Microsporum canis, Trichophyton rubrum*	Antileishmanial Antifungal	Mahmoudvand et al. (2015); Bouzabata et al. (2015)
EOs	*Nectandra megapotamica* (Sprengel) Mez, *Nectandra grandiflora* Nees, *Hesperozygis ringens* (Bentham) Epling, *Ocimum gratissimum* L., *Aloysia gratissima* (Gillies and Hooker) Troncoso, *Lippia sidoides* Chamisso	Coenagrionidae larvae: *Acanthagrion Selys, Homeoura Kennedy, Ischnura Charpentier, Oxyagrion Selys*	Larvicidal	Silva et al. (2014)

Dichloromethane-methanol extract, EO, the isolated: $4a\alpha,7\alpha,7a\beta$-nepetalactone	*Nepeta parnassica*	*Aedes (Stegomyia) cretinus* Edwards *Culex pipiens* pipiens biotype molestus Forskål	Repellent	Gkinis et al. (2014)
EOs	*Ocimum americanum* Linn *Zingiber officinale* Roscoe *Cymbopogon citratus* Stapf *C. nardus* Rendle *Zingiber cassumunar* Roxb	*Aedes aegypti (= Stegomyia aegypti)*	Insecticidal, repellent and irritant	Boonyuan et al. (2014)
EO	*Ocimum basilicum*	*Culex tritaeniorhynchus, Aedes albopictus Anopheles subpictus*	Larvicidal	Govindarajan et al. (2013b)
Methanol, acetone and petroleum ether extracts	*Ocimum basilicum Glycyrrhiza glabra*	*Culex pipiens* (Diptera: Culicidae)	Repellent	Hassan et al. (2015)
EO and 40 constituents	*Ocimum basilicum* L.	*Dermatophagoides farinae* Hughes		Perumalsamy et al. (2014)
EO	*Ocimum basilicum* L. *Mentha spicata* L. (Lamiaceae)	*Ephestia kuehniella* (Zeller) and *Plodia interpunctella* (Hübner) (Lepidoptera: Pyralidae)	Insecticidal	Eliopoulos et al. (2015)
EOs	*Ocimum basilicum* L. (four chemovariants), *O. tenuiflorum* L., *O. gratissimum* L., *O. kilimandscharicum* Guerke	*R. solani Choanephora cucurbitarum*	Antifungal	Padalia et al. (2014)
Ethanol solutions of five fractions obtained from EO	*Ocimum basilicum* L. (Lamiales: Lamiaceae)	*Lymantria dispar* L. (Lepidoptera: Lymantriidae)—2(nd) instar gypsy moth larvae	Antifeedant properties	Popović et al. (2013)
EOEOs	*Ocimum basilicum, Ocimum canum, Cymbopogon citratus*	*Plasmodium falciparum* *Anopheles funestus*	Larvicidal	Akono et al. (2014)
EO	*Ocimum gratissimum* L. leaf	*Aedes albopictus* Skuse (Diptera: Culicidae)	Larvicidal	Sumitha and Thoppil (2015)

(*Continued*)

Table 1.5 EOs with Pesticidial Activity (*cont.*)

Compound/Extract	Plant Species	Pest Species	Activity	References
EO and its major constituent: • carvacrol	*Origanum bilgeri* P.H. Davis (Lamiaceae)—aerial parts	*Rhipicephalus turanicus* Pomerantzev (Acari: Ixodidae)	Acaricidal	Koc et al. (2013)
EO	*Pachira glabra* Pasq.	*Sitophilus zeamais*	Insecticidal	Lawal et al. (2014)
EOs	*Pelargonium graveolens* *Artemisia arborescens*	*Rhysopertha dominica* *R. solani*	Insecticidal, antifungal	Bouzenna and Krichen (2013)
EOEOs and its major components: trans-nerolidol geraniol citronellol geranyl formate	*Pelargonium* spp., cultivars Bourbon, China, Egypt, Rober's Lemon Rose, and Frensham	*Stephanitis pyrioides* *Aedes aegypti*	Insecticidal, larvicidal and biting deterrent	Ali et al. (2013b)
EO and its main components: -3,4-Dimethoxytoluene,-2,4-Dimethoxytoluene,-β-caryophyllene, -*p*-Cresyl methyl ether,-caryophyllene oxide	*Phoenix dactylifera* L. (Arecaceae)	*Aedes aegypti*	Repellent	Demirci et al. (2013)
EOs	*Pinus brutia* *Pinus pinea*	*Micrococcus luteus* *B. subtilis Ephestia kuehniella* eggs *Lactuca sativa, Lepidium sativum, Portulaca oleracea*	Antimicrobial Contact toxicity, fumigant, Fitotoxic activities Antioxidant potential	Ulukanli et al. (2014b)
EOs	*Pinus nigra* (3 samples), *Pinus stankewiczii, Pinus brutia, Pinus halepensis, Pinus canariensis, Pinus pinaster, Pinus strobus*	*Aedes albopictus*	Larvicidal, Repellent	Koutsaviti et al. (2015)
EOEOs	*Pinus sylvestris Syzygium aromaticum*	*Aedes aegypti, Culex quinquefasciatus*	Larvicidal	Fayemiwo et al. (2014)
EO and its major component: 1,8-cineole	*Piper aduncum L.*	*Aedes aegypti*	Larvicidal	Oliveira et al. (2013)

EOEOs combined with Xentaei WG (Bta)	*Piper hispidinervum L.* *Syzygium aromaticum L.*	*Spodoptera frugiperda* (JE Smith) (Lepidoptera: Noctuidae)		Cruz et al. (2014)
EO and isolated compound: 1-butyl-3,4-methylenedioxybenzene	*Piper klotzschianum* (Piperaceae)	*Artemia salina* Leach nauplii and fourth-instar *Aedes aegypti* larvae	Larvicidal	do Nascimento et al. (2013)
EOEOs	*Piper subtomentosum* (leaves and inflorescences) *Piper septuplinervium* (aerial parts)	*Spodoptera frugiperda* second instar larvae	Insecticidal	Ávila Murilloa et al. (2014)
EO constituent: pogostone	*Pogostemon cablin* (Blanco) Benth	*Spodoptera litura* (Fabricius) *Spodoptera exigua* (Hübner)	Insecticidal	Huang et al. (2014)
EO	*Pogostemon cablin* (Blanco) Bentham leaves	*Blattella germanica* (L.)	Contact toxicity and repellent	Liu et al. (2015a)
EO and confertifolin	*Polygonum hydropiper*	*Anopheles stephensi, Culex quinquefasciatus*	Ovicidal, repellent, adulticidal, oviposition deterrent activity	Maheswaran et Ignacimuthu (2013)
EO and its components: confertifolin	*Polygonum hydropiper* L-leaves	*Aedes albopictus* L.	Larvicidal, ovicidal, repellent, oviposition deterrent and adulticidal activities	Maheswaran and Ignacimuthu (2014)
EO and confertifolin	*Polygonum hydropiper* L. (Polygonaceae)-leaves	*Aedes aegypti* L.	Ovicidal, repellent, oviposition deterrent activity	Maheswaran and Ignacimuthu (2015)
EO, ethanolic, methanolic and aqueous extracts	*Pseudocalymma alliaceum*-leaves	*Culex quinquefasciatus*—larvae	Larvicidal	Granados-Echegoyen et al. (2014)
EO	*Psoralea corylifolia* Linn.	*Culex quinquefasciatus* Say	Larvicidal, adulticidal and genotoxic	Dua et al. (2013)
EO	*Ruta chalepensis* L.-leaves	*Fusarium proliferatum, Fusarium pseudograminearum, Fusarium culmorum, Fusarium graminearum Fusarium polyphialidicum*	Antifungal	Bouajaj et al. (2014)
EO	*Ruta chalepensis L.* (Rutaceae)—wild and cultivated	*Aedes albopictus Skuse* (Diptera: Culicidae)	Larvicidal and repellent	Conti et al. (2013)
EO	*Ruta chalepensis* L. (Sapindales: Rutaceae)	*Aedes aegypti* L. *Anopheles quadrimaculatus Say*	Biting deterrent, repellent, larvicidal	Ali et al. (2013a)

(*Continued*)

Table 1.5 EOs with Pesticidial Activity (*cont.*)

Compound/Extract	Plant Species	Pest Species	Activity	References
EOs	*Ruta chalepensis, Zanthoxylum fagara, Thymus vulgaris*	Larvae of *Aedes aegypti*	Larvicidal	Pérez López et al. (2015)
EOs and its constituents: β-Eudesmol guaiol 13-epi-Manool Caryophyllene oxide Borneol Bornyl acetate β-Caryophyllene	*Salvia apiana* *Salvia elegans* *Salvia leucantha* *Salvia officinalis*	*Anopheles quadrimaculatus Aedes aegypti*	Biting-deterrent Larvicidal	Ali et al. (2015c)
EO	Schinus terebinthifolia	*Stegomyia aegypti* larvae	Structural demage of the larvae	Pratti et al. (2015)
EO constituent: 2-Isopropyl-5-methylcyclohexanone and structurally related derivatives	*Schizonepeta tenuifolia*	House dust, stored food mites	Acaricidal	Yang and Lee (2013)
EOs	*Siparuna guianensis*	*Aedes aegypti, Culex quinquefasciatus* (eggs, larvae, pupae, and adult) and *Aedes albopictus* (C6/36) cells	Oviposition-deterring activity, egg viability, repellent	Aguiar et al. (2015)
EO	*Syzygium aromaticum*	*Cacopsylla chinensis* (Yang and Li) (Hemiptera: Psyllidae)	LD50	Tian et al. (2015)
EO	*Syzygium aromaticum* L.	*Penicillium digitatum, Penicillium italicum*	Antifungal	Martínez and González (2013)
EOs	*Syzygium aromaticum* L., *Cinnamomum zeylanicum* L.	*Sitophilus zeamais* Motschulsky	Locomotory and respiratory responses and number of larvae per grain produced	Haddi et al. (2015)

EOs	*Tagetes lucida, Lippia alba, L. origanoides, Eucalyptus citriodora, Cymbopogon citratus, Cymbopogon flexuosus, Citrus sinensis, S. glutinosa, Cananga odorata*	*Aedes* (Stegomyia) *aegypti* Rockefeller larvae	Insecticidal	Vera et al. (2014)
EO	*Tagetes patula*	*Rhipicephalus sanguineus*	Acaricide	Politi et al. (2013)
EOs and its constituents: Beta-caryophyllene Caryophyllene oxide (−)-Beta-pinene (−)-Alpha-pinene (+)-Beta-pinene	*Tanacetum argenteum* (Lam.) Willd. subsp. *argenteum* (Lam.) *T. argenteum* (Lam.) Willd. *subsp. canum* (C. Koch) Grierson	*Aedes aegypti* (Diptera: Culicidae)	Larvicidal and biting deterrent	Ali et al. (2014)
EO and major constituents: • Geraniol • D-limonene • Isopimpinellin	*Toddalia asiatica* (L.) Lamc-roots	*Aedes albopictus*	Larvicidal	Liu et al. (2013b)
EOs	*Umbellularia californica, Laurus nobilis*	*Aedes aegypti*	Biting deterrent, larvicidal	Tabanca et al. (2013a)
EO	*Xylopia parviflora* (A. Rich.) Benth (Annonaceae)	*Callososbruchus maculatus* Fabricius (Coleoptera: Chrysomelidae: Bruchinae)	Fumigant	Babarinde et al. (2015)
EO and constituents: • α-Asarone • Menthol	*Youngia japonica*—aerial parts	*Aedes albopictus* larvae	Larvicidal	Liu et al. (2015c)
EO	*Zanthoxylum caribaeum*	*Rhodnius prolixus* fifth-instar nymphae	Bioassays	Nogueira et al. (2014a)
EO	*Zanthoxylum caribaeum* Lamarck (Rutaceae) leaves	*Rhipicephalus (Boophilus) microplus* females	Adult immersion test	Nogueira et al. (2014a,b)
EOs	*Zingiber officinale* (Zingiberaceae) *Piper cubeba* (Piperaceae)	*Callosobruchus chinensis* (Coleoptera: Bruchidae)	Repellent, insecticidal, antiovipositional, egg hatching	Chaubey (2013)
EO	*Zingiber purpureum Roscoe rhizomes*	*Tribolium castaneum* (Herbst) and *Lasioderma serricorne* (L.) adults	Contact toxicity, fumigant	Wang et al. (2015a)

5 Pesticides Biodecontamination by Bacterial Lactonases

Organophosphates are the largest class of known insecticides, several of which are potent nerve agents. Organophosphates have been widely used as insecticides and chemical warfare agents. The health risks associated with these agents have necessitated the need for better detoxification and bioremediation tools. Bacterial enzymes capable of hydrolyzing the lethal organophosphate nerve agents are of special interest (Tsai et al., 2012) as bioscavengers and biodecontaminants.

The *phosphotriesterases* (PTE), members of the amidohydrolase super family have been utilized to protect against organophosphate poisoning. PTE have a wide spectrum of biotechnological applications for detection and decontamination of insecticides and chemical warfare agents.

Serum paraoxonases PON1, PON2, and PON3 are lactonases/lactonyzing enzymes well recognized for their ability to hydrolyze arylesters, toxic oxon metabolites of organophosphate insecticides, and nerve agents. Dihydrocoumarin (DHC), long chain fatty acid lactones and acylhomoserine lactones (AHLs) are hydrolyzed by all three PONs and likely represent their natural substrates. Lactones are natural compounds, many of them with high biological activity, while organophosphates are human-made chemicals introduced in the 20th century. Therefore, the primary activity for which PON enzymes have evolved is lactonase, while the organophosphatase activity arose as a promiscuous activity during their evolution under the pressure of pesticides. Bacterial PTEs are members of the amidohydrolase super family and differ in their structure from the eukaryotic organophosphatases; PTEs are (beta/alpha)(8) barrels with an active site containing two transition metal ions, such as Co(2+), Mn(2+), or Zn(2+). PTE from *Pseudomonas diminuta* hydrolyzes paraoxon extremely efficiently; this enzyme was shown to hydrolyze also DHC and other lactones. At least three more bacterial lactonases, dubbed PTE-like lactonases (or PLL), have been identified to possess both lactonase and organophosphatase activities (Draganov, 2010).

Recently, a hyperthermophilic phosphotriesterase (SsoPox), from the Archaeon *Sulfolobus solfataricus*, has been isolated and found to possess a very high lactonase activity, associated with a very active site topology, and a unique hydrophobic channel with high affinity for the lactone substrate (Elias et al., 2008).

The recent specialization for utilization of pesticides reported for *P. diminuta* phosphotriesterase (pPTE) strongly suggests that this activity evolved from an enzyme endowed with promiscuous phosphotriesterase activity. Such a putative "generalist" enzyme was recently proposed to be a member of the new phoshotriesterase-like lactonase family (PLL). The promiscuous carboxylesterase and phosphodiesterase activities detected in pPTE and PLLs leads to the prediction of the existence in nature of PTE-like enzymes with predominant carboxylesterase or phosphodiesterase activities. On the basis of sequence similarity with the phosphotriesterase homology protein from *E. coli* and the carboxylesterase activity, it called phosphotriesterase-like carboxylesterase (MloPLC). The carboxylesterase activity is strictly dependent on divalent cations, and as such, MloPLC is the first phosphotriesterase-like metal-carboxylesterase characterized to date (Bhattacharyya and Jha 2012).

PTE variants were created through the manipulation of the substrate binding pockets to enhance catalytic activities for the detoxification of the more toxic S(P)-enantiomers of nerve agent analogues for GB, GD, GF, VX, and VR than the less toxic R(P)-enantiomers. Directed evolution and rational redesign of the active site of PTE isolated from the soil bacteria *P. diminuta* led to the identification of new variants with enhanced catalytic efficiency and stereoselectivity toward the hydrolysis of organophosphate neurotoxins. The catalytic activities of these newly identified PTE variants toward the S(P)-enantiomers of chromophoric analogues of GB, GD, GF, VX, and VR have been improved up to 15,000-fold relative to that of the wild-type enzyme (Tsai et al., 2012).

A combinatorial library of active site mutants was constructed by randomizing residues His-254, His-257, and Leu-303. The collection of mutant proteins was screened for the ability to hydrolyze a chromogenic analogue of the most toxic stereoisomer of the chemical warfare agent, soman. These studies demonstrate that substantial changes in substrate specificity can be achieved by relatively minor changes to the primary amino acid sequence.

6 Conclusions

Pesticides are represented by natural or chemical substances or mixtures of substances used for preventing, destroying, or controlling any pest (virucides, bactericides, fungicides, algaecides, herbicides, desiccants, insecticides, nematicides, molluscicides, rodenticides, avicides, piscicides). Despite their beneficial effects exhibited by the inhibitory effects against pests harmful for plants and animals, the chemical pesticides could also be toxic for other organisms and pollutants for the environment. Biopesticides, which are naturally occurring or derived materials from living organisms or their metabolites, have instead low negative effects as compared to chemical pesticides. The exploitation of inter-regn communication could lead to the development of novel and efficient biopesticides, with an extended spectrum of activity, but also of effective biodecontamination means of chemical pesticides. This ecological approach could therefore offer viable solutions for the implementation of a more sustainable agricultural system answering to the food security global issues.

References

Abbad, A., Kasrati, A., Jamali, C.A., Zeroual, S., Ba M'hamed, T., Spooner-Hart, R., Leach, D., 2014. Insecticidal properties and chemical composition of essential oils of some aromatic herbs from Morocco. Nat. Prod. Res. 28 (24), 2338–2341.

Abdullah, F., Subramanian, P., Ibrahim, H., Abdul Malek, S.N., Lee, G.S., Hong, S.L., 2015. Chemical composition, antifeedant, repellent, and toxicity activities of the rhizomes of galangal, *Alpinia galanga* against Asian subterranean termites, *Coptotermes gestroi* and *Coptotermes curvignathus* (Isoptera: Rhinotermitidae). J. Insect Sci. 15, 175.

Aguiar, R.W., dos Santos, S.F., da Silva Morgado, F., Ascencio, S.D., de Mendonça Lopes, M., Viana, K.F., Didonet, J., Ribeiro, B.M., 2015. Insecticidal and repellent activity of *Siparuna guianensis* Aubl. (Negramina) against *Aedes aegypti* and *Culex quinquefasciatus*. PLoS One 10 (2), e0116765.

Ajilogba, C.F., Babalola, O.O., 2013. Integrated management strategies for tomato *Fusarium wilt*. Biocontrol Sci. 18 (3), 117–127, 2013.

Akono, N.P., Baldovini, N., Mouray, E., Mambu, L., Belong, P., Grellier, P., 2014. Activity of *Ocimum basilicum*, *Ocimum canum*, and *Cymbopogon citratus*essential oils against *Plasmodium falciparum* and mature-stage larvae of *Anopheles funestus* s.s. Parasite 21, 33.

Alamir, A.E., Nenaah, G.E., Hafiz, M.A., 2015. Mathematical probit and logistic mortality models of the Khapra beetle fumigated with plant essential oils. Math. Biosci. Eng. 12 (4), 687–697.

Ali, A., Demirci, B., Kiyan, H.T., Bernier, U.R., Tsikolia, M., Wedge, D.E., Khan, I.A., Başer, K.H., Tabanca, N., 2013a. Biting deterrence, repellency, and larvicidal activity of *Ruta chalepensis* (Sapindales: Rutaceae) essential oil and its major individual constituents against mosquitoes. J. Med. Entomol. 50 (6), 1267–1274.

Ali, A., Murphy, C.C., Demirci, B., Wedge, D.E., Sampson, B.J., Khan, I.A., Baser, K.H., Tabanca, N., 2013b. Insecticidal and biting deterrent activity of rose-scented geranium (*Pelargonium* spp.) essential oils and individual compounds against *Stephanitis pyrioides* and *Aedes aegypti*. Pest Manag. Sci. 69 (12), 1385–1392.

Ali, A., Tabanca, N., Demirci, B., Baser, K.H., Ellis, J., Gray, S., Lackey, B.R., Murphy, C., Khan, I.A., Wedge, D.E., 2013c. Composition, mosquito larvicidal, biting deterrent and antifungal activity of essential oils of different plant parts of *Cupressus arizonica* var. Glabra (Carolina Sapphire). Nat. Prod. Commun. 8 (2), 257–260.

Ali, A., Tabanca, N., Kurkcuoglu, M., Duran, A., Blythe, E.K., Khan, I.A., Baser, K.H., 2014. Chemical composition, larvicidal, and biting deterrent activity of essential oils of two subspecies of *Tanacetum argenteum* (Asterales: Asteraceae) and individual constituents against *Aedes aegypti* (Diptera: Culicidae). J. Med. Entomol. 51 (4), 824–830.

Ali, A., Tabanca, N., Ozek, G., Ozek, T., Aytac, Z., Bernier, U.R., Agramonte, N.M., Baser, K.H., Khan, I.A., 2015a. EOs of *Echinophora lamondiana* (Apiales: Umbelliferae): a relationship between chemical profile and biting deterrence and larvicidal activity against mosquitoes (Diptera: Culicidae). J. Med. Entomol. 52 (1), 93–100.

Ali, A., Tabanca, N., Demirci, B., Blythe, E.K., Ali, Z., Baser, K.H., Khan, I.A., 2015b. Chemical composition and biological activity of four salvia essential oils and individual compounds against two species of mosquitoes. J. Agric. Food Chem. 63 (2), 447–456.

Ali, A., Wang, Y.H., Khan, I.A., 2015c. Larvicidal and biting deterrent activity of essential oils of *Curcuma longa*, Ar-turmerone, and Curcuminoids against *Aedes aegypti* and *Anopheles quadrimaculatus* (Culicidae: Diptera). J. Med. Entomol. 52 (5), 979–986.

Athanassiou, C.G., Kavallieratos, N.C., Evergetis, E., Katsoula, A.M., Haroutounian, S.A., 2013. Insecticidal efficacy of silica gel with *Juniperus oxycedrus* ssp. oxycedrus (Pinales: Cupressaceae) essential oil against *Sitophilus oryzae* (Coleoptera: Curculionidae) and *Tribolium confusum* (Coleoptera: Tenebrionidae). Econ. Entomol. 106 (4), 1902–1910.

Ávila Murilloa, M.C., Cuca Suareza, L.E., Cerón Salamanca, J.A., 2014. Chemical composition and insecticidal properties of essential oils of *Piper septuplinervium* and *P. subtomentosum* (Piperaceae). Nat. Prod. Commun. 9 (10), 1527–1530.

Azevedo, M.M., Almeida, C.A., Chaves, F.C., Campos-Takaki, G.M., Rozental, S., Bizzo, H.R., Alviano, C.S., Alviano, D.S., 2014. Effects of 7-hydroxycalamenene isolated from *Croton cajucara* essential oil on growth, lipid content and ultrastructural aspects of *Rhizopus oryzae*. Planta. Med. 80 (7), 550–556.

Babarinde, S.A., Akinyemi, A.O., Usman, L.A., Odewole, A.F., Sangodele, A.O., Iyiola, O.O., Olalere, O.D., 2014. Toxicity and repellency of *Hoslundia opposita* Vahl (Lamiaceae) leaves' essentialoil against rust-red flour beetle, *Tribolium castaneum* Herbst (Coleoptera: Tenebrionidae). Nat. Prod. Res. 28 (6), 365–371.

Babarinde, S.A., Pitan, O.O., Olatunde, G.O., Ajala, M.O., 2015. First report of toxicity of *Xylopiaparviflora* (A. Rich.) Benth (Annonaceae) root bark's essential oil against cowpea seed bruchid, *Callososbruchus maculatus* Fabricius (Coleoptera: Chrysomelidae: Bruchinae). Nat. Prod. Res. 29 (4), 349–352.

Basha, S.A., Sarma, B.K., Singh, D.P., Annapurna, K., Singh, U.P., 2006. Differential methods of inoculation of plant growth-promoting rhizobacteria induce synthesis of phenylalanine ammonia-lyase and phenolic compounds differentially in chickpea. Folia. Microbiol. (Praha). 51 (5), 463–468.

Benelli, G., Flamini, G., Fiore, G., Cioni, P.L., Conti, B., 2013. Larvicidal and repellent activity of the essential oil of *Coriandrum sativum* L. (Apiaceae) fruits against the filariasis vector *Aedes albopictus* Skuse (Diptera: Culicidae). Parasitol. Res. 112 (3), 1155–1161.

Bhattacharyya, P.N., Jha, D.K., 2012. Plant growth-promoting rhizobacteria (PGPR): emergence in agriculture. World J. Microbiol. Biotechnol. 28 (4), 1327–1350.

Boonyuan, W., Grieco, J.P., Bangs, M.J., Prabaripai, A., Tantakom, S., Chareonviriyaphap, T., 2014. Excito-repellency of essential oils against an *Aedes aegypti* (L.) field population in Thailand. J. Vector Ecol. 39 (1), 112–122.

Bossou, A.D., Mangelinckx, S., Yedomonhan, H., Boko, P.M., Akogbeto, M.C., De Kimpe, N., Avlessi, F., Sohounhloue, D.C., 2013. Chemical composition and insecticidal activity of plant essential oils from Benin against *Anopheles gambiae* (Giles). Parasit. Vectors 6, 337.

Bouajaj, S., Romane, A., Benyamna, A., Amri, I., Hanana, M., Hamrouni, L., Romdhane, M., 2014. Essential oil composition, phytotoxic and antifungal activities of *Ruta chalepensis* L. leaves from High Atlas Mountains (Morocco). Nat. Prod. Res. 28 (21), 1910–1914.

Bouzabata, A., Cabral, C., Gonçalves, M.J., Cruz, M.T., Bighelli, A., Cavaleiro, C., Casanova, J., Tomi, F., Salgueiro, L., 2015. *Myrtus communis* L. as source of a bioactive and safe essential oil. Food Chem. Toxicol. 75, 166–172.

Bouzenna, H., Krichen, L., 2013. *Pelargonium graveolens* L'Her. and *Artemisia arborescens* L. essential oils: chemical composition, antifungal activity against *Rhizoctonia solani* and insecticidal activity against *Rhysopertha dominica*. Nat. Prod. Res. 27 (9), 841–846.

Bovornnanthadej, T., Boonsoong, B., Taylor, D., Kainoh, Y., Koul, O., Bullangpoti, V., 2013. Effect of thymol on reproductive biology of *Helicoverpa armigera* Hübner (Lepidoptera: Noctuidae). Commun. Agric. Appl. Biol. Sci. 78 (2), 311–315.

Buchel, K.H., 1983. Chemistry of Pesticides. John Wiley & Sons, Inc, New York, USA.

Cervantes-Ceballos, L., Caballero-Gallardo, K., Olivero-Verbel, J., 2015. Repellent and anti quorum sensing activity of six aromatic plants occurring in Colombia. Nat. Prod. Commun. 10 (10), 1753–1757.

Chagas, A.C., Domingues, L.F., Fantatto, R.R., Giglioti, R., Oliveira, M.C., Oliveira, D.H., Mano, R.A., Jacob, R.G., 2014. *In* vitro and in vivo acaricide action of juvenoid analogs produced from the chemical modification of *Cymbopogon* spp. and *Corymbia citriodora* essential oil on the cattle tick *Rhipicephalus* (Boophilus) microplus. Vet. Parasitol. 205 (1–2), 277–284.

Chaubey, M.K., 2013. Biological activities of *Zingiber officinale* (Zingiberaceae) and *Piper cubeba* (Piperaceae) essential oils against pulse beetle, *Callosobruchus chinensis* (Coleoptera: Bruchidae). Pak. J. Biol. Sci. 16 (11), 517–523.

Chen, Q., Xu, S., Wu, T., Guo, J., Sha, S., Zheng, X., Yu, T., 2014. Effect of citronella essential oil on the inhibition of postharvest *Alternaria alternata* in cherry tomato. J. Sci. Food Agric. 94 (12), 2441–2447.

Chin-A-Woeng, T.F.C., de Priester, W., van der Bij, A.J., Lugtenberg, B.J.J., 1997. Description of the colonization of a gnotobiotic tomato rhizosphere by *Pseudomonas fluorescens* biocontrol strain WCS365, using scanning electron microscopy. Mol. Plant Microbe Interact. 10, 79–86.

Chin-A-Woeng, T.F.C., Bloemberg, G.V., van der Bij, A.J., van der Drift, K.M.G.M., Schripsema, J., Kroon, B., Scheffer, R.J., Keel, C., Bakker, P.A.H.M., Tichy, H.V., de Bruijn, F.J., Thomas-Oates, J.E., Lugtenberg, B.J.J., 1998. Biocontrol by phenazine-1-carboxamide-producing *Pseudomonas chlororaphis* PCL1391 of tomato root rot caused by *Fusarium oxysporum* f. sp. *radicis-lycopersici*. Mol. Plant Microbe Interact. 11, 1069–1077.

Chin-A-Woeng, T.F.C., Bloemberg, G.V., Lugtenberg, B.J.J., 2003. Phenazines and their role in biocontrol by *Pseudomonas* bacteria. New Phytologist 157, 503–523.

Chowhan, N., Singh, H.P., Batish, D.R., Kaur, S., Ahuja, N., Kohli, R.K., 2013. β-Pinene inhibited germination and early growth involves membrane peroxidation. Protoplasma 250 (3), 691–700.

Conti, B., Leonardi, M., Pistelli, L., Profeti, R., Ouerghemmi, I., Benelli, G., 2013. Larvicidal and repellent activity of essential oils from wild and cultivated *Ruta chalepensis* L. (Rutaceae) against *Aedes albopictus* Skuse (Diptera: Culicidae), an arbovirus vector. Parasitol. Res. 112 (3), 991–999.

Costa, D.C., Vermelho, A.B., Almeida, C.A., de Souza Dias, E.P., Cedrola, S.M., Arrigoni-Blank Mde, F., Blank, A.F., Alviano, C.S., Alviano, D.S., 2014. Inhibitory effect of linalool rich essential oil from *Lippia alba* on the peptidase and keratinase activities of dermatophytes. J. Enzyme Inhib. Med. Chem. 29 (1), 12–17.

Cruz, E.M., Costa, Jr., L.M., Pinto, J.A., Santos Dde, A., de Araujo, S.A., Arrigoni-Blank Mde, F., Bacci, L., Alves, P.B., Cavalcanti, S.C., Blank, A.F., 2013. Acaricidal activity of *Lippia gracilis* essential oil and its major constituents on the tick *Rhipicephalus* (Boophilus) microplus. Vet. Parasitol. 195 (1–2), 198–202.

Cruz, G.S., Wanderley-Teixeira, V., Oliveira, J.V., Correia, A.A., Breda, M.O., Alves, T.J., Cunha, F.M., Teixeira, A.A., Dutra, K.A., Navarro, D.M., 2014. Bioactivity of *Piper hispidinervum* (Piperales: Piperaceae) and *Syzygium aromaticum* (Myrtales: Myrtaceae) oils, with or without formulated Bta on the biology and immunology of *Spodoptera frugiperda* (Lepidoptera: Noctuidae). J. Econ. Entomol. 107 (1), 144–153.

de Assis Lage, T.C., Montanari, R.M., Fernandes, S.A., de Oliveira Monteiro, C.M., de Oliveira Souza Senra, T., Zeringota, V., da Silva Matos, R., Daemon, E., 2015. Chemical composition and acaricidal activity of the essential oil of *Baccharis dracunculifolia* De Candole (1836) and its constituents nerolidol and limonene on larvae and engorged females of *Rhipicephalus microplus* (Acari: Ixodidae). Exp. Parasitol. 148, 24–29.

de Lima, G.P., de Souza, T.M., de Paula Freire, G., Farias, D.F., Cunha, A.P., Ricardo, N.M., de Morais, S.M., Carvalho, A.F., 2013. Further insecticidal activities of essential oils from *Lippia sidoides* and Croton species against *Aedes aegypti* L. Parasitol. Res. 112 (5), 1953–1958.

de Mello, V., Prata, M.C., da Silva, M.R., Daemon, E., da Silva, L.S., Guimarães Fdel, G., de Mendonça, A.E., Folly, E., Vilela, F.M., do Amaral, L.H., Cabral, L.M., do Amaral Mda, P., 2014. Acaricidal properties of the formulations based on essential oils from *Cymbopogon winterianus* and *Syzygium aromaticum* plants. Parasitol. Res. 113 (12), 4431–4437.

Demirci, B., Tsikolia, M., Bernier, U.R., Agramonte, N.M., Alqasoumi, S.I., Al-Yahya, M.A., Al-Rehaily, A.J., Yusufoglu, H.S., Demirci, F., Başer, K.H., Khan, I.A., Tabanca, N., 2013. *Phoenix dactylifera* L. spathe essential oil: chemical composition and repellent activity against the yellow fever mosquito. Acta Trop. 128 (3), 557–560.

Deweer, C., Yaguiyan, A., Muchembled, J., Sahmer, K., Dermont, C., Halama, P., 2013. In vitro evaluation of dill seed essential oil antifungal activities to control *Zymoseptoria tritici*. Commun. Agric. Appl. Biol. Sci. 78 (3), 489–495.

Diallo, S., Crépin, A., Barbey, C., Orange, N., Burini, J.F., Latour, X., 2011. Mechanisms and recent advances in biological control mediated through the potato rhizosphere. FEMS Microbiol. Ecol. 75 (3), 351–364.

do Nascimento, J.C., David, J.M., Barbosa, L.C., de Paula, V.F., Demuner, A.J., David, J.P., Conserva, L.M., Ferreira, Jr., J.C., Guimarães, E.F., 2013. Larvicidal activities and chemical composition of essential oils from *Piper klotzschianum* (Kunth) C. DC. (Piperaceae). Pest Manag. Sci. 69 (11), 1267–1271.

Do Prado, G.P., Stefani, L.M., Da Silva, A.S., Smaniotto, L.F., Garcia, F.R., De Moura, N.F., 2013. *Alphitobius diaperinus* (Coleoptera: Tenebrionidae) susceptibility to *Cunila angustifolia* essential oil. J. Med. Entomol. 50 (5), 1040–1045.

Draganov, D.I., 2010. Lactonases with organophosphatase activity: structural and evolutionary perspectives. Chem. Biol. Interact. 6 (187(1–3)), 370–372.

Drum, C., 1980. Soil Chemistry of Pesticides. PPG Industries, Inc, USA.

Dua, V.K., Kumar, A., Pandey, A.C., Kumar, S., 2013. Insecticidal and genotoxic activity of *Psoralea corylifolia* Linn. (Fabaceae) against *Culex quinquefasciatus* Say, 1823. Parasit. Vectors 6, 30.

Dunlap, C., Delaney, I., Fenton, A., Lohrke, S., Moënne-Loccoz, Y., O'Gara, F., 1996. The biotechnology and application of *Pseudomonas* inoculants for the biocontrol of phytopathogens. In: Stacey, G., Mullin, B., Gresshoff, P.M. (Eds.), Biology of plant microbe interactions. International Society for Molecular Plant–Microbe Interactions, St Paul, MN, USA, pp. 441–448.

Elias, M., Dupuy, J., Merone, L., Mandrich, L., Porzio, E., Moniot, S., Rochu, D., Lecomte, C., Rossi, M., Masson, P., Manco, G., Chabriere, E., 2008. Structural basis for natural lactonase and promiscuous phosphotriesterase activities. J. Mol. Biol. 379 (5), 1017–1028.

Eliopoulos, P.A., Hassiotis, C.N., Andreadis, S.S., Porichi, A.E., 2015. Fumigant toxicity of essential oils from basil and spearmint against two major pyralid pests of stored products. J. Econ. Entomol. 108 (2), 805–810.

Ellse, L., Burden, F.A., Wall, R., 2013. Control of the chewing louse *Bovicola* (Werneckiella) ocellatus in donkeys, usingessential oils. Med. Vet. Entomol. 27 (4), 408–413.

Faghihzadeh Gorji, S., Faghihzadeh Gorji, S., Rajabloo, M., 2014. The field efficacy of garlic extract against *Dermanyssus gallinae* in layer farms of Babol, Iran. Parasitol. Res. 113 (3), 1209–1213.

Fayemiwo, K.A., Adeleke, M.A., Okoro, O.P., Awojide, S.H., Awoniyi, I.O., 2014. Larvicidal efficacies and chemical composition of essential oils of *Pinus sylvestris* and *Syzygium aromaticum* against mosquitoes. Asian Pac. J. Trop. Biomed. 4 (1), 30–34.

Fernandez, R.O., Pizarro, R.A., 1997. High performance liquid chromatographic analysis of *Pseudomonas aeruginosa* phenazines. J. Chromatog. A 771, 99–104.

Füller, T.N., Bertrand, C., Simon, A., Inchausti de Barros, I.B., Barbosa Neto, J.F., 2014. Elionurus muticus as an alternative source of citral from Pampa biome, Brazil. J. Oleo. Sci. 63 (11), 1109–1116.

Gallardo, A., Picollo, M.I., Mougabure-Cueto, G., 2015. Lethal activity of individual and mixed monoterpenoids of geranium essential oil on *Musca domestica*. Parasitol. Res. 114 (3), 1229–1232.

Galli, E., Silver, S., Witholt, B., 1992. Pseudomonas: molecular biology and biotechnology. American Society for Microbiology, Washington DC.

Giatropoulos, A., Pitarokili, D., Papaioannou, F., Papachristos, D.P., Koliopoulos, G., Emmanouel, N., Tzakou, O., Michaelakis, A., 2013. Essential oil composition, adult repellency and larvicidal activity of eight *Cupressaceae* species from Greece against *Aedes albopictus* (Diptera: Culicidae). Parasitol. Res. 112 (3), 1113–1123.

Gkinis, G., Michaelakis, A., Koliopoulos, G., Ioannou, E., Tzakou, O., Roussis, V., 2014. Evaluation of the repellent effects of *Nepeta parnassica* extract, essential oil, and its major nepetalactone metabolite against mosquitoes. Parasitol. Res. 113 (3), 1127–1134.

Godara, R., Parveen, S., Katoch, R., Yadav, A., Verma, P.K., Katoch, M., Kaur, D., Ganai, A., Raghuvanshi, P., Singh, N.K., 2014. Acaricidal activity of extract of *Artemisia absinthium* against *Rhipicephalus sanguineus* of dogs. Parasitol. Res. 113 (2), 747–754.

Gomes, S.P., Favero, S., 2013. Assessment of the insecticidal potential of *Eucalyptus urograndis* essential oil against *Rhodnius neglectus* Lent (Hemiptera: Reduviidae). Neotrop. Entomol. 42 (4), 431–435.

Gomes, G.A., Monteiro, C.M., Julião Lde, S., Maturano, R., Senra, T.O., Zeringóta, V., Calmon, F., Matos Rda, S., Daemon, E., Carvalho, M.G., 2014. Acaricidal activity of essential oil from *Lippia sidoides* on unengorged larvae and nymphs of *Rhipicephalus sanguineus* (Acari: Ixodidae) and *Amblyomma cajennense* (Acari: Ixodidae). Exp. Parasitol. 137, 41–45.

Govindarajan, M., Sivakumar, R., Rajeswary, M., Veerakumar, K., 2013a. Mosquito larvicidal activity of thymol from essential oil of *Coleus aromaticus* Benth. against *Culex tritaeniorhynchus*, *Aedes albopictus*, and *Anopheles subpictus* (Diptera: Culicidae). Parasitol. Res. 112 (11), 3713–3721.

Govindarajan, M., Sivakumar, R., Rajeswary, M., Yogalakshmi, K., 2013b. Chemical composition and larvicidal activity of essential oil from *Ocimum basilicum* (L.) against *Culex tritaeniorhynchus*, *Aedes albopictus* and *Anopheles subpictus* (Diptera: Culicidae). Exp. Parasitol. 134 (1), 7–11.

Granados-Echegoyen, C., Pérez-Pacheco, R., Soto-Hernández, M., Ruiz-Vega, J., Lagunez-Rivera, L., Alonso-Hernandez, N., Gato-Armas, R., 2014. Inhibition of the growth and development of mosquito larvae of *Culex quinquefasciatus* (Diptera: Culicidae) treated with extract from leaves of *Pseudocalymma alliaceum* (Bignonaceae). Asian Pac. J. Trop. Med. 7 (8), 594–601.

Gutterson, N., 1990. Microbial fungicides: recent approaches to elucidating mechanisms. Crit. Rev. Microbiol. 10, 69–91.

Haddi, K., Oliveira, E.E., Faroni, L.R., Guedes, D.C., Miranda, N.N., 2015. Sublethal exposure to clove and cinnamon essential oils induces hormetic-like responses and disturbs behavioral and respiratory responses in *Sitophilus zeamais* (Coleoptera: Curculionidae). J. Econ. Entomol. 108 (6), 2815–2822.

Hammami, I., Ben Hsouna, A., Hamdi, N., Gdoura, R., Triki, M.A., 2013. Isolation and characterization of rhizosphere bacteria for the biocontrol of the damping-off disease of tomatoes in Tunisia. C. R. Biol. 336 (11–12), 557–564.

Hassan, M.I., Hammad, K.M., Saeed, S.M., 2015. Repellent effect of *Ocimum basilicum* and *Glycyrrhiza glabra* extracts against the mosquito vector, *Culex pipiens* (Diptera: Culicidae). J. Egypt. Soc. Parasitol. 45 (2), 241–248.

Hsu, W.S., Yen, J.H., Wang, Y.S., 2013. Formulas of components of citronella oil against mosquitoes (*Aedes aegypti*). J. Environ. Sci. Health B 48 (11), 1014–1019.

Huang, S.H., Xian, J.D., Kong, S.Z., Li, Y.C., Xie, J.H., Lin, J., Chen, J.N., Wang, H.F., Su, Z.R., 2014. Insecticidal activity of pogostone against *Spodoptera litura* and *Spodoptera exigua* (Lepidoptera: Noctuidae). Pest Manag. Sci. 70 (3), 510–516.

Hynes, R.K., Leung, G.C., Hirkala, D.L., Nelson, L.M., 2008. Isolation, selection, and characterization of beneficial rhizobacteria from pea, lentil, and chickpea grown in western Canada. Can. J. Microbiol. 54 (4), 248–258.

Ivoke, N., Ogbonna, P.C., Ekeh, F.N., Ezenwaji, N.E., Atama, C.I., Ejere, V.C., Onoja, U.S., Eyo, J.E., 2013. Effects of grapefruit (Citrus paradisi MACF) (Rutaceae) peel oil against developmental stages of *Aedes aegypti* (Diptera: Culicidae). Southeast Asian J. Trop. Med. Public Health 44 (6), 970–978.

Izakmehri, K., Saber, M., Mehrvar, A., Hassanpouraghdam, M.B., Vojoudi, S., 2013. Lethal and sublethal effects of essential oils from *Eucalyptus camaldulensis* and *Heracleum persicum* against the adults of *Callosobruchus maculatus*. J. Insect. Sci. 13, 152.

Jaya, Singh, P., Prakash, B., Dubey, N.K., 2014. Insecticidal activity of *Ageratum conyzoides* L., *Coleus aromaticus* Benth. and *Hyptis suaveolens* (L.) Poit essential oils as fumigant against storage grain insect *Tribolium castaneum* Herbst. J. Food Sci. Technol. 51 (9), 2210–2215.

Jo, H.J., Park, K.M., Min, S.C., Na, J.H., Park, K.H., Han, J., 2013. Development of an anti-insect sachet using a polyvinyl alcohol-cinnamon oil polymer strip against *Plodia interpunctella*. J. Food Sci. 78 (11), e1713–e1720.

Karamaouna, F., Kimbaris, A., Michaelakis, A., Papachristos, D., Polissiou, M., Papatsakona, P., Tsora, E., 2013. Insecticidal activity of plant essential oils against the vine mealybug, *Planococcus ficus*. J. Insect Sci. 13, 142.

Kazemi, M., 2015. Effect of *Carum copticum* essential oil on growth and aflatoxin formation by *Aspergillus* strains. Nat. Prod. Res. 29 (11), 1065–1068.

Kedia, A., Prakash, B., Mishra, P.K., Dubey, N.K., 2014. Antifungal and antiaflatoxigenic properties of *Cuminum cyminum* (L.) seedessential oil and its efficacy as a preservative in stored commodities. Int. J. Food Microbiol. 168–169, 1–7.

Khater, H.F., 2014. Bioactivities of some essential oils against the camel nasal botfly, *Cephalopina titillator*. Parasitol. Res. 113 (2), 593–605.

Klauck, V., Pazinato, R., Stefani, L.M., Santos, R.C., Vaucher, R.A., Baldissera, M.D., Raffin, R., Boligon, A., Athayde, M., Baretta, D., Machado, G., DA Silva, A.S., 2014. Insecticidal and repellent effects of tea tree and andiroba oils on flies associated with livestock. Med. Vet. Entomol. 28 (Suppl. 1), 33–39.

Klauck, V., Pazinato, R., Radavelli, W.M., Volpato, A., Stefani, L.M., Santos, R.C., Vaucher, R.A., Boligon, A.A., Athayde, M.L., Da Silva, A.S., 2015. In vitro repellent effect of tea tree (*Melaleuca alternifolia*) and andiroba (*Carapa guianensis*) oils on *Haematobia irritans* and *Chrysomya megacephala* flies. Trop. Biomed. 32 (1), 160–166.

Koc, S., Oz, E., Cinbilgel, I., Aydin, L., Cetin, H., 2013. Acaricidal activity of *Origanum bilgeri* P.H. Davis (Lamiaceae) essential oil and its major component, carvacrol against adults *Rhipicephalus turanicus* (Acari: Ixodidae). Vet. Parasitol. 193 (1–3), 316–319.

Koster, M., van de Vossenberg, J., Leong, J., Weisbeek, P.J., 1993. Identification and characterization of the pupB gene encoding an inducible ferricpseudobactin receptor of *Pseudomonas putida* WCS358. Mol. Microbiol. 8, 591–601.

Koster, M., Ovaa, W., Bitter, W., Weisbeek, P., 1995. Multiple outer membrane receptors for uptake of ferric pseudobactins in *Pseudomonas putida* WCS385. Mol. Gen. Genet. 248, 735–743.

Koutsaviti, K., Giatropoulos, A., Pitarokili, D., Papachristos, D., Michaelakis, A., Tzakou, O., 2015. Greek Pinus essential oils: larvicidal activity and repellency against *Aedes albopictus* (Diptera: Culicidae). Parasitol. Res. 114 (2), 583–592.

Kumar, V., Kumar, A., Kharwar, R.N., 2007. Antagonistic potential of fluorescent pseudomonads and control of charcoal rot of chickpea caused by *Macrophomina phaseolina*. J. Environ. Biol. 28 (1), 15–20.

Kumar, P., Mishra, S., Malik, A., Satya, S., 2013. Housefly (*Musca domestica* L.) control potential of *Cymbopogon citratus* Stapf. (Poales: Poaceae) essential oil and monoterpenes (citral and 1,8-cineole). Parasitol. Res. 112 (1), 69–76.

Kumar, P., Mishra, S., Malik, A., Satya, S., 2014. Biocontrol potential of essential oil monoterpenes against housefly, *Musca domestica* (Diptera: Muscidae). Ecotoxicol. Environ. Saf. 100, 1–6.

La Torre, A., Caradonia, F., Gianferro, M., Molinu, M.G., Battaglia, V., 2014. Activity of natural products against some phytopathogenic. Commun. Agric. Appl. Biol. Sci. 79 (3), 439–449.

Lachance, S., Grange, G., 2014. Repellent effectiveness of seven plant essential yoils, sunflower oil and natural insecticides against horn flies on pastured dairy cows and heifers. Med. Vet. Entomol. 28 (2), 193–200.

Lage, T.C., Montanari, R.M., Fernandes, S.A., de Oliveira Monteiro, C.M., de Oliveira Souza Senra, T., Zeringota, V., Calmon, F., da Silva Matos, R., Daemon, E., 2013. Activity of essential oil of *Lippia triplinervis* Gardner (Verbenaceae) on *Rhipicephalus microplus* (Acari: Ixodidae). Parasitol. Res. 112 (2), 863–869.

Lawal, O.A., Ogunwande, I.A., Salvador, A.F., Sanni, A.A., Opoku, A.R., 2014. *Pachira glabra* Pasq. essential oil: chemical constituents, antimicrobial and insecticidal activities. J. Oleo. Sci. 63 (6), 629–635.

Lebouvier, N., Hue, T., Hnawia, E., Lesaffre, L., Menut, C., Nour, M., 2013. Acaricidal activity of essential oils from five endemic conifers of New Caledonia on the cattle tick *Rhipicephalus* (Boophilus) microplus. Parasitol. Res. 112 (4), 1379–1384.

Lima, T.C., da Silva, T.K., Silva, F.L., Barbosa-Filho, J.M., Marques, M.O., Santos, R.L., Cavalcanti, S.C., de Sousa, D.P., 2014. Larvicidal activity of Mentha × villosa Hudson essential oil, rotundifolone and derivatives. Chemosphere 104, 37–43.

Líska, D., Kolesár, D., 1982. Toxicological classification of pesticides. Czech. Med. 5 (3), 137–145.

Liu, X.C., Liu, Z.L., 2015. Analysis of the essential oil of *Illicium henryi* Diels root bark and its insecticidal activity against *Liposcelis bostrychophila* Badonnel. J. Food Prot. 78 (4), 772–777.

Liu, X.C., Li, Y.P., Li, H.Q., Deng, Z.W., Zhou, L., Liu, Z.L., Du, S.S., 2013a. Identification of repellent and insecticidal constituents of the essential oil of *Artemisia rupestris* L. aerial parts against *Liposcelis bostrychophila* Badonnel. Molecules 18 (9), 10733–10746.

Liu, X.C., Dong, H.W., Zhou, L., Du, S.S., Liu, Z.L., 2013b. Essential oil composition and larvicidal activity of *Toddalia asiatica* roots against the mosquito *Aedes albopictus* (Diptera: Culicidae). Parasitol. Res. 112 (3), 1197–1203.

Liu, X.C., Liang, Y., Shi, W.P., Liu, Q.Z., Zhou, L., Liu, Z.L., 2014a. Repellent and insecticidal effects of the essential oil of *Kaempferia galanga* rhizomes to *Liposcelis bostrychophila* (Psocoptera: Liposcelidae). J. Econ. Entomol. 107 (4), 1706–1712.

Liu, X.C., Liu, Q., Zhou, L., Liu, Z.L., 2014b. Evaluation of larvicidal activity of the essential oil of *Allium macrostemon* Bunge and its selected major constituent compounds against *Aedes albopictus* (Diptera: Culicidae). Parasit. Vectors. 7, 184.

Liu, X.C., Liu, Q., Chen, H., Liu, Q.Z., Jiang, S.Y., Liu, Z.L., 2015a. Evaluation of contact toxicity and repellency of the essential oil of *Pogostemon cablin* leaves and its constituents against *Blattella germanica* (Blattodae: Blattelidae). J. Med. Entomol. 20152 (1), 86–92.

Liu, X.C., Zhou, L., Liu, Q., Liu, Z.L., 2015b. Laboratory evaluation of larvicidal activity of the essential oil of *Allium tuberosum* roots and its selected major constituent compounds against *Aedes albopictus* (Diptera: Culicidae). J. Med. Entomol. 52 (3), 437–441.

Liu, X.C., Liu, Q., Chen, X.B., Liu, Q.Z., Liu, Z.L., 2015c. Larvicidal activity of the essential oil of *Youngia japonica* aerial parts and its constituents against *Aedes albopictus*. Z. Naturforsch C. 70 (1–2), 1–6.

Lucia, A., Zerba, E., Masuh, H., 2013. Knockdown and larvicidal activity of six monoterpenes against *Aedes aegypti* (Diptera: Culicidae) and their structure-activity relationships. Parasitol. Res. 112 (12), 4267–4272.

Lugtenberg, B.J.J., de Weger, L.A., Schippers, B., 1994. Bacterization to protect seed and rhizosphere against disease. BCPC Monograph 57, 293–302.

Lugtenberg, B.J.J., Kravchenko, L.V., Simons, M., 1999a. Tomato seed and root exudate sugars: composition, utilization by *Pseudomonas* biocontrol strains and role in rhizosphere colonization. Environ. Microbiol. 1, 439–446.

Lugtenberg, B.J.J., Dekkers, L.C., Bansraj, M., Bloemberg, G.V., Camacho, M., Chin-A-Woeng, T.F.C., van den Hondel, C., Kravchenko, L., Kuiper, I., Lagopodi, A.L., Mulders, I., Phoelich, C., Ram, A., Tikhonovich, I., Tuinman, S., Wijffelman, C., Wijfjes, A., 1999b. *Pseudomonas* genes and traits involved in tomato root colonization. De Wit, P.J.G.M., Bisseling, T., Stiekema, W.J. (Eds.), 1999 IC-MPMI Congress Proceedings: biology of plant–microbe interactions, 2, International Society for Molecular Plant–Microbe Interactions, St Paul, MN, USA, pp. 324–330.

Lutz, A., Sfara, V., Alzogaray, R.A., 2014. Repellence produced by monoterpenes on *Rhodnius prolixus* (Hemiptera: Reduviidae) decreases after continuous exposure to these compounds. J. Insect Sci. 14, 254.

Lynch Ianniello, I., Horenstein, M.B., Lábaque, M.C., Luna, A., Marin, R.H., Gleiser, R.M., 2014. Fly emergence from manure of Japanese quail fed thymol- or isoeugenol-supplemented diets. Poult. Sci. 93 (10), 2449–2456.

Ma, W.B., Feng, J.T., Jiang, Z.L., Wu, H., Ma, Z.Q., Zhang, X., 2014. Fumigant activity of eleven essential oil compounds and their selected binary mixtures against *Culex pipiens* pallens (Diptera: Culicidae). Parasitol. Res. 113 (10), 3631–3637.

Mahajan, M.S., Tan, M.W., Rahme, L.G., Ausubel, F.M., 1999. Molecular mechanisms of bacterial virulence elucidated using a *Pseudomonas aeruginosa–Caenorhabditis elegans* pathogenesis model. Cell 96, 47–56.

Mahakittikun, V., Soonthornchareonnon, N., Foongladda, S., Boitano, J.J., Wangapai, T., Ninsanit, P., 2014. A preliminary study of the acaricidal activity of clove oil, *Eugenia caryophyllus*. Asian Pac. J. Allergy Immunol. 32 (1), 46–52.

Maheswaran, R., Ignacimuthu, S., 2013. Bioefficacy of essential oil from *Polygonum hydropiper* L. against mosquitoes, *Anopheles stephensi* and *Culex quinquefasciatus*. Ecotoxicol. Environ. Saf. 97, 26–31.

Maheswaran, R., Ignacimuthu, S., 2014. Effect of *Polygonum hydropiper* L. against dengue vector mosquito *Aedes albopictus* L. Parasitol. Res. 113 (9), 3143–3150.

Maheswaran, R., Ignacimuthu, S., 2015. Effect of confertifolin from *Polygonum hydropiper* L. against dengue vector mosquitoes *Aedes aegypti* L. Environ. Sci. Pollut. Res. Int. 22 (11), 8280–8287.

Mahmoudvand, H., Ezzatkhah, F., Sharififar, F., Sharifi, I., Dezaki, E.S., 2015. Antileishmanial and cytotoxic effects of essential oil and methanolic extract of *Myrtus communis* L. Korean J. Parasitol. 53 (1), 21–27.

Manjari, M.S., Karthi, S., Ramkumar, G., Muthusamy, R., Natarajan, D., Shivakumar, M.S., 2014. Chemical composition and larvicidal activity of plant extracts from *Clausena dentata* (Willd) (Rutaceae) against dengue, malaria, and filariasis vectors. Parasitol. Res. 113 (7), 2475–2481.

Martínez, J.A., González, R., 2013. Essential oils from clove affect growth of *Penicillium* species obtained from lemons. Commun. Agric. Appl. Biol. Sci. 78 (3), 563–572.

Mayeku, W.P., Omollo, N.I., Odalo, O.J., Hassanali, A., 2014. Chemical composition and mosquito repellency of essential oil of *Conyza newii* propagated in different geographical locations of Kenya. Med. Vet. Entomol. 28 (3), 253–256.

Mazzola, M., Cook, R.J., Thomashow, L.S., Weller, D.M., Pierson, L.S., 1992. Contribution of phenazine antibiotic biosynthesis to the ecological competence of fluorescent Pseudomonads in soil habitats. Appl. Environ. Microbiol. 58, 2616–2624.

Mdoe, F.P., Cheng, S.S., Lyaruu, L., Nkwengulila, G., Chang, S.T., Kweka, E.J., 2014. Larvicidal efficacy of *Cryptomeria japonica* leaf essential oils against *Anopheles gambiae*. Parasit. Vectors 4 (7), 426.

Mejía-Garibay, B., Palou, E., López-Malo, A., 2015. Composition, diffusion, and antifungal activity of black mustard (*Brassica nigra*) essential oil when applied by direct addition or vapor phase contact. J. Food Prot. 78 (4), 843–848.

Montefuscoli, A.R., Werdin González, J.O., Palma, S.D., Ferrero, A.A., Fernández Band, B., 2014. Design and development of aqueous nanoformulations for mosquito control. Parasitol. Res. 113 (2), 793–800.

Monteiro, C.M., Araújo, L.X., Gomes, G.A., Senra, T.O., Calmon, F., Daemon, E., de Carvalho, M.G., Bittencourt, V.R., Furlong, J., Prata, M.C., 2014. Entomopathogenic nematodes associated with essential oil of *Lippia sidoides* for control of *Rhipicephalus microplus* (Acari: Ixodidae). Parasitol. Res. 113 (1), 189–195.

Myresiotis, C.K., Karaoglanidis, G.S., Vryzas, Z., Papadopoulou-Mourkidou, E., 2012. Evaluation of plant-growth-promoting rhizobacteria, acibenzolar-S-methyl andhymexazol for integrated control of *Fusarium* crown and root rot on tomato. Pest Manag. Sci. 68 (3), 404–411.

Nogueira, J., Vinturelle, R., Mattos, C., Tietbohl, L.A., Santos, M.G., Junior, I.S., Mourão, S.C., Rocha, L., Folly, E., 2014a. Acaricidal properties of the essential oil from *Zanthoxylum caribaeum* against *Rhipicephalus microplus*. J. Med. Entomol. 51 (5), 971–975.

Nogueira, J., Mourão, S.C., Dolabela, I.B., Santos, M.G., Mello, C.B., Kelecom, A., Mexas, R., Feder, D., Fernandes, C.P., Gonzalez, M.S., Rocha, L., 2014b. *Zanthoxylum caribaeum* (Rutaceae) essential oil: chemical investigation and biological effects on *Rhodnius prolixus* nymph. Parasitol. Res. 113 (11), 4271–4279.

Noosidum, A., Chareonviriyaphap, T., Chandrapatya, A., 2014. Synergistic repellent and irritant effect of combined essential oils on *Aedes aegypti* (L.) mosquitoes. J. Vector Ecol. 39 (2), 298–305.

Oliveira, G.L., Cardoso, S.K., Lara, Jr., C.R., Vieira, T.M., Guimarães, E.F., Figueiredo, L.S., Martins, E.R., Moreira, D.L., Kaplan, M.A., 2013. Chemical study and larvicidal activity against *Aedes aegypti* of essential oil of *Piper aduncum* L. (Piperaceae). An. Acad. Bras. Cienc. 85 (4), 1227–1234.

Owolabi, M.S., Padilla-Camberos, E., Ogundajo, A.L., Ogunwande, I.A., Flamini, G., Yusuff, O.K., Allen, K., Flores-Fernandez, K.I., Flores-Fernandez, J.M., 2014. Insecticidal activity and chemical composition of the *Morinda lucida* essential oil against pulse beetle *Callosobruchus maculatus*. Sci. World J. 2014, 784613.

Padalia, R.C., Verma, R.S., Chauhan, A., Goswami, P., Chanotiya, C.S., Saroj, A., Samad, A., Khaliq, A., 2014. Compositional variability and antifungal potentials of *Ocimum basilicum, O. tenuiflorum, O. gratissimum* and *O. kilimandscharicum* essential oils against *Rhizoctonia solani* and *Choanephora cucurbitarum*. Nat. Prod. Commun. 9 (10), 1507–1510.

Park, I.K., 2014. Fumigant toxicity of Oriental sweetgum (*Liquidambar orientalis*) and valerian (*Valeriana wallichii*) essential oils and their components, including their acetylcholinesterase inhibitory activity, against Japanese termites (*Reticulitermes speratus*). Molecules 19 (8), 12547–12558.

Pérez López, L.A., de la Torre, Y.C., Cirio, A.T., de Torres, N.W., Flores Suárez, A.E., Aranda, R.S., 2015. Essential oils from *Zanthoxylum fagara* Wild Lime, *Ruta chalepensis* L. and *Thymus vulgaris* L.: composition and activity against *Aedes aegypti* larvae. Pak. J. Pharm. Sci. 28 (5 Suppl.), 1911–1915.

Perumalsamy, H., Kim, J.Y., Kim, J.R., Hwang, K.N., Ahn, Y.J., 2014. Toxicity of basil oil constituents and related compounds and the efficacy of spray formulations to *Dermatophagoides farinae* (Acari: Pyroglyphidae). J. Med. Entomol. 51 (3), 650–657.

Pesticide Application and Safety Training for Applicators of Public Health Pesticides, 2016. Chapter 2. Available from: http://westnile.ca.gov/special/category_a/?page(Chapter2.htm, January 10, 2016

Phukerd, U., Soonwera, M., 2013. Larvicidal and pupicidal activities of essential oils from Zingiberaceae plants against *Aedes aegypti* (Linn.) and *Culex quinquefasciatus* say mosquitoes. Southeast Asian J. Trop. Med. Pub. Health 44 (5), 761–771.

Phukerd, U., Soonwera, M., 2014. Repellency of essential oils extracted from Thai native plants against *Aedes aegypti* (Linn.) and *Culex quinquefasciatus* (Say). Parasitol. Res. 113 (9), 3333–3340.

Pierson, III, L.S., Gaffney, T., Lam, S., Gong, F., 1995. Molecular analysis of genes encodi phenazine biosynthesis in the biological control bacterium *Pseudomonas aureofaciens* 30–84. FEMS Microbiol. Lett. 134, 299–307.

Politi, F.A., de Souza-Moreira, T.M., Rodrigues, E.R., de Queiroz, G.M., Figueira, G.M., Januário, A.H., Berenger, J.M., Socolovschi, C., Parola, P., Pietro, R.C.,

2013. Chemical characterization and acaricide potential of essential oil from aerial parts of *Tagetes patula* L. (Asteraceae) against engorged adult females of *Rhipicephalus sanguineus* (Latreille, 1806). Parasitol. Res. 112 (6), 2261–2268.

Popović, Z., Kostić, M., Stanković, S., Milanović, S., Sivčev, I., Kostić, I., Kljajić, P., 2013. Ecologically acceptable usage of derivatives of essential oil of sweet basil, *Ocimum basilicum*, as antifeedants against larvae of the gypsy moth, *Lymantria dispar*. J. Insect Sci. 13, 161.

Prakash, B., Singh, P., Yadav, S., Singh, S.C., Dubey, N.K., 2013. Safety profile assessment and efficacy of chemically characterized *Cinnamomum glaucescens* essential oil against storage fungi, insect, aflatoxin secretion and as antioxidant. Food Chem. Toxicol. 53, 160–167.

Pratti, D.L., Ramos, A.C., Scherer, R., Cruz, Z.M., Silva, A.G., 2015. Mechanistic basis for morphological damage induced by essential oil from Brazilian pepper tree, *Schinus terebinthifolia*, on larvae of *Stegomyia aegypti*, the dengue vector. Parasit. Vectors 8, 136.

Rizwan-ul-Haq, M., Aljabr, A.M., 2015. *Rhynchophorus ferrugineus* midgut cell line to evaluate insecticidal potency of different plant essential oils. In Vitro Cell Dev. Biol. Anim. 51 (3), 281–286.

Rocha, D.K., Matosc, O., Novoa, M.T., Figueiredo, A.C., Delgado, M., Moiteiro, C., 2015. Larvicidal activity against *Aedes aegypti* of *Foeniculum vulgare* essential oils from Portugal and Cape Verde. Nat. Prod. Commun. 10 (4), 677–682.

Ruiz, M.J., Juárez, M.L., Alzogaray, R.A., Arrighi, F., Arroyo, L., Gastaminza, G., Willink, E., Bardón Adel, V., Vera, T., 2014. Toxic effect of citrus peel constituents on *Anastrepha fraterculus* Wiedemann and *Ceratitis capitata* Wiedemann immature stages. J. Agric. Food Chem. 62 (41), 10084–10091.

Santana, O., Fe Andrés, M., Sanz, J., Errahmani, N., Abdeslam, L., González-Coloma, A., 2014. Valorization of essential oils from Moroccan aromatic plants. Nat. Prod. Commun. 9 (8), 1109–1114.

Saraf, M., Pandya, U., Thakkar, A., 2014. Role of allelochemicals in plant growth promoting rhizobacteria for biocontrol of phytopathogens. Microbiol. Res. 20 (169(1)), 18–29.

Sathantriphop, S., White, S.A., Achee, N.L., Sanguanpong, U., Chareonviriyaphap, T., 2014. Behavioral responses of *Aedes aegypti*, *Aedes albopictus*, *Culex quinquefasciatus*, and *Anopheles minimus* against various synthetic and natural repellent compounds. J. Vector Ecol. 39 (2), 328–339.

Senthilkumar, A., Jayaraman, M., Venkatesalu, V., 2013. Chemical constituents and larvicidal potential of *Feronia limonia* leaf essential oil against *Anopheles stephensi*, *Aedes aegypti* and *Culex quinquefasciatus*. Parasitol. Res. 112 (3), 1337–1342.

Shyma, K.P., Gupta, J.P., Ghosh, S., Patel, K.K., Singh, V., 2014. Acaricidal effect of herbal extracts against cattle tick *Rhipicephalus* (Boophilus) microplus using in vitro studies. Parasitol. Res. 113 (5), 1919–1926.

Silva, D.T., Silva, L.L., Amaral, L.P., Pinheiro, C.G., Pires, M.M., Schindler, B., Garlet, Q.I., Benovit, S.C., Baldisserotto, B., Longhi, S.J., Kotzian, C.B., Heinzmann, B.M., 2014. Larvicidal activity of Brazilian plant essential oils against *Coenagrionidae larvae*. J. Econ. Entomol. 107 (4), 1713–1720.

Simons, M., van der Bij, A.J., Brand, J., de Weger, L.A., Wijffelman, C.A., Lugtenberg, B.J.J., 1996. Gnotobiotic system for studying rhizosphere colonization by plant growth-promoting *Pseudomonas* bacteria. Mol. Plant–Microbe Interact. 9, 600–607.

Sinthusiri, J., Soonwera, M., 2014. Oviposition deterrent and ovicidal activities of seven herbal essential oils against female adults of housefly, *Musca domestica* L. Parasitol. Res. 113 (8), 3015–3022.

Slimane, B.B., Ezzine, O., Dhahri, S., Ben Jamaa, M.L., 2014. Essential oils from two Eucalyptus from Tunisia and their insecticidal action on *Orgyia trigotephras* (Lepidotera, Lymantriidae). Biol. Res. 47, 29.
Sparagano, O., Khallaayoune, K., Duvallet, G., Nayak, S., George, D., 2013. Comparing terpenes from plant essential oils as pesticides for the poultry red mite (*Dermanyssus gallinae*). Transbound Emerg. Dis. 60 (Suppl. 2.), 150–153.
Stappen, I., Wanner, J., Tabanca, N., Wedge, D.E., Ali, A., Khan, I.A., Kaul, V.K., Lal, B., Jaitak, V., Gochev, V., Girova, T., Stoyanova, A., Schmidt, E., Jirovetz, L., 2014. Chemical composition and biological effects of *Artemisia maritima* and *Artemisia nilagirica* essential oils from wild plants of western Himalaya. Planta. Med. 80 (13), 1079–1087.
Sugumar, S., Clarke, S.K., Nirmala, M.J., Tyagi, B.K., Mukherjee, A., Chandrasekaran, N., 2014. Nanoemulsion of eucalyptus oil and its larvicidal activity against *Culex quinquefasciatus*. Bull. Entomol. Res. 104 (3), 393–402.
Sumitha, K.V., Thoppil, J.E., 2015. Larvicidal efficacy and chemical constituents of *O. gratissimum* L. (Lamiaceae) essential oil against *Aedes albopictus* Skuse (Diptera: Culicidae). Parasitol. Res. 115 (2), 673–680.
Tabanca, N., Avonto, C., Wang, M., Parcher, J.F., Ali, A., Demirci, B., Raman, V., Khan, I.A., 2013a. Comparative investigation of *Umbellularia californica* and *Laurus nobilis* leaf essential oils and identification of constituents active against *Aedes aegypti*. J. Agric. Food Chem. 61 (50), 12283–12291.
Tabanca, N., Bernier, U.R., Ali, A., Wang, M., Demirci, B., Blythe, E.K., Khan, S.I., Baser, K.H., Khan, I.A., 2013b. Bioassay-guided investigation of two Monarda essential oils as repellents of yellow fever mosquito *Aedes aegypti*. J. Agric. Food Chem. 61 (36), 8573–8580.
Tabanca, N., Gao, Z., Demirci, B., Techen, N., Wedge, D.E., Ali, A., Sampson, B.J., Werle, C., Bernier, U.R., Khan, I.A., Baser, K.H., 2014. Molecular and phytochemical investigation of *Angelica dahurica* and *Angelica pubescentis* essential oils and their biological activity against *Aedes aegypti*, *Stephanitis pyrioides*, and *Colletotrichum* species. J. Agric. Food Chem. 62 (35), 8848–8857.
Thomashow, L.S., Weller, D.M., 1988. Role of a phenazine antibiotic from *Pseudomona fluorescensin* biological control of *Gaeumannomyces graminis* var. tritici. J. Bacteriol. 170, 3499–3508.
Tian, B.L., Liu, Q.Z., Liu, Z.L., Li, P., Wang, J.W., 2015. Insecticidal potential of clove essential oil and its constituents on *Cacopsylla chinensis* (Hemiptera: Psyllidae) in laboratory and field. J. Econ. Entomol. 108 (3), 957–961.
Toohey, J.I., Nelson, C.D., Krotkov, G., 1965. Toxicity of phenazine carboxylic acid to some bacteria, algae, higher plants, and animals. Can. J. Botany 43, 1151–1155.
Tsai, P.C., Fox, N., Bigley, A.N., Harvey, S.P., Barondeau, D.P., Raushel, F.M., 2012. Enzymes for the homeland defense: optimizing phosphotriesterase for the hydrolysis of organophosphate nerve agents. Biochemistry 51 (32), 6463–6475.
Turner, J.M., Messenger, A.J., 1986. Occurence, biochemistry and physiology of phenazine pigment production. Adv. Microb. Physiol. 27, 211–275.
Turusov, V.S., Rakitski , V.N., 1997. Classification of pesticides according to carcinogenicity to man. Vopr. Onkol. 43 (3), 299–303.
Udaya Shankar, A.C., Chandra Nayaka, S., Niranjan-Raj, S., Bhuvanendra Kumar, H., Reddy, M.S., Niranjana, S.R., Prakash, H.S., 2009. Rhizobacteria-mediated resistance against the blackeye cowpea mosaic strain of bean common mosaic virus in cowpea (*Vigna unguiculata*). Pest. Manag. Sci. 65 (10), 1059–1064.

Ulukanli, Z., Karabörklü, S., Bozok, F., Çenet, M., Oztürk, B., Balcilar, M., 2014a. Antimicrobial, insecticidal and phytotoxic activities of *Cotinus coggyria* Scop. essential oil (Anacardiaceae). Nat. Prod. Res. 28 (23), 2150–2157.

Ulukanli, Z., Karabörklü, S., Bozok, F., Ates, B., Erdogan, S., Cenet, M., Karaaslan, M.G., 2014b. Chemical composition, antimicrobial, insecticidal, phytotoxic and antioxidant activities of Mediterranean *Pinus brutia* and *Pinus pinea* resin essential oils. Chin. J. Nat. Med. 12 (12), 901–910.

Velivelli, S.L., Kromann, P., Lojan, P., Rojas, M., Franco, J., Suarez, J.P., Prestwich, B.D., 2015. Identification of mVOCs from *Andean rhizobacteria* and field evaluation of bacterial and mycorrhizal inoculants on growth of potato in its center of origin. Microb. Ecol. 69 (3), 652–667.

Vera, S.S., Zambrano, D.F., Méndez-Sanchez, S.C., Rodríguez-Sanabria, F., Stashenko, E.E., Duque Luna, J.E., 2014. Essential oils with insecticidal activity against larvae of *Aedes aegypti* (Diptera: Culicidae). Parasitol. Res. 113 (7), 2647–2654.

Wang, X., Li, Q., Shen, L., Yang, J., Cheng, H., Jiang, S., Jiang, C., Wang, H., 2014a. Fumigant, contact, and repellent activities of essential oils against the darkling beetle, *Alphitobius diaperinus*. J. Insect Sci. 14, 75.

Wang, Y., You, C.X., Wang, C.F., Yang, K., Chen, R., Zhang, W.J., Du, S.S., Geng, Z.F., Deng, Z.W., 2014b. Chemical constituents and insecticidal activities of the essential oil from *Amomum tsaoko* against two stored-product insects. J. Oleo. Sci. 63 (10), 1019–1026.

Wang, Y., Zhao, R., Yu, L., Zhang, Y., He, Y., Yao, J., 2014c. Evaluation of cinnamon essential oil microemulsion and its vapor phase for controlling postharvest gray mold of pears (*Pyrus pyrifolia*). J Sci Food Agric. 94 (5), 1000–1004.

Wang, D.C., Qiu, D.R., Shi, L.N., Pan, H.Y., Li, Y.W., Sun, J.Z., Xue, Y.J., Wei, D.S., Li, X., Zhang, Y.M., Qin, J.C., 2015a. Identification of insecticidal constituents of the essential oils of *Dahlia pinnata* Cav. against *Sitophilus zeamais* and *Sitophilus oryzae*. Nat. Prod. Res. 29 (18), 1748–1751.

Wang, Y., You, C.X., Yang, K., Wu, Y., Chen, R., Zhang, W.J., Liu, Z.L., Du, S.S., Deng, Z.W., Geng, Z.F., Han, J., 2015b. Bioactivity of essential oil of *Zingiber purpureum* Rhizomes and its main compounds against two stored product insects. J. Econ. Entomol. 108 (3), 925–932.

Weert de, S., Vermeiren, H., Mulders, I.H.M., Kuiper, I.H.M., Bloemberg, G.V., Vanderleyden, J., De Mot, R., Lugtenberg, B.J.J., 2002. Chemotaxis towards exudate components is an important trait for tomato root colonisation by *Pseudomonas fluorescens*. Mol. Plant–Microbe Interact. 15, 1173–1180.

Werdin González, J.O., Gutiérrez, M.M., Ferrero, A.A., Fernández Band, B., 2014. Essential oils nanoformulations for stored-product pest control—characterization and biological properties. Chemosphere 100, 130–138.

Wu, Y., Zhang, W.J., Wang, P.J., Yang, K., Huang, D.Y., Wei, J.Y., Tian, Z.F., Bai, J.F., Du, S.S., 2015. Contact toxicity and repellency of the essential oil of *Liriope muscari* (DECN.) bailey against three insect tobacco storage pests. Molecules 20 (1), 1676–1685.

Xie, Y., Huang, Q., Lei, C., 2013. Bioassay-guided isolation and identification of antitermitic active compound from the leaf of Chinese cedar (*Cryptomeria fortunei* Hooibrenk). Nat. Prod. Res. 27 (22), 2137–2139.

Xie, Y., Li, M., Huang, Q., Lei, C., 2014. Chemical composition and termiticidal activity of essential oils from different tissues of Chinese cedar (*Cryptomeria fortunei*). Nat Prod Commun. 9 (5), 719–722.

Xu, S., Yan, F., Ni, Z., Chen, Q., Zhang, H., Zheng, X., 2014. In vitro and in vivo control of *Alternaria alternata* in cherry tomato by essential oil from *Laurus nobilis* of Chinese origin. J. Sci. Food Agric. 94 (7), 1403–1408.

Yang, J.Y., Lee, H.S., 2013. Changes in acaricidal potency by introducing functional radicals and an acaricidal constituent isolated from *Schizonepeta tenuifolia*. J. Agric. Food Chem. 61 (47), 11511–11516.

Yang, K., You, C.X., Wang, C.F., Guo, S.S., Li, Y.P., Wu, Y., Geng, Z.F., Deng, Z.W., Du, S.S., 2014. Composition and repellency of the essential oils of *Evodia calcicola* Chun ex Huang and *Evodia trichotoma* (Lour.) Pierre against three stored product insects. J. Oleo Sci. 63 (11), 1169–1176.

You, C.X., Guo, S.S., Zhang, W.J., Yang, K., Wang, C.F., Geng, Z.F., Du, S.S., Deng, Z.W., Wang, Y.Y., 2015. Chemical constituents and activity of *Murraya microphylla* essential oil against *Lasioderma serricorne*. Nat. Prod. Commun. 10 (9), 1635–1638.

Zacharia, J.T., 2011. Identity, physical and chemical properties of pesticides. In: Stoytcheva, M (Ed.), Pesticides in the Modern World—Trends in Pesticides Analysis. InTech.

Zamora, D., Klotz, S.A., Meister, E.A., Schmidt, J.O., 2015. Repellency of the components of the essential oil, Citronella, to *Triatoma rubida*, *Triatoma protracta*, and *Triatoma recurva* (Hemiptera: Reduviidae: Triatominae). J. Med. Entomol. 52 (4), 719–721.

Zandi-Sohani, N., Hojjati, M., Carbonell-Barrachina, ÁA, 2013. Insecticidal and repellent activities of the essential oil of *Callistemon citrinus* (Myrtaceae) against *Callosobruchus maculatus* (F.) (Coleoptera: Bruchidae). Neotrop. Entomol. 42 (1), 89–94.

Zhang, N., Tang, L., Hu, W., Wang, K., Zhou, Y., Li, H., Huang, C., Chun, J., Zhang, Z., 2014a. Insecticidal, fumigant, and repellent activities of sweet wormwood oil and its individual components against red imported fire ant workers(Hymenoptera: Formicidae). J. Insect Sci. 14., 241.

Zhang, W.J., You, C.X., Yang, K., Chen, R., Wang, Y., Wu, Y., Geng, Z.F., Chen, H.P., Jiang, H.Y., Su, Y., Lei, N., Ma, P., Du, S.S., Deng, Z.W., 2014b. Bioactivity of essential oil of *Artemisia argyi* Lévl. Et Van. and its main compounds against *Lasioderma serricorne*. J. Oleo Sci. 63 (8), 829–837.

Zhang, W.J., Yang, K., You, C.X., Wang, Y., Wang, C.F., Wu, Y., Geng, Z.F., Su, Y., Du, S.S., Deng, Z.W., 2015. Bioactivity of *essential* oil from *Artemisia stolonifera* (Maxim.) Komar and its main compounds against two stored-product insects. J. Oleo. Sci. 64 (3), 299–307.

Zhu, L., Tian, Y., 2013. Chemical composition and larvicidal activity of essential oil of *Artemisia gilvescens* against *Anopheles anthropophagus*. Parasitol. Res. 112 (3), 1137–1142.

2

NEW PESTICIDES: A CUTTING-EDGE VIEW OF CONTRIBUTIONS FROM NANOTECHNOLOGY FOR THE DEVELOPMENT OF SUSTAINABLE AGRICULTURAL PEST CONTROL

Krishnendu Sinha*,, Jyotirmoy Ghosh†, Parames C. Sil***

**Bose Institute, Division of Molecular Medicine, Kolkata, West Bengal, India; **Jhargram Raj College, Department of Zoology, Jhargram, West Bengal, India; †Banwarilal Bhalotia College, Chemistry Department, Asansol, West Bengal, India*

1 Introduction

The term "nano" in "nanotechnology" has been originated from the Greek word meaning "dwarf" (Rai and Ingle, 2012). Accurately, the word "nano" means one-billionth part of a metre (i.e., 10^{-9}). The term nanotechnology is usually used for materials having size range between 1 and 100 nm. It is also obvious that these materials should exhibit different properties from bulk (i.e., micrometric and larger) materials due to their size. Usually these differences in properties include chemical reactivity, physical strength, magnetism, electrical conductance, and optical effects. The term "nanobiotechnology" is a multidisciplinary combination of nanotechnology, biotechnology, material science, chemical processing, system engineering, nanocrystals, and nanobiomaterials (Huang et al., 2007). Researchers in biology and chemistry field are actively engaged in the synthesis of organic, inorganic, hybrid, and metal nanomaterials including different kinds of nanoparticles having unusual optical, physical, biological properties (Rai and Ingle, 2012). Due to these unusual properties, nanoparticles have tremendous applications in various

New Pesticides and Soil Sensors. http://dx.doi.org/10.1016/B978-0-12-804299-1.00003-5

fields including electronic, nanomedicine, pharmaceuticals, biomaterial engineering, and agriculture (Elibol et al., 2003). Nanotechnology is one of the emerging fields and it has the prospective to change the current scenario of the agricultural and food industry with the help of newly developed methods. These includes the treatment of plant diseases, improving the ability of plants to absorb nutrients, nanobased kits mediated rapid detection of pathogens, and so on. Currently developed nanobiosensors and other smart delivery systems have enormous application in agriculture field. This will help the agricultural industry to contest against different crop pathogens. Nanostructured catalysts will be developed in near future and it will increase the efficacy of commercially available pesticides and insecticides (Joseph and Morrison, 2006). In Asia, the existing global population is near about 7 billion. A major population of this area faces daily food shortages due to environmental impacts on agriculture including droughts, storms, and flood (Joseph and Morrison, 2006). On the other hand, agricultural production also constrained by a number of abiotic and biotic factors like insect pests, diseases, and weeds cause substantial damage to agricultural production. Literature suggests that pests cause 5–10% in wheat, 25% loss in rice, 35% in oilseeds, 30% in pulses, 20% in sugar cane, and 50% in cotton (Dhaliwal et al., 2010). These also infest the food and other stored products. These products include storage structures and packages, bins, causing huge amount of loss to the stored food and also deterioration of food quality. Study by Pimentel (2009) analyzed that worldwide insect pests caused a tremendous damage in the agricultural output. Side by side, plant pathogens and weeds are also severely influencing the agricultural output and thus require immediate attention (Pimentel, 2009). The crop loss was estimated to be US $2000 billion per year. This will be discussed in details later in this chapter. So, in these scenarios developing countries like India, the crop yield can be maximized by developing new pest-resistant and drought-crops (Joseph and Morrison, 2006).

Integrated pest management (IPM) is the utmost prevalent approach to lessen the usage of pesticide. US Academy of Sciences in 1969 was formalized the term "IPM". IPM is considered as a resolution to evade the side effects of pesticide. It combines the use of different pest control strategies, for example, cultural, resistant varieties, biological, and chemical control. IPM is more complex than the other pest management methods for the farmer to contrivance, because it requires expertise in monitoring and understanding the basic mechanism of pest dynamics, besides the cooperation of among all the farmers for the operative employment of IPM (Peshin et al., 2009; Dhawan and Peshin, 2009;

Pimentel, 2009; Rai and Ingle, 2012). In 1960s, IPM was promoted as a pest control stratagem and at that time, there were only few IPM technologies available for field application (Roy et al., 2009). In the 1970s, a new area on IPM was discovered and extensive research on the management of insect pest generated some original products and knowledge which help in the successful implementation of IPM in crops like cotton, rice, sugar cane, and vegetables. However, IPM technology was not successful to that extent. In practice the dramatic reduction in pesticide, use could not be achieved without significant decline in crop yields as a result of adoption of IPM (Peshin et al., 2009; Pimentel, 2009). It is mainly an ecologically based strategy. It focuses on long-term solution of the pests through a combination of techniques, such as biological control, habitat manipulation, and modification of agronomic practices and use of resistant varieties. Integration of multiple pest suppression techniques is considered to have the highest probability of sustaining long-term crop protection. While applying pest control tactics, including pesticides precautions have to take to minimize risks to the human health, beneficial and nontarget organisms, and environment (Peshin et al., 2009; Pimentel, 2009; Rai and Ingle, 2012). In near future, the field of nanotechnology will fetch essential new products and approaches to succour crop production. With the advancement of research in the field of nanotechnologies, genomics, and microelectronics, new diagnostic tools for animal and plant diseases have been discovered that dramatically improves our capability to detect and monitor the spread of plant and animal diseases. Nanotechnologies have already discovered new and improved way to deliver pesticides through encapsulation and controlled release procedures. Pesticides can be applied more easily and safely in combination with the use of nanoemulsions. Smart nanotechnology-based sensors, applied to the field in near future may early detect the disease and monitors the soil conditions to improve application of fertilizers, water, and pesticides (Joseph and Morrison, 2006). Though, the potential risks must be investigated and weighed against the benefits before there practical application because new technology brings new risk (Beddington, 2010).

Currently, the application of agricultural fertilizers, antibiotics, pesticides, and nutrients is limited to spray method or drench application to soil or plants or through feed or injection systems to animals (Srilatha, 2011). Usually, the delivery of pesticides or medicines is provided as "preventative" treatment. However, it also can be provided once the disease causing organism has multiplied which causes the expression of symptoms (Ravi, 2010). In this context, nanotechnologies have a huge potential and offer a great opportunity to develop new products against pests (Caraglia et al., 2011). Nanotechnology improves and enhances its performance and acceptability by increasing effectiveness, safety, patient adherence, as well as ultimately reducing health care costs (Anwunobi and Emeje, 2011). Nanoscale devices are capable to detect and treat nutrient deficiency, an infection, or other health problem, long before symptoms were visibly evident. This chapter aims to compile up-to-date knowledge on the nanotechnology based new age pesticides.

2 New Generation Pesticides

Nanotechnology principally deals with the introduction of novel nanomaterials that can lead to revolutionary new structures and devices with the help of extremely sophisticated biological tools (Srilatha, 2011). In this rapidly developing field, the integration of biologically active species (like enzymes, metabolites, or whole cells) with nanostructures leading to hybrid systems which find several applications in many fields comprising agriculture (Bailey et al., 2010). Nowaday's pesticides are typically applied through drench or spray application to plants or soil as either as "preventative" treatment, or after a disease establishes (Ravi, 2010; Srilatha, 2011). In this circumstance, nanotechnology can provide great chance to develop new pesticides (Caraglia et al., 2011; Srilatha, 2011). Actually nanotechnology improves the performance and acceptability of a traditional or novel pesticides by increasing its effectiveness, targeted action, safety, disease adherence, along with eventually reducing the management costs (Anwunobi and Emeje, 2011). Along with the advancement of nanotechnology, nanoscale devices are being proposed that have the potentials to sense and treat an infection at a very beginning stage, actually long before symptoms were apparent at the macroscale (Srilatha, 2011). This type of treatment using nanotechnology is possible if the affected area is targeted with a greater awareness of the hazards, which is associated with the use of synthetic organic insecticides and for that reason, exploration of appropriate alternative products for pest control becomes an urgent need (Ravi, 2010). Nanoparticles is, therefore, thought to be needed to reduce the number of unnecessary problems associated with agriculture (Srilatha, 2011). Development of targeted pesticide delivery will improve efficacy of the pesticide through reductions in dosing intervals, and diminishing its environmental toxicities (Srilatha, 2011; Zhao et al., 2011). We can use nanoparticles for the preparation of new generation of pesticides, insect repellents, and insecticides (Barik et al., 2008; Prasad et al., 2014;

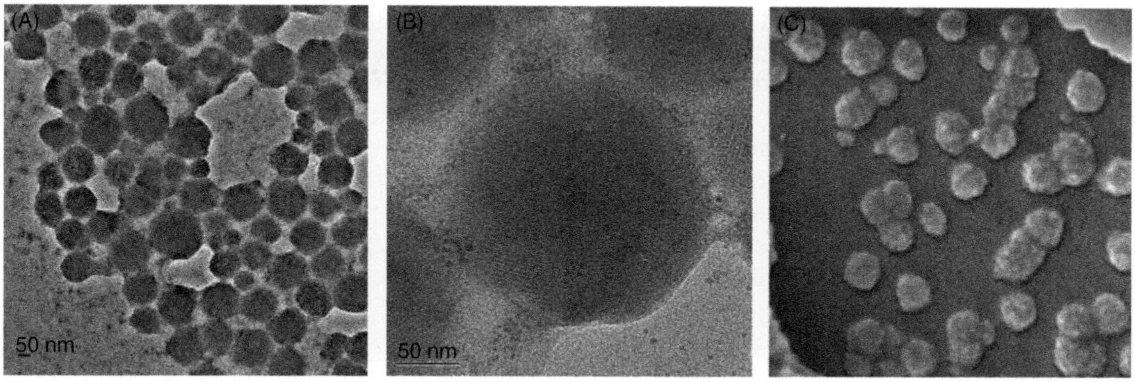

Figure 2.1. Mesoporous silica nanoparticles (MSNs). (A–B) TEM micrograph, (C) SEM micrograph.

Gajbhiye et al., 2009a). Although many preparation methods for nanoparticles can be modified to create nanocomposites and nanostructured films, completely novel approaches are required for the preparation of some types of specific nanostructures (Pandurangappa and Lakshminarasappa, 2011; Srilatha, 2011). In this section, we are going to give a glimpse of few such new generation pesticides.

Well-engineered nanoparticles can serve as "magic sphere" which can accommodate pesticides, herbicides, chemicals, or genetic materials, and can be the target to a precise parts of plant to release their content in a targeted manner (Pérez-de-Luque and Rubiales, 2009). Porous hollow silica nanoparticles (PHSNs) or mesoporous silica nanoparticles (MSNs) have engrossed the attention of nanotechnologists due to their prospective applications (Fig. 2.1). These relatively inert nanomaterials have features like high surface area, variable pore volume, and stability under specific physicochemical conditions. Also these pore networks are tightly ordered and extremely homogeneous in size (Douroumis, 2011; Srilatha, 2011). MSNs are well known as a candidate for drug delivery system and have been extensively investigated in recent years although at the beginning these particles were used only for controlled delivery of various hydrophilic or hydrophobic active agents. However, extensive studies discovered advanced surface properties (such as surface functionalization and PEGylation) in the MSNs and rendered them as a promising drug delivery system (Douroumis, 2011); into isolated plant cells, MSNs are also used in delivering chemicals and DNA. MSNs can withstand extensive surface modifications and also serve as a container for the spatiotemporal delivery of pesticides. They are also very good agent for targeted DNA delivery. For this, the coating on these particles activates the plant system to take the particles via the cell walls. It has been found that MSNP/DNA complexes enhanced receptor-mediated endocytosis efficiency through mannose receptors. These results give an indication of the use of MSNP both as a potential gene carrier to antigen presenting cells and pesticides carrier in the future (Park et al., 2008; Srilatha, 2011). These pesticides can be directed very precisely to the target cells of target pest species adopting the similar principle as aforementioned of gene delivery. These could prove themselves extremely effective in sustainable agro ecosystem. Pesticide validamycin loaded PHSNs can be considered for efficient delivery system for its controlled release (Prasad et al., 2014). This type of controlled release behavior of the hollow silica nanoparticles provides the possibility of employing it as a promising carrier for pesticide controlled delivery in agriculture because immediate, as well as prolonged release of pesticide is needed for plants (Prasad et al., 2014; Liu et al., 2006). As per Barik et al. (2008) another silica derivative, nanosilica, can also be effectively used as a nanopesticide, more precisely as nanoinsecticide. To understand the action on nanosilica the cuticular chemistry of insects must be known. Insects use a variety of cuticular lipids, which help them to maintain their cuticular barrier and thus stop desiccation-related death. When the nanosilica is applied on plant surface, they got rapidly absorbed by the cuticular lipids of insect coat due to their hydrophobic nature. This causes death of the insect by physical means like destroying the hydrophobic coat. It can, therefore, be said that modified surface charged hydrophobic nanosilica (~3–5 nm) could be successfully implemented to manage a variety of ectoparasites of animals and agricultural insect pests (Prasad et al., 2014; Ulrichs et al., 2005b). Besides silica, polyethylene-glycol (PEG) coated nanoparticles are useful in pest management. The insecticidal activity of these nanoparticles loaded with garlic essential oil are well documented against the adult of stored products pest *Tribolium castaneum* with an efficacy up to 80% against control. This high efficacy value is probably due to the unique feature of the nanoparticle, which ensure slow but persistent release of the active components from these nanoparticles (Yang et al., 2009a). Amorphous nanosilica, found in various natural sources (like epidermis of vegetables, burnt pretreated rice hulls, the shell wall of phytoplankton, straw at thermoelectric plants, and volcanic soil, etc.) shows promising potential as a biopesticide (Barik et al., 2008; Prasad et al., 2014). The silica NPs undergo physiosorbtion by the cuticular lipids and were reported to cause the death of insects purely applying physical means of disrupting protective barrier (Barik et al., 2008). Neither photosynthesis nor respiration, were altered by the application of

NPs on the leaf and stem surface in several groups of crop and horticultural plants. Besides, gene expression alteration in insect trachea did not occur because of their application and thus, nanoparticles were qualified for the approval as the nanobiopesticide. World Health Organization (WHO) also considers the use of amorphous silica as a safe nanobiopesticide for humans. A recent report suggests that silica NPs caused 100% mortality in rice weevil, *Sitophilus oryzae* (Debnath et al., 2011). Furthermore, silica nanoparticles (3–5 nm), modified by hydrophobic charge on the surface, were successfully utilized to regulate a range of agricultural insect pests and veterinary importance animal ectoparasites (Ulrichs et al., 2005a). This particle has also been successfully applied as a thin film on seeds to reduce the fungal growth and boost cereal germination (Ghormade et al., 2011; Robinson and Salejova-Zadrazilova, 2010). It is well known that nuclear polyhedrosis virus (BmNPV) infects silkworms, *Bombax mori*, and is the cause for the heavy losses in the silk industry. Studies in detail suggest that BmNPV infection enhances the level of certain lipids in silkworms. Although lipase treatment, a viable option for controlling BmNPV, could be a solution, studies showed that this treatment interfered in the hormonal balance and could not be applied to premolting stage (Yao et al., 2006). Plant–stem derived nanosilica has been reported to be capable of reducing certain classes of native lipoproteins present in the silkworm larval hemolymph (Barik et al., 2008). Nanoparticles can easily circulate in lepidopteran system and would be not as much harmful in the hemocoel in this regard (Ulrichs et al., 2005a). Application of nanosilica of the size of 40–60 nm to BmNPV afflicted silkworms increased the survival rate from 0% to 30% (Ghormade et al., 2011; Goswami et al., 2010; Ulrichs et al., 2005a). In addition to the silkworm, where an upsurge in host lipids was exploited for pathogen growth, this model could successfully be used for regulating other insect, animal, and human diseases. For example, Barik et al. (2008) reported that nanosilica also could control malaria by causing alterations in host lipid profiles (Ghormade et al., 2011; Ulrichs et al., 2005a).

After a discussion of inert silica nanoparticles now we are going to glimpse of active metal nanoparticles (Fig. 2.2). In this context, nanosilver has come under much consideration due to their novel material properties and diminutive size. Their efficacy is greatly depended on their size, shape, and composition (Rosarin and Mirunalini, 2011). Due to its unique properties, use of nanosilver in agriculture is a well-known phenomenon. Many studies are there which shows the reaction of plants when they contact with nanosilver (Srilatha, 2011). Nanosilver in the form of solution have significant effect in reducing the occurrence of

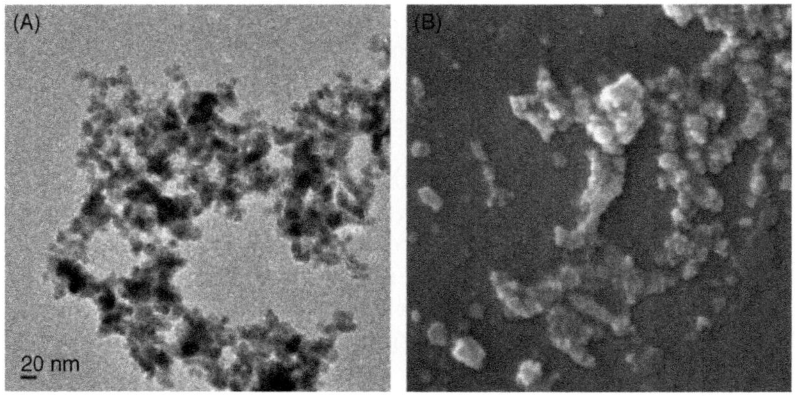

Figure 2.2. Metal nanoparticles. (A) TEM micrograph, (B) SEM micrograph.

root diseases. These studies validate the beneficial role of a colloidal nanosilver solution on the health and growth of several plants (Srilatha, 2011). Along with nanosilver, the applications of an array of metal oxide nanoparticles like zinc oxide, aluminium oxide, and titanium dioxide also proven to be effective in field study (Srilatha, 2011). For example, *S. oryzae* (rice weevil) and baculovirus BmNPV (*Bombyx mori* nuclear polyhedrosis virus) cause significant damage to the rice crop and causes disease like grasserie in silk worm (e.g., *B. mori*), respectively. Both the damage can be significantly controlled by the metal oxide nanoparticles (Goswami et al., 2010; Prasad et al., 2014). It is described in details later in this chapter. Nanostructured alumina has proven its potent insecticidal activity against two major cosmopolitan pest of the stored grain, namely *Rhyzopertha dominica* (F.) and *S. oryzae* L. (Stadler et al., 2010). When wheat was treated with nanoaluminium, substantial mortality was there after a period of 3 days. This study proved the efficacy of nanoaluminium over the available insecticides as these aluminium is actually cheaper and user friendly (Prasad et al., 2014). Besides these silica and metal nanoparticles, carbon based nanoparticles, the vertically-aligned multiwalled carbon nanotubes (VACNTs) and functionalized fullerenes Bucky balls are gaining importance in agro researches. This is because of their exceptional combination of chemical and mechanical properties along with biocompatibility (Srilatha, 2011). Functionalized fullerenes Bucky balls and carbon nanotubes or CNT have biorecognition property, which could be used at nanoscale. Now, coming to another nanomaterial called nanofibers, which are produced by electro spinning. These 100-nm diameter nanofibers can be used as excellent absorbent of pesticides, which can be used for exact spaciotemporal application (Mousavi and Rezaei, 2011;

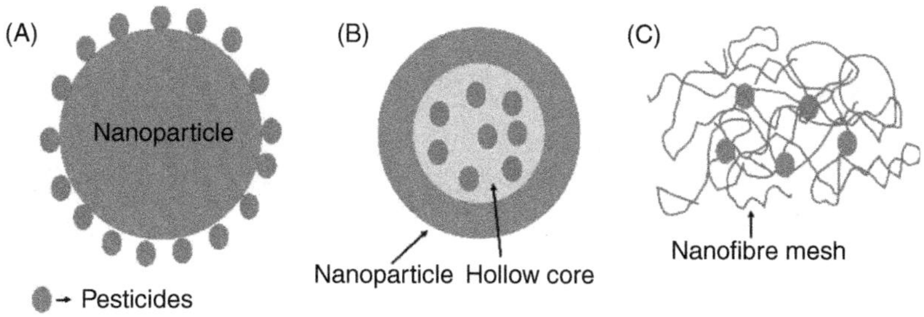

Figure 2.3. Pesticide loaded nanostructure. (A) Nanoparticle loaded with pesticides at the surface, (B) pesticides loaded inside porous panoparticles, (C) nanofiber mesh loaded with pesticides.

Lang, 2003) (Fig. 2.3). Nanofibers also helped to encapsulate chemical pesticides, which intensifies the strength of pesticides and prevent smattering of chemicals in the environment and thus prevent pollution. Upon degradation by various means like chemical or biological, loaded pesticides are gradually released in the soil (Mousavi and Rezaei, 2011).

Now we are going to discuss a different kind of nanomaterials, the nanoemulsion. Nanoemulsion is a complex systems entailing of water, surfactant and oil phase. The resulting colloidal solution is kinetically stable and optically isotropic. It has a droplet size, which is in 20–200 nm range. Presently, due to wide range of nanoparticle sizes nanoemulsions are widely used in different branches of applied science including agriculture (Srilatha, 2011; Salim et al., 2011). Nanoemulsions are generally characterized based on few criteria like particle size, surface morphology, viscosity, and refractive index though they are usually unstable (Shakeel et al., 2009). This instability can be bypassed by eliminating the aqueous dispersions. Thus, it forms a dry solid (Mehrotra et al., 2010). Property of the nanoemulsions depends on the composition, as well as mode of preparation (Gutiérrez et al., 2008; Srilatha, 2011). Nanoemulsions in turn delays degradation of pesticides by encapsulating it inside (Srilatha, 2011). Wang et al. (2007) discussed that oil in water, that is, nanoemulsion is cheap and advantageous for pesticides formulations and also effective against several pest insect species (Wang et al., 2009). Likewise, solid lipid nanoparticles loaded with essential oil are also useful in such cases (Liu et al., 2006; Prasad et al., 2014). Usually plants provide nontoxic phytochemicals, namely essential oils and secondary metabolites, which have immense biological efficacy. However, these are usually unstable in soil and water (Isman, 2000). A major concern is that in case of essential oils, in the presence of light, air, high temperatures, and moisture, their chemical instability cause quick evaporation and degradation of some of their active components.

3 Safe Carriers: New-Generation Nanocides

Nanocides are pesticides encapsulated at nanoscale. Packaging of nanoscale active materials inside a tiny "envelope" or "shell" could be considered as a more sophisticated encapsulation approach for the formulation of nanoscale pesticides. "Nanocapsules" are usually composed of thin external layers, (considered as shells) having huge space inside (Fig. 2.3B) (Joseph and Morrison, 2006). At present, the methods of both controlled release and encapsulation are playing a major role in controlling the use of various pesticides, herbicides, as well as fertilizers in agriculture worldwide. Nanoencapsulation is the method of encapsulation of the so-called nanomaterial and is probably the most promising technology used to protect host plants against insect pests. Nanocapsules are generally composed of polymers and this technology helps to formulate nanocide containing the pesticides inside the shell. In this preparation, the chemical is protected by the shell and remains safe from the damage induced by the external agents. Besides, it improves the solubility of the active material and helps to enhance the penetration power through the target tissues. By adjusting the external factors (e.g., pH), the chemicals inside the shells can be released through the controlled opening which makes these capsules more attractive toward the balanced unloading of the materials as they reach target places of a particularly defined conditions (Chinnamuthu and Boopathi, 2009; Pérez-de-Luque and Rubiales, 2009). Nanoencapsulation is a procedure through which several chemicals viz. insecticides are gradually but proficiently released for the control of insect pest to a specific host plant (Prasad et al., 2014). Nanoencapsulation allows proper delivery and the absorption of the DNA along with several other chemicals into plant tissues to protect the host plants against insect pests (Ding and Shah, 2009; Vidhyalakshmi et al., 2009). Several release mechanisms like diffusion, dissolution, and osmotic pressure with definite pH used in nanoencapsulation (Prasad et al., 2014). Engineered encapsulated pesticides are being developed so that it can have discharge coupled to an environmental trigger (Prasad et al., 2014). Along with the revolutionary change of controlled release, reformulation of pesticides in microcapsules can also encompass increase solubility, protection, lessen active ingredient's contact with the agricultural workers. Other environmental advantages, such as plummeting run-off rates are also to be compared. A number of food corporations and agro-companies developed and patented these nano- and microformulations with potential applications in veterinary medicine, pesticides, vaccines, and nutritionally enhanced food. Some nanoscale active ingredients containing pesticides are already available in the market and more new formulations of the same or improved types would be expected in near future as a result of the ongoing research of several of the leading agrochemical firms of the world. As an example, we could say that the potential usefulness of the nanotechnology in the formulation of pesticides has already been recognized by the world's fourth ranking agrochemical corporation BASF of Germany. This company has been conducting basic research involving particles of the size of 10–150 nm for a period of time. A patent application has also been filed for the pesticides involving these particles. As it has been mentioned earlier, the pesticide containing the nanoformulation dissolves more easily in water; its stability is also more compared to the normal ones and by controlling external factors, the killing-capacity of the chemical for can be optimized. Another patent application in the form of an emulsion on agrochemicals has also been filed by the Bayer Crop Science of Germany. The active ingredient of that emulsion is comprised of nanoscale droplets whose dimension falls within the range of 10–400 nm. The company refers this invented emulsion as a "microemulsion concentrate" and claims that it possesses various advantages like decreased application rate, "a more reliable, rapid, and extended long-term activity", and so on. Like Bayer Crop Science, another company, namely Syngenta, claims that its Banner MAXX fungicide and Primo MAXX Plant Growth Regulator contain extremely tiny particles having the size of about 100 nm. These chemicals are highly miscible in water and mix themselves very efficiently so that they neither settle down in the spray tank nor separate themselves from water for up to one year. Besides, this product prevents spray tank filters from clogging as well. In addition, the fungicides of "microemulsion concentrate" could be safely absorbed into the plant's system so that they cannot be washed off by the irrigation or natural rain (Prasad et al., 2014). Here it is worth mentioning that herbicide could be applied only when necessary with the combination of a smart delivery system, resulting in less harm to agricultural workers and more production of crops. Formulations are also made by many other companies using nanoparticles of comparatively larger size (within the size ranges of 100–250 nm). Since their solubility increase in water effectively than the existing ones, their respective activities also increased. Some other companies make suspensions of either water or oil-based nanoscale particles (nanoemulsions) that contain uniform suspensions of herbicidal or pesticidal nanoparticles (size ranging from 200 to 400 nm). An encapsulated product from Syngenta, world's largest agrochemical corporation (Karate ZEON) is a fast release microencapsulated product. It contains the active compound namely lambda-cyhalothrin (a natural pyrethrins based synthetic insecticide), which breaks open only on contact with leaves (Prasad et al., 2014). Whereas "gutbuster" (another encapsulated product) breaks open and release the contents only in alkaline environments, for instance the stomach of several specific insects (Taylor et al., 2005). In this aspect, liposomes and polymers can be considered as good candidates. Many companies make liposomes for years and find applications mainly in pharmaceuticals and cosmetics. Although not that elaborately, its applications to food technology and agriculture have also been reported (Taylor et al., 2005). These are shaped by dispersal of polar lipids in aqueous solvents and are identified as spherical bilayer vesicles. The polar lipids used for this purpose are of the sizes ranging from nanometer to micrometer. The functionalities and properties of liposomes depend both on extrinsic, as well as intrinsic parameters. Some important factors controlling those are pH, temperature, ionic strength, phospholipid composition, and concentration. Besides, the liposome's stability and the compound's release are controlled largely by the characteristics of the entrapped compounds (Teixeira et al., 2005). However, the major concern regarding the stability of the liposomes still remains, as they are only kinetically stable, means, they remain stable only for a limited duration but not for long time. Hence, their main use has been limited within the food industry. Nowaday, polymers become the elementary components for nanocapsules that are strongly held together by covalent bonds. This makes the polymer more stable and robust than liposomes (Prashanth and Tharanathan, 2007; Holister et al., 2003). Use of polymers is more advantageous for making nanocapsules as their sizes and shapes can be controlled more efficiently using polymers. Besides, the polymers containing nanocapsules are more efficient to be functionalized with different substances, resulting the addition of new suitable target properties. Chitosan and chitin derivatives seem to be very attractive in the field of research associated with the nanocapsules containing natural polymers (Prashanth and Tharanathan, 2007). They are basically polysaccharides made of linear glucose residues linked in β-1,4-configuration. These polymers are the second most common (cellulose is the first) in nature. They are rigid having unbranched structures and mostly found in crustaceans. Fungi and bacteria also contain these polymers but to a lesser extent. Chitosans can be used to encapsulate and delivery drug as they have the property of being transformed into thin membranous films. They can facilitate the drug transport across cellular membranes because of their good muco adhesive properties, suggesting their possible use in agrochemical industry (Pérez-de-Luque and Rubiales, 2009). In agriculture, chitosan are best known for their antimicrobial properties. In addition to eliciting defense responses in plants, their oligomers also show antifungal and antibacterial activity. Besides, insecticidal properties of these derivatives have also been reported (Scrinis and Lyons, 2007; Torney, 2009b). Nanoparticles loaded with an active substance with and/or its external modification allow guidance and/or accumulation into a specific area inside the living organism where the chemical will be discharged. These basic principles of nanoparticles insertion can also be translated into plants. Here attention should be made to design the appropriate carriers for the agrochemicals so that they can travel through the plant and the charge is released after they have penetrated inside particular tissues or when a specific condition has been achieved. Research and the related experimentation along these lines are just at the stage of beginning. Studies associated with penetration and nanoparticles translocation inside the entire plants have not been reported yet and believed to be under way.43. The chemical would be expected to be released after accumulation inside bacterial cells or by the action of fungal lytic enzymes. Here, activation of nanoparticles by the enzymes secreted by the parasite; like, pectin methyl esterases, for example, in the case of parasitic plants like *Orobanche* spp. could take place (Losner-Goshen et al., 1998). The concept is that, in this system, the nanoparticles would act like an artificial immune system, can deliver the toxic substances only when and where they are needed for plants, although the parasite still remains underground. Besides, infinite possibilities exist for plant breeding and genetic transformation using nanotechnology. It was possible to prevent crop damage if such a system could be developed where a nanoparticle carrying DNA or RNA could trigger the defence responses in plants after being activated by an invading pathogen or parasitic weed. RNA of internal resistant gene (e.g., peroxidases and glucanases) could be used against parasitic weeds control (Pérez-de-Luque et al., 2006; Hamamouch et al., 2005). Also small interfering RNA (siRNA) and oligonucleotides may be used to disrupt the pathogenic processes of an explicit pest (Toub et al., 2006). For example, siRNA could be delivered at infection points, directing known genes of the parasitic plants involved in pathogenesis (González-Verdejo et al., 2007; Westwood et al., 2009; Yoder et al., 2009). Another application of this nanotechnology might be hyperthermia, meaning the delivery of lethal amounts of heat to the desired system. It implies the use of paramagnetic nanoparticles as needed and is being studied as an anticancer therapeutic (Xie et al., 2008). The principle of this process is that, the temperature increases around these nanoparticles when they are exposed to electromagnetic waves. This excess heat is located only to those cells, which contain the nanoparticles and because of elevated temperatures, they would eventually die.

With advancement of the field, pest like viruses are now coming under consideration of agrobiologists for their unique properties like quick spreading, especially in the plant vascular systems. They are applied systemically in the infected plant and with the help of insects, it is transported long distances. Researchers are trying to transform them for beneficial purposes (Pérez-de-Luque and Rubiales, 2009). In short, viruses are perfect natural nanomachines, which are able to carry substances inside their capsids. Nanobiotechnology researchers accepted this idea and began investigation on them, particularly on plant viruses as carriers in the field of pharmacology and medicine (Singh et al., 2007; Loo et al., 2007; Steinmetz and Evans, 2007). Scientists are also using viruses for single-generation transformation of crops with specific herbicide resistance encoded genes (Baulcombe, 1999). The capsids of the viruses are robust and it exhibits interesting features as carriers and delivery systems because of the protein coat on them could protect the nucleic acid inside. The capsid size ranges from nanometer to micrometer [cowpea chlorotic mottle virus (CPMV)] to 140 nm [chilo iridescent virus (CIV)-nanometer; bacteriophage M13-micrometer]. Besides, many viruses self-assemble their capsid in vitro and can also change their shape and size depending on the external factors (like pH) leading to open or close nanopores and allow the entry or release of desired substances (Steinmetz and Evans, 2007).

4 Nanobiosensors for Pesticide Detection and Degradation

For the protection of crops and seeds, numerous pesticides are commonly used in agriculture. However, these applied pesticide residues are not destroyed completely and may remain on or inside foods. These substances can be carcinogenic, mutagenic, or cytotoxic and might also cause environmental impact, as well as public health risks. That is why proper detection of pesticides residue is of our prior concern. In this aspect, different sensors are playing a great role. Sensors, being various sophisticated instruments, usually respond to different physicochemical and biological aspects. Those responses are transferred into signals or outputs in such a manner so that it render harmless to the human and help to detect contaminants (like microbes, pests, nutrient content, and plant stress) arises as a result of external factors like insect or pathogen pressure, lack of nutrients, drought, temperature, and so on (Prasad et al., 2014). Although biosensors have been discovered long time back (1970s, glucose monitors), very few were commercialized as there is a lag of commercialization of biosensor laboratory research and innumerable research papers on biosensors (Prasad et al., 2014). Application of nanomaterials in biosensing has few advantages over conventional system. These are like further miniaturization, less requirement of sample, measurement of more variables, better sensitivity, quicker detection rates, real time read-outs and so on. Due to fast response time and high sensitivity of nanomaterials, they have been widely used as the electrochemical biosensors. The crucial point in construction of steady and robust electrode materials for biosensor depends on the effective immobilization of biomolecules without shifting its bioactivity (Srilatha, 2011). Thus, developed biosensor can be perfect tool for ready monitoring of pesticides like organophosphate pesticides (OPs) and nerve agents. In this aspect a short discussion on acetylcholinesterase (AChE) would be helpful as it is the prime target of the OPs and nerve agents. AChE renders active neurotransmitter acetylcholine (ACh) to its inactive choline form by catalyzing the hydrolysis ACh. Inhibition of AChE will help in the accumulation of ACh in the synaptic cleft. This will ultimately lead to hyperactivity and dysregulation of neural functions. Usually, nanomaterials are used for the development of AChE-based pesticide sensing devices using the following three different methods. In the first method, nanomaterials, possessing peroxidase- or oxidase-like activities, are used as catalysts to catalyze the oxidation of various substrates [including 2,2′-azino-bis(3-ethylbenzothiazoline-6-sulfonic acid) diammonium salt and 3,3,5,5-tetramethylbenzidine (TMB) by enzyme-generated hydrogen peroxide (H_2O_2)] for the detection of ACh and AChE inhibitors using colorimetric or fluorescence techniques (Du et al., 2008b). Second method is based on the enhanced detection of the signal of a particular reaction, especially in the electrochemical detection protocols, these materials are used as enzyme carriers for loading a large amount of AChE (Du et al., 2008b). For this specific purpose, the enzyme is deposited on the working electrode surface in a typical configuration and the AChE activity is then monitored by adding the substrate to the solution followed by measuring the redox current of the enzymatic products. Electrode materials (including nanomaterials) are used to immobilize large quantities of enzyme to improve the performance of the AChE-based electrochemical methods. It provides a favorable microenvironment to maintain the enzyme activity to facilitate the oxidation of the enzymatic products. Finally, nanomaterials are employed as the direct signal sources in the third method. The versatility of the array of nanobiosensor to both biological and chemical contaminants may be extended by its ability to integrate enzymes for catalytic detection. Now coming to the OPs, as environmental concerns related to OPs are raised continuously to critical levels due to unnecessary use of OPs in agriculture. Conventional analytical techniques, like GC and HPLC were used to detect OPs in the environment. However, their usages were limited as these are of high cost, time consumption, and need highly trained labors. Providentially, with great advancements in nanotechnology, different nanomaterials with unique chemical and physical properties have been widely employed to develop nanosensors for OPs. Along with the technique described aforementioned, metal oxide nanoparticles, graphene, quantum dots, coordination polymers, nanocrystal, and other functionalized/nonfunctionalized nanomaterials appearing to be sensitive, rapid, and user friendly resolutions. A zirconium oxide NPs (~50 nm) based immunoassay with a sensitive detection limit (0.02 nM) of OPs using phosphorylated enzyme AChE as a potential biomarker has recently been developed by Wang et al. (2009). Besides, Ramanathan et al. (2009) also developed a biosensor based on organophosphate array. In that technique, a pH-responsive fluorophore was encapsulated in silica NPs (100–500 nm) and conjugated to organophosphate hydrolase (OPH) and patterned to a waveguide surface. Silica NPs encapsulated OPH was found to be stable for about 60 days and retained a detection limit (34 μM) of parts per million for paraoxon. An AChE coated iron oxide magnetic NPs (30 nm) was also developed in which carbon nanotubes and zirconium oxide was bound to NPs (31.5 nm) composite on the screen printed electrode surface for the detection of dimethoate, an organophosphorus pesticide with a sensitivity of 50 pg/L (Ghormade et al., 2011). OPs can selectively interact with some of the advanced materials [like metalorganic frameworks (MOFs)], to yield measurable signals on the basis of the electron transfer reaction involved. A number of factors (availability of a stable framework structure, ultra highporosity, a high internal surface area, porevolume, thermal/chemical stability, selectivity, and their nontoxic nature) should be positively considered for the feasibility of MOFs. The use of MOFs is, therefore, projected for expansion in the construction of next generation pesticide sensors. Molecularly imprinted polymer (MIP) sensors are another kind of sensors that consist of highly cross-linked polymers with shared advantages of synthetic recognition platforms and biological recognition elements (Audrey et al., 2012). These sensors display excellent thermal, chemical, and mechanical stability and they can also be tailored to meet specific requirements. Despite of such advantages, draw backs like poor signal transduction, lack of stability, and so on are to be considered and as suggested by some authors, these shortcomings of MIPs can be overcome by attaching them with other molecules so as to improve the chemical affinity and to obtain as specific signal (Audrey et al., 2012). Another powerful method, surface-enhanced Raman scattering (SERS) has been used for a long time as a technique for chemical and biological sensing (Kim et al., 2015). It is highly sensitive and practical over time scales. Along with portable Raman spectrometers, this technique is highly attractive as real-time sensors in the field. Based on SERC, Kim et al. (2015) reported a simple, rapid, cheap, and very sensitive method of detecting trace level of two pesticides, chlorpyrifos (CPF; one of the most widely used pesticides associated with neurotoxicity, asthma, carcinogenicity, reproductive, and developmental toxicity and suspected endocrine disruptor) and TBZ which is a fungicide. It is likely to be carcinogenic at high level of exposure, and extremely toxic to aquatic life (Kim et al., 2015).

For pesticides detection both unimolecular, as well as array type of nanosensors are being developed currently. Electrical potential, color, and fluorescence changes are measured to probe interaction of the target with the help of a biosensor. Simultaneous measurements of multiple biomolecules fixed on a particular substrate are allowed in array technologies. To detect organochlorine pesticide, such as DDT at a concentration as low as 27 ng/mL, 30 nm gold NPs based dipstick competitive immunoassay (an unimolecular array systems) is proven to be helpful (Lisa et al., 2009). The gold NP based dipstick technique is also suitable for the rapid on-site testing of several other pesticides (Lisa et al., 2009). A gold NPs (40 nm) based portable one-step strip assay has been developed by Guo et al. (2009) in which simultaneous screening without any equipment could be performed for two pesticides (carbofuran and triazophos) within 8–10 min (Guo et al., 2009; Hatton et al., 2008). These unique nanoparticles (gold NPs) are capable of agglomeration in association with color production and that property is used for pesticide detection. Besides, cadmium telluride quantum dots (CdTe QDs) semiconductor fluorescent NPs were used in a fluoroimmunoassay to detect the herbicide, 2,4-dichlorophenoxyacetic acid (2,4-D) (Vinayaka et al., 2009). Detection of up to 250 pg/L of 2,4-D was possible using this technique. Kaushik et al. (2009) fabricated a nucleic acid sensor for the detection of pyrethroid, cypermethrin, and permethrin by immobilizing single standard calf thymus DNA onto a chitosan nanobiocomposite film of iron oxide NPs (Fe_3O_4, 22 nm), deposited onto indium-tin-oxide coated glass surface (Kaushik et al., 2009). Under refrigerated conditions, this disposable nanobiocomposite bioelectrode was found to be stable for long time (about two months) and could detect cypermethrin and permethrin rapidly (N50 s) even at 0.0025 ppm concentration.

A multiresidue retention problem found in the environment is caused by the widespread use of various pesticides and their mixtures in the agricultural fields. Thus, simultaneous identification of several pesticides in a complex sample is needed. Multianalyte immunoassay is able to simultaneously discriminate at least two analytes in a single run. In this assay, a bispecific monoclonal antibody (McAb), for both was labeled with nanogold in comparison to the nanogold labeled antibodies as detector reagents. Various advantages, like high sample throughput, low consumption of reagent and time (Fu et al., 2007; Kricka, 1992) are the major benefit in this technique. The pesticides, carbofuran and triazophos, were successfully detected using this assay.

The key challenge for the commercialization of the biosensors with the application of biotechnology depends mainly on the development of the biosensors, which are specific, fast, simple, and low cost. In addition, combination of nanotechnology and microfluidic devices, which allow the flow of the required liquid in microvolumes quantity through proper channels, will promote further miniaturization, as well as rapid sampling. Another interesting aspect in this regard is the cantilever nanomechanical devices, with springboard like-mechanism. When the target molecule binds with a reporter molecule, which is attached to the cantilever, then the presence of specific target molecules can be detected by these nanomechanical devices. It is nice to think that cantilever arrays can give rise to a sensitive nanosensor electronic "nose" or "tongue" for the detection of specific molecules applying nanomechanical devices. At this stage, we would say that the development of multianalyte array sensors, microfluidic devices and cantilever arrays of this particular area of nanotechnology to make easy environmental monitoring will be worked out successfully in future (Ghormade et al., 2011).

It is evident that different types of nanoparticles, like QDs, AuNPs, and so on, have been used for the development of electrochemical enzyme based biosensors in recent years. For the amperometric detection of trichlorfon, an enzyme biosensor has been developed using poly(N-vinyl-2-pyrrolidone) (PVP)-capped CdS QDs (Li et al., 2006). The electrode surface containing PVP-QD nanostructures creates a favorable microenvironment, which can lead to a highly sensitive (the detection limit is 4.8×10^{-8} M) and stable electrochemical environment for the detection of the enzymatically generated thiocholine products. Another kind of nanoparticles used for the particular enzyme biosensors are gold nanoparticles (AuNPs). A major advantage for the biosensors preparation using these particles lies to their unique properties of providing a suitable microenvironment for immobilization of biomolecules, which retains their bioactivity. Furthermore, direct electron transfer between immobilized redox molecules and the electrode surface are facilitated by AuNPs (Pingarrón et al., 2008).

Recently an electrochemical biosensor has been developed for the detection of monocrotophos and methyl parathion based on colloidal AuNP modified sol–gel interface technique (Audrey et al., 2012; Du et al., 2008a). Here, the assembled AuNPs on a sol–gel derived silicate network favors the interface enzymatic hydrolysis reaction, increases the sensitivity of the amperometric response and provides a conductive pathway to electron transfer. This biosensor is stable and retains 90% of its initial current response even after a 30-day storage period. Recently, an efficient biosensor has been developed in which the unique properties of AuNPS with those of QDs are combined. This newly developed electrochemical system based on CdTe QDs-AuNPs electrode was found to be more sensitive than those based on QDs or AuNPs alone and has been used for the detection of monocrotophos (Audrey et al., 2012; Du et al., 2008b; Xia et al., 2014).

5 Nanotechnology and Insect Pest Management

However, insects comprise the major portion of these agricultural pest populations. Insects are cosmopolitan and it consist approximately two thirds of the known animal species in the world. Insects infest on all kinds of plants including crop plants, medicinal plants, forest trees, and weeds along with the stored products in godowns, storage structures, and bins. This renders great harm to the stored food and its quality. For the security of their food, insects usually inflict injury to plants and stored desirable products in two ways, either directly or indirectly. According to the amount of damage, insects can be grouped into three major categories. Insects causing less than 5% damage are not considered as pests. On the other hand, the insects which cause damage between the limit 5–10% are considered as minor pests whereas insects that cause damage above the limit 10% are designated as major pests

(Dhaliwal et al., 2010). Among the worldwide loss of agricultural products, insects secured the top rank among plant pathogens and weeds. Both of them are responsible for approximately 13% loss where insects are responsible for 14% causing a loss upto US $2000 billion per year (Pimentel, 2009). Limitations like environmental degradation, generation of resistance over long period and less efficiency of traditional methods lead to investigate new and modern approaches for management of insect pest. These difficulties for the development of the efficient and potential approaches for the management of insect pest in agriculture can be overcome by the applications of nanotechnology, that is, by using nanomaterials in agriculture. As discussed throughout the text nanotechnology has been used widely to control different pest populations. Insect pest management could be implicated through the formulations of pesticides and insecticides based on nanomaterial (Vinutha et al., 2013). However, bioconjugated nanoparticles with the property of slow and sustainable release could also be implicated in such scenario. The basic aspect of nanotechnology lies in the potential of precisely forming matter to the specificity in the atomic level. Thus, the opportunity for enhancing the properties like efficacy and specificity are the major benefit of employing nanobased insecticides. Along with the chemical-based methods nanoparticle-mediated gene transfer proving itself promising. Insect resistant plant can be raised by delivering DNA materials to the host plant (Torney, 2009b; Vinutha et al., 2013). Synthesized silver nanoparticles (SNP) using an aqueous leaf extract of *Tinospora cordifolia* exhibited significant pediculocidal and larvicidal activity. It is proven very effective against the head louse *Pediculus humanus* and fourth instars larvae of *Culex-quinque fasciatus* and *Anopheles subpictus* (Jayaseelan et al., 2011). High-pressure homogenization using 2.5% surfactant and 100% glycerol used to develop encapsulated citronella oil nanoemulsion. These droplets are stable and they also increase the retention of the oil and slow release of the same. Now here a decrease in release rate by nanoemulsification can lengthen mosquito protection time (Sakulku et al., 2009). Garlic essential oil, when loaded in nanoparticles has been reported efficacious against *Tribolium castaneum* Herbst (Yang et al., 2009b). Ingredients of nanotubes possess the ability to stick to the surface hair of insect pests while aluminosilicate filled nanotube can stick to plant surfaces and have the ability to enter the body and influences certain physiological functions by this process. Thus, various nanoinsecticides are getting importance and being used efficiently in agriculture (Owolade et al., 2008; Patil, 2009; Ragaei and Sabry, 2014). Nowaday, trials are on going to compare the efficacy available pesticides and their nanoformulation. For instance, nanosulfur has been found ten times more effective for control of mites and nanohexaconazole has been found five times more effective in controlling pathogens as compared to its water dispersible powder (WDP) formulations generally used till date. The production of a nicotine carboxylate nanoemulsion made with the help of a series of fatty acids (C10–C18) and surfactant was reported by Casanova et al. (2005); Ragaei and Sabry (2014). A monomodal distribution of size was shown by the oil-in-water nanoemulsion with mean particle sizes of 100 nm. Recently, the bioactivity of the insecticide formulations was also evaluated by assessing the lethal time 50 (LT50) in adults of *Drosophila melanogaster*. It has been observed that with increasing size of the fatty acids, the encapsulation efficiency was decreased. In addition, the same trend was found in the bioactivity. When the chain length was decreased, better bioactivity was detected (Ragaei and Sabry, 2014).

Now coming to another example of oleander aphids, *Aphis nerii*. The management of oleander aphid has been found to be depended on the synthetic insecticides. However, long-term use of insecticides causes resistance in this pest to the pesticides. Presently, nanoparticles have received much attention for controlling the pests, *A. nerii* (Elek et al., 2010; Guan et al., 2008). Rouhani et al. (2012) assessed the insecticidal activities of Ag and Ag–Zn nanoparticles on the *A. nerii*. They found that these nanoparticles were an effective in the control of *A. nerii* (Rouhani et al., 2012). They showed increase in nanopesticide concentrations results in significant increase in the insect mortality. Also, there is another prime advantage of using these nanoparticles. This is the low risk of developing resistance over a long-term usage. Nanometer-sized Ag particles, has been suggested to possess different physical and chemical properties from their macroscale counterparts. This differences, in turn commonly affect the interaction of different biological structures and physiological processes (Kim et al., 2009; Nel et al., 2006).

The effectiveness of metal nanoparticles against plants pathogens, insects, and pests were confirmed by a number of previous studies and suggests that these particles can be used as an effective tool in the preparation of various new formulations like insecticides, pesticides, insect repellants, and so on (Barik et al., 2008; Gajbhiye et al., 2009b; Goswami et al., 2010; Owolade et al., 2008; Rai and Ingle, 2012). Insect mortality effect of Ag nanoparticles was reported to be slightly higher than that of Ag–Zn nanoparticles. It was found that ZnO–TiO_2–Ag nanoparticles have insecticidal activity on *Frankliniella occidentalis* Pergande (Rouhani et al., 2012). It is also been reported that the toxicity of the imidacloprid (IMI) increased upon coated with nanoparticles (Guan et al., 2008). Guan et al. (2008), also showed that adult stage of *Martianus dermestoides* Chevrolat (Coleoptera: Tenebrionidae) is more sensitive to 50% nano-SDS/Ag/TiO_2-IMI in comparison to the 95% IMI (Guan et al., 2008; Rouhani et al., 2012). Rouhani et al. (2012) also showed that the insecticidal effect of $ZnOTiO_2$–Ag increased with the increasing amount of Ag (Guan et al., 2008; Rouhani et al., 2012). Rouhani et al. (2012) also suggest the possibility of using Ag nanoparticles can be used as prized tools in the management programs of *A. nerii* (Guan et al., 2008; Rouhani et al., 2012). Torney (2009a) appraised the role of nanotechnology in nanoparticle mediated gene (DNA) transfer which can be used to deliver genetic materials and other desired chemicals into plant tissues. These in turn can lead to the development of protection from insect pests in plants. Wang et al. (2007) suggested that the oil in water nanoemulsions could be considered as useful materials for formulation of pesticides and could act as effective agents against various insect pests used in agriculture (Wang et al., 2007). A similar report by Liu et al. also showed that essential oil-loaded solid lipid nanoparticles were effective in the nanopesticide formulations (Bhattacharyya et al., 2010; Liu and Du, 2004). Nanosilica can also be used as nanoinsecticide (Barik et al., 2008). Surface charged modified hydrophobic nanosilica (~3–5 nm) could be used successfully for controlling a variety of agricultural insect pests, as well as animal ectoparasites, which have significant veterinary importance (Ulrichs et al., 2005a). The mechanism nanosilica action on insects solely depends on physical means and described in details before in this chapter. Insecticidal activity of polyethylene glycol-coated nanoparticles loaded with garlic essential oil was investigated by Yang et al. (2009b) against adult *Tribolium castaneum* insect found in stored products. The efficacy of control of adult *T. castaneum* has been observed to be about 80%, and is considered to be due to the slow and tenacious release of the active components from the nanoparticles. To control grasserie and rice weevil disease in silkworm (*B. mori*) caused by baculovirus BmNPV (*B. mori* nuclear polyhedrosis virus) and *S. oryzae*, respectively, aluminum oxide (ANP), SNP, zinc oxide, and titanium dioxide play a significant role (Goswami et al., 2010). Based on the bioassay performed on the solid and liquid formulations of the aforementioned nanoparticles, they applied such formulations on rice and kept them in a plastic box with 20 adults of *S. oryzae* and observed the effects for 7 days. Maximum effectiveness of hydrophilic SNP was observed on the first day. From the second day, more than 90% mortality was observed following SNP and

ANP treatment. After the completion of 7 days of exposure, 86 and 95% mortality were observed with hydrophobic and hydrophilic SNP and at the same time, nearly 70% of the insects were found to be killed, when the rice was treated with lipophilic SNP. ANP treatment lead to 100% mortality. Likewise, Goswami et al. (2010) showed that there was significant decrease in viral load in the larvae of *B. mori* affected with grasserie disease, followed by the treatment with ethanolic suspension of hydrophobic alumino-silicate nanoparticles (Goswami et al., 2010). Bhattacharyya et al. (2010) nicely described the contribution of nanotechnology in revolutionizing agriculture, including the management of pest problems in the near future. With the help of nanotechnology, "green revolution" will be accelerated in next two decades. Nanoencapsulation, a major contributor in nanotechnology, is currently used as an important and promising approach for the protection of host plants against insect pests. Nanoencapsulation with nanoparticles in form of pesticide is better candidate than larger particles for proper absorption of the chemical into the plants (Scrinis and Lyons, 2007). The insecticidal activity of nanostructured alumina was studied for the first time against two major insect pests in stored food supplies viz. *S. oryzae* L. and *Rhyzopertha dominica* (F.) (Stadler et al., 2010). Significant mortality has been observed in nanostructured alumina-treated wheat after continuous exposure for 3 days. Therefore, nanostructured alumina is a better option than commercially available insecticides and may provide a reliable and cheap alternative for insect pest control. Research in this field may provide a new direction for nanoparticle-based technologies in pest management (Rai and Ingle, 2012).

Along with the previous discussion, it is noteworthy to mention that insect group contains many nanostructured materials for their unique survival strategies and evolution. Here a brief knowledge about these would be beneficial for pest management and also to understand their biology. Naturally occurring nanostructures can be potentially rich sources of various products that meet certain stipulations (Watson and Watson, 2004). However, much focus has not been laid on that field yet and the nanotechnology based emerging industries have made very little use of such technology available freely in nature (Bhattacharyya et al., 2010; Ehrlich et al., 2008). Ordered hexagonal packed array of structures in the wings of cicada (*Psaltoda claripennis* Ashton, for example) and termite (Rhinotermitidae family, for example) can be mentioned as a good example in this area (Ragaei and Sabry, 2014; Zhang et al., 2006). The size of these naturally occurring nanoparticles has been shown to be in the nanometer range, usually vary from 200 to 1000 nm. The structures have been reported to have a rounded shape at the apex and protrude approximately 150–350 nm out from the surface plane. Aerodynamic efficiency of the insect can be increased by these particular wing nanoparticles. Insects are known to possess temperature dependent ferromagnetic resonance and these magnetic nanoparticles can act as geomagnetic sensors in social insects (Ragaei and Sabry, 2014). For example, honeybees have been shown to use this geomagnetic field information for orientation, homing, and foraging (Ragaei and Sabry, 2014). However, the exact mechanism of the detection of the geomagnetic field by the animals is still not clearly known although it has been indicated by a number of observations that the geomagnetic field could interact with the intracellular biomineralized magnetite on its intensity and direction. Observing the behavior of different species of insects in the presence of magnetite particles, influenced by the geomagnetic field, is the initial step toward the demonstration of the involvement of biogenic magnetite in geomagnetic field detection (Bhattacharyya et al., 2010; Ishay et al., 2008). The ant *Formica rufa* Linnaeus has been shown to use information from the geomagnetic field for orientation during the foraging process. The ant *Solenopsis invicta* Buren also behaves in an identical manner (Slowik et al., 1997). Electron microscope studies on the behavior of several species of ants clearly demonstrated magnetic signals with the help of magnetite nanoparticles (Abraçado et al., 2005; Bhattacharyya et al., 2010). It is worth mentioning that magnetite particles are present in the head, antennae, thorax, and abdomen in the stingless bee *Schwarziana quadripunctata* Lepeletier (Bhattacharyya et al., 2010; Luacano et al., 2006). Reports also showed the presence of ferromagnetic material in *Apis mellifera* Linnaeus abdomens and identified as suitable for magnetic reception (Desoil et al., 2005). In order to understand the physiological response of bees to a magnetic field, the biogenic magnetic properties of the honeybee *A. mellifera* were investigated in detail (Bhattacharyya et al., 2010; Billen, 2006; Hsu et al., 2007). The magnetizations of bee abdomens and separately on heads and thoraxes were measured as the functions of field and temperature (Bhattacharyya et al., 2010; Esquivel, 2007). The results revealed both the antiferromagnetic responses of the ferrihydrite cores of the iron storage protein ferritin, as well as the ferromagnetic responses of nanoscale magnetite (Fe_3O_4) particles (Bhattacharyya et al., 2010; Dawson, 2008). Reports also suggest the presence of large magnetite particles (c. 30 nm or more), which have the capacity of retention of remanence magnetization at room temperature in the abdomens, although these particles were absent in the heads and thoraxes. Besides, for the detection of natural magnetism, fire ant (*S. invicta*) workers, queens, and alates were analyzed by magnetic resonance imaging (MRI) and it was found that all ferromagnetic materials are magnetic nanoparticles solely responsible for localization of specific direction for food and host of insects. Nanostructure components were also reported to be present in compound eyes of insects. The bright color components in the wings of butterflies has been to be nothing but nanoparticles. Recently, Guan et al. (2008) reported the construction of a novel photodegradable insecticide involving nanoparticles. There are many naturally occurring volatile phytochemicals and nanoparticles of insects, which are dedicated for plant–insect interaction. Similarly, electrospun silk fibroin-based fibers with an average diameter of 700 nm is being produced from silkworm, more precisely from aqueous silk solutions, helps to produce single wall carbon nanotubes (SWNT) for efficient insecticide delivery system (Bhattacharyya et al., 2010).

6 Conclusions

Natotechnology revolutionizing many field of applied science including agriculture. In agriculture, it has many interdisciplinary roles summarized in Fig. 2.4. It is providing us with solutions in the field of fertilizers, pest management, new variety of plant generations, and so on. Nanotechnology has revolutionized the

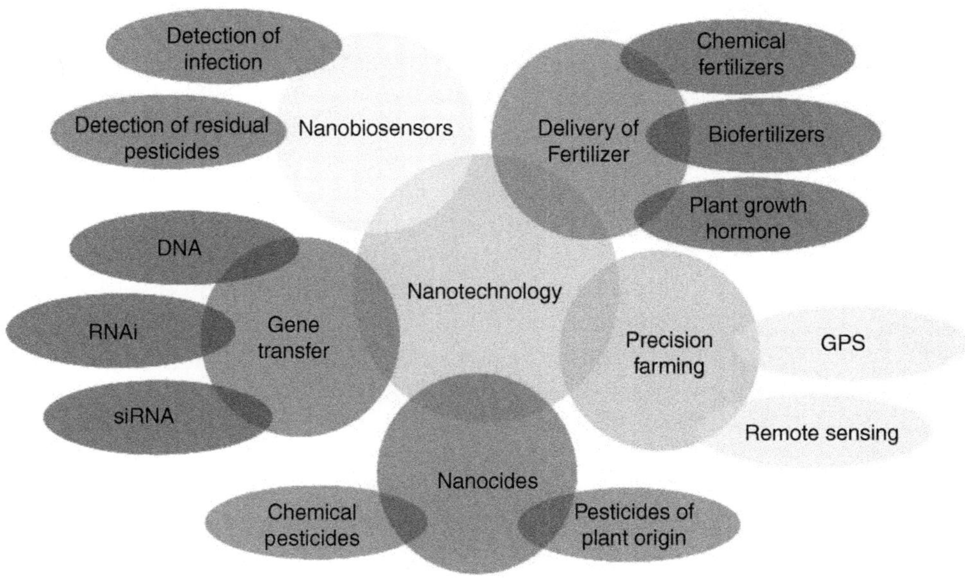

Figure 2.4. Nanotechnology in agriculture.

existing technologies used in insect pest management using traditional methods. Insect resistant varieties could be developed by nanoparticle-mediated gene transfer. Thus, without affecting the, nature nanotechnology can be used in insect pest management. Different forms of nanoproducts are being used for pest managements using unique properties of nanoparticles like high reactivity, miniscule size, and so on. Chemical pesticide pollutes both the top-soil and the ground water but nanotechnologically modified pesticides have proven them useful in many aspects like slow and targeted release of the pesticides. This in turn lowers the overall pesticides load and thus damage of vulnerable agroecosystems. Management of agro-ecosystem by traditional is laborious and also economically depressing. Properties of nanopesticides will definitely reduce such burden. Besides directly acting as pesticides or carrying those nanomaterials are being widely used for biosensing process. It is proving itself in the detection of trace amount of pesticidal or microbial contaminations in the field, as well as in the postharvest stages. Thus, integration of nanosensors with IPM will ultimately make the process more efficient and less hazardous. Nanotechnology is going to revolutionize the traditional farming in the near future using a technique other than that discussed previously. By promoting thoughtful farming practices with "precision farming" in the near future we can optimize the use of natural resources. Precision farming will maximize the annual crop yields and will minimize inputs like pesticides, herbicides, and so on. It works through scanning of the environmental variables and helps us to apply highly target actions in a broad scale. Precision farming takes the help of modern computing system, tiny sensors, satellite mediated global positioning systems and remote-sensing devices for the measurement of extremely localized environmental conditions. This highly advanced approach helps to determine the growing efficiency of crops and can precisely identify the location and nature of various complications. Thus, in many ways precision farming will check the pollution of agro-ecosystem by checking the generation of agricultural waste. In near future it will greatly enhanced the net production and will augment the decision-making process during irrigation, pest control, fertilization, and even in the harvesting, by many folds (Rai and Ingle, 2012). However, the technology is labor-consuming, expensive, and need great expertise to analyze the available data. Despite these positive aspects, the use of nanonanomaterials in agro ecosystem needs proper and extreme careful evaluation. Also with the advancement of nanotechnology growing concern about the side-effects are being evaluated with nanotoxicology. Studies are going on but more and more reproducible revisions are required for the measurement of the actual toxicity and behavior of the ecosystem to the nanomaterials. Also to check the effect of the nanomaterials in respect to the living object is highly required. All these concerns arising also from the same properties, which are responsible for the effectiveness of the nanomaterials like the highly reactive surfaces of nanomaterials, owing to the increased surface-to-volume ratio. But nowadays the dark sides of nanomaterials are coming in front of us (Bakshi et al., 2014; Sarkar et al., 2014). Nowadays studies are coming out showing the deleterious effect of nanoparticles like silica, titanium dioxide, iron, copper, cobalt–chromium nanoparticles (de Oliveira et al., 2014; Yamashita et al., 2011; Sarkar et al., 2011, 2014; Sarkar and Sil, 2014; Bhabra et al., 2009). Metallic nanoparticles reduce the growth of seedling (Lee et al., 2012; Lin and Xing, 2008). Ma et al. (2013) showed that ZnO nanoparticles also harms nontarget beneficial organisms like bacteria, algae, and different invertebrates and thus render great harm the ecosystem (Ma et al., 2013). Hence, these studies are showing that along with beneficial effects there are lots to think about the side effects. Nanoparticles might be ecotoxic and thus before releasing a naïve product to the nature there must be rigorous checking about their toxicity. Thus, including all, there are of immense possibility in near future to use the nanotechnology in the agricultural science but we must be extremely careful because they also can disturb the delicate balance of the nature.

Acknowledgment

Authors are grateful to Mr. Abhijit Sarkar for providing the TEM and SEM micrographs of MSN and metal nanoparticles.

References

Abraçado, L., Esquivel, D., Alves, O., Wajnberg, E., 2005. Magnetic material in head, thorax, and abdomen of *Solenopsis substituta* ants: a ferromagnetic resonance study. J. Magn. Reson. 175, 309–316.

Anwunobi, A., Emeje, M., 2011. Recent applications of natural polymers in nanodrug delivery. J. Nanomed. Nanotechnol. S 4, 002.

Audrey, S., Beatriz, P.-S., Jean-Louis, M., 2012. Biosensors for pesticide detection: new trends. American Journal of Analytical Chemistry 3.

Bailey, K.L., Boyetchko, S.M., Längle, T., 2010. Social and economic drivers shaping the future of biological control: a Canadian perspective on the factors affecting the development and use of microbial biopesticides. Biol. Control 52, 221–229.

Bakshi, M., Singh, H., Abhilash, P., 2014. The unseen impact of nanoparticles: more or less. Curr. Sci. 106, 350–352.

Barik, T., Sahu, B., Swain, V., 2008. Nanosilica—from medicine to pest control. Parasitol. Res. 103, 253–258.

Baulcombe, D.C., 1999. Fast forward genetics based on virus-induced gene silencing. Curr. Opin. Plant Biol. 2, 109–113.

Beddington, J., 2010. Food security: contributions from science to a new and greener revolution. Phil. Trans. R. Soc. B 365 (1537), 61–71.

Bhabra, G., Sood, A., Fisher, B., Cartwright, L., Saunders, M., Evans, W.H., Surprenant, A., Lopez-Castejon, G., Mann, S., Davis, S.A., 2009. Nanoparticles can cause DNA damage across a cellular barrier. Nat. Nanotechnol. 4, 876–883.

Bhattacharyya, A., Bhaumik, A., Rani, P.U., Mandal, S., Epidi, T.T., 2010. Nano-particles-A recent approach to insect pest control. Afr. J. Biotechnol. 9, 3489–3493.

Billen, J., 2006. Signal variety and communication in social insects. In: Proceedings of the section experimental and applied entomology-Netherlands entomological society. CiteSeer, 9.

Caraglia, M., Rosa, G., Abbruzzese, A., Leonetti, C., 2011. Nanotechnologies: new opportunities for old drugs. The Case of Aminobisphosphonates. J Nanomed. Biotherap. Discov. 1, 103e.

Casanova, H., Araque, P., Ortiz, C., 2005. Nicotine carboxylate insecticide emulsions: effect of the fatty acid chain length. J. Agric. Food Chem. 53, 9949–9953.

Chinnamuthu, C., Boopathi, P.M., 2009. Nanotechnology and agroecosystem. Madras Agric. J. 96, 17–31.

Dawson, K., 2008. Bionano interactions—a rational approach to the interaction between nanoscale materials and living matter. NanoBioEurope 8, 1–2.

de Oliveira, J.L., Campos, E.V.R., Bakshi, M., Abhilash, P., Fraceto, L.F., 2014. Application of nanotechnology for the encapsulation of botanical insecticides for sustainable agriculture: prospects and promises. Biotechnol. Adv. 32, 1550–1561.

Debnath, N., Das, S., Seth, D., Chandra, R., Bhattacharya, S.C., Goswami, A., 2011. Entomotoxic effect of silica nanoparticles against *Sitophilus oryzae* (L.). J. Pest Sci. 84, 99–105.

Desoil, M., Gillis, P., Gossuin, Y., Pankhurst, Q., Hautot, D., 2005. Definitive identification of magnetite nanoparticles in the abdomen of the honeybee *Apis mellifera*. J. Phys. Conf. Ser. 17, 45.

Dhaliwal, G., Jindal, V., Dhawan, A., 2010. Insect pest problems and crop losses: changing trends. Indian J. Ecol. 37, 1–7.

Dhawan, A. K., Peshin, R., 2009. Integrated pest management: concept, opportunities and challenges. Integrated pest management: innovation-development process, vol. 1. Springer, Netherlands, pp. 51–81.

Ding, W., Shah, N.P., 2009. Effect of various encapsulating materials on the stability of probiotic bacteria. J. Food Sci. 74, M100–M107.

Douroumis, D., 2011. Encapsulation of water insoluble drugs in mesoporous silica nanoparticles using supercritical carbon dioxide. J. Nanomed. Nanotechnol. 2, 111.

Du, D., Chen, S., Cai, J., Zhang, A., 2008a. Electrochemical pesticide sensitivity test using acetylcholinesterase biosensor based on colloidal gold nanoparticle modified sol–gel interface. Talanta 74, 766–772.

Du, D., Chen, W., Cai, J., Zhang, J., Qu, F., Li, H., 2008b. Development of acetylcholinesterase biosensor based on CdTe quantum dots modified cysteamine self-assembled monolayers. J. Electroanal. Chem. 623, 81–85.

Ehrlich, H., Janussen, D., Simon, P., Bazhenov, V.V., Shapkin, N.P., Erler, C., Mertig, M., Born, R., Heinemann, S., Hanke, T., 2008. Nanostructural organization of naturally occurring composites-Part II: Silica-chitin-based biocomposites. Journal of Nanomaterials 2008, 54.

Elek, N., Hoffman, R., Raviv, U., Resh, R., Ishaaya, I., Magdassi, S., 2010. Novaluron nanoparticles: formation and potential use in controlling agricultural insect pests. Coll. Surf. A 372, 66–72.

Elibol, O., Morisette, D., Akin, D., Denton, J., Bashir, R., 2003. Integrated nanoscale silicon sensors using top–down fabrication. Appl. Phys. Lett. 83, 4613–4615.

Esquivel, D.M.S., 2007. Magnetic nanoparticles in social insects: are they the geomagnetic sensors. Entomological Society of America 2007 Annual Meeting.

Fu, Z., Liu, H., Yang, Z., Ju, H., 2007. Recent developments in multianalyte immunoassay. Curr. Trends Biotechnol. Pharm. 1, 1–17.

Gajbhiye, M., Kesharwani, J., Ingle, A., Gade, A., Rai, M., 2009a. Fungus-mediated synthesis of silver nanoparticles and their activity against pathogenic fungi in combination with fluconazole. Nanomed. Nanotechnol. Biol. Med. 5, 382–386.

Gajbhiye, M., Kesharwani, J., Ingle, A., Gade, A., Rai, M., 2009b. Fungus-mediated synthesis of silver nanoparticles and their activity against pathogenic fungi in combination with fluconazole. Nanomedicine 5, 382–386.

Ghormade, V., Deshpande, M.V., Paknikar, K.M., 2011. Perspectives for nano-biotechnology enabled protection and nutrition of plants. Biotechnol. Adv. 29, 792–803.

González-Verdejo, C., Dita, M., di Pietro, A., Moreno, M.T., Barandiarán, X., Rubiales, D., González-Melendi, P., Pérez-de-Luque, A., 2007. Identification and expression analysis of a MYB family transcription factor in the parasitic plant Orobanche ramosa. Ann. Appl. Biol. 150, 123–130.

Goswami, A., Roy, I., Sengupta, S., Debnath, N., 2010. Novel applications of solid and liquid formulations of nanoparticles against insect pests and pathogens. Thin Solid Films 519, 1252–1257.

Guan, H., Chi, D., Yu, J., Li, X., 2008. A novel photodegradable insecticide: preparation, characterization and properties evaluation of nano-Imidacloprid. Pest. Biochem. Physiol. 92, 83–91.

Guo, Y.-R., Liu, S.-Y., Gui, W.-J., Zhu, G.-N., 2009. Gold immunochromatographic assay for simultaneous detection of carbofuran and triazophos in water samples. Anal. Biochem. 389, 32–39.

Gutiérrez, J., González, C., Maestro, A., Sole, I., Pey, C., Nolla, J., 2008. Nano-emulsions: new applications and optimization of their preparation. Curr. Opin. Colloid Interface Sci. 13, 245–251.

Hamamouch, N., Westwood, J.H., Banner, I., Cramer, C.L., Gepstein, S., Aly, R., 2005. A peptide from insects protects transgenic tobacco from a parasitic weed. Transgenic Res. 14, 227–236.

Hatton, R.A., Miller, A.J., Silva, S., 2008. Carbon nanotubes: a multi- functional material for organic optoelectronics. J. Mater. Chem. 18, 1183–1192.

Holister, P., Harper, T.E., Vas, C.R., 2003. Nanotubes white paper. CMP Científica.

Hsu, C.-Y., Ko, F.-Y., Li, C.-W., Fann, K., Lue, J.-T., 2007. Magnetoreception system in honeybees (*Apis mellifera*). PLoS One 2, e395–e1395.

Huang, J., Li, Q., Sun, D., Lu, Y., Su, Y., Yang, X., Wang, H., Wang, Y., Shao, W., He, N., 2007. Biosynthesis of silver and gold nanoparticles by novel sundried *Cinnamomum camphora* leaf. Nanotechnology 18, 105104.

Ishay, J.S., Barkay, Z., Eliaz, N., Plotkin, M., Volynchik, S., Bergman, D.J., 2008. Gravity orientation in social wasp comb cells (*Vespinae*) and the possible role of embedded minerals. Naturwissenschaften 95, 333–342.

Isman, M.B., 2000. Plant essential oils for pest and disease management. Crop Prot. 19, 603–608.

Jayaseelan, C., Rahuman, A.A., Rajakumar, G., Vishnu Kirthi, A., Santhoshkumar, T., Marimuthu, S., Bagavan, A., Kamaraj, C., Zahir, A.A., Elango, G., 2011. Synthesis of pediculocidal and larvicidal silver nanoparticles by leaf extract from heartleaf moonseed plant, *Tinospora cordifolia* Miers. Parasitol. Res. 109, 185–194.

Joseph, T., Morrison, M., 2006. Nanotechnology in agriculture and food. Nanoforum Report. Institute of Nanotechnology.

Kaushik, A., Solanki, P.R., Ansari, A.A., Malhotra, B.D., Ahmad, S., 2009. Iron oxide-chitosan hybrid nanobiocomposite based nucleic acid sensor for pyrethroid detection. Biochem. Eng. J. 46, 132–140.

Kim, S.W., Kim, K.S., Lamsal, K., Kim, Y.J., Kim, S.B., Jung, M., Sim, S.J., Kim, H.S., Chang, S.J., Kim, J.K., Lee, Y.S., 2009. An in vitro study of the antifungal effect of silver nanoparticles on oak wilt pathogen *Raffaelea* sp. J. Microbiol. Biotechnol. 19, 760–764.

Kim, A., Barcelo, S.J., Li, Z., 2015. SERS-based pesticide detection by using nanofinger sensors. Nanotechnology 26, 015502.

Kricka, L., 1992. Multianalyte testing. Clin. Chem. 38, 327–328.

Lang, S., 2003. Waste fiber can be recycled into valuable products using new technique of electrospinning. Cornell Researchers Report.

Lee, W.-M., Kwak, J.I., An, Y.-J., 2012. Effect of silver nanoparticles in crop plants *Phaseolus radiatus* and *Sorghum bicolor*: media effect on phytotoxicity. Chemosphere 86, 491–499.

Li, X.H., Xie, Z., Min, H., Li, C., Liu, M., Xian, Y., Jin, L., 2006. Development of quantum dots modified acetylcholinesterase biosensor for the detection of trichlorfon. Electroanalysis 18, 2163–2167.

Lin, D., Xing, B., 2008. Root uptake and phytotoxicity of ZnO nanoparticles. Environ. Sci. Technol. 42, 5580–5585.

Lisa, M., Chouhan, R., Vinayaka, A., Manonmani, H., Thakur, M., 2009. Gold nanoparticles based dipstick immunoassay for the rapid detection of dichlorodiphenyltrichloroethane: an organochlorine pesticide. Biosens. Bioelectron. 25, 224–227.

Liu, X.Y., Du, N., 2004. Zero-sized effect of nano-particles and inverse homogeneous nucleation principles of freezing and antifreeze. J. Biol. Chem. 279, 6124–6131.

Liu, F., Wen, L.-X., Li, Z.-Z., Yu, W., Sun, H.-Y., Chen, J.-F., 2006. Porous hollow silica nanoparticles as controlled delivery system for water-soluble pesticide. Mater. Res. Bull. 41, 2268–2275.

Loo, L., Guenther, R.H., Lommel, S.A., Franzen, S., 2007. Encapsidation of nanoparticles by red clover necrotic mosaic virus. J. Am. Chem. Soc. 129, 11111–11117.

Losner-Goshen, D., Portnoy, V.H., Mayer, A.M., Joel, D.M., 1998. Pectolytic activity by the haustorium of the parasitic plant *Orobanche* L. (*Orobanchaceae*) in host roots. Ann. Bot. 81, 319–326.

Luacano, M.J., Cernicchiaro, G., Wajnberg, E., Esquivel, D.M., 2006. Stingless bee antennae: a magnetic sensory organ? Biometals 19, 295–300.

Ma, H., Williams, P.L., Diamond, S.A., 2013. Ecotoxicity of manufactured ZnO nanoparticles—a review. Environ. Pollut. 172, 76–85.

Mehrotra, A., Nagarwal, R.C., Pandit, J.K., 2010. Fabrication of lomustine loaded chitosan nanoparticles by spray drying and in vitro cytostatic activity on human lung cancer cell line L132. J. Nanomed. Nanotechnol. 1, 103.

Mousavi, S.R., Rezaei, M., 2011. Nanotechnology in agriculture and food production. J. Appl. Environ. Biol. Sci. 1, 414–419.

Nel, A., Xia, T., Madler, L., Li, N., 2006. Toxic potential of materials at the nanolevel. Science 311, 622–627.

Owolade, O., Ogunleti, D., Adenekan, M., 2008. Titanium dioxide affects disease development and yield of edible cowpea. EJEAF Chem. 7, 2942–2947.
Pandurangappa, C., Lakshminarasappa, B., 2011. Optical absorption and photoluminescence studies in gamma-irradiated nanocrystalline CaF_2. J. Nanomed. Nanotechnol. 2, 2.
Park, I.Y., Kim, I.Y., Yoo, M.K., Choi, Y.J., Cho, M.H., Cho, C.S., 2008. Mannosylated polyethylenimine coupled mesoporous silica nanoparticles for receptor-mediated gene delivery. Int. J. Pharm. 359, 280–287.
Patil, S., 2009. Economics of agri poverty: nano-bio solutions. Indian Agricultural Research Institute, New Delhi, Indian, 56.
Pérez-de-Luque, A., Rubiales, D., 2009. Nanotechnology for parasitic plant control. Pest Manag. Sci. 65, 540–545.
Pérez-de-Luque, A., González-Verdejo, C.I., Lozano, M.D., Dita, M.A., Cubero, J.I., González-Melendi, P., Risueño, M.C., Rubiales, D., 2006. Protein cross-linking, peroxidase and β-1, 3-endoglucanase involved in resistance of pea against *Orobanche crenata*. J. Exp. Bot. 57, 1461–1469.
Peshin, R., Bandral, R.S., Zhang, W., Wilson, L., Dhawan, A.K., 2009. Integrated pest management: a global overview of history, programs and adoption. Integrated pest management: innovation-development process. Springer.
Pimentel, D., 2009. Integrated pest management: innovation-development process. Integrated Pest Management: Innovation-Development Process, pp. 89–111.
Pingarrón, J.M., Yanez-Sedeno, P., González-Cortés, A., 2008. Gold nanoparticle-based electrochemical biosensors. Electrochim. Acta 53, 5848–5866.
Prasad, R., Kumar, V., Prasad, K.S., 2014. Nanotechnology in sustainable agriculture: present concerns and future aspects. Afr. J. Biotechnol. 13, 705–713.
Prashanth, K.H., Tharanathan, R., 2007. Chitin/chitosan: modifications and their unlimited application potential—an overview. Trends Food Sci. Technol. 18, 117–131.
Ragaei, M., Sabry, A.-K.H., 2014. Nanotechnology for insect pest control. Int. J. Sci. Environ. Technol. 3, 528–545.
Rai, M., Ingle, A., 2012. Role of nanotechnology in agriculture with special reference to management of insect pests. Appl. Microbiol. Biotechnol. 94, 287–293.
Ramanathan, M., Luckarift, H.R., Sarsenova, A., Wild, J.R., Ramanculov, E.K., Olsen, E.V., Simonian, A.L., 2009. Lysozyme-mediated formation of protein–silica nano-composites for biosensing applications. Colloids Surf. B 73, 58–64.
Ravi, S.P., 2010. Evaluation of insecticidal efficacy of *Calotropis procera* and *Annona squamosa* ethanol extracts against *Musca domestica*. J. Biofertil. Biopestic.
Robinson, D., Salejova-Zadrazilova, G., 2010. Observatory NANO (2010). Nanotechnologies for nutrient and biocide delivery in agricultural production. Working paper version.
Rosarin, F.S., Mirunalini, S., 2011. Nobel metallic nanoparticles with novel biomedical properties. J. Bioanal. Biomed. 3, 085–091.
Rouhani, M., Samih, M.A., Kalantari, S., 2012. Insecticide effect of silver and zinc nanoparticles against *Aphis nerii* Boyer De Fonscolombe (Hemiptera: Aphididae). Chil. J. Agri. Res. 72, 590–594.
Roy, S., Gurusubramanian, G., Mukhopadhyay, A., 2009. Variation of resistance to endosulfan in tea mosquito bug, *Helopeltis theivora* Waterhouse (Heteroptera: Miridae) in the tea plantation of the Sub-Himalayan Dooars, northern West Bengal, India. J. Bacteriol. Res. 1, 029–035.

Sakulku, U., Nuchuchua, O., Uawongyart, N., Puttipipatkhachorn, S., Soottitantawat, A., Ruktanonchai, U., 2009. Characterization and mosquito repellent activity of citronella oil nanoemulsion. Int. J. Pharm. 372, 105–111.

Salim, N., Basri, M., Abdul Rahman, M.B., Kuang, D.A., Basri, H., Salleh, A.B., 2011. Phase behavior, formation and characterization of palm-based esters nanoemulsion formulation containing ibuprofen. J. Nanosci. Nanotechnol. 2, 113.

Sarkar, A., Sil, P.C., 2014. Iron oxide nanoparticles mediated cytotoxicity via PI3K/AKT pathway: role of quercetin. Food Chem. Toxicol. 71, 106–115.

Sarkar, A., Das, J., Manna, P., Sil, P.C., 2011. Nano-copper induces oxidative stress and apoptosis in kidney via both extrinsic and intrinsic pathways. Toxicology 290, 208–217.

Sarkar, A., Ghosh, M., Sil, P.C., 2014. Nanotoxicity: oxidative stress mediated toxicity of metal and metal oxide nanoparticles. J. Nanosci. Nanotechnol. 14, 730–743.

Scrinis, G., Lyons, K., 2007. The emerging nano-corporate paradigm: nanotechnology and the transformation of nature, food and agri-food systems. Int. J. Sociol. Food Agri. 15, 22–44.

Shakeel, F., Ramadan, W., Shafiq, S., 2009. Solubility and dissolution improvement of aceclofenac using different nanocarriers. J. Bioequiv. Availab. 1, 39–43.

Singh, P., Prasuhn, D., Yeh, R.M., Destito, G., Rae, C.S., Osborn, K., Finn, M., Manchester, M., 2007. Bio-distribution, toxicity and pathology of cowpea mosaic virus nanoparticles in vivo. J. Control. Release 120, 41–50.

Slowik, T., Green, B., Thorvilson, H., 1997. Detection of magnetism in the red imported fire ant (*Solenopsis invicta*) using magnetic resonance imaging. Bioelectromagnetics 18, 396–399.

Srilatha, B., 2011. Nanotechnology in agriculture. J. Nanomed. Nanotechnol. 2, 123.

Stadler, T., Buteler, M., Weaver, D.K., 2010. Novel use of nanostructured alumina as an insecticide. Pest Manag. Sci. 66, 577–579.

Steinmetz, N.F., Evans, D.J., 2007. Utilisation of plant viruses in bionanotechnology. Org. Biomol. Chem. 5, 2891–2902.

Taylor, T.M., Weiss, J., Davidson, P.M., Bruce, B.D., 2005. Liposomal nanocapsules in food science and agriculture. Crit. Rev. Food Sci. Nutr. 45, 587–605.

Teixeira, M., Alonso, M.J., Pinto, M.M., Barbosa, C.M., 2005. Development and characterization of PLGA nanospheres and nanocapsules containing xanthone and 3-methoxyxanthone. Eur. J. Pharma. Biopharma. 59, 491–500.

Torney, F., 2009a. Nanoparticle mediated plant transformation. Emerging technologies in plant science research. Interdepartmental Plant Physiology Major Fall Seminar Series. Physics p. 696.

Torney, F., 2009b. Nanoparticle mediated plant transformation: emerging technologies in plant science research. Proceedings of the Interdepartmental Plant Physiology Major Fall Seminar Series, (IPPM'09), Iowa State University.

Toub, N., Malvy, C., Fattal, E., Couvreur, P., 2006. Innovative nanotechnologies for the delivery of oligonucleotides and siRNA. Biomed. Pharmacother. 60, 607–620.

Ulrichs, C., Krause, F., Rocksch, T., Goswami, A., Mewis, I., 2005a. Electrostatic application of inert silica dust based insecticides onto plant surfaces. Commun. Agri. Appl. Biol. Sci. 71, 171–178.

Ulrichs, C., Mewis, I. Goswami, A., 2005b. Crop diversification aiming nutritional security in West Bengal: biotechnology of stinging capsules in nature's water-blooms. Ann. Tech. Issue State Agri. Technol. Service Assoc. ISSN, 1–18.

Vidhyalakshmi, R., Bhakyaraj, R., Subhasree, R., 2009. Encapsulation "The future of probiotics"—a review. Adv. Biol. Res. 3, 96–103.

Vinayaka, A., Basheer, S., Thakur, M., 2009. Bioconjugation of CdTe quantum dot for the detection of 2,4-dichlorophenoxyacetic acid by competitive fluoroimmunoassay based biosensor. Biosens. Bioelectron. 24, 1615–1620.

Vinutha, J., Bhagat, D., Bakthavatsalam, N., 2013. Nanotechnology in the management of polyphagous pest *Helicoverpa armigera*. J. Acad. Indus. Res. 1, 606–608.

Wang, L., Li, X., Zhang, G., Dong, J., Eastoe, J., 2007. Oil-in-water nanoemulsions for pesticide formulations. J. Colloid Interface Sci. 314, 230–235.

Wang, H., Wang, J., Choi, D., Tang, Z., Wu, H., Lin, Y., 2009. EQCM immunoassay for phosphorylated acetylcholinesterase as a biomarker for organophosphate exposures based on selective zirconia adsorption and enzyme-catalytic precipitation. Biosens. Bioelectron. 24, 2377–2383.

Watson, G.S., Watson, J.A., 2004. Natural nano-structures on insects—possible functions of ordered arrays characterized by atomic force microscopy. Appl. Surf. Sci. 235, 139–144.

Westwood, J.H., Roney, J.K., Khatibi, P.A., Stromberg, V.K., 2009. RNA translocation between parasitic plants and their hosts. Pest Manag. Sci. 65, 533–539.

Xia, N., Wang, Q., Liu, L., 2014. Nanomaterials-based optical techniques for the detection of acetylcholinesterase and pesticides. Sensors 15, 499–514.

Xie, J., Chen, K., Lee, H.-Y., Xu, C., Hsu, A.R., Peng, S., Chen, X., Sun, S., 2008. Ultrasmall c (RGDyK)-coated Fe_3O_4 nanoparticles and their specific targeting to integrin αvβ3-rich tumor cells. J. Am. Chem. Soc. 130, 7542–7543.

Yamashita, K., Yoshioka, Y., Higashisaka, K., Mimura, K., Morishita, Y., Nozaki, M., Yoshida, T., Ogura, T., Nabeshi, H., Nagano, K., 2011. Silica and titanium dioxide nanoparticles cause pregnancy complications in mice. Nat. Nanotechnol. 6, 321–328.

Yang, F.-L., Li, X.-G., Zhu, F., Lei, C.-L., 2009a. Structural characterization of nanoparticles loaded with garlic essential oil and their insecticidal activity against *Tribolium castaneum* (Herbst)(Coleoptera: Tenebrionidae). J. Agri. Food Chem. 57, 10156–10162.

Yang, F.L., Li, X.G., Zhu, F., Lei, C.L., 2009b. Structural characterization of nanoparticles loaded with garlic essential oil and their insecticidal activity against *Tribolium castaneum* (Herbst) (Coleoptera: Tenebrionidae). J. Agri. Food Chem. 57, 10156–10162.

Yao, H.-P., Wu, X.-F., Gokulamma, K., 2006. Antiviral activity in the mulberry silkworm, *Bombyx mori* L. J. Zhejiang Univ. Sci. A 7, 350–356.

Yoder, J.I., Gunathilake, P., Wu, B., Tomilova, N., Tomilov, A.A., 2009. Engineering host resistance against parasitic weeds with RNA interference. Pest Manag. Sci. 65, 460–466.

Zhang, G., Zhang, J., Xie, G., Liu, Z., Shao, H., 2006. Cicada wings: a stamp from nature for nanoimprint lithography. Small 2, 1440–1443.

Zhao, Y., Haney, M.J., Mahajan, V., Reiner, B.C., Dunaevsky, A., Mosley, R.L., Kabanov, A.V., Gendelman, H.E., Batrakova, E.V., 2011. Active targeted macrophage-mediated delivery of catalase to affected brain regions in models of Parkinson's disease. J. Nanomed. Nanotechnol. 10, 3.

3

NANOPESTICIDES: PREPARATION, TARGETING, AND CONTROLLED RELEASE

Josef Jampílek*, Katarína Král'ová**

**Comenius University, Department of Pharmaceutical Chemistry, Faculty of Pharmacy, Bratislava, Slovakia; **Comenius University, Institute of Chemistry, Faculty of Natural Sciences, Bratislava, Slovakia*

1 Introduction

Symptoms resembling plant damages caused by pathogens can be induced by abiotic (nonliving) factors, such as nutrient deficiency and soil or air pollution. Frequently diseases are a major source of plant damage that can be caused by a number of plant pathogenic (disease-causing) organisms. Thus, it is essential to first determine the cause of symptoms of plant wilting. According to definition of the US Environmental Protection Agency, a pesticide is any substance or mixture of substances intended for preventing, destroying, repelling, or mitigating any pest (Afifi et al., 2010). Pesticides, such as insecticides, acaricides, rodenticides, nematicides, molluscicides, fungicides, and herbicides (or weed killers) are commonly used in agriculture to improve crop yield and efficiency and in general protect plants from damaging influences, such as weeds, plant diseases, or insects. It was found that some of used pesticides are toxic for environment; moreover, some of them are hazardous or even toxic for human and other animals, and thus they were restricted by state or international authorities. Since the development of effective and safe pesticides is difficult and expensive, new technologies have been tested. Nanoscale science and nanotechnology have been demonstrated to have a great potential in providing novel and improved solutions (Sasson et al., 2007; Chen and Yada, 2011; Gopal et al., 2012; Chowdappa and Gowda, 2013; Kah et al., 2013; Sekhon, 2014; Agrawal and Rathore, 2014; Kah and Hofmann, 2014), and thus the number of contributions increases exponentially (Rai et al., 2015;

New Pesticides and Soil Sensors. http://dx.doi.org/10.1016/B978-0-12-804299-1.00004-7

Dolez, 2015; Alghuthaymi et al., 2015; Unsworth et al., 2015; Jampílek and Kráľová, 2015).

Nanotechnology is regarded as one of the key technologies of the 21st century. Nanosize materials change their physical and chemical properties; a variety of industrial, pharmaceutical, and medical products have been improved and innovated in such a way (Hussain et al., 2005; Borm et al., 2006; Fröhlich, 2013; Dolez, 2015; Unsworth et al., 2015). Nanotechnology application in agriculture and the food sector is relatively recent compared to its use in pharmacy (drug delivery) (Garcia et al., 2010; Sekhon, 2014). The use of nanotechnologies can significantly contribute to sustainable intensification of agricultural production, because they can facilitate not only protection of plants against pesticides but also monitoring of plant growth, secure rising of global food production, guarantee enhanced food quality, and minimize the waste (Sonkaria et al., 2012; Pérez-de-Luque and Hermosín, 2013; Prasad et al., 2014; Jampílek and Kráľová, 2015). Food and agricultural production are among the most important fields of nanotechnology application (Kuzma and VerHage, 2006; Coles and Frewer, 2013; Raliya et al., 2013; Chen et al., 2014).

According to the adopted recommendation on the definition of a nanomaterial by the European Commission the term "nanomaterial" means "a natural, incidental, or manufactured material containing particles, in an unbound state or as an aggregate or as an agglomerate and where, for 50% or more of the particles in the number size distribution, one or more external dimensions is in the size range 1–100 nm. In specific cases and where warranted by concerns for the environment, health, safety, or competitiveness the number size distribution threshold of 50% may be replaced by a threshold between 1 and 50%. By derogation from the aforementioned, fullerenes, graphene flakes, and single wall carbon nanotubes with one or more external dimensions below 1 nm should be considered as nanomaterials" (European Commission, 2015).

In general, it can be stated that the ability of nanoparticles (NPs) "to permeate anywhere" connects primarily with their particle size and shape (Hagens et al., 2007; Buzea et al., 2007; Keck and Müller, 2013; Nehoff et al., 2014). Three categories of NPs were defined based on particle size: (1) *ultrafine particles*, <100 nm in diameter (largely consisting of primary combustion products); (2) *accumulation-mode particles* between 100 nm and 2.5 μm in diameter (from aggregation of ultrafine particles or vapors); and (3) *coarse-mode particles* >2.5 μm in diameter (largely mechanically generated particles) (Sioutas et al., 2005).

Based on aforementioned particle size definitions, a concept of a classification system was suggested that classify NPs not only according to their particle sizes but also according to biodegradability (ability of a compound to be degrade in organism/environment) into four classes: (1) size >100 nm and biodegradable; (2) size >100 nm and nonbiodegradable; (3) size <100 nm and biodegradable; (4) size <100 nm and nonbiodegradable (Keck and Müller, 2013).

NPs are characterized by large surface area that is able to bind, absorb and transport compounds. Besides their extremely small particle size (that causes easy permeability through any biomembrane), they are used for carrying compounds (Nehoff et al., 2014). Therefore, nanosystems consist of two basic components: an active ingredient and a nanocarrier that stabilizes the active ingredient in the nanoform. Nanoformulations usually consist of several surfactants, polymers, or inorganic (e.g., metal) NPs in the nanometer size range and therefore cannot be considered as a single entity (Perlatti et al., 2013). Current NP platforms can be classified into three major categories including: (1) inorganic-based (solid) NPs (nonbiodegradable), for example, nanocrystals, shells, quantum dots based on gold, silver, copper, iron, various semiconductors, ceramic (silica-based NPs), and carbon nanotubes or fullerenes; (2) organic-based NPs (frequently biodegradable), for example, liposomes, solid lipid NPs, polymeric NPs, micelles, and capsules; and (3) hybrid NPs (combination of inorganic and organic components). Most frequently organic-based NPs consist of water-soluble biodegradable biocompatible polymers, such as polylactide homopolymers, poly(lactide-*co*-glycolide), poly(propylene glycol), poly(ε-caprolactone), poly(amidoamine), polyacrylamide, and polysorbate 80-coated poly(butylcyanoacrylate), or from natural compounds, such as chitosan, lignin, phospholipids (and other lipids), lecithin, starch, cellulose (and its derivatives), and alginates. The formulations based on biodegradable organic-based matrices allow designing controlled release nanocarriers. The surface of prepared nanocarriers can be modified by various other molecules or specific compounds, and by this approach aqueous solubility (lipophilicity or hydrophilicity) can be modified, and targeted biodistribution can be ensured (De Jong and Borm, 2008; Perlatti et al., 2013; Passeleu-Le Bourdonnec et al., 2013; Onoue et al., 2014; Lu et al., 2014).

According to Thornton (2010), the use of nanotechnology in agriculture will enhance not only the management and conservation of inputs in crops but also in animal production and fisheries, which ultimately will be reflected in improved agricultural practices. In the food industry, NPs are applied in new packaging materials, development of new functional foods, and control of food quality by nanosensors detecting pathogens, as well as in purification of water (Boom, 2011; Senturk et al., 2013). The effectivity of active compounds, such are insecticides, fungicides, and herbicides can be enhanced if they are applied in the nanoscale form, including functionalized nanocapsules (Zhao et al. 2012). The application of nanotechnology in agriculture enables targeted delivery of active ingredients accompanied with their controlled release and monitoring of conditions of cultivated crops, including the impact of environmental stresses, when field-sensing systems are used. Nanoparticle-mediated DNA and gene delivery can result in improved plant traits against environmental stresses and diseases (Joseph and Morrison, 2006; Knauer and Bucheli, 2009; Manimegalai et al., 2011; Sekhon, 2014).

The examples of the most frequent applied nanopesticides (nanoinsecticides, nanoherbicides, nanofungicides, and nanonematicides), as well as the most frequent nanoformulations based on encapsulation of active ingredients into biodegradable organic-based matrix systems and silica-based nanocarriers or silver- and copper-based nanoformulations are mentioned later. Special attention is devoted to ecotoxicology and safety of nanoformulations.

2 Nanoinsecticides

Insect pests are a major issue in agriculture, as they destroy crops and infest stored food and food products. The loss is also caused by deterioration in quality of food and transmission of plant diseases (Neethirajan and Jayas, 2011; Ragaei and Sabry, 2014). Synthetic chemical insecticides occupy predominant position in control strategies. These mostly hazardous chemicals exert unwarranted toxicity and lethal effects on nontarget organisms, develop physiological resistance in target and cause adverse environmental effect. Therefore, nanotechnology would provide green and efficient alternatives for the management of insect pests in agriculture without harming the nature (Bhattacharyya et al., 2010; Rai and Ingle, 2012). Formulations that target the pests specifically and in turn, prevent pollution, for example, the "gut buster" (i.e., the encapsulated product) breaks open only when it comes in contact with the alkaline environment like the gut of the insects (Prasad et al., 2014).

The botanical insecticides include those based on active agents isolated from plant extracts, as well as essential oils derived from certain plants. The use of botanical insecticides associated with nanotechnology offers considerable potential for increasing agricultural productivity, while at the same time reducing impacts on the environment and human health (de Oliveira et al., 2014). For example, the formulation of water dispersible amorphous permethrin NPs with the mean particle size of 151 nm showed higher larvicidal activity (LC_{50} = 0.117 mg/L) against *C. quinquefasciatus* than bulk permethrin (LC_{50} = 0.715 mg/L), indicating that permethrin NPs may be a good choice as a potent and selective larvicide for this insect (Anjali et al., 2010). On the other hand, the 24 h LC_{50} of permethrin NPs prepared by solvent evaporation from an oil-in-water volatile microemulsion against *Aedes aegypti* (6.3 μg/L) was approximately threefold lower than that of regular, microparticular permethrin (19.9 μg/L). The nanoscale formulation did not show toxicity against nontarget organisms (e.g., *Escherichia coli* (ATCC 13534 and 25922), *Bacillus subtilis, Lycopersicum esculentum, Cucumis sativus,* and *Zea mays*). Unlike to regular microparticular permethrin that showed in the *Allium cepa* test a mitotic index (MI) of 46.8% and chromosomal aberration of 0.6% no significant differences were observed in 0.13 mg/L nanopermethrin exposure as compared to the control (MI of 52.0 and 55.03% and chromosomal aberration of 0.2 and 0%, respectively) (Kumar et al., 2013).

Bhagat et al. (2013) tested a nanogel prepared from a pheromone methyl eugenol using a low-molecular mass gelator, such as all-*trans* tri(*p*-phenylenevinylene) bis-aldoxime. This formulation was found to be suitable for an effective management of *Bactrocera dorsalis,* a prevalent harmful pest for a number of fruit crops, including guava (*Psidium guajava*).

Nanoformulations used as insecticides require a nanocarrier system enabling the controlled release of the active compound situated in the core, so that the adequate concentration of this active compound could be preserved during the whole period of insect growth (i.e., from the larval stage to the imaginal stage). For example, the sustainable nanocarrier system was prepared by Bang et al. (2011) using a coating process, in which the basic liposomes of etofenprox or alpha-cypermethrin were coated with chitosan. The coating layer in chitosan-coated nanoliposomes becomes thicker and the sustainable release period of etofenprox and alpha-cypermethrin entrapped in the core gets longer with increasing coating material concentration and intrinsic surface charge. The insecticidal efficacy of liposome-based formulations was described also by Hwang et al. (2011) and Kang et al. (2012). Chitosan-coated nanoformulations of pyrifluquinazon that modifies insect behavior by rapid feeding cessation, so that insects starve to death, were prepared and investigated on mortality of the green peach aphid, *Myzus persicae* by Kang et al. (2012). Nanoformulation of pyrifluquinazon loaded in chitosan 3000 exhibited an effective controlled-release feature and was more potent at 14 days after treatment, while the best lethal efficiency of the bulk pyrifluquinazon appeared at 2 days after treatment at 50 and 25 ppm. Also, NPs composed of a chitosan nanocarrier and a metabolite from entomopathogenic fungi *Nomuraea rileyi* showed higher pesticidal activity against the pest *Spodoptera litura* than the corresponding uncoated fungal metabolite and fungal spores (Chandra et al., 2013).

Nanoencapsulation techniques enabled not only development of in-built pesticides for crops but also in-built switches to control the release and subsequent availability of pesticides. These NP pesticides have improved the capacity for absorption into plants and may not be washed off as readily, thereby increasing their effectiveness (Scrinis and Lyons, 2007; Lyons et al., 2012). Kuzma and VerHage (2006) described, for instance, a smart pesticide that releases its active ingredient only when inhaled by insects. For example, nanoencapsulated essential oil of *Carum copticum* (L.) Benth. & Hook. f. ex C.B. Clarke showed antifeedant activity on *Plutella xylostella* larvae, causing a significant decrease in nutritional indices, such as relative consumption rate, relative growth rate, efficacy of conversion of ingested food and efficacy of conversion of digested food with increasing oil concentration; a significant decrease of digestibility was observed in 72 h after feeding (Jamal et al., 2013).

An interesting experiment was performed by Pant et al. (2014); in order to increase the activity of eucalyptus oil (*Eucalyptus globulus*) as a pesticide the researchers utilized the aqueous filtrate of deoiled cakes of karanja (*Pongamia glabra*) and jatropha (*Jatropha curcas*) obtained after extracting oil for biodiesel preparation by making nanoemulsion for the control of the stored product pest *Tribolium castaneum*. The nanoemulsion containing aqueous filtrate was found to be more toxic (LC_{50} = 0.16 mg/L) than the nanoemulsion without the aqueous filtrate (LC_{50} = 5.49 mg/L), and the loss of eucalyptus oil by volatilization in the nanoemulsion containing the aqueous filtrate was reduced.

NPs loaded with neem (*Azadirachta indica*) extracts formulated as colloidal suspension and (spray-dried) powder showed 100% larval mortality against *P. xylostella*, and their release profile was based on swelling and relaxation of the polymer or polymer erosion (Forim et al., 2013).

Polyethylene glycol (PEG) NPs loaded with garlic essential oil have been successfully tested against store-product pests like *T. castaneum* insect (Yang et al., 2009). The control efficacy against adult *T. castaneum* remained over 80% after 5 months, presumably due to the slow and persistent release of the active components from the NPs, while the control efficacy of free garlic essential oil at the similar concentration (640 mg/kg) was only 11%.

Insecticide formulations with PEG-based amphiphilic copolymers, from which the release of the active ingredient in water followed first order kinetics and was significantly slower than from commercial formulations, were prepared, for example, with beta-cyfluthrin (Loha et al., 2012), carbofuran (Pankaj et al., 2012), imidacloprid (Adak et al., 2012), thiamethoxam (Sarkar et al., 2012), and thiram (Kaushik et al., 2013). The period related to the availability of insecticide can be adjusted using PEG of different molecular weight, because the release rates increase with increasing PEG molecular weight.

On the other hand, Memarizadeh et al. (2014a) prepared imidacloprid NPs by direct encapsulation to linear–dendritic ABA triblock copolymer composed of poly(citric acid) (PCA) as A block and PEG as B block. Molecular self-assembly of PCA–PEG–PCA copolymer allowed encapsulating imidacloprid, and the resulting formulation improved the insecticidal efficiency of the pesticide, decreased the dosage and the frequency of the pesticide use and increased the length of effectiveness. Photodegradable and biocompatible indoxacarb NPs prepared by encapsulation of indoxacarb to linear–dendritic ABA-type copolymers PCA–PEG–PCA with TiO_2 NPs via supramolecular interactions also significantly decreased the essential dosage of the pesticide for pest control (Memarizadeh et al., 2014b).

The nanocapsules can be designed to release the active ingredient in specific environmental conditions or physiological environments, for example, the stomach of an insect. These smart pesticides could provide more precise, controlled and effective use of pesticides and therefore potentially reduce the overall quantities of pesticide used (Lyons and Scrinis, 2009).

Guan et al. (2008) directly encapsulated imidacloprid microcrystals with nature chitosan and sodium alginate through layer-by-layer self-assembly. The release rate of imidacloprid microcrystals decreased with an increase in the number of layers of microcapsules, and the decrease in the multilayer permeability was attributed to the increase in shell thickness and close of the pores existing in the deposited polysaccharide layers with further layer deposition, suggesting that the release of imidacloprid NPs can be effectively controlled by varying the number of self-assembled chitosan/alginate layers.

Saini et al. (2014) evaluated the in vitro insecticidal activity of pyridalyl nanosuspension prepared using sodium alginate against larvae of *Helicoverpa armigera* in comparison with bulk material and commercial formulation. The average micelle particle size of different formulations was approximately 138 nm; the nanocapsules had spherical shape and physical stability. It was found that the insecticidal activity of the pyridalyl nanosuspension increased remarkably with LC_{50} values of 40 μg/mL in comparison to LC_{50} values of bulk pyridalyl (90 μg/mL) and the commercial product (250 μg/L). The bioassay results obtained using the leaf dip method showed that the nanoformulation was two- and sixfold more effective as stomach poison against *H. armigera* than the technical product and the commercial formulation, respectively.

Balaji et al. (2015) prepared water-dispersive nanoformulation of a poor water-soluble insect repellent, diethylphenyl acetamide (DEPA) by PEG polymerization followed by the phase inversion temperature emulsification method, which could serve as an effective alternate in controlling the expansion of the Japanese encephalitis vector *Culex tritaeniorhynchus*. Polymeric nanomicelles of DEPA with the hydrodynamic mean diameter of 154 nm showed characteristic core–shell structure of micelle and eightfold lower median lethal concentration (48 h) for *C. tritaeniorhynchus* 3rd instar larvae (52 μg/L) in comparison with that of bulk DEPA (416 μg/L).

Foster et al. (2014) described an interesting laser-based photoacoustic and photothermal nanotheranostic platform that can be used for detection and physical destruction of small organisms and carriers of pathogens, such as malaria vectors, spiders, bed bugs, fleas, ants, locusts, grasshoppers, phytophagous mites, or other arthropod pests. The researchers demonstrated that laser-induced thermal and accompanying nano- and microbubble phenomena can injure or kill *Caenorhabditis elegans* and mosquitoes fed by carbon nanotubes, gold nanospheres, gold nanoshells, or magnetic NPs at laser energies that are safe for humans, and photoacoustic effect can be used to control NP delivery.

Stadler et al. (2010) reported the insecticidal effect of nanostructured alumina on two globally important stored insect pests *Sitophilus oryzae* and *Rhyzopertha dominica*, which was reflected in significant mortality rate on treated wheat after 3 days of continuous exposure.

3 Nanoherbicides

Development of a target specific herbicide molecule encapsulated in NP is aimed at a specific receptor in the roots of target weeds, which enter into the roots system of the weeds and translocate to parts that inhibit glycolysis of food reserves in the root system, ultimately making the specific weed plant to starve for food and get killed (Nair et al., 2010; Ali et al., 2014; Jampílek and

Kráľová, 2015). The control of parasitic weeds with nanoencapsulated herbicides reduces the phytotoxicity of herbicides on crops (Pérez-de-Luque and Diego, 2009).

NP formulations of poly(ε-caprolactone) containing the herbicide atrazine were shown to be effective for the control of the target *Brassica* species; NPs reduced the mobility of atrazine in the soil and they were able to reduce the genotoxicity of the herbicide, thereby reducing the risk of harm to the environment and human (Pereira et al., 2014). Poly(ε-caprolactone) nanocapsules containing ametryn and atrazine showed lower toxicity also to the alga *Pseudokirchneriella subcapitata* compared to the herbicides alone indicating their potential in agricultural applications (Clemente et al., 2014).

Similarly, results of Nishisaka et al. (2014) who observed less chromosome damage in nanoparaquat treated samples compared to conventional paraquat herbicide indicate that nanoencapsulation is a viable option as an attempt to minimize damage caused by bulk paraquat. NPs prepared from chitosan and sodium tripolyphosphate (TPP) could be considered as an effective herbicidal formulation characterized by lower cytotoxicity and genotoxicity than bulk paraquat, and this formulation is suitable for safer control of weeds in agriculture. The benefit of these encapsulated paraquat formulations is reduced environmental impact with simultaneous preservation of herbicidal effectiveness (Grillo et al., 2014). The incorporation of paraquat to alginate/chitosan NPs altered the release profile of the herbicide, as well as its interaction with the soil, indicating that this system could be an effective means of reducing negative impact caused by paraquat (Silva et al., 2011). Similarly, also clomazone release profile showed a significant difference in release behavior of the pure herbicide in solution when compared with the herbicide loaded in alginate NPs (Silva et al., 2010).

Silver NPs (AgNPs)–chitosan encapsulated paraquat was evaluated against *Eichhornia crassipes* from the aspect of controlled release and improved herbicidal activity (Namasivayam and Aruna, 2014). The controlled release study showed 90% of release at 24 h, and the distinct improved herbicidal activity was observed against *E. crassipes* due to the formation of necrotic lesions at all the tested concentrations of the nanoformulation. Moreover, the nanoformulation did not affect soil macro and micronutrients, soil enzymes, soil microflora seedling emergence, and plant growth parameters of *Vigna mungo* plants.

Hollow-shell particles that were formed from manganese (II) carbonate core–shell NPs coated with suitable water soluble polymers, such as sodium polystyrene sulfonate and polyallylamine hydrochloride were used by Kanimozhi and Chinnamuthu (2012) for loading the selective preemergence herbicide pendimethalin programmed to release smartly based upon the requirements.

The formulation prepared by the addition of emulsion components (long-chain fatty acid methyl esters + long-chain alkylpolyglucosides + organosilicone + water) into the 41% (w/w) glyphosate isopropylamine formed polymerized multiconnected network structure. The dilution of the formulation with water led to the destruction of the polymerized network, thus forming dispersed NPs of the nanoemulsion formulation. Such optimum entrapped glyphosate isopropylamine with the nanoemulsion could entail improved physicochemical characteristics of the nanoemulsion formulation (Lim et al., 2012). Similarly, an environmentally friendly nanoemulsion system for application of water-soluble herbicide glyphosate isopropylamine was prepared by Jiang et al. (2012). The nanoemulsion system with particle sizes of the diameter of less than 200 nm showed significantly lower surface tension than a commercial formulation (Roundup), and its ED_{50} (0.40 kg a.e./ha) in controlling the weed *Eleusine indica* was lower than that of Roundup (0.48 kg a.e./ha). This indicates that a nanoemulsion system can be used to increase penetration and uptake of glyphosate isopropylamine. On the other hand, the nanoemulsion formulations of glyphosate isopropylamine displayed a significantly lower spray deposition on creeping foxglove (2.9–3.5 ng/cm^2), slender button weed (2.6–2.9 ng/cm^2), and buffalo grass (1.8–2.4 ng/cm^2) than Roundup (3.7–5.1 ng/cm^2) even though the visible injury rates of weeds treated with the nanoemulsion formulations were statistically equivalent to those relating to Roundup. Consequently, it was hypothesized that the significant difference in spray deposition with equal injury rates can be attributed to enhanced bioactivity of the nanoemulsion formulations (Lim et al., 2013).

By hybridization of the phenoxy herbicides into zinc–aluminium-layered double hydroxide interlamellar new nanohybrids of 2-chloro-(2-CPA) and 2,4,5-trichlorophenoxyacetic acids (2,4,5-T) were prepared (Sarijo et al., 2010a). Basal spacing expansion from 8.9 Å in the layered double hydroxide to 18.5 and 26.2 Å in these nanohybrids suggested that phenoxy herbicides were successfully intercalated into the layered double hydroxide inorganic interlayers. The release data for the whole process followed the pseudosecond-order equation, and the release process was found to be pH-dependent, in the order of pH $12 > 3 > 6.25$. These results indicate that application of Zn–Al-layered double hydroxide is suitable as the matrix of the controlled release formulation of agrochemicals, such as 2-CPA and 2,4,5-T. The inorganic Zn–Al layered double hydroxide was also used by Hussein et al. (2005) as a matrix, hosting 2,4-dichlorophenoxyacetic acid (2,4-D) by self-assembly technique. Initially the release of the guest 2,4-D into aqueous solutions containing chloride, carbonate, and distilled water was rapid followed by a more sustained release thereafter, and this behavior was dependent on the type of anions and their concentrations in the release medium (aqueous solution). The mechanism of release consists in the ion exchange process between the 2,4-D anion intercalated into the interlamellar host and carbonate or chloride and/or hydroxyl anions in the aqueous solution.

In another paper Sarijo et al. (2010b) demonstrated that the release of phenoxy herbicide agrochemicals from the nanohybrid formulations can be tuned by choosing the right combination of exchangeable anions, both incoming and outgoing. The release of 2-CPA, 4-CPA, and 2,4,5-T from their nanohybrids into aqueous solutions containing various anions was found to be controlled by pseudosecond-order rate expression and the percentage of saturated release decreased in the order of carbonate >sulfate >chloride for the release media and 2-CPA > 4-CPA > 2,4,5-T for the anionic guests.

Solid lipid nanoparticles (SLNs) containing the herbicides atrazine and simazine were prepared and characterized by de Oliveira et al. (2015). SLNs were found to modify the release profiles of the herbicides in water. The formulations of NPs containing the herbicides were effective in pre- and postemergence treatment of the target species *Raphanus raphanistrum*, but they did not affect plant growth of nontarget organism *Z. mays*. Guo et al. (2014) investigated controlled release of acetochlor from poly(butyl methacrylate-diacetone acrylamide)-based formulation and found that improved herbicide incorporation and slower release were linked to potential interactions between the herbicide and the polymer.

4 Nanofungicides

Fungi cause crop losses worldwide. Fungal diseases have a significant economic impact on plant yield and quality, thus managing such diseases is an essential component of production for most crops. A fungicide is a specific type of pesticide that controls fungal disease by specifically inhibiting or killing the fungus that causes the disease. Not all diseases caused by fungi can be adequately controlled by fungicides. These include the vascular wilt fungal diseases *Fusarium* and *Verticillium*. Fungicides are used to control a disease during the establishment and development of a crop, to increase productivity of a crop and to reduce blemishes and to improve the storage life and the quality of harvested plants. Therefore, fungicides are extensively used in agriculture system to control soilborne, seedborne, or airborne fungal pathogens (McGrath, 2004). The ever-increasing number of different kinds of fungicides and their wide-spread use in modern agriculture caused a concern about their possible interaction with nontarget organisms that are directly or indirectly involved in the maintenance of soil fertility (Yadav and Aggarwal, 2014). Therefore, as in other classes of nanopesticides, also development of nanofungicides has been focused on design and production of nanoformulations respecting the environment (Jampílek and Kráľová, 2015).

Polymerization of citric acid onto the surface of oxidized multiwall carbon nanotubes led to hybrid materials grafted by poly(citric acid) that were not only soluble in water but also able to trap water-soluble pesticides, such as zineb or mancozeb and showed a superior toxic influence on *Alternaria alternata* fungi in comparison with bulk pesticide (Sarlak et al., 2014).

Biodegradable chitosan–lactide copolymer was applied as a hydrophobic carrier for pyraclostrobin, a new broad-spectrum foliar fungicide in the strobilurin chemical class (Xu et al., 2014). The fungicide loaded in NPs was protected from light and by varying the feed mass ratio of copolymer to pyraclostrobin from 50:1 to 5:1 the size of pesticide-loaded NPs could be adjusted between 77 and 128 nm. The pyraclostrobin-loaded NPs showed an initial burst and subsequent sustained and pH-controlled release profile. Compared to 25% pyraclostrobin emulsifiable concentrate, the NPs demonstrated better fungicidal activity against *Colletotrichum gossypii* at long incubation time, which further exhibited sustained release characteristic.

Kumar et al. (2015) developed a nanoform of hexaconazole (with particle size 100 nm) using PEG-400 as the surface-stabilizing agent. Hexaconazole NPs were more potent in comparison to that of bulk hexaconazole. Hydrolytic and thermal stability studies confirmed its stability at par with the conventional formulation of fungicide. Impact of nanohexaconazole on soil nitrifiers was tested in vitro, and there were no significant adverse effect in their numbers observed as compared to conventional registered formulation, proving the safety of the nanofungicide.

Antifungal properties of AgNPs have been exploited to a great extent against a broad range of human pathogens (Morones et al., 2005; Tian et al., 2007; Oves et al., 2013; Prakash et al., 2013). However, the full potential of AgNPs is still largely unexplored for crop protection, and presently there has been a growing interest to utilize their antifungal properties for plant disease management

(Karimi et al., 2012). Earlier findings have advocated the toxicity of AgNPs on fungal hyphae and conidial development (Kim et al., 2009; He et al., 2011). In recent years, in vitro assays showed the strong inhibitory effects of biosynthesized AgNPs against various fungal plant pathogens, such as *A. alternata, Sclerotinia sclerotiorum, Macrophomina phaseolina, Rhizoctonia solani, Botrytis cinerea, Curvularia lunata* (Krishnaraj et al., 2012), *Fusarium oxysporum* (Gopinath and Velusamy, 2013), *Colletotrichum coccodes, Monilinia* sp., and *Pyricularia* sp. (Lee et al., 2013a).

Spherical AgNPs with the size range from 10 to 20 nm exhibited strong antifungal activity against *Bipolaris sorokiniana*, the spot blotch pathogen of wheat, and a detached leaf bioassay revealed that the germination of conidia was totally inhibited when leaves were treated with AgNPs. Moreover, histochemical staining revealed a significant role of the treatment with AgNPs in inducing lignin deposition in vascular bundles (Mishra et al., 2014). The effectiveness of AgNPs against plant pathogenic fungi like *B. sorokiniana* and *Magnaporthe grisea* was also proved by Jo et al. (2009) and against the most important plant pathogenic fungi like *Fusarium* sp. and *Phoma* sp. by Gajbhiye et al. (2009).

Kim et al. (2012a) confirmed considerable antifungal activity of nanosized silver colloidal solutions against plant pathogenic fungi, such as *Alternaria solani, Cylindrocarpon destructans, Fusarium* sp., *Pythium aphanidermatum, Pythium spinosum, Cladosporium cucumerinum, Didymella bryoniae, Glomerella cingulata, Monosporascus cannonballus*, and *Stemphylium lycopersici* by in vitro experiments. Treatment with a 100 ppm concentration of AgNPs resulted in growth inhibition more than 90%.

Park et al. (2006) prepared a nanosized silica–silver formulation consisting of nanosilver combined with silica molecules and water soluble polymer that showed antifungal activity against the plant infecting fungi *R. solani, B. cinerea, M. grisea, Pythium ultimum*, and *Colletotrichum gloeosporioides* at 3.0 ppm with varied degrees and effectively controlled powdery mildews of pumpkin even at 0.3 ppm in both field and greenhouse tests. The pathogens disappeared from the infected leaves 3 days after spraying, and the plants remained healthy. In contrast, a number of bacteria were not significantly affected at 10 ppm level but were completely inhibited by 100 ppm of nanosized silica–silver.

Copper-based agents have been used as agricultural fungicides for a long time. In the last years, copper NPs capable of killing fungi that infect important agricultural crops were synthesized, and these NPs could be used as next generation agricultural pesticides. Copper is an essential micronutrient for plants, and the excess of copper NPs taken up by plants can by detoxified by benign fungi occurring in the roots of plants (Vitanovic, 2012; Anjum et al., 2015).

The activity of CuNPs with the particle size in the range of 3–10 nm coated with capping agent cetyltrimethylammonium bromide was found to be superior to that of the commercially available fungicide Bavistin against four plant pathogenic fungi *C. lunata, A. alternata, F. oxysporum,* and *Phoma destructiva* (Kanhed et al., 2014). Though *C. lunata* and *A. alternata* exhibited resistance to Bavistin, they were sensitive to the aforementioned CuNPs. The antifungal activity of CuNPs decreased in following order: *C. lunata* > *A. alternata* > *P. destructiva.* The findings of Kanhed et al. (2014) confirmed that the antifungal activity of CuNPs predestine them to control plant pathogenic fungi in agriculture, however, they can be also used as effective disinfectants in poultry and animal husbandry.

The antifungal properties of Cu–chitosan NPs against phytopathogenic fungi, namely *A. alternata, M. phaseolina,* and *R. solani* were investigated at various concentrations ranging from 0.001 to 0.1%. In an in vitro model Cu-chitosan NPs were found to be most effective at 0.1% concentration and showed 89.5, 63.0, and 60.1% growth inhibition of *A. alternata, M. phaseolina,* and *R. solani*; at the same concentration they showed maximum of 87.4% inhibition rate of spore germination of *A. alternata* (Saharan et al., 2013).

Giannousi et al. (2013) tested the activity of CuO, Cu_2O NPs, and Cu/Cu_2O nanocomposites of particle size 11–55 nm in the field on tomato (*L. esculentum*) plants against *Phytophthora infestans* by assessing the fungal infection on the leaves in comparison with the performance of the registered commercially used copper-based products. It was found that the prepared copper-based NPs are more effective than the marketed fungicides and can be applied in a lower formulated product and active ingredient rate without any deleterious effect on plants.

AgNPs and copper-based NPs as potential nanopesticides and their mechanism of action and toxicological profiles are discussed in detail in separate chapters later dealing with nanosilver and nanocopper formulations.

5 Nanonematicides

Nematodes are common soilborne organisms. Plant–parasitic nematodes are known to cause significant damage of crops. For many years, nematodes were controlled using inexpensive chemical nematicides that effectively kill nematodes in soil. Recently most nematicides have been banned or restricted by the US Environmental Protection Agency as environmental toxins. Since nematicides are expensive to develop, new approaches have been tested, including application of NPs (Lambert and Bekal, 2002).

Uniform spherical nanocapsules of lansiumamide B with the mean particle size of 38.5 nm prepared by the microemulsion polymerization method showed nematicidal activity against *Bursaphelenehus xylophilus* and second-stage juveniles (J2) of *Meloidogyne incognita* with the LC_{50} values of 2.14 and 19.36 mg/L, respectively, at 24 h after treatment. Moreover, treatment with lansiumamide B nanocapsules, lansiumamide B, and ethoprophos led to a decrease in the disease progression by 68.42, 36.84, and 26.32%, respectively, and a decline in the average number of root knots of *Ipomoea aquatica* by 83.94, 78.03, and 63.66%, respectively, indicating that the nematicide nanoformulation performed more efficient and longer effective maintenance against plant parasitic nematodes (Yin et al., 2012).

As potential nematicides, also AgNPs stabilized by a starch were evaluated. These AgNPs inactivated the root-knot nematode *M. incognita* in 6 h by >99% in vitro. Treatment with 150 μg/mL AgNPs of infested turfgrass and soil composite with *Meloidogyne graminis* reduced the population of nematode in the soil samples by 92 and 82% after 4 and 2 days exposures in comparison with the nontreated soil samples (Cromwell et al., 2014). Ardakani (2013) investigated application of 800, 400, and 200 mg/mL AgNPs (with particle size 20 nm) to *M. incognita*, which resulted in 100% J2 immobility and mortality. The LC_{50} value was found to be 100 mg/mL. AgNPs used at 0.02, 0.01, 0.005, 0.0025, 0.00125, and 0.0007% concentrations (w/w) completely controlled *M. incognita*; however, treatment with 0.02, 0.01, and 0.005% of AgNPs was toxic to tomato plants and significantly reduced tomato root and stem length and fresh weights in comparison with the control.

6 Nanoformulations

6.1 Controlled Release Formulations

Nanoformulations, similarly to other pesticide or drug formulations, are designed to increase the apparent solubility of poorly soluble active ingredients and to release the active ingredient in a slow/targeted manner and/or to protect the active ingredient against premature degradation (Kawabata et al., 2011; Margulis-Goshen and Magdassi, 2012). In controlled release formulations (CRFs) for pesticide delivery most frequently nanospheres, nanocapsules, hydrophilic nanogels and micelles are used. The benefit of such formulations is that the application of smaller amount of active compound per area is sufficient, as long as the formulation may provide an optimal concentration delivery for the target pesticide for longer times. Since reapplications are not necessary, they decrease the costs and reduce phytotoxicity and environmental damage to other untargeted organisms and even the crops themselves (Margulis-Goshen and Magdassi, 2012). Wilkins (2004) described chemical and physical methods for preparation of CRFs. A chemical bond (usually a covalent one) formed between the active ingredient and a carrier, such as a polymer or a porous inorganic matrix, is the basis of chemical methods. In some cases, a biocide can be immobilized in the network of the cross-linked polymer.

Using physical methods, a mixture of a biocide and a polymer could be made, or a membrane formed by polymeric chains can isolate a bioactive compound from the external environment by nanoencapsulation. Nanoencapsulation can enhance the dispersion of hydrophobic pesticides in aqueous media and allows a controlled release of the active ingredient. Such smart delivery systems are characterized by high selectivity, without hindering the bioactive agents to target the pathogen (Peteu et al., 2010). Moreover, insoluble compounds in preparations of NP pesticides can be relatively readily dispersed in solution, the interaction with the target insect could be more effective, and the risk of environment contamination is reduced. It is important for CRFs that they must remain inactive until the active compound is released.

The benefits of polymer encapsulated formulations in comparison with nonencapsulated commercial formulations are extended activity (Shaviv, 2000; Rudzinski et al., 2002), reduced evaporative (Nisar et al., 2009), degradation losses (Adak et al., 2012) and leaching (Garratt and Kennedy, 2006), and these formulations are especially advantageous when a half-life of a potent pesticide is too short (Mohanraj and Chen, 2006; Bajpai et al., 2007). Increasing/decreasing human health hazards ranging from respiratory exposure to penetration/permeation through the skin remain open to question, because nanoformulations have considerably different properties than bulk pesticides (Hagens et al., 2007; Crosera et al., 2009; Bouwmeester et al., 2009; Barcelo and Farré, 2012; Choi et al., 2013; Kawamura et al., 2014; Brenner, 2014; Vaculíková et al., 2015; Cao et al., 2015).

The release mode of a bioactive compound is closely connected with the chemical nature of the formulation and can proceed via diffusion and disassembling of polymeric nanomatrices containing the bioactive compound after contact with water and a subsequent release of this compound. In nanoformulations, in which polymer—pesticide bonds occur, a hydrolysis reaction is needed for the release of the active ingredient, and the release is affected by the strength of these chemical bonds, the chemical properties of both molecules and by the size and the structure of the macromolecule.

Encapsulation technology has been widely used in the pharmaceutical drug delivery field, because CRFs prepared using the encapsulation technology protect the drug, maintain the concentration of the drug within an optimum range by adjusting the release of active components and provide the sustainability of the effect. In such preparations, hydrophobic or hydrophilic materials can be entrapped, for example, by liposomes formed by lecithin (a carrier system and surfactant consisting of a mixture of phospholipids) inside and in micelles under aqueous conditions (Calvo et al., 1997; Ogawa et al., 2003; De Jong and Borm, 2008; Liu and Park, 2009; Svenson and Prudhomme, 2012; Zhang et al., 2013; Lu et al., 2014; Nehoff et al., 2014; Onoue et al., 2014; Safari and Zarnegar, 2014; Yang et al., 2014; Demetzos, 2015). In such CRFs drugs are protected, the released amount of the active component is automatically adjusted, which results in maintaining the drug concentration within an optimum range and ensuring the sustainability of the effect for a certain period of time. Similar CRFs prepared by encapsulation technology can be successfully used also in agriculture, because they can reduce the amount of agricultural chemicals used, enhance the stability of unsteady core materials, suppress sharp odors of releasing materials and secure biocompatibility to carrier systems having a minimum size distribution.

Biodegradability, nontoxicity and adsorption abilities of chitosan predestined it to be a valuable carrier for controlled delivery of agrochemicals. A chitosan matrix is able to function as a protective reservoir for the encapsulated active ingredients, protecting ingredients from the surrounding environment when they are in the chitosan domain and controlling their release (Kashyap et al., 2015). For example, Hwang et al. (2011) used etofenprox as a core material for the CRF, which was encapsulated with a coating material, such as chitosan or lecithin. In the liposome, hydrophilic groups of lecithin were situated in its outer part, and hydrophobic groups of lecithin were located in inner part of liposome, where also the active hydrophobic ingredient etofenprox was situated. Since an outer layer of the formed liposome had a negative charge under acidic conditions, chitosan with a positive charge under acidic conditions was used for the coating, and consequently, the resulting etofenprox CRF showed a hydrophilic property ensuring its good miscibility with water. It was reported that CRFs of etofenprox with a wide size range from 200 to 600 nm could be prepared using coating (Bang et al., 2009).

By blending botanical insecticide capsaicin and a new chitosan derivate prepared by grafting ricinoleic acid anhydride on carboxymethyl chitosan, NPs of spherical shape with negative surface charge in water were formed showing loading efficiency of up to 0.86 that provided efficient protection for capsaicin and extended its release period (Feng and Zhang, 2011).

Stabilized polymeric NPs for controlled and efficient release of bifenthrin prepared using polyvinylpyrrolidone, polyvinyl alcohol, poly(acrylic acid)-β-poly(butyl acrylate) and poly(styrene)-β-poly(ethylene oxide) showed steric stability caused by the corona structure of the hydrophilic block of the polymers preventing NPs aggregation (Liu et al., 2008).

Release from the commercial formulation 025 SC was faster than with the CRFs of beta-cyfluthrin prepared using PEG-based amphiphilic copolymers; the rate of release of encapsulated beta-cyfluthrin from nanomicellar aggregates was reduced by increasing the molecular weight of PEG. It could be noted that the release was diffusion controlled with a half-release time from c. 4 to 8 days in water from different formulations, and the period of optimum availability of beta-cyfluthrin ranged from c. 1.5 to 20 days (Loha et al., 2011).

Aouada et al. (2011) comprehensively described the use of biodegradable hydrogels as a potential delivery vehicle for the controlled release of pesticides. For example, polyacrylamide–methylcellulose hydrogels presented high loading capacity of paraquat pesticide, up to 82% of paraquat, in relation to the amount of paraquat available in the loading solution. It could be noted that the release of pesticides entrapped in a hydrogel occurs only after water penetrates the network to swell the polymer and dissolve the pesticides, followed by diffusion along the aqueous pathways to the surface of the device. Thus, the release of chemicals is closely related to the swelling characteristics of hydrogels, which, in turn, is a key function for the chemical architecture of hydrogels. In aforementioned paraquat preparations pesticide diffusion capacity out of hydrogel was dependent on the swelling of the matrix and the density of the network chains, that is, methylcellulose/acrylamide ratio and pore sizes, and the release of paraquat became slower when the methylcellulose and acrylamide concentrations increased.

Garrido-Herrera et al. (2006) prepared controlled release systems of isoproturon, imidacloprid, and cyromazine by gelling sodium alginate with calcium ions and using different amounts of bentonite and activated carbon as modifying agents. Based on evaluation of the kinetic experiments related to pesticide release in water it could be concluded that (1) imidacloprid formulations showed higher release rates than isoproturon formulations, (2) the release rate of isoproturon and imidacloprid is reduced when bentonite and/or activated carbon samples are used as modifying agents of alginate isoproturon/imidacloprid formulations as compared to the control and to the alginate formulation without modifying agents, and (3) the application of the highest percentage of activated carbon in the formulation leads to the highest decrease in the release rate. In the diffusion-caused release of isoproturon and imidacloprid from the various alginate-based CRFs into water the sorption capacity of modifying agents for pesticides and formulations permeability were the most influencing factors.

As mentioned previously, in various polymeric nanomaterials, the controlled release proceeds via diffusion. Regardless of whether the bioactive compound is dissolved (micro- or nanospheres) or encapsulated (micro- or nanocapsules), this process neither depends on the chemical structure of the formulation constituents (Allan et al., 1971) nor on intermolecular interactions, and the rate control is based on the interactions between the carrier and the biocide (Perlatti et al., 2013). Consequently, the stronger is the interaction, the slower is the release rate.

In some formulations, the bioactive compound is covalently bound to the polymeric matrix, and the release is conditioned by disturbance of chemical interaction that usually occurs via hydrolysis and affects many polymer-pesticide bonds in a chain reaction. As aforementioned, the release is then affected by the strength of those chemical bonds, the chemical properties of both molecules and by the size and the structure of the macromolecule formed (Perlatti et al., 2013; Allan et al., 1971). The higher biocompound solubility in water, the faster reaction occurs.

Organoclays as sorbents of pesticides have shown their usefulness as pesticide supports to prolong the efficacy of soil-applied pesticides and to reduce large transport losses that usually affect pesticides applied in an immediately available form. Celis et al. (2002) investigated the Wyoming montmorillonite saturated with Fe(III) ions and Arizona montmorillonite saturated with hexadecyltrimethylammonium as carriers for slow release of hexazinone with the goal to decrease herbicide leaching losses. The researchers found that the slowest breakthrough of hexazinone in soil columns determined for loosely bound hexazinone–Arizona montmorillonite formulation was associated with the greatest amounts of herbicide released from the clay particles. These findings indicated that aforementioned clay particles could be used as slow release formulations suitable for prevention of ground water contamination. Organoclay-based formulations of 2,4-D using hexadecyltrimethylammonium-treated Arizona montmorillonites displayed slow release properties in water and reduced herbicide leaching through soil columns, while maintaining a herbicidal efficacy similar to that of the free (technical) 2,4-D (Hermosin et al., 2006). Lvov et al. (2008) developed halloysite aluminosilicate nanotubes with a 15 nm lumen, 50 nm external diameter and the length of 800 ± 300 nm as an entrapment system for loading, storage, and controlled release of anticorrosion agents and biocides. By variation of internal fluidic properties, formation of nanoshells over the nanotubes and creation of smart caps at the tube ends it is possible to develop further means of controlling the fate of release, and halloysite tubes could be used as additives in biocide and protective coatings. Clay nanotubes (halloysites) were developed as carriers of pesticides with extended release and better contact with plants, enabling the reduction of the amount of pesticides by 70–80%, which is then reflected in reduction of costs and the impact on water streams (Ditta, 2012).

6.2 Silica-Based Nanoformulations

Silica-based NPs are widely used in nanotechnology in the biomedical sector, because they are easy to prepare and inexpensive to produce. Their specific surface characteristics, porosity, and capacity for functionalization make them good tools for biomolecule detection and separation, providing solid media for delivery systems and for agent protectors. They are used as safe for human organism and biocompatible with many active ingredients and additives (Ku et al., 2010; Bitar et al., 2012; Tang and Cheng, 2013; Liao et al., 2014; Liu et al., 2014; Marzaioli et al., 2014; Nehoff et al., 2014; Jampílek et al., 2015; Vaculíková et al., 2015). Silica-based NPs also found application in agriculture, since silica materials can offer distinct advantages over other materials, as they provide more mechanically stable structures than polymeric materials (Torney et al., 2007) and have structural flexibility in forming nanomaterials with high-capacity loading of active ingredients (Lou et al., 2008). The release of various agrochemicals from silica-based nanomaterials was investigated including nonporous silica NPs (Ao et al., 2013), mesoporous silica NPs (Popat et al., 2012; Wanyika et al., 2012; Wanyika, 2013) and hollow-core silica-shell NPs (Tan et al., 2012; Liu et al., 2006; Qian et al., 2013). The core of hollow-core silica shell NPs provides higher loading capacity of active ingredients than nonporous and mesoporous silica NPs. This type of NPs could be prepared by post loading and preloading techniques. While post loading is based on diffusion of active compounds into the interior space via immersion (e.g., Tan et al., 2012) or high-pressure supercritical fluid (e.g., Liu et al., 2006), the preloading technique is based on the solubilization of active substances in template materials prior to formation of silica shells (Stőber et al., 1968; Xu et al., 2003; Qian et al., 2013; Jampílek et al., 2015). The preloading technique is more advantageous, because it reduces the possibility of attachment of active ingredients at the external surfaces of the shells, thus increasing the flexibility to protect and release active compounds. Wibowo et al. (2014) reported that the sustained release of fipronil from oil-core silica-shell nanocapsules in vitro was tunable through the control of the silica-shell thickness (i.e., 8–44 nm), and the insecticidal effect of the fipronil-encapsulated silica nanocapsules against economically important subterranean termites could be controlled by tuning the shell thickness.

Mesoporous silica NPs have proven to be promising supports for enzyme immobilization enabling the enzymes to retain their activity, thereby affording them greater potential for wide applications in biocatalysis and energy (Popat et al., 2011). Surface modified hydrophobic nanosilica (nano-Si) has been successfully used to control a range of agricultural insect pests (Barik et al., 2008; Rahman et al., 2009).

Uniconazole-loaded porous hollow silica NPs prepared by simple immersing and supercritical fluid drug loading both demonstrated sustained release properties and had improved retardation effects on rice growth, and the latter showed better-controlled release ability with a slower release rate. These NPs exhibited a stronger retardation capacity than free uniconazole by being applied into soil before seedling transplantation (Tan et al., 2012). Porous hollow silica NPs loaded with validamycin were found to be an effective transfer system for pesticides that are soluble in water for the release under controlled conditions. A multistaged release pattern was observed probably due to the different adsorption locations of validamycin on porous hollow silica NPs indicating that this type of silica-based NPs could be used as a promising carrier in agriculture, especially for pesticide controlled delivery, whose immediate, as well as prolonged release is needed (Liu et al., 2006). Properly functionalized lipophilic silica-based NPs have already been tested to control agricultural insect pests. Physiosorption is the mode of action of nano-Si. It gets absorbed through insect cuticular lipids and damages the protective wax layer (consisting of various fatty acids and lipids) that acts as an effective barrier for evaporation of water, which ultimately results in insect's death by desiccation, hence leading to insect's death by physical means (Mewis and Ulrichs, 2001; Ulrichs et al., 2005).

Avermectin, a pesticide that is known to block neurotransmission in insects by inhibiting a chloride channel is inactivated by UV light on the fields with half-life of 6 h only (Ghormade et al., 2011). The encapsulation capacity of porous hollow silica NPs with the shell thickness of c. 15 nm and the pore diameter of 4–5 nm with respect to avermectin was found to be 625 g/kg; porous hollow silica NPs protected avermectin from UV degradation and allowed its slow release reaching for about 30 days (Li et al., 2007). This indicates that they could be used as carriers in the sustained-release pattern applications of various photosensitive components.

Similarly, in the preparation of a nanoconjugate derived from kasugamycin with amino-modified silica (particle size in the range from 53 to 315 nm), kasugamycin was found to be effectively protected against photodegradation and reduction of particle size, and increased temperature and acidity contributed to a faster release of the active ingredient. This nanoconjugate displayed a better and more sustained bactericidal efficacy against *E. coli* than bulk kasugamycin (Ding et al., 2014).

Also novel functionalized microcapsules with high loading efficiency of prochloraz (about 30% w/w) prepared using silica-based NPs cross-linked with alginate and some beneficial elements to crops were found to protect prochloraz effectively against degradation under UV irradiation and alkaline conditions, showing sustainable release for at least 60 days and likely increasing disease resistance due to the element on the surface (Zhang et al., 2014).

Loading of an agricultural biocide imidacloprid used for termite control into the mesoporous silica NPs with different pore sizes, morphologies, and mesoporous structures showed that specifically MCM-48 type mesoporous silica NPs with a three-dimensional (3D) open network structure and high surface area displayed the highest adsorption capacity compared to other types of silica NPs and the release of imidacloprid from these NPs was found to be controlled over 48 h (Popat et al., 2012).

The study of the controlled release of herbicides 2,4-D and picloram anchored on hexagonal mesoporous silica NPs modified with carboxylic acid, in which the carboxylic group was chemically bonded to an inorganic structure and the material presented a nanometric structure with spheres <50 nm and porous diameter of 10 nm, showed that the controlled release of picloram from the nanocarrier was less than that of bulk 2,4-D (Prado et al., 2011).

Formulations of alpha-pinene and linalool (terpenes prohibiting feeding in several lepidopterous insects) with silica NPs enhanced the antifeedant potential of the individual terpenes against tobacco cutworm (*S. litura*) and castor semilooper (*Achaea janata*), while producing longer shelf life for the terpenes. In these formulations the presence of H-bonds between terpenes and silica nanocarriers were demonstrated, and the enhancement of biological activity against *S. litura* up to 25-fold was observed (Usha Rani et al., 2014).

Both laboratory and field tests demonstrated that the insecticidal toxicity of chlorfenapyr nanoformulation prepared using dispersible silica-based NPs as a carrier was twice as higher as that of the microformulation (Song et al., 2012). The insecticidal toxicity tests were performed using cotton bollworm larvae (3 mg/larva) as a model insect and carried out by the diet incorporation method, and effects of nano- and microformulations against diamondback moth (*P. xylostella*) were investigated on *Brassica chinensis* field.

According to Goswami et al. (2010), also amorphous nano-Si alone was found to be a potent and safe pesticide against two stored grain pests *S. oryzae* and *T. castaneum* and two field pests *Lipaphis pseudobrassicae* and *S. litura*. The insecticidal property of nano-Si could be connected with its ability of absorption into the cuticular layer of insect pests that otherwise acts as a barrier for protection of insect pests against pesticides (Barik et al., 2008). Moreover, due to small particle size (3–5 nm), modified surface charge and hydrophobicity, nano-Si could be successfully utilized to manage a variety of ectoparasites of animals and agricultural insect pests (Ulrichs et al., 2005).

Diatomaceous earths, composed mainly of amorphous silica and derived from fossilized phytoplankton (Subramanyam and Roesli, 2000; Mewis and Ulrichs, 2001) have been also successfully evaluated against several stored-product pest species (Vassilakos et al., 2006; Athanassiou et al., 2007; Iatrou et al., 2010), and it was found that their effectiveness against insects increased if they possessed high amorphous silica content with uniform size distribution (Korunik, 1997). The entomotoxicity of silica NPs was tested against rice weevil, *S. oryzae*, by Debnath et al. (2011) who found that amorphous silica NPs were highly effective against this insect pest, causing more than 90% mortality, indicating the effectiveness of silica NPs to control insect pests. Maize plants treated with nano-Si (20–40 nm) showed significantly higher resistance against phytopathogens, such as *F. oxysporum* and *Aspergillus niger* than those treated with bulk silica, especially at 10 and 15 kg/ha, and they showed a higher expression of phenolic compounds and a lower expression of stress-responsive enzymes against both the fungi (Suriyaprabha et al., 2014).

Ebeid et al. (2013) tested local raw nanonized diatomaceous earth with and without a commercial pesticide Challenger 36% SC against adults, 4th and 2nd nymphal instars of alfalfa grasshopper, *Heteracris littoralis*, and found that the mean duration of adults at all applied concentration levels (0.25, 0.5, and 1.0%) of both treatments did not exceed 12 days compared to 31 days in the control. Silica NPs were found to induce great irregularity or malformation in the mouthparts and the mid-gut morphology, causing shortening of adult longevity, and it can be assumed that the killing action could be attributed to the reduction in food uptake and digestibility as a result of silica treatments.

Thus, it could be concluded that silica-based NPs in any formulation could be applied as a safe pest control agent. The monodispersed mesoporous silica NPs with the size of 20 nm and with interconnected pores with the approximate diameter of 3 nm did not have negative effects on seed germination. It was shown that, when these silica-based NPs were transported to different plant organs, symplastic and apoplastic pathways were used for their penetration into the roots. Then they were transported to the aerial parts (stems and leaves) of the plants via the conducting tissues of the xylem (Sun et al., 2014). These findings show that mesoporous silica NPs can be used as a new delivery means enabling transport of biomolecules of different sizes into plants.

6.3 Formulations of Nanosilver

The application of nanotechnology techniques to agricultural crop inputs is one of the proposed tools for "sustainable intensification" as the future of agricultural production (Gruère et al., 2011). Reducing the volume of pesticide use could be achieved for example through adding silver nanoparticles (AgNPs) to pesticides to make them more effective in targeting pests with a smaller pesticide volume (Suppan, 2013). Products that claim to kill germs based on the use of AgNPs are viewed by the US Environmental Protection Agency as pesticides, that is, products with pesticide components that therefore require authorization (Bachmann, 2007). Due to the ability to destroy bacteria and other microorganisms, the entry of unbound AgNPs in the environment represents a risk that useful bacteria and aquatic organisms will be destroyed as well. The toxic impact of metal NPs, including AgNPs, on plants is connected with chemical toxicity based on their chemical composition (e.g., release of toxic metal ions) and with stress or stimuli caused by the surface, size, and shape of these NPs (Masarovičová and Kráľová, 2013; Masarovičová et al., 2014). Although baseline risk comes from the amount of silver in the environment – the amount of silver ions, NPs can then add to that risk, whether by facilitating ions' behavior or disrupting cell activity on their own (Lubick, 2008).

The antimicrobial activity of silver is much higher than that of other metals, such as mercury, copper, lead, chromium, and tin.

Silver(I) oxide can produce free silver ions in the presence of oxygen, thus the antimicrobial activity of silver depends on the active surface of silver. The antifungal activity of silver ions is connected with disruption of transmembrane energy metabolism and the membrane electron transport chain by formation of insoluble compounds in the cell wall due to the inactivation of cell wall thiol groups, with mutations in fungal DNA by displacing the hydrogen bonds, with dissociation of the enzyme complexes that are essential for the respiratory chain by silver ions and with disruption of membrane bounded enzymes and lipids resulting in the cell lysis and reduced membrane permeability (Velmurugan et al., 2009).

Thus, it may be anticipated that a bacterial cell in contact with AgNPs takes in silver ions that inhibit a respiratory enzyme(s), facilitating the generation of reactive oxygen species and consequently damaging the cell. Sulfur-containing proteins in the membrane or inside the cells and phosphorus-containing elements like DNA are likely to be the preferential sites for AgNPs binding (McDonnell and Russell, 1999). Due to AgNPs treatment, disruption of membrane morphology may cause a significant increase in permeability, leading to uncontrolled transport through the plasma membrane and, finally, to cell death (Sondi and Salopek-Sondi, 2004). Moreover, AgNPs prevent the expression of proteins associated with ATP production (Yamanka et al., 2005).

Due to their biocide properties, the AgNPs are used in indoor paints against clinically important bacteria, and it was also found that incorporation of nanosilver (nano-Ag) is a viable method for prolonging the effective life of gypsum plaster inoculated with the fungus *Cladosporium* (Shirakawa et al., 2013). According to Mishra and Singh (2015), biosynthesized AgNP-based biopesticides could revolutionize the agricultural sector in the future and can be used as nanoweapon against phytopathogens. However, increased attention must be devoted to the impact of risk factors associated with their usage on the environment.

It is reported that the bactericidal effect of AgNPs decreases as their size increases, and it is also affected by the shape of the particles (Pal et al., 2007; Panáček et al., 2006). Although most studies have utilized spherical particles, truncated triangular shaped particles are reported to have greater bactericidal effect compared to that of spherical and rod shaped particles (Pal et al., 2007).

Kim et al. (2008) evaluated the antifungal efficacy of colloidal nano-Ag solution against rose powdery mildew. Nano-Ag colloid is more adhesive on bacterial and fungal cell surface and can act as a better fungicide because of its well-dispersed and stabilized AgNPs solution. The colloidal solutions of metal NPs were found to inhibit the growth of *A. cepa* roots due to their ability to penetrate into cells and interact with their components and, thus, to inhibit mitosis, and the cytotoxicity of NPs decreased in the following order: Cu ≥ Zn ≥ Ag ≥ Fe (Konotop et al., 2014). Although the foliar pathway is even less-known than the soil-root pathway, significant inputs of NPs on plant foliage may be expected due to deposition of atmospheric particles or application of NP-containing pesticides. Larue et al. (2014) provided first evidence for the entrapment of AgNPs by the cuticle and penetration in the leaf tissue through stomata, the diffusion of Ag in leaf tissues and oxidation of AgNPs and complexation of Ag(I) ions by thiol-containing molecules.

Sundaravadivelan and Padmanabhan (2014) reported about effective larvicidal and pupicidal activity of AgNPs with particle size about 10–20 nm synthesized from an entomopathogenic fungi *Trichoderma harzianum* extracellular filtrate which can be used as an ideal ecofriendly and inexpensive approach for the control of dengue vector *A. aegypti.*

AgNPs with particle size ranging from 25 to 55 nm prepared using algae *Chroococcus dispersus* and *Chlorella vulgaris* were tested against the plant pathogenic bacteria, *Pseudomonas flavescens* and *Erwinia amylovora* and plant pathogenic fungi, *Fusarium solani, F. oxysporum, R. solani, Helminthosporium* sp., *A. alternata,* and *S. sclerotiorum.* Antibacterial activity was obtained by the resultant nano-Ag, and the inhibition zones were ranged from 35 to 55 mm. The antibacterial activity of AgNPs was found to be four to fivefold higher than that obtained by the chemical antibiotics ampicillin, gentamycin, and streptomycin, and their antifungal activity was even ninefold higher than that of the generic antibiotics (Hafez and Kabeil, 2013).

Sooresh et al. (2011) prepared AgNP-pesticide core–shell conjugate, using a pyrethroid pesticide. The conjugate was intended to be used as an active agent against arthropod vectors, such as mosquitoes. Exposition of this conjugate to mosquitoes for a 24 h resulted in mortality at 9×10^{-4} mol/L, and silver was detected in the hemolymph of mosquitoes exposed to this conjugate indicating that the nanoconjugate did not inactivate the primary function of the pesticide and was effective in killing mosquitoes at low concentrations. Cubic crystalline AgNPs with the mean particle size ranging between 10–45 nm and 5–15 nm prepared using *Couroupita guianensis* leaf and fruit extracts (LAgNPs and FAgNPs, respectively) were evaluated by Vimala et al. (2015) against IV instar larvae of *A. aegypti.* The larvicidal effect after 24 h of treatment depended on the applied dose, and extensive mortality rate was observed (LC_{50} = 2.1 ppm for LAgNPs and LC_{50} = 2.09 ppm for FAgNPs), being by one order more effective than ethyl acetate and methanol extracts of leaves and fruit.

In the study of the larvicidal and antimicrobial activities of AgNPs synthesized from fresh leaves, dry leaves, and green berries of *Solanum nigrum* (spherical to polyhedral shape and of 50–100 nm with the average size of 57 nm) against larvae of *C. quinquefasciatus* and *Anopheles stephensi* and four human pathogenic and five fish pathogenic bacteria, the highest mortality was observed at 10 ppm against *A. stephensi* with LC_{50} values of 1.33, 1.59, 1.56 ppm and LC_{90} values of 3.97, 7.31, 4.76 ppm for AgNPs prepared using dry leaves, fresh leaves, and berries of *S. nigrum*, respectively. The antibacterial activity of AgNPs against fish pathogenic bacteria was found to be better than against human pathogenic bacteria, and no abnormalities were recorded in the nontarget organisms like *Toxorhynchites* larvae (mosquito predator), *Diplonychus annulatum* (predatory water-bug) and *Chironomus circumdatus* larvae (chironomid) that were also exposed to respective lethal concentrations of dry NPs estimated for mosquito larvae (Rawani et al., 2013).

Nano-Ag pulse treatments increased vase life, water uptake rate, and fresh weight of *Rosa hybrida* and reduced the number of bacteria, water loss, stomatal conductance, and transpiration rate; the increased vase life was explained by suppressing stomatal opening, decreasing transpiration from leaves and inhibiting bacterial proliferation (Rafi and Ramezanian, 2013).

Soni and Prakash (2012) evaluated the effect of fungus-mediated AgNPs on mosquito control strategy. AgNPs were synthesized in the presence of *Chrysosporium keratinophilum*, *Verticillium lecanii*, and *F. oxysporum* f. sp. *pisi* and evaluated against the adult mosquito of filariasis vector *C. quinquefasciatus*. AgNPs synthesized using *C. keratinophilum* and *V. lecanii* were found to be more effective against *C. quinquefasciatus* than those generated with the help of *F. oxysporum* f. sp. *pisi*.

AgNPs synthesised with *Rhizophora mucronata* leaf extract with the average size of 60–95 nm showed larvicidal activity against *A. aegypti* and *C. quinquefasciatus* with LC_{50} values 0.585 and 0.891 mg/L for *A. aegypti* and *C. quinquefasciatus* species, respectively (Gnanadesigan et al., 2011).

In vitro examination of the ability of nano-Ag aqueous liquids to control the growth of green onion infected with *Sclerotium cepivorum* was performed by Jung et al. (2010). AgNPs with the average particle size 7–25 nm were applied in the concentration of silver 1, 3, 5, 7, 10, 25, 50, and 100 ppm, and it was found that the nano-Ag liquid samples showed more than 90% inhibition rates at a concentration of 7 ppm. In field experiments the application of 10, 25, 50, and 100 ppm nano-Ag at the base of each plant 4 times each week for up to 4 weeks showed that the onion treated with nano-Ag liquid had more weight than nontreated or control plants, and soil component analysis showed that AgNPs did not decrease the soil ingredients and were safe for controlling different fungi from an environmental perspective, too.

6.4 Formulations of Nanocopper and Copper Oxide

Nanoscale copper particles (nano-Cu) are used in many antimicrobial formulations and products for their antimicrobial activity. They may enter deliberately and/or accidentally into terrestrial environments including soils. In the soil-plant system, the plant can be an indirect nontarget organism of the soil-associated nano-Cu that may in turn affect plant-based products and their consumers. The uncontrolled generation and inefficient metabolism of reactive oxygen species through different reactions are the major factors underpinning the overall nano-Cu consequences in both the systems (Anjum et al., 2015).

CuO NPs were found to be more toxic than bulk CuO or dissolved Cu(II) ions to *Landoltia (Spirodela) punctata* (Shi et al., 2011) and *Z. mays* (Wang et al., 2012). Using transmission electron microscopy and energy-dispersive X-ray spectroscopy techniques it was found that CuO NPs were present in xylem sap of maize plants, and they were transported from roots into the shoots through the xylem. On the other hand, it was found that CuO NPs could be also translocated from shoots back into the roots through phloem, and during this translocation they could be reduced from Cu(II) to Cu(I) indicating that bioaccumulation and biotransformation of CuO NPs in maize could have significant implications on the potential risk of NPs and food safety (Wang et al., 2012).

The phytotoxic effect of CuNPs on *Cucurbita pepo* plants was reflected in significant reduction of growth and transpiration rate relative to untreated controls (Musante and White, 2012; Hawthorne et al., 2012). Application of 1000 mg/L of CuO NPs to *C. sativus* seedlings led to a significant biomass decrease (by 25% compared to the control), and the size and concentration of CuO NPs affected the bioavailability and oxidative stress potential of plants exposed to the NPs. CuO NPs caused a statistically significant increase in superoxide dismutase, catalase, and peroxidase activities at 100 mg/L concentration level. Moreover, they greatly adhered to the root cell wall, and NPs were also observed in the root cells (Kim et al., 2012b). Increased lipid peroxidation, as well as increased catalase and superoxide dismutase activities due to treatment with CuNPs were observed also in *Elodea densa* plants (Nekrasova et al., 2011).

CuO NPs were found to induce DNA damage in agricultural and grassland plants. Under controlled laboratory conditions significant accumulation of oxidatively modified, mutagenic DNA lesions (7,8-dihydro-8-oxoguanine; 2,6-diamino-4-hydroxy-5-formamidopyrimidine; 4,6-diamino-5-formamidopyrimidine) and strong plant growth inhibition were observed for radish (*Raphanus sativus*), perennial ryegrass (*Lolium perenne*), and annual ryegrass (*Lolium rigidum*) (Atha et al., 2012).

CuO NPs inhibited root growth of buckwheat (*Fagopyrum esculentum*) seedlings; the root morphological features and NP incorporation into the root epidermal cells at a high dose of NPs showed completely different patterns compared to those for the controls. Genotoxic effects of CuO NPs on early growth of buckwheat were estimated as well (Lee et al., 2013b).

Manceau et al. (2008) reported that in common wetland plants *Phragmites australis* and *Iris pseudacorus* which were grown in the natural environment in Cu-contaminated soils, transformation of Cu into metallic NPs occurred in the roots, as well as near the roots of these plants, evidently with the assistance by endomycorrhizal fungi.

Most standard copper fungicides form relatively insoluble deposit of copper compounds on the surface of treated plants. However, the solubility of Cu compounds in modern fungicide formulations is much higher resulting in much faster release of Cu ions and significantly higher amount of ions that penetrate into plant tissue. This increases biological efficacy against pathogens, but the ions that enter the plant tissue without being complexed with other molecules, can cause severe phytotoxic effect to the plant (Kurnik et al., 2010).

The nano-Cu was found to suppress the growth of *Xanthomonas axonopodis* pv. *punicae*, the incident of pomegranate (*Punica granatum*) bacterial blight, at 0.2 ppm, that is, at concentration >10,000-fold lower than that usually recommended for Cu-oxychloride. After 48 h of incubation at 28°C the bacterial cell wall of *X. axonopodis* pv. *punicae* treated with 0.2 ppm CuNPs was completely disrupted, while in the control the cell wall remained intact; cell wall disruption due to CuNPs induced a strong decrease in the number of viable cells of *X. axonopodis* pv. *punicae*. It was suggested that the antibacterial property of nano-Cu can be attributed mainly to NPs adhesion to the bacterial cell surface because of their opposite electrical charges, resulting in a reduction reaction at the bacterial cell wall (Mondal and Mani, 2012). Moreover, reduced number or no water-soaked areas developing on leaves infiltrated with *X. axonopodis* pv. *punicae* treated with nano-Cu was observed, and suppression of water-soaked lesions in bean and rice leaves sprayed with CuNPs after inoculation with *Xanthomonas campestris* pv. *phasolei* and *Xanthomonas oryzae* pv.

oryzae, respectively, was estimated as well (Mondal, 2009; Mondal et al., 2010).

CuNPs with the mean size c. 9 nm and approximately spherical shape exhibited antimicrobial activity against *E. coli*, *B. subtilis*, and *Staphylococcus aureus*, and although an oxide layer was formed on the CuNPs, they demonstrated better antimicrobial activity toward *B. subtilis*. The greater bactericidal effect could be connected with greater affinity of CuNPs to surface-active groups (amines and carboxyl groups) of *B. subtilis*. The released Cu(II) ions can subsequently bind with DNA molecules what results in disorder of the helical structure (Ruparelia et al., 2008). Similarly, CuNPs showed antimicrobial activity against five bacterial strains (*S. aureus*, *E. coli*, *Micrococcus luteus*, *Klebsiella pneumoniae*, *Pseudomonas aeruginosa*) and three fungal strains (*Aspergillus flavus*, *A. niger*, *Candida albicans*) (Ramyadevi et al., 2012).

7 Ecotoxicology of Nanomaterials and Related Regulations

Ecotoxicology is a multidisciplinary field that integrates toxicology and ecology; it is focused on the study of the effects of toxic compounds on biological organisms, especially at the population, community, and ecosystem level (Butler, 1978). Ecotoxicology of nanomaterials deals with toxicity of NPs that are able to retain their particle size, properties, and reactivity after entering environment, that is, it investigates the actual behavior of NPs in real environment in relation to other particles and contaminants. For now, the predominant reason that NPs aggregate after entering environment is their impaired stability. Nevertheless, mechanisms of toxic effects/impacts of NPs and factors responsible for their toxicity should be investigated. Various NPs have different mechanisms of actions that can differ under particular conditions. The most frequent mechanisms of toxic effects are damage of membranes, generation of reactive oxygen species and genotoxicity. The ecotoxicology of NPs has an increasing importance due to the increasing use of products containing NPs. For example, the toxicity of AgNPs depends on both intrinsic factors (particle shape, size, surface area, surface charge of NPs) and abiotic factors (pH, ionic strength, water hardness, presence of organic matter). An increased risk of toxicity can be observed for nonbiodegradable materials, which can remain in the body, accumulate and stimulate the immune system. When particles are degradable, after their elimination from the body, the body returns back to its normal state. In general, toxicity trials should be performed not only for bulk pesticide but also for nanocarrier and final nanoformulation. Especially toxicological investigation should be performed for nonbiodegradable materials due to risks of accumulation and persistence in soil, plants, and mammals, which may subsequently result in various pathological processes (Buzea et al., 2007; Handy et al., 2008; De Jong and Borm, 2008; Barcelo and Farré, 2012; Keck and Müller, 2013; Brenner, 2014; Vaculíková et al., 2015).

Based on these facts, codification and unification of regulation requirements for preparation and application of NPs especially in relation to nature, environment, and health is strongly needed. Many countries around the world have been trying to figure out how to give appropriate oversight to the development of the technology but without being so overbearing as to make the technology not viable. This is a constant challenge, and the various countries that have taken this on and tried to do the best job that they can are to be credited. There is a good deal of variability from country to country (Newsome, 2014). In addition to national regulation, there are other activities occurring more broadly between regulatory agencies around the world. The Organisation for Economic Co-operation and Development (OECD) Working Party on Manufactured Nanomaterials (WPMN), which is comprised primarily of regulators from various countries, is looking to share information among the countries about regulatory actions and voluntary programs and the data they have or need for discussions relating to regulatory decisions (OECD, 2013a,b).

The European Commission Directorate for Health & Consumers issued a final opinion regarding the definition of the term "nanomaterial" (SCENIHR, 2010) followed by opinion on AgNPs (SCENIHR, 2014) and opinion on the determination of Potential Health Effects of Nanomaterials Used in Medical Devices (SCENIHR, 2015). The European Food Safety Authority issued guidance draft on risk assessment for nanotechnologies used in food and feed applications (EFSA, 2011). The European Commission has initiated a public consultation on Registration, Evaluation, Authorisation and Restriction of Chemicals (REACH) annexes, and has concluded that REACH is a good tool but is open to how supporting documents inform on the preparation of dossiers for nanomaterials (REACH, 2013). More guidances are needed to make it more clear to registrants what information is sought and how to account for the volume thresholds. Nevertheless, those thresholds are not appropriate for nanomaterials because nanomaterials may be far more active than bulk forms of the same substances (Newsome, 2014; Dolez, 2015).

The U.S. Environmental Protection Agency (EPA) is actively involved in assessing nanomaterials in commerce, for industrial purposes at least. The EPA issued a proposal to use the provisions of the Federal Insecticide, Fungicide, and Rodenticide Act (FIFRA) to collect information on the use of nanomaterials in pesticide products (EPA, 2011); it also issued a conditional registration for a nanopesticide (EPA, 2010). Dr. Steve Suppan, a lead author in the global report of the International Assessment of Agricultural Science and Technology for Development, a multistakeholder project, the executive summary of which was approved by 58 governments in April 2008, published recently a very critical contribution about the EPA regulating policy in the term of the use of nanomaterials in pesticides (Suppan, 2015). In June 2014, the U.S. Food and Drug Administration (FDA) issued three final guidance documents reflecting FDA's current thinking on certain issues related to the use of nanotechnology in FDA-regulated products (FDA, 2014a,b,c). These guidelines are being issued as part of FDA's ongoing implementation of recommendations from FDA's 2007 Nanotechnology Task Force Report. Other relevant documents can be found on FDA website, see Nanotechnology Fact Sheet (FDA, 2015). The U.S. National Institute for Occupational Safety and Health (NIOSH) issued Occupational Exposure to Carbon Nanotubes and Nanofibers (NIOSH, 2013).

8 Conclusions

The characteristics of a successful modern crop protection chemical are: (1) to remain active in the environment (sun, heat, rain), (2) to penetrate the noxious organism (fungus, insect, nematode) and to be transported to the target, (3) to resist defense of the pest/pathogen, (4) to remain benign to plants and mammals, (5) to be cost effective to formulate and manufacture, preferably possessing a new mode of action, and (6) to provide economic returns and social benefits (Smith et al., 2008). As discussed previously, nanosize materials change their physical and chemical properties in comparison with bulk material and have improved and innovated a variety of pharmaceutical, medical, industrial, and agriculture products. On the other hand, materials being innocuous in bulk form often become toxic when they reach nanosize. These adverse cellular effects have been attributed to the high chemical surface reactivity of NPs (Filipponi and Sutherland, 2013). Therefore, increased attention must be devoted to the impact of risk factors associated with their usage on the environment and possible adverse effects on nontarget organisms and humans (in general mammals). The aforementioned proliferation of regulation demonstrates the increasing importance of nanotechnologies to agriculture. The development of agronanotechnologies, along with biotechnologies, could serve as a springboard from which to revolutionize agriculture to feed a rapidly growing world population and to help improve living conditions in the developing world (Watson et al., 2011).

References

Adak, T., Shakil, N.A., Walia, S., 2012. Development of controlled release formulations of imidacloprid employing novel nano-ranged amphiphilic polymers. Environ. Sci. Health B. 47, 217–225.

Afifi, F.U., Hajjo, R.M., Battah, A.H., 2010. Medicinal plants, pesticide residues, and analysis. In: Nollet, L.M.L., Rathore, H.S. (Eds.), Handbook of Pesticides: Methods of Pesticide Residues Analysis. CRC Press, Taylor & Francis Group, Boca Raton, pp. 401–434.

Agrawal, S., Rathore, P., 2014. Nanotechnology pros and cons to agriculture: a review. Int. J. Curr. Microbiol. App. Sci. 3, 43–55.

Ali, M.A., Rehman, I., Iqbal, A., Din, S., Rao, A.Q., Latif, A., Samiullah, T.R., Azam, S., Husnain, T., 2014. Nanotechnology: a new frontier in agriculture. Adv. Life Sci. 1, 129–138.

Alghuthaymi, M.A., Almoammar, H., Rai, M., Said-Galiev, E., Abd-Elsalam, K.A., 2015. Myconanoparticles: synthesis and their role in phytopathogens management. Biotechnol. Biotechnol. Equip. 29, 221–236.

Allan, G.G., Chopra, C.S., Neogi, A.N., Wilkins, R.M., 1971. Design and synthesis of controlled release pesticide-polymer combinations. Nature 234, 349–351.

Anjali, C.H., Khan, S.S., Margulis-Goshen, K., Magdassi, S., Mukherjee, A., Chandrasekaran, N., 2010. Formulation of water-dispersible nanopermethrin for larvicidal applications. Ecotoxicol. Environ. Saf. 73, 1932–1936.

Anjum, N.A., Adam, V., Kizek, R., Duarte, A.C., Pereira, E., Iqbal, M., Luktkin, A.S., Ahmad, I., 2015. Nanoscale copper in the soil–plant system—toxicity and underlying potential mechanisms. Environ. Res. 138, 306–325.

Ao, M.M., Zhu, Y.C., He, S., Li, D.G., Li, P.L., Li, J.Q., Cao, Y.S., 2013. Preparation and characterization of 1-naphthylacetic acid-silica conjugated nanospheres for enhancement of controlled-release performance. Nanotechnology 24, 1–8.

Aouada, F.A., de Moura, M.R., Capparelli Mattoso, L.H., 2011. Biodegradable hydrogel as delivery vehicle for the controlled release of pesticide. In: Stoytcheva, M. (Ed.), Pesticides—Formulations, Effects, Fate. InTech, Rijeka, pp. 81–102.

Ardakani, A.S., 2013. Toxicity of silver, titanium and silicon nanoparticles on the root-knot nematode, *Meloidogyne incognita*, and growth parameters of tomato. Nematology 15, 671–677.

Atha, D.H., Wang, H.H., Petersen, E.J., Cleveland, D., Holbrook, R.D., Jaruga, P., Dizdaroglu, M., Xing, B.S., Nelson, B.C., 2012. Copper oxide nanoparticle mediated DNA damage in terrestrial plant models. Environ. Sci. Technol. 46, 1819–1827.

Athanassiou, C.G., Kavallieratos, N.G., Peteinatos, G.G., Petrou, S.E., Boukouvala, M.C., Tomanovic, Z., 2007. Influence of temperature and humidity on insecticidal effect of three diatomaceous earth formulations against larger grain borer (Coleoptera: Bostrychidae). J. Econ. Entomol. 100, 599–603.

Bachmann, A., 2007. Synthetic nanoparticles and the precautionary principle. An ethical analysis. Available from: http://www.ekah.admin.ch/fileadmin/ekah-dateien/dokumentation/gutachten/e-Gutachten-Synthetische-Nanopartikel-2007.pdf

Bajpai, J., Mishra, S., Bajpai, A.K., 2007. Dynamics of controlled release of potassium nitrate from a highly swelling binary polymeric blend of alginate and carboxymethyl cellulose. J. Appl. Polym. Sci. 106, 961–972.

Balaji, A.P.B., Mishra, P., Kumar, R.S.S., Mukherjee, A., Chandrasekaran, N., 2015. Nanoformulation of poly(ethylene glycol) polymerized organic insect repellent by PIT emulsification method and its application for Japanese encephalitis vector control. Colloid Surf. B Biointerfaces 128, 370–378.

Bang, S.H., Yu, Y.M., Hwang, I.C., Park, H.J., 2009. Formation of size–controlled nano carrier systems by self–assembly. J. Microencapsul. 26, 722–733.

Bang, S.H., Hwang, I.C., Yu, Y.M., Kwon, H.R., Kim, D.H., Park, H.J., 2011. Influence of chitosan coating on the liposomal surface on physicochemical properties and the release profile of nanocarrier systems. J. Microencapsul. 28, 595–604.

Barcelo, D., Farré, M., 2012. Analysis and Risk of Nanomaterials in Environmental and Food Samples. Elsevier, Amsterdam.

Barik, T.K., Sahu, B., Swain, V., 2008. Nanosilica—from medicine to pest control. Parasitol. Res. 103, 253–258.

Bhagat, D., Samanta, S.K., Bhattacharya, S., 2013. Efficient management of fruit pests by pheromone nanogels. Sci. Rep. 3, 1294–1301.

Bhattacharyya, A., Bhaumik, A., Rani, P.U., Mandal, S., Epidi, T., 2010. Nanoparticles—a recent approach to insect pest control. Afr. J. Biotechnol. 9, 3489–3493.

Bitar, A., Ahmad, N.M., Fessi, H., Elaissari, A., 2012. Silica-based nanoparticles for biomedical applications. Drug Discov. Today 17, 1147–1154.

Boom, R.M., 2011. Nanotechnology in food production. In: Frewer, L.J., Norde, W., Fischer, A.R.H., Kampers, F.W.H. (Eds.), Nanotechnology in the agri-food sector: implications for the future. Wiley-VCH, Weinheim, pp. 39–58.

Borm, P.J.A., Robbins, D., Haubold, S., Kuhlbusch, T., Fissan, H., Donaldson, K., Schins, R., Stone, V., Kreyling, W., Lademann, J., Krutmann, J., Warheit, D., Oberdoster, E., 2006. The potential risks of nanomaterials: a review carried out for ECETOC. Part. Fibre Toxicol. 3, 11–45.

Bouwmeester, H., Dekkers, S., Noordam, M.Y., Hagens, W.I., Bulder, A.S., de Heer, C., ten Voorde, S.E., Wijnhoven, S.W., Marvin, H.J., Sips, A.J., 2009. Review of health safety aspects of nanotechnologies in food production. Regul. Toxicol. Pharmacol. 53, 52–62.

Brenner, S., 2014. The Clinical Nanomedicine Handbook. CRC Press, Taylor & Francis Group, Boca Raton.

Butler, G.C., 1978. Principles of Ecotoxicology. John Wiley & Sons, New York.

Buzea, C., Pacheco, I., Robbie, K., 2007. Nanomaterials and nanoparticles: sources and toxicity. Biointerphases 2, MR17–MR71.

Calvo, P., Remunan–Lopez, C., Vila–Jato, J.L., Alonso, M.J., 1997. Novel hydrophilic chitosan–polyethylene oxide nanoparticles as protein carrier. J. Appl. Polym. Sci. 63, 125–132.

Cao, L., Chen, B., Zheng, L., Wang, D., Liu, F., Huang, Q., 2015. Assessment of potential dermal and inhalation exposure of workers to the insecticide imidacloprid using whole-body dosimetry in China. J. Environ. Sci. 27, 139–146.

Celis, R., Hermosin, M.C., Carrizosa, M.J., Cornejo, J., 2002. Inorganic and organic clays as carriers for controlled release of the herbicide hexazinone. J. Agric. Food Chem. 50, 2324–2330.

Chandra, J.H., Raj, L.F.A.A., Namasivayam, S.K.R., Bharani, R.S.A., 2013. Improved pesticidal activity of fungal metabolite from *Nomureae rileyi* with chitosan nanoparticles. International Conference on Advanced Nanomaterials and Emerging Engineering Technologies (ICANMEET); Chennai, India, July 24–27, 2013, pp. 387–390.

Chen, H., Yada, R., 2011. Nanotechnologies in agriculture: new tools for sustainable development. Trends Food Sci. Technol. 22, 585–594.

Chen, H., Seiber, J.N., Hotze, M., 2014. ACS select on nanotechnology in food and agriculture: a perspective on implications and applications. J. Agric. Food Chem. 62, 1209–1212.

Chowdappa, P., Gowda, S., 2013. Nanotechnology in crop protection: status and scope. Pest Manag. Hortic. Ecosyst. 19, 131–151.

Choi, H., Moon, J.K., Kim, J.H., 2013. Assessment of the exposure of workers to the insecticide imidacloprid during application on various field crops by a hand-held power sprayer. J. Agric. Food Chem. 61, 10642–10648.

Clemente, Z., Grillo, R., Jonsson, M., Santos, N.Z., Feitosa, L.O., Lima, R., Fraceto, L.F., 2014. Ecotoxicological evaluation of poly(epsilon-caprolactone) nanocapsules containing triazine herbicides. J. Nanosci. Nanotechnol. 14, 4911–4917.

Coles, D., Frewer, L.J., 2013. Nanotechnology applied to European food production: a review of ethical and regulatory issues. Trends Food Sci. Technol. 34, 32–43.

Cromwell, W.A., Yang, J., Starr, J.L., Jo, Y.K., 2014. Nematicidal effects of silver nanoparticles on root-knot nematode in bermudagrass. J. Nematol. 46, 261–266.

Crosera, M., Bovenzi, M., Maina, G., Adami, G., Zanette, C., Florio, C., Filon Larese, F., 2009. Nanoparticle dermal absorption and toxicity: a review of the literature. Int. Arch. Occup. Environ. Health 82, 1043–1055.

de Oliveira, J.L., Campos, E.V.R., Bakshi, M., Abhilash, P.C., Fraceto, L.F., 2014. Application of nanotechnology for the encapsulation of botanical insecticides for sustainable agriculture: prospects and promises. Biotechnol. Adv. 32, 1550–1561.

de Oliveira, J.L., Campos, E.V.R., da Silva, C.M.G., Pasquoto, T., Lima, R., Fraceto, L.F., 2015. Solid lipid nanoparticles co-loaded with simazine and atrazine: preparation, characterization, and evaluation of herbicidal activity. J. Agric. Food Chem. 63, 422–432.

Debnath, N., Das, S., Seth, D., Chandra, R., Bhattacharya, S.C., Goswami, A., 2011. Entomotoxic effect of silica nanoparticles against *Sitophilus oryzae* (L.). J. Pestic. Sci. 84, 99–105.

De Jong, W.H., Borm, P.J., 2008. Drug delivery and nanoparticles: applications and hazards. Int. J. Nanomed. 3, 133–149.

Demetzos, C., 2015. Advanced drug delivery nanosystems: perspectives and regulatory issues. Adv. Exp. Med. Biol. 822, 195–198.

Ding, G.L., Li, D.G., Liu, Y., Guo, M.C., Duan, Y.H., Li, J.Q., Cao, Y.S., Preparation and characterization of kasuga-silica-conjugated nanospheres for sustained antimicrobial activity, *J. Nanopart. Res.* 16, 2014, Article Number: 2671 (10 pages).

Ditta, A., How helpful is nanotechnology in agriculture?, *Adv. Nat. Sci.: Nanosci. Nanotechnol.* 3, 2012, Article Number: 033002 (10 pages).

Dolez, P.I., 2015. Nanoengineering: Global Approaches to Health and Safety Issues. Elsevier, Amterdam.

Ebeid, A.R., Abdel, A.A., Gesraha, M.A., 2013. Impact of diatomaceous earth (silica nano-particles) on alfalfa grasshopper, *Heteracris littoralis* (Rambur) (Orthopetra: Acrididae) under laboratory conditions. Egypt. J. Biol. Pest Control. 23, 325–330.

EFSA, 2011. Guidance on the risk assessment of the application of nanoscience and nanotechnologies in the food and feed chain. EFSA Journal 9, 2140 (36 pages). Available from: http://www.efsa.europa.eu/en/consultations/call/scaf110114.pdf

EPA, 2010. Pesticide news story: EPA announces conditional registration of nanosilver pesticide product. Available from: http://www.epa.gov/oppfead1/cb/csb_page/updates/2011/nanosilver.html

EPA, 2011. Pesticides; policies concerning products containing nanoscale materials; opportunity for public comment. Available from: http://www.epa.gov/pesticides/regulating/prepub-nanopest.pdf

European Commission, 2015. Definition of a nanomaterial. Available from: http://ec.europa.eu/environment/chemicals/nanotech/faq/definition_en.htm

FDA, 2014a. Considering whether an FDA—regulated product involves the application of nanotechnology. Available from: http://www.fda.gov/downloads/RegulatoryInformation/Guidances/UCM401695.pdf

FDA, 2014b. Safety of nanomaterials in cosmetic products. Available from: http://www.fda.gov/Cosmetics/GuidanceRegulation/GuidanceDocuments/ucm300886.htm

FDA, 2014c. Assessing the effects of significant manufacturing process changes, including emerging technologies, on the safety and regulatory status of food ingredients and food contact substances, including food ingredients that are color additives. Available from: http://www.fda.gov/Food/GuidanceRegulation/GuidanceDocumentsRegulatoryInformation/ucm300661.htm

FDA, 2015. Nanotechnology fact sheet. Available from: http://www.fda.gov/ScienceResearch/SpecialTopics/Nanotechnology/ucm402230.htm

Feng, B.H., Zhang, Z.Y., 2011. Carboxymethyl chitosan grafted ricinoleic acid group for nanopesticide carriers. Adv. Mat. Res. 236–238, 1783–1788.

Filipponi, L., Sutherland, D., 2013. Nanotechnologies: principles, applications, implications and hands-on activities. European Union, Luxembourg. Available from: https://ec.europa.eu/research/industrial_technologies/pdf/nano-hands-on-activities_en.pdf

Forim, M.R., Costa, E.S., da Silva, G.F.M.F., Fernandes, J.B., Mondego, J.M., Boica, A.L., 2013. Development of a new method to prepare nano-/microparticles loaded with extracts of *Azadirachta indica*, their characterization and use in controlling *Plutella xylostella*. J. Agric. Food Chem. 61, 9131–9139.

Foster, S.R., Galanzha, E.I., Totten, D.C., Benes, H., Reis, R.J.S., Zharov, V.P., 2014. Photoacoustically-guided photothermal killing of mosquitoes targeted by nanoparticles. J. Biophotonics 7, 465–473.

Fröhlich, E., 2013. Cellular targets and mechanisms in the cytotoxic action of non-biodegradable engineered nanoparticles. Curr. Drug Metab. 14, 976–988.

Gajbhiye, M., Kesharwani, J., Ingle, A., Gade, A., Rai, M., 2009. Fungus mediated synthesis of silver nanoparticles and its activity against pathogenic fungi in combination of fluconazole. Nanomedicine 5, 282–286.

Garcia, M., Forbe, T., Gonzalez, E., 2010. Potential applications of nanotechnology in the agro-food sector. Food Sci. Technol. 30, 573–581.

Garratt, J., Kennedy, A., 2006. Use of models to assess the reduction in contamination of water bodies by agricultural pesticides through the implementation of policy instruments: a case study of the voluntary initiative in the UK. Pest Manag. Sci. 62, 1138–1149.

Garrido-Herrera, F.J., Gonzales-Pradas, E., Fernandez-Pérez, M., 2006. Controlled release of isoproturon, imidacloprid, and cyromazine from alginate–bentonite-activated carbon formulations. J. Agric. Food Chem. 54, 10053–10060.

Ghormade, V., Deshpande, M.V., Paknikar, K.M., 2011. Perspectives for nano-biotechnology enabled protection and nutrition of plants. Biotechnol. Adv. 29, 792–803.

Giannousi, K., Avramidis, I., Dendrinou-Samara, C., 2013. Synthesis, characterization and evaluation of copper based nanoparticles as agrochemicals against *Phytophthora infestans*. RSC Adv. 3, 21743–21752.

Gnanadesigan, M., Anand, M., Ravikumar, S., Maruthupandy, M., Vijayakumar, V., Selvam, S., Dhineshkumar, M., Kumaraguru, A.K., 2011. Biosynthesis of silver nanoparticles by using mangrove plant extract and their potential mosquito larvicidal property. Asian Pacific J. Tropic. Med. 4, 799–803.

Gopal, M., Kumar, R., Goswami, A., 2012. Nano-pesticides—a recent approach for pest control. J. Plant Protect. Sci. 4, 1–7.

Gopinath, V., Velusamy, P., 2013. Extracellular biosynthesis of silver nanoparticles using *Bacillus* sp. GP-23 and evaluation of their antifungal activity towards *Fusarium oxysporum*. Spectrochim. Acta A Mol. Biomol. Spectrosc. 106, 170–174.

Goswami, A., Roy, I., Sengupta, S., Debnath, N., 2010. Novel applications of solid and liquid formulations of nanoparticles against insect pests and pathogens. Thin Solid Films 519, 1252–1257.

Grillo, R., Pereira, A.E., Nishisaka, C.S., de Lima, R., Oehlke, K., Greiner, R., Fraceto, L., 2014. Chitosan/tripolyphosphate nanoparticles loaded with paraquat herbicide: an environmentally safer alternative for weed control. J. Hazard. Mat. 278, 163–171.

Gruère, G., Narrod, C., Abbott, M., 2011. Agriculture, Food and water nanotechnologies for the poor: opportunities and constraints, international food policy research institute, policy brief 19. Available from: http://www.ifpri.org/sites/default/files/publications/bp019.pdf

Guan, H.N., Chi, D.F., Yu, J.M., Li, X.C., 2008. A novel photodegradable insecticide: preparation, characterization and properties evaluation of nano-imidacloprid. Pestic. Biochem. Physiol. 92, 83–91.

Guo, Y.Z., Yang, Q., Yan, W., Li, B., Qian, K., Li, T., Xiao, W., He, L., 2014. Controlled release of acetochlor from poly (butyl methacrylate-diacetone acrylamide) based formulation prepared by nanoemulsion polymerisation method and evaluation of the efficacy. Int. J. Environ. Anal. Chem. 94, 1001–1012.

Hafez, E.E., Kabeil, S.S., 2013. Antimicrobial activity of nano-silver particles produced by micro algae. J. Pure Appl. Microbiol. 7, 35–42.

Hagens, W.I., Oomen, A.G., de Jong, W.H., Cassee, F.R., Sips, A.J.A.M., 2007. What do we (need to) know about the kinetic properties of nanoparticles in the body? Regul. Toxicol. Pharmacol. 49, 217–229.

Handy, R.D., Owen, R., Valsami-Jones, E., 2008. The ecotoxicology of nanoparticles and nanomaterials: current status, knowledge gaps, challenges, and future needs. Ecotoxicology 17, 315–325.

Hawthorne, J., Musante, C., Sinha, S.K., White, J.C., 2012. Accumulation and phytotoxicity of engineered nanoparticles to *Cucurbita pepo*. Int. J. Phytorem. 14, 429–442.

He, L., Liu, Y., Mustapha, A., Lin, M., 2011. Antifungal activity of zinc oxide nanoparticles against *Botrytis cinerea* and *Penicillium expansum*. Microbiol. Res. 166, 207–215.

Hermosin, M.C., Celis, R., Facenda, G., Carrizosa, M.J., Ortega-Calvo, J.J., Cornejo, J., 2006. Bioavailability of the herbicide 2,4-D formulated with organoclays. Soil Biol. Biochem. 38, 2117–2124.

Hussein, M.Z., Yahaya, A.H., Zainal, Z., Kian, L.H., 2005. Nanocomposite-based controlled release formulation of an herbicide, 2,4-dichlorophenoxyacetate encapsulated in zinc–aluminium-layered double hydroxide. Sci. Technol. Adv. Mat 6, 956–962.

Hussain, S.M., Hess, K.L., Gearhart, J.M., Geiss, K.T., Schlager, J.J., 2005. In vitro toxicity of nanoparticles in BRL 3A rat liver cells. Toxicol. In Vitro 19, 975–983.

Hwang, I.C., Kim, T.H., Bang, S.H., Kim, K.S., Kwon, H.R., Seo, M.J., Youn, Y.N., Park, H.J., Yasunga-Aoki, C., Yu, Y.M., 2011. Insecticidal effect of controlled release formulations of etofenprox based on nano-bio technique. J. Fac. Agri. Kyushu Univ. 56, 33–40.

Iatrou, S.A., Kavallieratos, N.G., Palyvos, N.E., Buchelos, C.T., Tomanovic, S., 2010. Acaricidal effect of different diatomaceous earth formulations against *Tyrophagus putrescentiae* (Astigmata: Acaridae) on stored wheat. J. Econ. Entomol. 103, 190–196.

Jamal, M., Moharramipour, S., Zandi, M., Negahban, M., 2013. Efficacy of nanoencapsulated formulation of essential oil from *Carum copticum* seeds on feeding behavior of *Plutella xylostella* (Lep.: Plutellidae). J. Entomol. Soc. Iran 33, 23–31.

Jampílek, J., Kráľová, K., 2015. Application of nanotechnology in agriculture and food industry, its prospects and risks. Ecol. Chem. Eng. S. 22, 321–361.

Jampílek, J., Záruba, K., Oravec, M., Kuneš, M., Babula, P., Ulbrich, P., Brezaniová, I., Opatřilová, R., Třiska, J., Suchý, P., Preparation of silica nanoparticles loaded with nootropics and their in vivo permeation through blood–brain barrier, *BioMed Res. Int.* 2015, Article ID 812673 (9 pages).

Jiang, L.C., Basri, M., Omar, D., Rahman, M.B.A., Salleh, A.B., Rahman, R.N.Z.R.A., Selamat, A., 2012. Green nano-emulsion intervention for water-soluble glyphosate isopropylamine (IPA) formulations in controlling *Eleusine indica* (*E. indica*). Pest. Biochem. Physiol. 102, 19–29.

Jo, Y.K., Kim, B.H., Jung, G., 2009. Antifungal activity of silver ions and nanoparticles on phytopathogenic fungi. Plant Dis. 93, 1037–1043.

Joseph, T., Morrison, M., 2006. Nanoforum report: nanotechnology in agriculture and food, European nanotechnology gateway. Available from: ftp://ftp.cordis.europa.eu/pub/nanotechnology/docs/nanotechnology_in_agriculture_and_food.pdf

Jung, J.H., Kim, S.W., Min, J.S., Kim, Y.J., Lamsal, K., Kim, K.S., 2010. The effect of nano-silver liquid against the white rot of the green onion caused by *Sclerotium cepivorum*. Mycobiology 38, 39–45.

Kah, M., Beulke, S., Tiede, K., Hofmann, T., 2013. Nanopesticides: state of knowledge, environmental fate, and exposure modelling. Crit. Rev. Env. Sci. Tech. 43, 1823–1867.

Kah, M., Hofmann, T., 2014. Nanopesticide research: current trends and future priorities. Env. Int. 63, 224–235.

Kang, M.A., Seo, M.J., Hwang, I.C., Jang, C., Park, H.J., Yu, Y.M., Youn, Y.N., 2012. Insecticidal activity and feeding behavior of the green peach aphid, *Myzus persicae*, after treatment with nano types of pyrifluquinazon. J. Asia Pac. Entomol. 15, 533–541.

Kanhed, P., Birla, S., Gaikwas, S., Gade, A., Seabra, A.B., Rubilar, O., Duran, N., Rai, M., 2014. In vitro antifungal efficacy of copper nanoparticles against selected crop pathogenic fungi. Mat. Lett. 115, 13–17.

Kanimozhi, V., Chinnamuthu, C.R., 2012. Engineering core/hallow shell nanomaterials to load herbicide active ingredient for controlled release. Res. J. Nanosci. Nanotechnol. 2, 58–69.

Karimi, N., Minaei, S., Almassi, M., Shahverdi, A.R., 2012. Application of silver nano-particles for protection of seeds in different soils. Afr. J. Agric. Res. 7, 1863–1869.

Kashyap, P.L., Xiang, X., Heiden, P., 2015. Chitosan nanoparticle based delivery systems for sustainable agriculture. Int. J. Biol. Macromol. 77, 36–51.

Kaushik, P., Shakil, N.A., Kumar, J., Singh, M.K., Yadav, S.K., 2013. Development of controlled release formulations of thiram employing amphiphilic polymers and their bioefficacy evaluation in seed quality enhancement studies. J. Environ. Sci. Health B 48, 677–685.

Kawabata, Y., Wada, K., Nakatani, M., Yamada, S., Onoue, S., 2011. Formulation design for poorly water-soluble drugs based on biopharmaceutics classification system: basic approaches and practical applications. Int. J. Pharm. 420, 1–10.

Kawamura, S., Kato, T., Nakaoka, M., Fantel, A.G., 2014. Dermal developmental toxicity of *N*-phenylimide herbicides in rats. Birth. Defects Res. B Dev. Reprod. Toxicol. 101, 162–167.

Keck, C.M., Müller, R.H., 2013. Nanotoxicological classification system (NCS)—a guide for the risk-benefit assessment of nanoparticulate drug delivery systems. Eur. J. Pharm. Biopharm. 84, 445–448.

Kim, H.S., Kang, H.S., Chu, G.J., Byun, H.S., 2008. Antifungal effectiveness of nanosilver colloid against rose powdery mildew in greenhouses. Solid State Phenom. 135, 15–18.

Kim, S.W., Kim, K.S., Lamsal, K., Kim, Y.J., Kim, S.B., Jung, M., Sim, S.J., Kim, H.S., Chang, S.J., Kim, J.K., Lee, Y.S., 2009. An in vitro study of the antifungal effect of silver nanoparticles on oak wilt pathogen *Raffaelea* sp. J. Microbiol. Biotechnol. 19, 760–764.

Kim, S.W., Jung, J.H., Lamasal, K., Kim, Y.S., Min, J.S., Lee, Y.S., 2012a. Antifungal effects of silver nanoparticles (AgNPs) against various plant pathogenic fungi. Mycobiology 40, 53–58.

Kim, S., Lee, S., Lee, I., 2012b. Alteration of phytotoxicity and oxidant stress potential by metal oxide nanoparticles in *Cucumis sativus*. Water Air Soil Pollut. 223, 2799–2806.

Knauer, K., Bucheli, T.D., 2009. Nano-materials: research needs in agriculture. Rev. Suisse Agric. 41, 337–341.

Konotop, Y.O., Kovalenko, M.S., Ulynets, V.Z., Meleshko, A.O., Batsmanova, L.M., Taran, N.Y., 2014. Phytotoxicity of colloidal solutions of metal-containing nanoparticles. Cytol. Genet. 48, 99–102.

Korunik, Z., 1997. Rapid assessment of the insecticidal value of diatomaceous earths without conducting bioassays. J. Stored Prod. Res. 33, 219–229.

Krishnaraj, C., Ramachandran, R., Mohan, K., Kalaichelvan, P.T., 2012. Optimization for rapid synthesis of silver nanoparticles and its effect on phytopathogenic fungi. Spectrochim. Acta A Mol. Biomol. Spectrosc. 93, 95–99.

Ku, S., Yan, F., Wang, Y., Sun, Y., Yang, N., Ye, L., 2010. The blood–brain barrier penetration and distribution of PEGylated fluorescein-doped magnetic silica nanoparticles in rat brain. Biochem. Biophys. Res. Commun. 394, 871–876.

Kumar, R.S.S., Shiny, P.J., Anjali, C.H., Jerobin, J., Goshen, K.M., Magdassi, S., Mukherjee, A., Chandrasekaran, N., 2013. Distinctive effects of nano-sized permethrin in the environment. Environ. Sci. Pollut. Res. 20, 2593–2602.

Kumar, R., Nair, K.K., Alam, M.I., Gogoi, R., Singh, P.K., Srivastava, C., Gopal, M., Goswami, A., 2015. Development and quality control of nanohexaconazole as an effective fungicide and its biosafety studies on soil nitifiers. J. Nanosci. Nanotechnol. 15, 1350–1356.

Kurnik, V., Gaberšek, V., Lešnik, M., 2010. Influence of copper fungicide/fertilizer formulations applied during the blooming period on a fruit set of apples. Agricultural 7, 23–30.

Kuzma, J., VerHage, P., 2006. Nanotechnology in agriculture and food production: anticipated applications. Washington, DC. Available from: http://www.nanotechproject.org/process/assets/files/2706/94_pen4_agfood.pdf

Lambert, K., Bekal, S., 2002. (Revised 2009). Introduction to plant-parasitic nematodes. The plant health instructor. Available from: http://www.apsnet.org/edcenter/intropp/PathogenGroups/Pages/IntroNematodes.aspx

Larue, C., Castillo-Michel, H., Sobanska, S., Cecillon, L., Bureau, S., Barthes, V., Ouerdane, L., Carriere, M., Sarret, G., 2014. Foliar exposure of the crop *Lactuca sativa* to silver nanoparticles: evidence for internalization and changes in Ag speciation. J. Hazard. Mat. 264, 98–106.

Lee, K.J., Park, S.H., Govarthanan, M., Hwang, P.H., Seo, Y.S., Cho, M., Lee, W.H., Lee, J.Y., Kamala-Kannan, S., Oh, B.T., 2013a. Synthesis of silver nanoparticles using cow milk and their antifungal activity against phytopathogens. Mat. Lett. 105, 128–131.

Lee, S., Chung, H., Kim, S., Lee, I., The genotoxic effect of ZnO and CuO nanoparticles on early growth of buckwheat, *Fagopyrum esculentum, Water Air Soil Pollut.* 224, 2013b, Article Number: 1668 (1 page).

Li, Z.Z., Chen, J.F., Liu, F., Liu, A.Q., Wang, Q., Sun, H.Y., Wen, L.X., 2007. Study of UV-shielding properties of novel porous hollow silica nanoparticle carriers for avermectin. Pest Manag. Sci. 63, 241–246.

Liao, Y.T., Liu, C.H., Yu, J., Wu, K.C.W., 2014. Liver cancer cells: targeting and prolonged-release drug carriers consisting of mesoporous silica nanoparticles and alginate microspheres. Int. J. Nanomed. 9, 2767–2778.

Lim, C.J., Basri, M., Omar, D., Rahman, M.B.A., Salleh, A.B., Rahman, R.N.Z.R.A., 2012. Physicochemical characterization and formation of glyphosate-laden nano-emulsion for herbicide formulation. Ind. Crop. Prod. 36, 607–613.

Lim, C.J., Basri, M., Omar, D., Rahman, M.B.A., Salleh, A.B., Rahman, R.N.Z.R.A., 2013. Green nanoemulsion-laden glyphosate isopropylamine formulation in suppressing creeping foxglove (*A. gangetica*), slender button weed (*D. ocimifolia*) and buffalo grass (*P. conjugatum*). Pest Manag. Sci. 69, 104–111.

Liu, F., Wen, L.X., Li, Z.Z., Yu, W., Sun, H.Y., Chen, J.F., 2006. Porous hollow silica nanoparticles as controlled delivery system for water soluble pesticide. Mat. Res. Bull. 41, 2268–2275.

Liu, Y., Tong, Z., Prudhomme, R.K., 2008. Stabilized polymeric nanoparticles for controlled and efficient release of bifenthrin. Pest Manag. Sci. 64, 808–812.

Liu, N., Park, H.J., 2009. Chitosan–coated nanoliposome as vitamin E carrier. J. Microencapsul. 26, 235–242.

Liu, D., Lin, B., Shao, W., Zhu, Z., Ji, T., Yang, C., 2014. In vitro and in vivo studies on the transport of PEGylated silica nanoparticles across the blood–brain barrier. ACS Appl. Mater. Interfaces 6, 2131–2136.

Loha, K.M., Shakil, N.A., Kumar, J., Singh, M.K., Adak, T., Jain, S., 2011. Release kinetics of beta-cyfluthrin from its encapsulated formulations in water. J. Environ. Sci. Health B 46, 201–206.

Loha, K.M., Shakil, N.A., Kumar, J., Singh, M., Srivastava, C., 2012. Bio-efficacy evaluation of nanoformulations of β-cyfluthrin against *Callosobruchus maculatus* (Coleoptera: Bruchidae). J. Environ. Sci. Health B 47, 687–691.

Lou, X.W., Archer, L.A., Yang, Z.C., 2008. Hollow micro-/nanostructures: synthesis and applications. Adv. Mater. 20, 3987–4019.

Lu, C.T., Zhao, Y.Z., Wong, H.L., Cai, J., Peng, L., Tian, X.Q., 2014. Current approaches to enhance CNS delivery of drugs across the brain barriers. Int. J. Nanomed. 9, 2241–2257.

Lubick, N., 2008. Nanosilver toxicity: ions, nanoparticles—or both? Environ. Sci. Technol. 42, 8617–18617.

Lvov, Y.M., Shchukin, D.G., Möhwald, H., Price, R.R., 2008. Halloysite clay nanotubes for controlled release of protective agents. ACS Nano 2, 814–820.

Lyons, K., Scrinis, G., 2009. Under the regulatory radar? Nanotechnologies and their impacts for rural Australia. In: Merlan, F., Raftery, D. (Eds.), Tracking Rural Change: Community, Policy and Technology in Australia. ANU Press, Abilene, New Zealand and Europe, pp. 151–171.

Lyons, K., Scrinis, G., Whelan, J., 2012. Nanotechnology, agriculture, and food. In: Maclurcan, D., Radywyl, N. (Eds.), Nanotechnology and Global Sustainablity. CRC Press, Boca Raton, pp. 117–140.

Manceau, A., Nagy, K.L., Marcus, M.A., Lanson, M., Geoffroy, N., Jacquet, T., Kirpichtchikova, T., 2008. Formation of metallic copper nanoparticles at the soil-root interface. Environ. Sci. Technol. 42, 1766–1772.

Manimegalai, G., Kumar, S.S., Sharma, C., 2011. Pesticide mineralization in water using silver nanoparticules. Int. J. Chem. Sci. 9, 1463–1471.

Margulis-Goshen, K., Magdassi, S., 2012. Nanotechnology: an advanced approach to the development of potent insecticides. In: Ishaaya, I., Horowitz, A.R., Palli, S.R. (Eds.), Advanced Technologies for Managing Insect Pests. Springer, Dordrecht, pp. 295–314.

Marzaioli, V., Aguilar-Pimentel, J.A., Weichenmeier, I., Luxenhofer, G., Wiemann, M., Landsiedel, R., Wohlleben, W., Eiden, S., Mempel, M., Behrendt, H., Schmidt-Weber, C., Gutermuth, J., Alessandrini, F., 2014. Surface modifications of silica nanoparticles are crucial for their inert versus proinflammatory and immunomodulatory properties. Int. J. Nanomed. 9, 2815–2832.

Masarovičová, E., Kráľová, K., 2013. Metal nanoparticles and plants. Ecol. Chem. Eng. S 20, 9–22.

Masarovičová, E., Kráľová, K., Zinjarde, S.S., 2014. Metal nanoparticles in plants. Formation and action. In: Pessarakli, M. (Ed.), Handbook of Plant and Crop Physiology, third ed. CRC Press, Taylor & Francis Group, Boca Raton, pp. 683–731.

McDonnell, G., Russell, A.D., 1999. Antiseptics and disinfectants: activity, action, and resistance. Clin. Microbiol. Rev. 19, 147–179.

McGrath, M.T., 2004. The plant health instructor: what are fungicides. Available from: http://www.apsnet.org/edcenter/intropp/topics/Pages/fungicides.aspx

Memarizadeh, N., Ghadamyari, M., Adeli, M., Talebi, K., 2014a. Preparation, characterization and efficiency of nanoencapsulated imidacloprid under laboratory conditions. Ecotoxicol. Environ. Saf. 107, 77–83.

Memarizadeh, N., Ghadamyari, M., Adeli, M., Talebi, K., 2014b. Linear-dendritic copolymers/indoxacarb supramolecular systems: biodegradable and efficient nano-pesticides. Environ. Sci. Processes Impacts 16, 2380–2389.

Mewis, I., Ulrichs, C., 2001. Action of amorphous diatomaceous earth against different stages of the stored product pests *Tribolium confusum*, *Tenebrio molitor*, *Sitophilus granaries* and *Plodia interpunctella*. J. Stored Prod. Res. 37, 153–164.

Mishra, S., Singh, B.R., Singh, A., Keswani, C., Naqvi, A.H., Singh, H.B., 2014. Biofabricated silver nanoparticles act as a strong fungicide against *Bipolaris sorokiniana* causing spot blotch disease in wheat. PLoS One 9, e97881.

Mishra, S., Singh, H.B., 2015. Biosynthesized silver nanoparticles as a nanoweapon against phytopathogens: exploring their scope and potential in agriculture. Appl. Microbiol. Biotechnol. 99, 1097–1107.

Mohanraj, V.J., Chen, Y., 2006. Nanoparticles—a review. Tropic. J. Pharm. Res. 5, 561–573.

Mondal, K.K., 2009. Suppression of common bacterial blight in mungbean by phylloplane resident *Pseudomonas fluorescens* strain MBPF-01 alone and in combination with nanocopper. Indian Phytopathol. 62, 445–448.

Mondal, K.K., Bhar, L.M., Mani, C., 2010. Combined efficacy of *Pseudomonas fluorescens* strain MBPF-01 and nanocopper against bacterial leaf blight in rice. Indian Phytopathol. 63, 266–268.

Mondal, K.K., Mani, C., 2012. Investigation of the antibacterial properties of nanocopper against *Xanthomonas axonopodis* pv. *punicae*, the incitant of pomegranate bacterial blight. Ann. Microbiol. 62, 889–893.

Morones, J.R., Elechiguerra, J.L., Camacho, A., Holt, K., Kouri, J.B., Ramírez, J.T., Yacaman, M.J., 2005. The bactericidal effect of silver nanoparticles. Nanotechnology 16, 2346–2354.

Musante, C., White, J.C., 2012. Toxicity of silver and copper to *Cucurbita pepo*: differential effects of nano and bulk-size particles. Environ. Toxicol. 27, 510–517.

Nair, R., Varghese, S.H., Nair, B.G., Maekawa, T., Yoshida, Y., Sakthi, K.D., 2010. Nanoparticulate material delivery to plants. Plant Sci. 179, 154–163.

Namasivayam, S.K.R., Aruna, A., 2014. Evaluation of silver nanoparticles-chitosan encapsulated synthetic herbicide paraquate (AgNp–CS–PQ) preparation for the controlled release and improved herbicidal activity against *Eichhornia crassipes*. Res. J. Biotechnol. 9, 19–27.

Neethirajan, S., Jayas, D.S., 2011. Nanotechnology for the food and bioprocessing industries. Food Biprocess Technol. 4, 39–47.

Nehoff, H., Parayath, N.N., Domanovitch, L., Taurin, S., Greish, K., 2014. Nanomedicine for drug targeting: strategies beyond the enhanced permeability and retention effect. Int. J. Nanomed. 9, 2539–2555.

Nekrasova, G.F., Ushakova, O.S., Ermakov, A.E., Uimin, M.A., Byzov, I.V., 2011. Effects of copper(II) ions and copper oxide nanoparticles on *Elodea densa* Planch. Russ. J. Ecol. 42, 458–463.

Newsome, R., 2014. 2013 IFT International Food Nanoscience Conference: Proceedings. Compr. Rev. Food. Sci. Food Saf. 13, 190–228.

NIOSH, 2013. Occupational exposure to carbon nanotubes and nanofibers. Available from: http://www.cdc.gov/niosh/docs/2013-145/

Nisar, K., Kumar, J., Shakil, N.A., Walia, S., Parmar, B.S., 2009. Controlled release formulations of acephate: water and soil release kinetics. J. Environ. Sci. Health B 44, 533–537.

Nishisaka, C., Grillo, R., Sanches, G., Fraceto, L., Lima, R., 2014. Analysis of the effects of pesticides and nanopesticides on the environment. BMC Proc. 8 (Suppl. 4), P100.

OECD, 2013a. Regulatory frameworks for nanotechnology in foods and medical products: summary results of a survey activity. OECD Science, Technology and Industry Policy Papers, No. 4. Organisation for Economic Co-operation and Development. OECD Publishing. Available from: http://dx.doi.org/10.1787/5k47w4vsb4s4-en

OECD, 2013b. OECD working party on nanotechnology (WPN): vision statement. science and nanotechnology policy. Organisation for Economic Co-operation and Development. Available from: http://www.oecd.org/sti/nano/oecdworkingpartyonnanotechnologywpnvisionstatement.htm

Ogawa, S., Decker, E.A., McClements, D.J., 2003. Influence of environmental conditions on the stability of oil in water emulsions containing droplets stabilized by lecithin–chitosan membranes. J. Agric. Food Chem. 51, 5522–5527.

Onoue, S., Yamada, S., Chan, H.K., 2014. Nanodrugs: Pharmacokinetics and safety. Int. J. Nanomed. 9, 1025–1037.

Oves, M., Khan, M.S., Zaidi, A., Ahmed, A.S., Ahmed, F., Ahmad, E., Sherwani, A., Owais, M., Azam, A., 2013. Antibacterial and cytotoxic efficacy of extracellular silver nanoparticles biofabricated from chromium reducing novel OS4 strain of *Stenotrophomonas maltophilia*. PLoS ONE 8, e59140.

Pal, S., Tak, Y.K., Song, J.M., 2007. Does the antibacterial activity of silver nanoparticles depend on the shape of the nanoparticle? A study of the Gram-negative bacterium *Escherichia coli*. Appl. Environ. Microbiol. 73, 1712–1720.

Panáček, A., Kvítek, L., Prucek, R., Kolář, M., Večeřová, R., Pizúrová, N., Sharma, V.K., Nevěčná, T., Zbořil, R., 2006. Silver colloid nanoparticles: synthesis, characterization, and their antibacterial activity. J. Phys. Chem. B 110, 16248–16253.

Pankaj, Shakil, N.A., Kumar, J., Singh, M.K., Singh, K., 2012. Bioefficacy evaluation of controlled release formulations based on amphiphilic nano-polymer of carbofuran against *Meloidogyne incognita* infecting tomato. J. Environ. Sci. Health B 47, 520–528.

Pant, M., Dubey, S., Patanjali, P.K., Naik, S.N., Sharma, S., 2014. Insecticidal activity of eucalyptus oil nanoemulsion with karanja and jatropha aqueous filtrates. Int. J. Biodeterior. Biodegrad. 91, 119–127.

Park, H.J., Kim, S.H., Kim, H.J., Choi, S.H., 2006. A new composition of nanosized silica-silver for control of various plant diseases. Plant Pathol. J. 22, 295–302.

Passeleu-Le Bourdonnec, C., Carrupt, P.A., Scherrmann, J.M., Martel, S., 2013. Methodologies to assess drug permeation through the blood–brain barrier for pharmaceutical research. Pharm. Res. 30, 2729–2756.

Pereira, A.E., Grillo, R., Mello, N.F., Rosa, A.H., Fraceto, L.F., 2014. Application of poly(epsilon-caprolactone) nanoparticles containing atrazine herbicide as an alternative technique to control weeds and reduce damage to the environment. J. Hazard. Mat. 268, 207–215.

Pérez-de-Luque, A., Diego, R., 2009. Nanotechnology for parasitic plant control. Pest Manag. Sci. 65, 540–545.

Pérez-de-Luque, A., Hermosín, M.C., 2013. Nanotechnology and its use in agriculture. In: Bagchi, D., Bagchi, M., Moriyama, H., Shahidi, F. (Eds.), Bio-nanotechnology: A Revolution in Food, Biomedical and Health Sciences. Wiley-Blackwell, West Sussex, pp. 299–405.

Perlatti, B., de Souza Bergo, P.L., das Graças Fernandes da Silva, M.F., Fernandes, J.B., Forim, M.R., 2013. Polymeric nanoparticle-based insecticides: a controlled release purpose for agrochemicals. In: Trdan, S. (Ed.), Insecticides—Development of Safer and More Effective Technologies. Intech, Rijeka, pp. 523–550.

Peteu, S.F., Oancea, F., Sicuia, O.A., Constantinescu, F., Dinu, S., 2010. Responsive polymers for crop protection. Polymers 2, 229–251.

Popat, A., Hartono, S.B., Stahr, F., Liu, J., Qiao, S.Z., Lu, G.Q., 2011. Mesoporous silica nanoparticles for bioadsorption, enzyme immobilisation, and delivery carriers. Nanoscale 3, 2801–2818.

Popat, A., Liu, J., Hu, Q.H., Kennedy, M., Peters, B., Lu, G.Q., Qiao, S.Z., 2012. Adsorption and release of biocides with mesoporous silica nanoparticles. Nanoscale 4, 970–975.

Prado, A.G.S., Moura, A.O., Nunes, A.R., 2011. Nanosized silica modified with carboxylic acid as support for controlled release of herbicides. J. Agric. Food Chem. 59, 8847–8852.

Prakash, P., Gnanaprakasam, P., Emmanuel, R., Arokiyaraj, S., Saravananc, M., 2013. Green synthesis of silver nanoparticles from leaf extract of *Mimusops elengi*, Linn. for enhanced antibacterial activity against multi drug resistant clinical isolates. Colloids Surf. B Biointerfaces 108, 255–259.

Prasad, R., Kumar, V., Prasad, K.S., 2014. Nanotechnology in sustainable agriculture: present concerns and future aspects. Afr. J. Biotechnol. 13, 705–713.

Qian, K., Shi, T.Y., He, S., Luo, L.X., Liu, X.L., Cao, Y.S., 2013. Release kinetics of tebuconazole from porous hollow silica nano-spheres prepared by miniemulsion method. Micropor. Mesopor. Mat. 169, 1–6.

Rafi, Z.N., Ramezanian, A., 2013. Vase life of cut rose cultivars "Avalanche" and "Fiesta" as affected by nano-silver and S-carvone treatments. South Afr. J. Bot. 86, 68–72.

Ragaei, M., Sabry, A.H., 2014. Nanotechnology for insect pest control. Int. J. Sci. Environ. Technol. 3, 528–545.

Rahman, A., Seth, D., Mukhopadhyaya, S.K., Brahmachary, R.L., Ulrichs, C., Goswami, A., 2009. Surface functionalized amorphous nanosilica and microsilica with nanopores as promising tools in biomedicine. Naturwissenschaften 96, 31–38.

Rai, M., Ingle, A., 2012. Role of nanotechnology in agriculture with special reference to management of insect pests. Appl. Microbiol. Biotechnol. 94, 287–293.

Rai, M., Ribeiro, C., Mattoso, L., Duran, N., 2015. Nanotechnologies in Food and Agriculture. Springer, Heidelberg.

Raliya, R., Tarafdar, J.C., Gulecha, K., Choudhary, K., Ram, R., Mal, P., Saran, R.P., 2013. Review article; scope of nanoscience and nanotechnology in agriculture. J. Appl. Biol. Biotechnol. 1, 41–44.

Ramyadevi, J., Jeyasubramanian, K., Marikani, A., Rajakumar, G., Rahuman, A.A., 2012. Synthesis and antimicrobial activity of copper nanoparticles. Mat. Lett. 71, 114–116.

Rawani, A., Ghosh, A., Chandra, G., 2013. Mosquito larvicidal and antimicrobial activity of synthesized nano-crystalline silver particles using leaves and green berry extract of *Solanum nigrum* L. (Solanaceae: Solanales). Acta Trop. 128, 613–622.

REACH, 2013. Reach and nanomaterials. European Commission, Brussels. Available from: http://ec.europa.eu/enterprise/sectors/chemicals/reach/nanomaterials/

Rudzinski, W.E., Dave, A.M., Vaishnav, U.H., Kumbar, S.G., Kulkarni, A.R., Aminabhavi, T.M., 2002. Hydrogels as controlled release devices in agriculture. Des. Monomers Polym. 5, 39–65.

Ruparelia, J.P., Chatterjee, A.K., Duttagupta, S.P., Mukherji, S., 2008. Strain specificity in antimicrobial activity of silver and copper nanoparticles. Acta Biomater. 4, 707–716.

Safari, J., Zarnegar, Z., 2014. Advanced drug delivery systems: nanotechnology of health design. Rev. J. Saudi Chem. Soc. 18, 85–99.

Saharan, V., Mehrotra, A., Khatik, R., Rawal, P., Sharma, S.S., Pal, A., 2013. Synthesis of chitosan based nanoparticles and their in vitro evaluation against phytopathogenic fungi. Int. J. Biol. Macromol. 62, 677–683.

Saini, P., Gopal, M., Kumar, R., Srivastava, C., 2014. Development of pyridalyl nanocapsule suspension for efficient management of tomato fruit and shoot borer (*Helicoverpa armigera*). J. Environ. Sci. Health B 49, 344–351.

Sarijo, S.H., Hussein, M.Z., Yahaya, A.H., Zainal, Z., Yarmo, M.A., 2010a. Synthesis of phenoxyherbicides-intercalated layered double hydroxide nanohybrids and their controlled release property. Curr. Nanosci. 6, 199–205.

Sarijo, S.H., Hussein, M.Z., Yahaya, A.H.J., Zainal, Z., 2010b. Effect of incoming and outgoing exchangeable anions on the release kinetics of phenoxyherbicides nanohybrids. J. Hazard. Mat. 182, 563–569.

Sarkar, D.J., Kumar, J., Shakil, N.A., Walia, S., 2012. Release kinetics of controlled release formulations of thiamethoxam employing nano-ranged amphiphilic PEG and diacid based block polymers in soil. J. Environ. Sci. Health Tox. Hazard. Subst. Environ. Eng. 47, 1701–1712.

Sarlak, N., Taherifar, A., Salehi, F., 2014. Synthesis of nanopesticides by encapsulating pesticide nanoparticles using functionalized carbon nanotubes and application of new nanocomposite for plant disease treatment. J. Agric. Food Chem. 62, 4833–4838.

Sasson, Y., Levy-Ruso, G., Toledano, O., Ishaaya, I., 2007. Nanosuspensions: emerging novel agrochemical formulations. In: Ishaaya, I., Nauen, R., Horowitz, A.R. (Eds.), Insecticides Design Using Advanced Technologies. Springer-Verlag, Berlin, Heidelberg, pp. 1–39.

SCENIHR, 2010. Scientific basis for the definition of the term "nanomaterial". Brussels, Available from: http://ec.europa.eu/health/scientific_committees/emerging/docs/scenihr_o_032.pdf

SCENIHR, 2014. Opinion on nanosilver: safety, health and environmental effects and role in antimicrobial resistance. Brussels. Available from: http://ec.europa.eu/health/scientific_committees/emerging/docs/scenihr_o_039.pdf

SCENIHR, 2015. Opinion on the guidance on the determination of potential health effects of nanomaterials used in medical devices. Brussels. Available from: http://ec.europa.eu/health/scientific_committees/emerging/docs/scenihr_o_045.pdf

Scrinis, G., Lyons, K., 2007. The emerging nano-corporate paradigm: nanotechnology and the transformation of nature, food and agri-food systems. Int. J. Sociol. Food Agri. 15, 22–44.

Sekhon, B.S., 2014. Nanotechnology in agri-food production: an overview. Nanotechnol. Sci. Appl. 7, 31–53.

Senturk, A., Yalcyn, B., Otles, S., 2013. Nanotechnology as a food perspective. J. Nanomater. Mol. Nanotechnol. 2, 6.

Shaviv, A., 2000. Advances in controlled release of fertilizers. Adv. Agron. 71, 1–49.

Shi, J.Y., Abid, A.D., Kennedy, I.M., Hristova, K.R., Silk, W.K., 2011. To duckweeds (*Landoltia punctata*), nanoparticulate copper oxide is more inhibitory than the soluble copper in the bulk solution. Environ. Pollut. 159, 1277–1282.

Shirakawa, M.A., Gaylarde, C.C., Sahao, H.D., Lima, J.R.B., 2013. Inhibition of *Cladosporium* growth on gypsum panels treated with nanosilver particles. Int. Bioterior. Biodegrad. 85, 57–61.

Silva, M.D., Cocenza, D.S., de Melo, N.F.S., Grillo, R., Rosa, A.H., Fraceto, L.F., 2010. Alginate nanoparticles as a controlled release system for clomazone herbicide. Quimica Nova 33, 1868–1873.

Silva, M.D., Cocenza, D.S., Grillo, R., de Melo, N.F.S., Tonello, P.S., de Oliveira, L.C., Cassimiro, D.L., Rosa, A.H., Fraceto, L.F., 2011. Paraquat-loaded alginate/chitosan nanoparticles: preparation, characterization and soil sorption studies. J. Hazard. Mat. 190, 366–374.

Sioutas, C., Delfino, R.J., Singh, M., 2005. Exposure assessment for atmospheric ultrafine particles (UFPs) and implications in epidemiologic research. Environ. Health Perspect. 113, 947–955.

Smith, K., Evans, D.A., El-Hiti, G.A., 2008. Role of modern chemistry in sustainable arable crop protection. Phil. Trans. R. Soc. B 363, 623–637.

Sondi, I., Salopek-Sondi, B., 2004. Silver nanoparticles as antimicrobial agent: a case study on *E. coli* as a model for Gram-negative bacteria. J. Colloid Interface Sci. 275, 177–182.

Song, M.R., Cui, S.M., Gao, F., Liu, R.Y., Fan, C.L., Lei, T.Q., Liu, D.C., 2012. Dispersible silica nanoparticles as carrier for enhanced bioactivity of chlorfenapyr. J. Pestic. Sci. 37, 258–260.

Soni, N., Prakash, S., 2012. Fungal-mediated nano silver: an effective adulticide against mosquito. Parasit. Res. 111, 2091–2098.

Sonkaria, S., Ahn, S.H., Khare, V., 2012. Nanotechnology and its impact on food and nutrition: a review. Recent Pat. Food Nutr. Agric. 4, 8–18.

Sooresh, A., Kwon, F., Tayor, R., Pietrantonio, P., Pine, M., Sayes, C.M., 2011. Surface functionalization of silver nanoparticles: novel applications for insect vector control. ACS Appl. Mater. Interfaces 3, 3779–3787.

Stadler, T., Butelert, M., Weaver, D.K., 2010. Novel use of nano-structured alumina as an insecticide. Pest Manag. Sci. 66, 577–579.

Stöber, W., Fink, A., Bohn, E., 1968. Controlled growth of monodisperse silica spheres in the micron size range. J. Colloid. Interface Sci. 26, 62–69.

Subramanyam, B., Roesli, R., 2000. Inert dusts. In: Subramanyam, Bh., Hagstrum, D.W. (Eds.), Alternatives to Pesticides in Stored-Product IPM. Kluwer Academic Publishers, Dordreecht, pp. 321–380.

Sun, D., Hussain, H.I., Siegele, R., Cresswell, T., Kong, L., Cahill, D.M., 2014. Uptake and cellular distribution, in four plant species, of fluorescently labeled mesoporous silica nanoparticles. Plant Cell Rep. 33, 1389–1402.

Sundaravadivelan, C., Padmanabhan, M.N., 2014. Effect of mycosynthesized silver nanoparticles from filtrate of *Trichoderma harzianum* against larvae and pupa of dengue vector *Aedes aegypti* L. Environ. Sci. Pollut. Res. 21, 4624–4633.

Suppan, S., 2013. Nanomaterials in soil. Our future food chain? IATP. Washington, DC. Available from: http://www.iatp.org/files/2013_04_23_Nanotech_SS.pdf

Suppan, S., 2015. Suing EPA for failure to regulate nano-pesticides. Available from: http://www.iatp.org/blog/201504/suing-epa-for-failure-to-regulate-nano-pesticides-0

Suriyaprabha, R., Karunakaran, G., Kavitha, K., Yuvakkumar, R., Rajendran, V., Kannan, N., 2014. Application of silica nanoparticles in maize to enhance fungal resistance. IET Nanobiotechnol. 8, 133–137.

Svenson, S., Prudhomme, R.K., 2012. Multifunctional Nanoparticles for Drug Delivery Applications: Imaging, Targeting, and Delivery, Nanostructure Science and Technology. Springer-Verlag, New York.

Tan, W.M., Hou, N., Pang, S., Zhu, X.F., Li, Z.H., Wen, L.X., Duan, L.S., 2012. Improved biological effects of uniconazole using porous hollow silica nanoparticles as carriers. Pest Manag. Sci. 68, 437–443.

Tang, L., Cheng, J., 2013. Nonporous silica nanoparticles for nanomedicine application. Nano Today 8, 290–312.

Thornton, P.K., 2010. Livestock production: recent trends, future prospects. Phil. Trans. R. Soc. B. 365, 2853–2867.

Tian, J., Wong, K.K., Ho, C.M., Lok, C.N., Yu, W.Y., Che, C.M., Chiu, J.F., Tam, P.K., 2007. Topical delivery of silver nanoparticles promotes wound healing. ChemMedChem 2, 129–136.

Torney, F., Trewyn, B.G., Lin, V.S.Y., Wang, K., 2007. Mesoporous silica nanoparticles deliver DNA and chemicals into plants. Nat. Nanotechnol. 2, 295–300.

Ulrichs, C., Mewis, I., Goswami, A., 2005. Crop diversification aiming nutritional security in West Bengal—biotechnology of stinging capsules in nature's water-blooms. Ann. Tech. Issue of State Agri Technologists Service Association. ISSN, 1–18.

Unsworth, J.B., Corsi, C., Van Emon, J.M., Farenhorst, A., Hamilton, D.J., Howard, C.J., Hunter, R., Jenkins, J.J., Kleter, G.A., Kookana, R.S., Lalah, J.O., Leggett, M., Miglioranza, K.S., Miyagawa, H., Peranginangin, N., Rubin, B., Saha, B., Shakil, N.A., Developing global leaders for research, regulation, and stewardship of crop protection chemistry in the 21st century. *J. Agric. Food Chem.* 13, 2015, 52–60.

Usha Rani, P., Madhusudhanamurthy, J., Sreedhar, B., 2014. Dynamic adsorption of alpha-pinene and linalool on silica nanoparticles for enhanced antifeedant activity against agricultural pests. J. Pestic. Sci. 87, 191–200.

Vaculíková, E., Plachá, D., Jampílek, J., 2015. Toxicology of drug nanocarriers. Chem. Listy 109, 346–352.

Vassilakos, T.N., Athanassiou, C.G., Kavallieratos, N.G., Vayias, B.J., 2006. Influence of temperature on the insecticidal effect of *Beauveria bassiana* in combination with diatomaceous earth against *Rhyzopertha dominica* and *Sitophilus oryzae* on stored wheat. Biol. Control 38, 270–281.

Velmurugan, N., Gnana Kumar, G., Sub Han, S., 2009. Synthesis and characterization of potential fungicidal silver nano-sized particles and chitosan membrane containing silver particles. Iran. Polym. J. 18, 383–392.

Vimala, R.T.V., Sathishkumar, G., Sivaramakrishnan, S., 2015. Optimization of reaction conditions to fabricate nano-silver using *Couroupita guianensis* Aubl. (leaf & fruit) and its enhanced larvicidal effect. Spectochim. Acta Mol. Biomol. Spetrosc. 135, 110–115.

Vitanovic, E., 2012. Use of Cu fungicides in vineyards and olive groves. In: Dhanasekaran, D., Thajuddin, N., Panneerselvam, A. (Eds.), Fungicides for Plant and Animal Diseases. InTech, Rijeka, pp. 279–298.

Wang, Z., Xie, X., Zhao, J., Liu, X., Feng, W., White, J.C., Xing, B., 2012. Xylem- and phloem-based transport of CuO nanoparticles in maize (*Zea mays* L.). Environ. Sci. Technol. 46, 4434–4441.

Wanyika, H., Gatebe, E., Kioni, P., Tang, Z., Gao, Y., 2012. Mesoporous silica nanoparticles carrier for urea: potential applications in agrochemical delivery systems. J. Nanosci. Nanotechnol. 12, 2221–2228.

Wanyika, H., Sustained release of fungicide metalaxyl by mesoporous silica nanospheres. *J. Nanopart. Res.* 15, 2013, 1831 (9 pages).

Watson, S.B., Gergely, A., Janus, E.R., 2011. Where is "Agronanotechnology" heading in the United States and European Union? Nat. Res. Environ. 26, 8–12.

Wibowo, D., Zhao, C.X., Peters, B.C., Middelberg, A.P., 2014. Sustained release of fipronil insecticide in vitro and in vivo from biocompatible silica nanocapsules. J. Agric. Food Chem. 62, 12504–12511.

Wilkins, R.M., 2004. Controlled release technology, agricultural. In: Seidel, A. (Ed.), Kirk Othmer Encyclopedia of Chemical Technology. fifth ed. John Wiley & Sons, New Jersey.

Xu, H., Yan, F., Monson, E.E., Kopelman, R., 2003. Room-temperature preparation and characterization of poly(ethylene glycol)-coated silica nanoparticles for biomedical applications. J. Biomed. Mater. Res. A 66, 870–879.

Xu, L., Cao, L.D., Li, F.M., Wang, X.J., Huang, Q.L., 2014. Utilization of chitosan-lactide copolymer nanoparticles as controlled release pesticide carrier for pyraclostrobin against *Colletotrichum gossypii* Southw. J. Dispers. Sci. Technol. 35, 544–550.

Yadav, A., Aggarwal, A., 2014. Effect of Benomyl and Dithane M-45 on mycoflora, mycorrhizae and growth enhancement of *Helianthus annuus* L. N.Y. Sci. J. 7, 7–15.

Yamanka, M., Hara, K., Kudo, J., 2005. Bactericidal actions of silver ions solution on *Escherichia coli* studying by energy filtering transmission electron microscopy and proteomic analysis. Appl. Environ. Microbiol. 71, 7589–7593.

Yang, F.L., Li, X.G., Zhu, F., Lei, C.L., 2009. Structural characterization of nanoparticles loaded with garlic essential oil and their insecticidal activity against *Tribolium castaneum* (Herbst) (Coleoptera: Tenebrionidae). J. Agric. Food Chem. 57, 10156–10162.

Yang, Z., Kang, S.G., Zhou, R., 2014. Nanomedicine: de novo design of nanodrugs. Nanoscale 6, 663–677.

Yin, Y.H., Guo, Q.M., Han, Y., Wang, L.J., Wan, S.Q., 2012. Preparation, characterization and nematicidal activity of lansiumamide B nano-capsules. J. Integr. Agric. 11, 1151–1158.

Zhao, M., Liu, L., Her, R., Kalantar, T., Schmidt, D., Mathieson, T., Tolley, M., Yau, K., Wensing, S., Zhang, Q., Zettler, M., Li, Z.S., Zweifel, D., 2012. Nano-sized delivery for agricultural chemicals. In: Tiddy, G., Tan, R. (Eds.), NanoFormulation. Royal Society of Chemistry. Cambridge, pp. 256–265.

Zhang, Y., Chan, H.F., Leong, K.W., 2013. Advanced materials and processing for drug delivery: the past and the future. Adv. Drug Deliv. Rev. 65, 104–120.

Zhang, W.B., He, S., Liu, Y., Geng, Q.Q., Ding, G.L., Guo, M.C., Deng, Y.F., Zhu, J.L., Li, J.Q., Cao, Y.S., 2014. Preparation and characterization of novel functionalized prochloraz microcapsules using silica-alginate-elements as controlled release carrier materials. ACS Appl. Mater. Interfaces 6, 11783–11790.

4

NANOPESTICIDES: A NEW PARADIGM IN CROP PROTECTION

Paul Cătălin Balaure, Dragoş Gudovan, Iulia Gudovan

University "Politehnica" of Bucharest, Faculty of Applied Chemistry and Materials Science, "Costin Nenitzescu" Department of Organic Chemistry, Bucharest, Romania

1 Introduction

The global problem of food security and how can nanotechnology help with crop protection.

Scientists have raised alarm about the rate of global population growth, which in a half-century between 1950 and 2000 has increased from 2.1 billion to 6.1 billion (Carvalho, 2006). Although the growth rate showed a descending trend over the last decades, decreasing from 2.1% by the end of the 1960s to 1.2% in the present, world population is estimated to raise from about 7.3 billion now to 9.7 billion by 2050 (Department of Economic and Social Affairs, Population Division, 2015). With an ever-increasing world population there is a corresponding growing demand for food. As the planet's environmental resources are limited, the steady population growth inevitably resulted in an unbalance: the population has been growing at a faster rate than the planted area (Funk and Brown, 2009) so that the per capita harvested area continuously decreased since 1961 leading to the food crisis the world is facing nowadays. According to the latest report on the state of the food insecurity in the world released last year by the Food and Agriculture Organization of the United Nations (FAO), there are about 795 million undernourished people in the world representing 14.3% of world's population (Food and Agriculture Organization of the United Nations, International Fund for Agricultural Development, World Food Programme, 2015). The most worrying form of undernutrition is protein-energy malnutrition (PEM) or protein-calorie malnutrition (PCM). This potentially lethal condition is characterized by rapid weight loss due to insufficient protein uptake. PEM

New Pesticides and Soil Sensors. http://dx.doi.org/10.1016/B978-0-12-804299-1.00005-9

in young children results in growth failure. There are two types of malnutrition: wasting or acute malnutrition where although height is normal for age, weight is low for both age and height, and stunting or chronic malnutrition where despite a normal weight for height, weight and height are both low for age. Wasting and stunting condition means that weight for age, weight for height, and height for age are all low. According to the United Nations Children's Fund (UNICEF), the global wasting rate was 7.5% (1 in 13 children in the world) meaning that 50 million children were wasted in 2014, 16 million of them suffering of severe wasting (UNICEF, World Health Organization, World Bank Group, 2016). Due to the uneven distribution of food supplies around the globe, the huge majority of undernourished people that is, 780 million people leave in developing countries which also have the highest population growth rates [developing countries will account for about 95% of the global population increase (Cohen, 2005)] and at the same time are the poorest economies in the world. The worst situation is encountered in the Sub-Saharan Africa where undernourishment has a prevalence of 23.2%. Although the undernourishment prevalence in this area went down by 10% compared to 1990, in fact this fall in percentage did not keep pace with population increase so that the number of undernourished people and children has risen. It is clear that a more rapid increase of the world agricultural production and a more equitable and fair distribution of food are vitally required in order to eradicate hunger.

FAO estimated that average pre- and postharvest losses caused by pests (weeds, insects, rodents, and diseases) range from 20% to 40% depending on the type of the crop and on the geographical area. In temperate climates most damages are produced by weeds and diseases, while insects have a greater impact in subtropical and tropical regions. Crop losses reflect the inefficiency of crop protection methods and again the highest crop losses are registered in Central Africa (52% of the potential yield) (Organization for Economic Co-operation and Development, 2010).

There are several ways to control pests and to mitigate crop damages they cause. A sustainable crop protection should rely on the concept of integrated pest management (IPM) which means the utilization of all suitable methods including biological controls, cultural controls, mechanical controls, and chemical controls in order to keep the population of damaging organisms below the economic injury levels without adversely affecting the ecological balance and the environmental health. Biological control means to control a pest population with the aid of its natural enemies. Mechanical control destroys pests using physical methods by preventing pest entry or making the environment unsuitable for pest development. Several types of mechanical devices, such as plows, disks, mowers, cultivators, bed conditioners, barriers, fences, nets, screens, and traps are used. Cultural control is based on disruption of the normal relationship between the pest and its host thereby pest survival, growth, and reproduction becoming less likely. Cultural control embraces cultural practices and source reduction (sanitation). There are a lot of cultural practices that can prevent and/or suppress pest infestation, for example, selection of crop varieties, timing of planting and harvesting, crop rotation, use of trap crops, and use of mulches. Sanitation aims to deprive pests of their sources of food, water, or other necessities by removing weed plants, crop wastes, and diseased plants and by maintaining a border free of pests and pests mating sites around the crop area. Another way to combat pest damages is to increase host resistant to pests by genetic control. Chemical control involves the use of pesticides which are chemical substances either synthesized or of natural origin that kill, control, drive away, or modify the behavior of a pest.

Pesticides including herbicides, fungicides, insecticides, rodenticides, and so on are widely used due to their effectiveness, the ease of application, availability, and their relatively low cost compared to other control methods. However, pesticides have also a series of major drawbacks. Nontargeted useful species like insect polinators, birds, or natural enemies of pests can be threatened by the application of nonselective pesticides. Pesticides affect the ecological balance and if they destroy useful species that control pests the result will be in fact a proliferation of damaging species. Moreover, persistent lipophilic pesticides that are not broken down in the environment may enter the food chain. Moving unchanged up the food chain they tend to accumulate in adipose (fatty) tissues. As a result, the concentration of the pesticides retained by the organisms increases at each chain food level (bioaccumulation), eventually becoming a serious threat for animals and humans health. Furthermore, pesticides can be ineffective because they do not reach the target organism, being washed off or taken away by wind thereby spreading out in the environment and contaminating soil and groundwater in nontargeted areas. Another factor that can affect efficiency is the stability of the pesticide formulation and of the active ingredients (AIs). Environmental factors, such as temperature, humidity, light, and the presence of decomposing microorganisms cause pesticides degradation before reaching their targets. In fact it estimated that up to 90% of the applied pesticides are lost during- and postapplication (Ghormade et al., 2011). Improper timing of application meaning that the pesticide is applied at the wrong stage of pest development also leads to ineffective pest control. All these factors unduly increase the costs of pest management due to the use of much larger amounts of pesticides than those really needed to effectively control pests which in turn negatively impacts the environment by reducing soil biodiversity, reducing nitrogen fixation, and increasing bioaccumulation of pesticides in humans and other living organisms. Nevertheless, it should not be omitted that in response to frequent pesticide applications, pests may develop resistance to pesticides.

Nanotechnology can help mitigate the drawbacks associated with the classical pesticide formulation and application technologies. Any pesticide formulation intentionally including nanosized entities (up to 1000 nm) and claiming new properties arising from size are referred to herein as "nanopesticide" (Kah et al., 2013; Kah and Hofmann, 2014). Due to the small size and huge surface area-to-volume ratio, nanopesticides are expected to exhibit unique useful features as compared to their bulk counterparts. Nanoformulation can increase solubility and dispersion of lipophilic pesticides in water. Using appropriate surface active agents stable aqueous nanodispersions of lipohilic pesticides can be prepared thereby increasing pesticide bioavailability on one hand and avoiding the use of toxic organic solvents on the other hand. Such stable aqueous nanodispersions could be used for simultaneous application of two or more incompatible pesticides that would react with each other in solution. However, in a stable nanodispersion chemical reaction between incompatible pesticides is prevented at least temporarily since pesticides are shielded away from one another (Carvalho, 2006; Storm et al., 2001). Moreover, nanoencapsulation provides the possibility to control the rate of pesticide release and, hence, to maintain the effective pesticide concentration over a longer period of time. On the other hand, nanoencapsulation also protects pesticides from being prematurely degraded. Nanodelivery systems can be engineered so that they overcome the various natural environmental and biological barriers keeping classical pesticide formulations from reaching their intended targets. Site-specific delivery of pesticides would greatly improve their efficiency simultaneously reducing potential pollution from undelivered components (Chen et al., 2015). Smart multifunctional delivery systems provide spatial and temporal control on the process of pesticide release that may be triggered by specific environmental features thereby imparting to these systems the characteristics of remotely regulated, preprogrammed systems. Consequently, such smart nanosized delivery systems allow a more judicious use of pesticides since the amount of pesticides required for efficient pest control is significantly reduced, the costs associated with pesticide production and pesticide waste management are decreased, and at the same time the probability of resistance emerging decreases too. Nanocomposites made up of clusters of photocatalitically-active TiO_2 deposited on the surface of pesticide loaded microcapsules reduce environmental risks by promoting photocatalytic degradation of pesticide residuals that were not taken up by their biological targets (Kah et al., 2013; Guan et al., 2011). Last but not least, nanotechnology can be used to control pesticide losses due to runoff and leaching. Loss control pesticides (LCPs) can be prepared using special additives that increase adhesive properties causing nanocarriers to get stuck to crop leaves thereby reducing pesticide losses and environmental contamination (Jia et al., 2014; Xiang et al., 2014). The advantages of nanoformulation of pesticides are illustratively depicted in Fig. 4.1.

To highlight the advantages of nanopesticides we have chosen from the literature two recent and relevant achievements in the field.

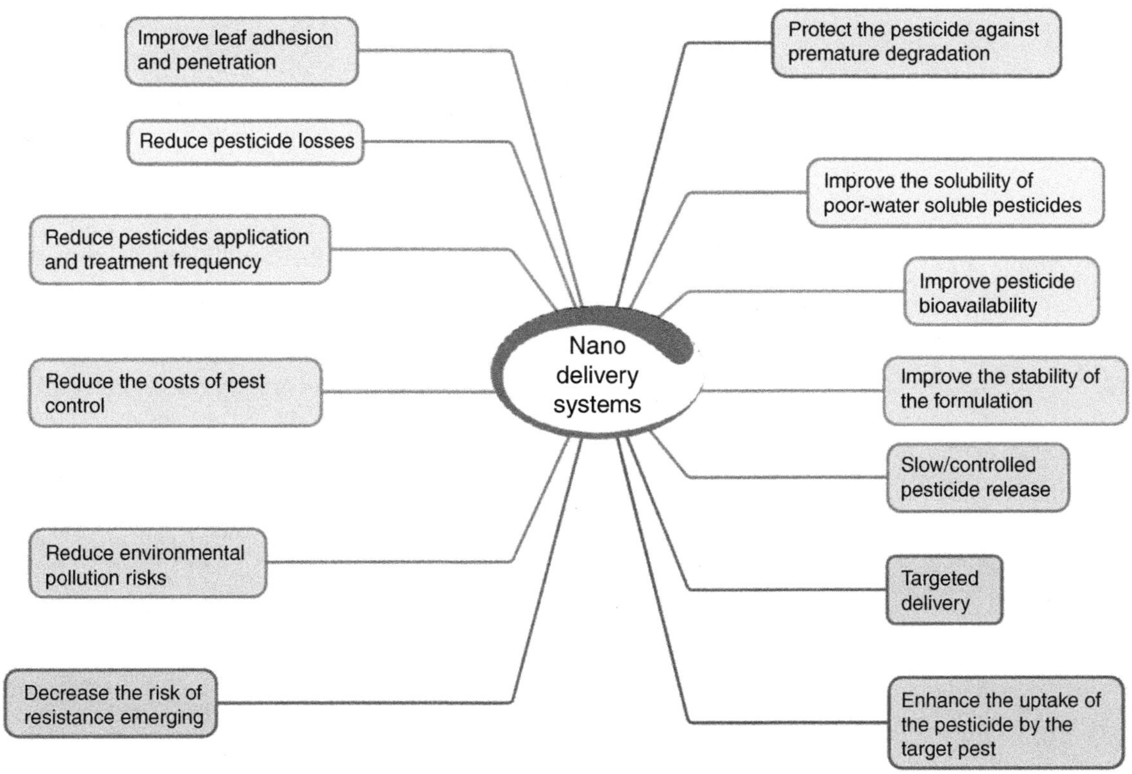

Figure 4.1. Benefits of nanoformulation of pesticides.

The first one refers to a pH-responsive nanocarrier used for targeted delivery of pesticides in plants. Chen et al. (2015), synthesized a smart nanodelivery system based on an amphiphilic polysuccinimide star copolymer. Stimuli-responsive polymeric nanomaterials have been intensively studied due to their unique capability to trigger the release of their payload in sharp response to some changes in the microenvironment conditions. For instance, taking advantage of the slightly acidic nature of tumors as compared to healthy tissues, smart nanodevices have been designed for targeted site-specific delivery of anticancer drugs. However, as compared to the huge number of papers reporting on biomedical applications of smart nanodelivery systems, there are only a few works dealing with the application of such systems for site-specific delivery of pesticides and nutrients. The synthesis of the pH-sensitive, biodegradable polymeric nanocarrier developed by Chen et al. is presented in Fig. 4.2. The first step in the synthesis of amphiphilc star polypeptides consisted in the 2,4,6-triaminopyrimidine (TAP) initiated anionic ring opening polymerization of benzylic-protected L-aspartic acid *N*-carboxyanhydride (NCA-Bn-L-Asp). Next, the protecting benzyl ester groups were removed by acid hydrolysis yielding the intermediates three-armed star polymers, TAP-$[\text{poly(Bn-L-Asp)}]_3$. On treatment with thionyl chloride in refluxing dichloromethane (DCM), the latter were eventually converted into the three-arm star copolymers of poly(aspartic acid-*co*-succinimide), TAP-$[\text{poly(L-Asp-}co\text{-SI)}]_3$. When placed in water, these amphiphilic star copolymers self assemble forming core/shell type nanostructures, with an inner core consisting of the hydrophobic polysuccinimide segments surrounded by the hydrophilic corona of polyaspartate segments (Fig. 4.3). The authors used naphthaleneacetic acid (NAA), which is a synthetic plant hormone in the auxin family as a model pesticide. NAA was encapsulated into the hydrophobic core of the nanoparticles and release studies were carried out in buffered media of various pH values. A pH-dependent release of the encapsulated pesticide from the prepared star copolymers was revealed. The release rate was controlled by the hydrolysis reaction converting the hydrophobic succinimide segments into hydrophilic ones (aspartates) with concomitant nanocarrier disassembly and payload release. The hydrolysis reaction was ineffective at pH values below 8.0 and, consequently the nanocarrier stability was not affected up to pH 8.0. This behavior could be nicely exploited to selectively deliver pesticides to the plant phloem since this tissue, which is specialized in the transport of photosynthates and nutrients in vascular plants has a characteristic pH (8.0–8.5) which is higher than that of the surrounding plant tissue. Moreover, to

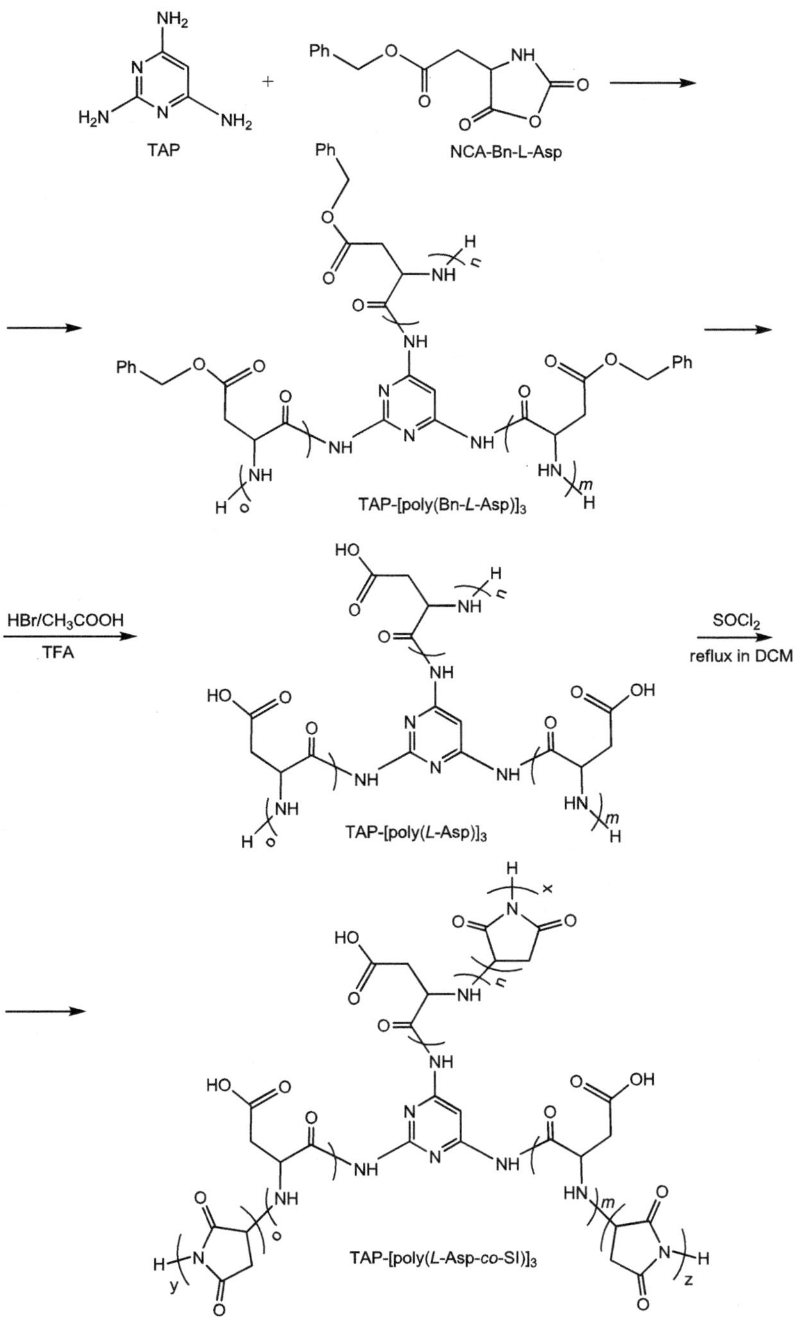

Figure 4.2. Synthesis of pH-responsive three-arm star copolymers of poly(aspartic acid-*co*-succinimide) (Chen et al., 2015).

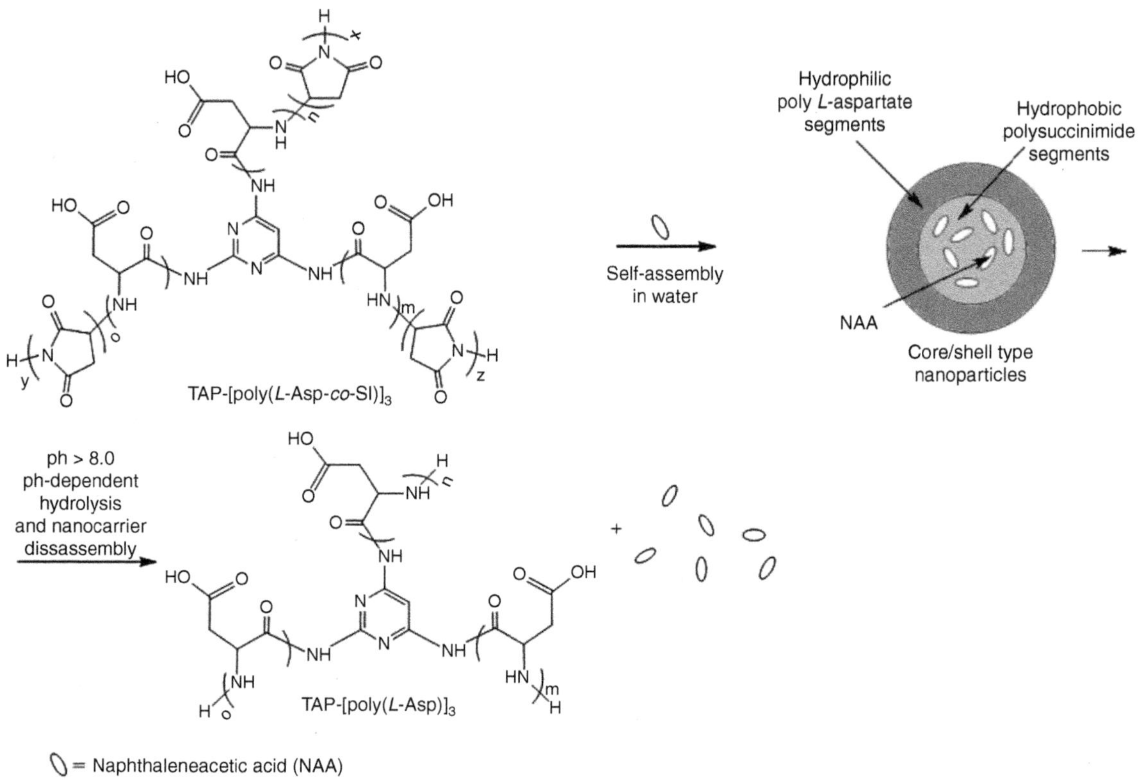

Figure 4.3. pH-responsive pesticide delivery system in plants (Chen et al., 2015).

assess the toxicity of TAP-[L-Asp$_{26}$-*co*-SI$_{17}$]$_3$ the authors performed a viability test using fluorescein diacetate (FdA) and propidium iodide (PI) double staining. Viable cells with intact intracellular enzymes content are able to hydrolyze the membrane permeable nonfluorescent FdA into the membrane nonpermable green fluorescent fluorescein and, hence, the cytoplasm will exhibit green fluorescence. On the other hand, dead cells with damaged plasma membranes will uptake the membrane impermeable dye PI which entering cell nucleus binds to the DNA resulting in an enhanced red fluorescence. The authors used citrus leaves for this double-staining assay. Citrus leaves were first incubated for 1 h in TAP-[L-Asp$_{26}$-*co*-SI$_{17}$]$_3$ copolymer solution at room temperature, and then were incubated with staining solution for 2 min. The results obtained demonstrated that the TAP-[L-Asp$_{26}$-*co*-SI$_{17}$]$_3$ star copolymer is nontoxic to citrus plant even at high concentrations (242 μg/mL).

The second example illustrates how the adhesion of pesticides on crop leaves can be increased by using either organic polymeric

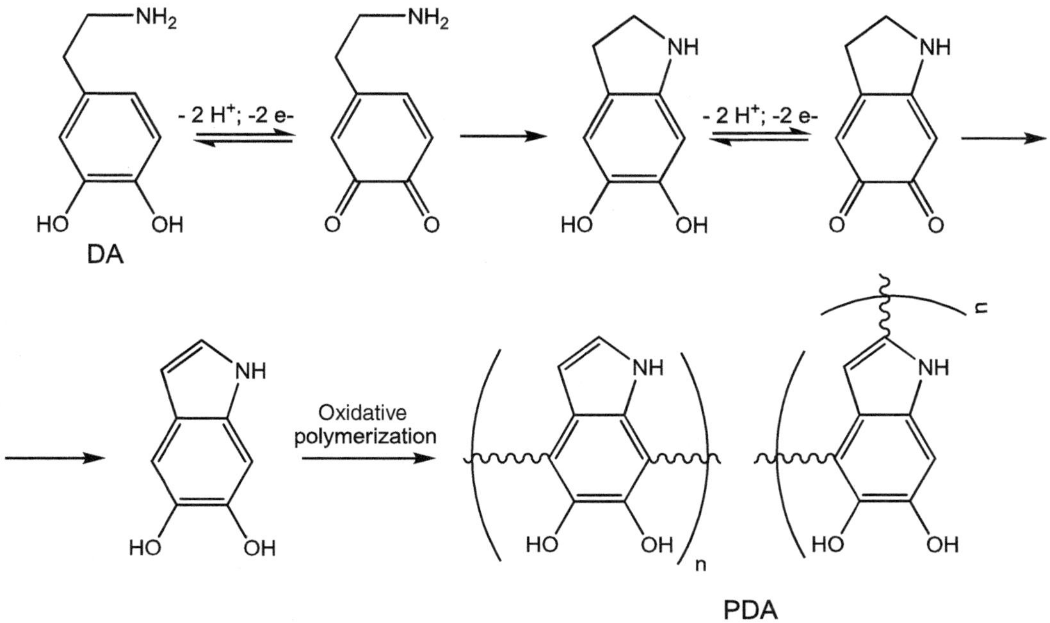

Figure 4.4. Oxidative self-polymerization of dopamine (DA) (Postma et al., 2009; d'Ischia et al., 2009).

nanomaterials (Jia et al., 2014) or inorganic nanoclays (Xiang et al., 2014). Polydopamine (PDA) is a natural adhesive, and avermectin (Av) is a natural pesticide with antihelminthic and insecticidal properties. It is known that in basic media dopamine (DA) readily undergoes oxidative self-polymerization (Fig. 4.4) forming an adherent PDA coating that readily sticks to almost any surface (Postma et al., 2009; d'Ischia et al., 2009). Jia et al. (2014) nicely exploited this DA property to encapsulate Av. Using the emulsion interfacial polymerization technique, the authors have prepared Av loaded adhesive PDA microcapsules. The interfacial emulsion polymerization is a soft chemical template synthesis in which oil drops containing Av serve as soft template. Briefly, a surfactant stabilized oil-in-water emulsion was prepared by pouring the oily phase consisting of Av dissolved in *n*-butanol into an aqueous tris(hydroxymethyl)aminomethane (TRIS) buffer (pH = 8.5) that contains the hexadecyl trimethylammonium chloride (CTAC) surfactant. Next, DA was added, the mixture was vigorously stirred for 24 h at room temperature, and eventually the prepared microcapsules were harvested by centrifugation. The adhesive Av loaded PDA microcapsules showed improved residence time on crop surfaces and excellent sustained release properties.

Xiang et al. (2014) reported the synthesis of a loss control pesticide based on another type of natural material, that is, attapulgite—a sort of hydrated magnesium aluminum silicate. Attapulgite has a nanorod structure with intrinsic aggregation tendency. Therefore, prior to utilization of this natural nanoclay, attapulgite has been subjected to a high-energy electron beam (HEEB) treatment in order to improve dispersion and hence the loading capacity. Through the HEEB treatment, the pristine aggregated bunches of attapulgite were taken apart and converted into a nanoporous network (Cai et al., 2009). The organophosphate insecticide chlorpyrifos (CPF) was used by the authors as a model pesticide. An oil-in-water emulsion of CPF was prepared using Tween 80 as an emulsifier. Next, several samples of HEEB irradiation modified attapulgite obtained at different electron beam fluences were added to obtain the loss control chlorpyrifos (LCC) emulsions. The authors proved not only the increased loading capacity as compared to natural unmodified attapulgite (NA) of the attapulgite samples irradiated with HEEB (HIA), but also the improved adhesion performances of LCC emulsions on leaf surface and at the same time the reduced leaching loss through the soil. All these characteristic recommend such pesticide–attapulgite nanocomposites as promising solutions to reduce both the pesticide loss and the pollution risk.

However, nanoformulations of pesticides may also have some deleterious effects that have been insufficiently studied yet especially in the case of organic nanocarriers (Kah and Hofmann, 2014). For instance, the increased protection against premature degradation conferred by the nanoencapsulation of pesticides may come at the cost of an increased persistence of the AI in the environment. Important issues that still remain to be addressed are the following ones: (1) the extent to which a nanocarrier can facilitate the transport of the AI in soil; (2) how much can a nanoformulation increase the bioavailability of the AI to nontarget organisms; (3) the release profile; and (4) fate of the nanocarriers in the environment, plant, and soils (Kah and Hofmann, 2014).

2 Types of Pesticide Nanocarriers

Nanopesticide formulations can be classified according to several criteria. For instance, they can be classified according to their intended purpose as: (1) formulations that increase the solubility of poorly-water soluble pesticides; (2) formulations that slow down the release rate of the encapsulated pesticide; (3) formulations able to achieve targeted delivery and to provide protection against premature degradation (Kah et al., 2013).

Herein nanoformulations will be divided into different categories based on the chemical nature of the nanocarrier, such as organic polymer-based formulations, lipid-based formulations, nanosized metals and metal oxides, clay based nanomaterials, layered double hydroxides (LDH), silica nanoparticles, and so on. Furthermore, depending on the particular manufacturing method nanoparticles falling into any of the aforementioned classes can have various structures and morphologies with different properties like nanocapsules, nanospheres, micelles, nanogels, nanofibers, nanoliposomes, solid lipid nanoparticles (SLNs), and so on. Fig. 4.5 illustrates the various types of nanopesticide delivery systems classified by chemistry and structure along with representative examples of both natural and synthetic encapsulated AIs.

3 Polymer-Based Nanopesticide Delivery Systems

3.1 Nanocapsules

Nanocapsules are vesicular or reservoir type structures comprising an inner central cavity surrounded by a polymer coating or membrane (Soppimath et al., 2001; Balaure and Grumezescu, 2014). The internal cavity, which confines the AI may be either hydrophilic or hydrophobic. In the former case, the structure is also referred to as a polymersome, the aqueous cavity being surrounded by a bilayer of an amphiphilic di- or triblock (ABA) copolymer coating, or by a monolayer membrane of an amphiphilic triblock copolymer (ABA), where A and B stand for the hydrophilic, and the hydrophobic segments, respectively. Unlike nanocapsules which can entrap only hydrophobic AIs, polymersomes can encapsulate both hydrophilic AIs which are solubilized in the aqueous inner cavity and hydrophobic AIs which are confined within the amphiphilic membrane through hydrophobic interactions with the hydrophobic B blocks.

Polymeric nanocapsules can be fabricated from preformed polymers or alternatively during the polymerization of suitable monomers. Both methods have been used to prepare pesticide-loaded nanocapsules.

3.1.1 Preparation of Pesticide-Loaded Polymeric Nanocapsules Starting With Monomers

Methyl methacrylate (MMA)—styrene (St) copolymer nanocapsules containing the natural AI lansiumamide B (LB) have been prepared by Yin et al. (2012) LB isolated from kernels of *Clausena lansium* was dissolved together with the two monomers in a little amount of petroleum ether and chloroform. Next, this solution

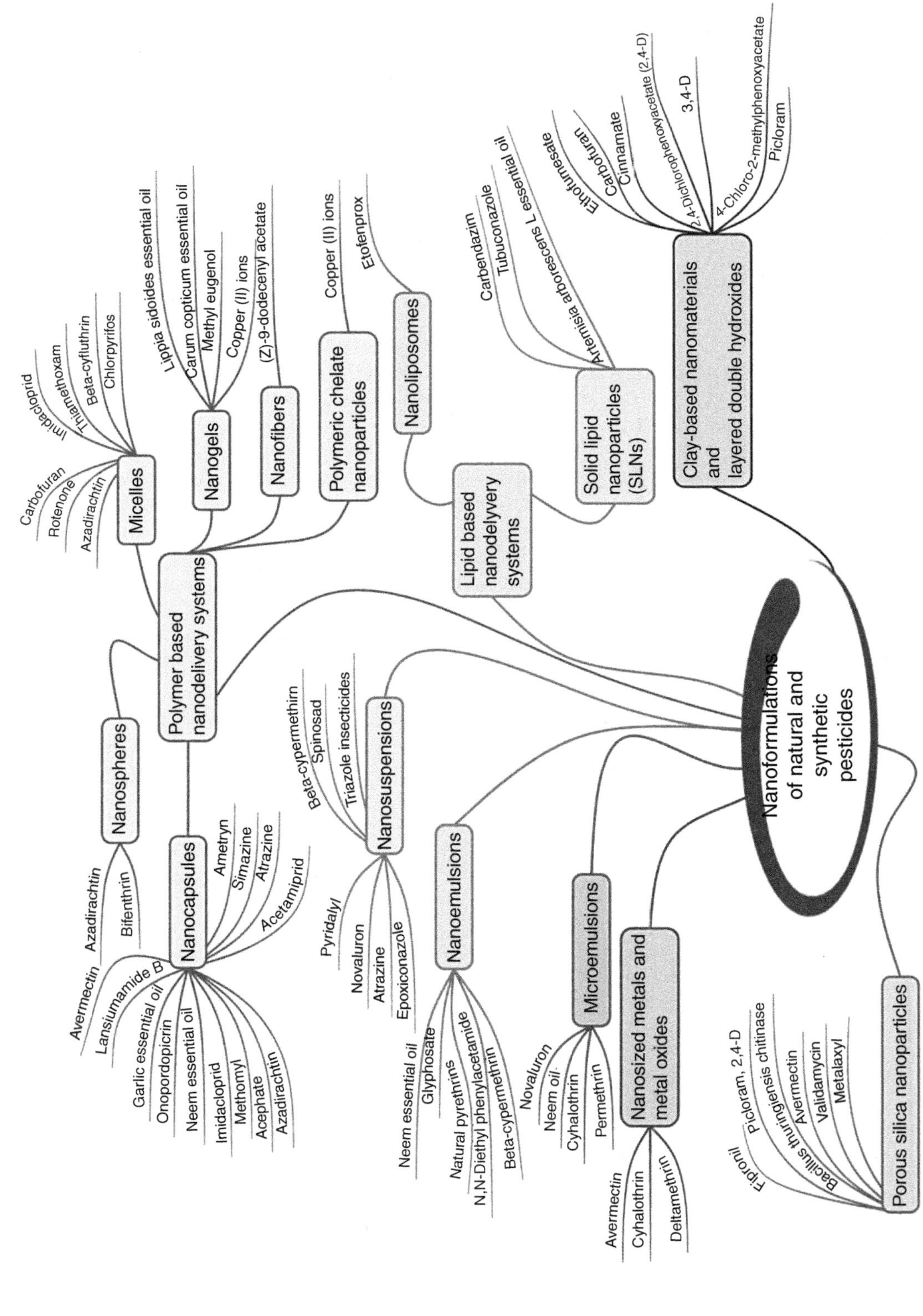

Figure 4.5. Types of nanocarriers for delivery of natural and synthetic pesticides.

was emulsified by ultrasonication in an aqueous solution of the anionic emulsifier sodium dodecyl sulfate (SDS) and the cosurfactant, *n*-amyl alcohol. Then, the radical polymerization initiator azoisobutyronitrile (AIBN) was added to the clarify emulsion and the reaction mixture was heated in 70°C water bath for 3 h under magnetic stirring. Eventually, a translucent aqueous suspension containing LB-loaded poly(MMA-*co*-St) nanocapsules (NCLB) was obtained. The authors reported remarkable improvement of the nematicidal activity of LB through nanoencapsulation. The nematicidal activity of NLCB was assessed using the sterilization soil cultivation method in a flowerpot test. Briefly, leaves of *Ipomoea aquatica* (water spinach) were planted in the sterilized matrix soil and sand (1200 cm^3) contained in each test pot. Afterward, each pot was infected with nematodes, which have been applied in doses of about 500 nematodes per pot. LB and NCLB aqueous dispersions were prepared in a concentration of 200 mg/L and 10 mL of these dispersions were introduced in each pot. Water treatment was used as blank control. These pot experiments were replicated four times. Twenty days after infestation, plants were excavated, washed and the root-knot nematodes were counted. The average number of root knots in the treatment of NCLB was 7.25 as compared to 19.5 in the treatment of LB.

Another example, that is, the preparation of Av-loaded adhesive PDA nanocapsules by interfacial emulsion self-polymerization of DA (Jia et al., 2014) has been already presented in the introductory part.

3.1.2 Preparation of Pesticide-Loaded Polymeric Nanocapsules From Preformed Polymers

There are several methods to prepare pesticide-loaded nanocapsules from preformed polymers, such as nanoprecipitation, emulsion-solvent diffusion, emulsion-solvent evaporation, layer by layer (LbL) self-assembly, ionic gelation, polyelectrolyte complexation, and melt-dispersion techniques.

Biodegradable polyesters and polysaccharides have been mostly used.

Using an oil-in-water (O/W) emulsion-solvent evaporation technique (Zhou et al., 2010), Pereira et al. (2014) have prepared poly(ε-caprolactone) (PCL) nanocapsules containing the herbicide atrazine. In brief, atrazine was dissolved in the water miscible organic solvent acetone, while the polymer was dissolved in the water immiscible organic solvent methylene chloride and myritol was added into the latter solution. The organic phase was produced by mixing and sonicating the above two solutions for 1 min. Then, the aqueous phase containing polyvinyl alcohol (PVA) as a hydrophilic surfactant was added and the O/W emulsion was sonicated for 8 min. Eventually, organic solvents were removed in a rotary evaporator. The resulted formulation contained 1 mg/mL of atrazine. The authors tested the nanoparticle formulation with target plant (*Brassica* sp.) and nontarget maize (*Zea mays*) and proved that in this case nanoencapsulation did not alter the action mechanism of the herbicide, the nanoformulation being active only against the target organism. Moreover, the nanoencapsulated herbicide was shown to be more effective against the target organism as compared to the naked herbicide proving an increase in bioavailability. Using soil column experiments, the authors demonstrated that atrazine was more evenly distributed at different heights in the soil column when applying the nanocapsule formulation as compared to free herbicide application. In the case of the free herbicide, the highest atrazine concentration was found in the upper part of the soil column indicating a greater retention of the herbicide by the colloids present in the soil, which results in reduced bioavailability and increased environmental contamination. The surfactants used to encapsulate atrazine in PCL nanocapsules also mitigate herbicide sorption to soil colloids thereby contributing to the enhanced bioavailability of the nanocapsule-formulated atrazine and at the same time reducing soil pollution. Furthermore, nanoencapsulation reduced the genotoxicity of atrazine and, hence, the risk associated with occupational exposure to atrazine. The authors concluded that the formulation developed appears as an attractive alternative to control weeds due to the sustained release profile allowing a decrease in application frequency, minimization of soil sorption, which reduces environmental risk, and increased bioavailability which increases treatment efficiency.

The sensitivity of azadirachtin (Aza)—the main component responsible for the pesticidal activity of neem products—to light, humidity, temperature, and environmental pH, requires its protection through nanoencapsulation.

PCL nanocapsules loaded with neem (*Azadirachta indica* or Indian Lilac) products that is, neem extracts and oil have been prepared by Forim et al. (2013) through a modified nanoprecipitation method. First, the authors prepared an O/W nanoemulsion by addition of the internal oily phase consisting of neem oil, neem extract, and sorbitan monostearate into water under vigorous agitation. Next, a solution of the PCL polymer in a water-miscible organic solvent (acetone) was injected in the above emulsion under moderate magnetic stirring by means of a peristaltic pump. If necessary, an aqueous solution of Tween 80 was added after a while. Eventually, the nanoparticle suspension was concentrated under vacuum. Using this concentrated nanoparticle suspension, the authors have prepared microparticles containing azadiractin-loaded PCL nanocapsules through the dry spraying technique. Stability assessments showed that 7 days of UV exposure resulted in only 55 and 10% Aza photodegradation in the case of nanoparticles in colloidal suspension and in powder, respectively, while Aza in nonencapsulated neem oil was completely degraded. The first-instar larvae of *Plutella xylostella* (cabbage moth) showed 100% mortality at day 9 after treatment with the colloidal suspension of nanoparticles loaded with neem oil and extracts.

Kumara et al. (2014) prepared alginate (ALG) nanocapsules loaded with the neonicotinoid insecticide imidacloprid (IMI) by double emulsion technique. IMI was dissolved under sonication in an aqueous solution of sodium ALG, which was further emulsified into methylene chloride containing dioctyl sodium sulfosuccinate as an emulsifier. By further dispersion of the obtained water-in-oil (W/O) simple emulsion into an aqueous solution of PVA under sonication, a water-in-oil-in-water (W/O/W) double emulsion was prepared. Next, an aqueous calcium chloride solution was added gradually to the magnetically stirred double emulsion. The mixture was kept stirring for an additional 18 h. Then, methylene chloride was removed under vacuum and the formed nanoparticles were harvested by ultracentrifugation. To evaluate the efficiency of their IMI nanoformulation, the authors conducted field studies on crop pests, more specific on leafhopper, a species of insects that suck plant sap. To this end, four different plots all of one square meter in size and each one containing ten healthy plants were used. One plot was the reference or control plot (untreated). Equal volumes of aqueous dispersions of the plain pesticide, the dummy nanoparticles, and the pesticide-loaded nanoparticles prepared at the same concentration of the dispersed component were uniformly applied by spraying on each of the remaining three plots. After treatment, at predefined time intervals, leaf infestation was estimated by counting the leafhopper population found on three leaves from the bottom, middle, and top of one plant randomly selected from each plot. The results showed that dummy nanoparticles had no effect on the leafhopper population. The nanoencapsulated IMI was found to be more effective than the free insecticide. Moreover, the authors have performed also toxicity studies revealing that nanoformulated IMI was significantly less toxic than the commercial pesticide.

Aiming to reduce the negative environmental impact caused by pesticides, Guan et al. (2008) have developed a new photodegradable nanoinsecticide. An efficient way to reduce environmental pollution is the breaking down of the pollutant residues by in situ generation of very reactive hydroxyl radicals which in the presence of oxygen are able to trigger a cascade of oxidative processes resulting in the mineralization of the organic compounds under mild conditions (advanced oxidation processes; AOPs). TiO_2 is a semiconductor material, which has photocatalytic activity. Absorption of photons with energies that match the bandgap of the semiconductor produces conduction band electrons and valence band holes. These charge carriers are able to promote, reduction (electrons), and oxidation (holes) processes. Holes having an extremely positive oxidation potential are able to oxidize almost all substances including water to produce highly reactive hydroxyl radicals. Hence, under irradiation with near UV light, the chemical species adsorbed on the surface of a TiO_2 particle may undergo AOPs, resulting in mineralization. The synthesis of the photodegradable nanoinsecticide was accomplished in several steps. In the first step, the authors have prepared IMI microcrystals using the antisolvent precipitation technique ("bottom up" approach). In brief, an aqueous solution of hydroxypropyl methylcellulose (HPMC) stabilizer was added with stirring into a previously prepared solution of IMI in acetone and the resulted dispersion was further lyophilized. In the second step, the IMI microcrystals were encapsulated through the LbL self-assembly of a polyelectrolyte multilayer film of the biodegradable and biocompatible polysaccharides chitosan (CHI) and ALG. The first layer was obtained by adsorbing the positively charged polyelectrolyte (CHI). The process was continued by the adsorption onto the first layer of an oppositely charged polyelectrolyte layer (ALG), and repeated identically with alternate adsorptions of positively and negatively charged polyelectrolytes until the desired multilayer film IMI $(CHI/ALG)_n$ was obtained. The photocatalyst was prepared as follows. Silver nitrate was used as silver source to prepare silver doped TiO_2 nanocomposites. The amount of silver nitrate required to obtain nanocomposites containing 1.5% Ag was added to an aqueous dispersion of TiO_2 previously aged by sonication for 30 min. The reductant 2-meracptoethanol was added next to eventually yield the Ag/TiO_2 nanocomposite. Then, the surface of Ag/TiO_2 was modified with SDS as an anionic surfactant to complete the synthesis of the nanophotocatalyst $SDS/Ag/TiO_2$. Eventually, the $SDS/Ag/TiO_2$ photocatalyst was adsorbed in dark under stirring over IMI $(CHI/ALG)_n$. Photocatalytic studies showed 97% degradation of the IMI in samples exposed to irradiation by natural light for 7 days. Release profile studies revealed that the rate release is tunable by adjusting the number of self-assembled CHI/ALG layers. Moreover, the photodegradable insecticide nano-TiO_2/Ag/SDS-IMI $(CHI/ALG)_5$ was proved to be more toxic against *Martianus dermestoides* (LC_{50} = 9.86 mg/L) than the bare IMI (LC_{50} = 13.45 mg/L).

A controlled-release nanoformulation of the neonicotinoid insecticide acetamipirid has been developed by the group of Kumar et al. (2015). They obtained acetamipirid-loaded ALG-CHI nanocapsules using the ionic pregelation and polyelectrolyte complexation method. In brief, acetamipirid was dissolved in an aqueous solution of sodium ALG under sonication for 15 min. Then, an aqueous solution of calcium chloride was added dropwise to the aforementioned solution under stirring when a Ca/ALG pregel was formed. The stirring was continued for the next 30 min and then, an aqueous CHI solution was dropped into the above calcium ALG pregel while stirring. As a result of the ionic interactions between positively charged ammonium groups of CHI and negatively charged carboxylate groups of ALG, a polyionic complex ALG–CHI was formed. Stirring was kept for 30 min and eventually, the nanocapsules were collected by centrifugation of the colloidal suspension. A loading efficiency of 62% was achieved. Release studies from acetamipirid-loaded ALG–CHI nanocapsules after applying in different soil media, revealed improved controlled-release performances as compared to commercially available formulations of acetamipirid, the best results being obtained for acidic soils.

Sun et al. (2014) have developed an elegant way to encapsulate the hydrophilic carbamate insecticide methomyl. Methomyl is a broad-spectrum insecticide but its aqueous solutions undergo rapid decomposition on aeration, in sunlight, or in alkaline media. Therefore, nanoencapsulation is required to avoid its premature degradation. The authors prepared an amphiphilic, photocross-linkable carboxymethyl chitosan (Az-CMCS) polymer by reacting an ethanolic solution of azidobenzaldehyde (Az) previously prepared as depicted in Fig. 4.6 with an aqueous solution of carboxymethyl chitosan (CMCS). Methomyl was dissolved in an aqueous solution of Az-CMCS, the pH was adjusted to 4.0 and the solution was sonicated for 3 min. Under these conditions, the amphiphatic polymer self-assembled into methomyl-loaded nanocapsules with an aqueous core. The shell surrounding the aqueous core bears hydrophobic aryl azide moieties which are known photoreactive reagents that upon exposure to UV radiation generate reactive nitrene intermediates that can initiate insertion into C—H bonds or can dimerize thereby promoting cross-linking (Hayashi et al., 1992; Yin et al., 2010; Preston and Wilson, 2013) (Fig. 4.6). The release rate was shown to be dependent on the cross-linking degree: the higher the cross-link density, the slower the release rate. The biological activity of nanoencapsulated methomyl was

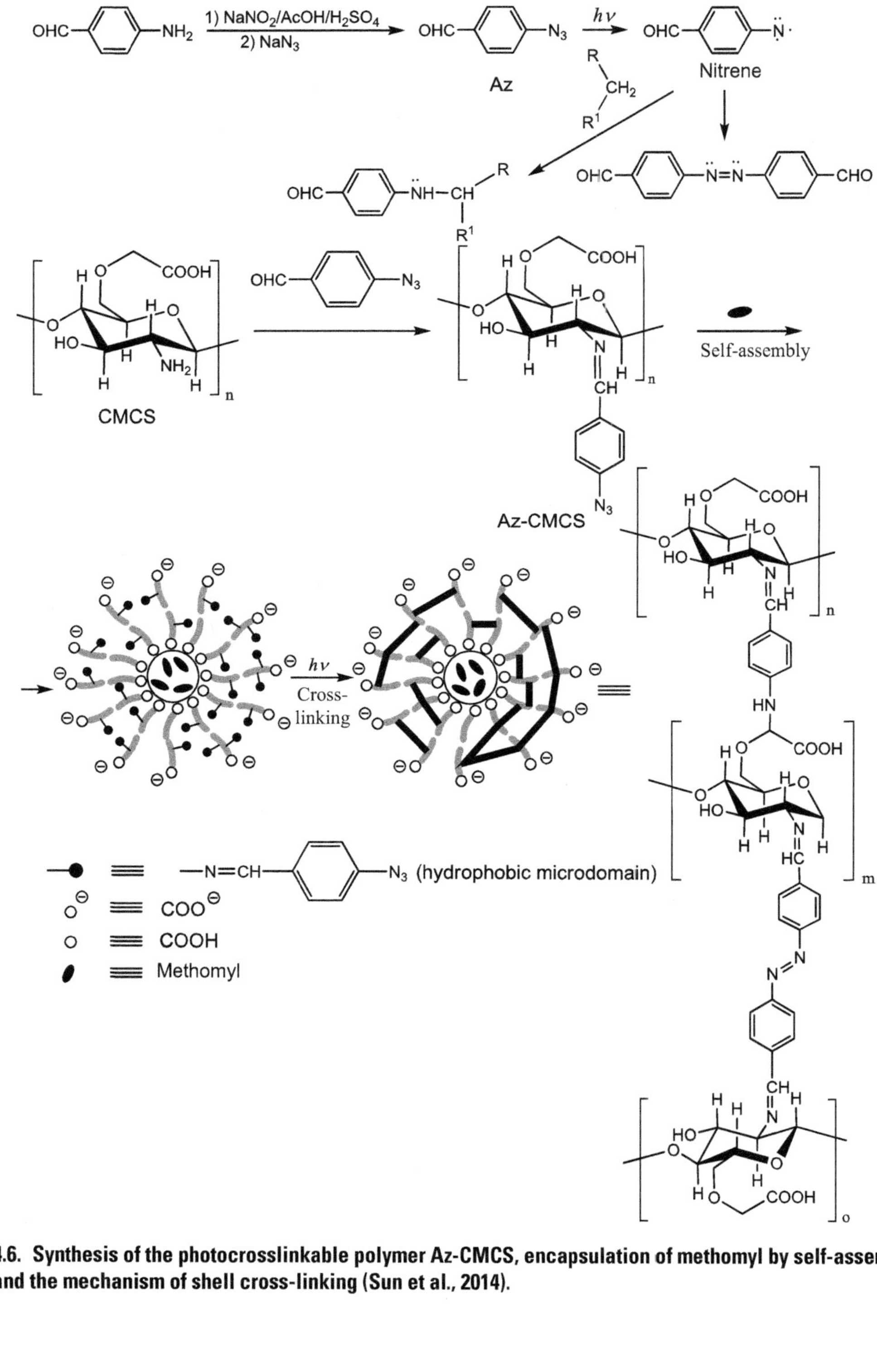

Figure 4.6. Synthesis of the photocrosslinkable polymer Az-CMCS, encapsulation of methomyl by self-assembly in water, and the mechanism of shell cross-linking (Sun et al., 2014).

tested against armyworm larvae using methomyl water solution as a control. The nanoformulated insecticide maintained 100% rate mortality at day 7 after application, while the mortality rate of the aqueous solution of methomyl fell to zero in less than three days. The authors suggested that the attractive interaction between the negatively charged methomyl-loaded nanoparticles and the positively charged surface of the leaves would help to control pests for extended periods of time.

Amphiphilic triblock copolymers have been also used for fabrication of pesticide-loaded nanocapsules. For instance, an extract of *Onopordon leptolepis* DC containing the antifungal and antibacterial sesquiterpene onopordopicrin was loaded into nanocapsules of polyethylene glycol–polybutylene adipate–polyethylene glycol (PEG–PBA–PEG) prepared by the emulsion-solvent diffusion method (Esmaeili and Saremnia, 2012). The authors dissolved the amphiphilic triblock copolymer PEG–PBA–PEG, the onopordopicrin extract, and olive oil in acetone and the oily organic phase was added dropwise into water under stirring. The resulted suspension was sequentially sonicated, filtered through cellulose acetate, cooled to −70°C, and freeze–dried. Memarizadeh et al. (2014) encapsulated IMI within an ABA type triblock linear dendritic copolymer through molecular self-assembly. The ability of linear dendritic poly(citric acid)–poly(ethylene glycol)–poly(citric acid) (PCA–PEG–PCA) amphiphilic triblock copolymer to self-assemble in aqueous solutions forming nanoparticles and fibers of different sizes and shapes is known (Tavakoli Naeini et al., 2010). The authors took advantage of this interesting property to encapsulate IMI. Briefly, an acetone solution of IMI was mixed with an ethanol solution of the PCA–PEG–PCA triblock copolymer (for the structure of the linear dendritic triblock copolymer see Fig. 4.7). The resulted solution was mixed for 8 h and next, free IMI was removed by dialysis. Certain volumes of the remaining solutions were diluted using water, and, respectively, ethanol as solvents. Depending on the size of the hydrophilic PCA blocks, the solvent used, the concentration of the solution, and the time the self-assembly process was allowed to proceed, aggregates of various dimensions ranging from 10 nm to several mm, and of different morphological sorts like fiber-like, globular, and tubular-shaped could be obtained. The authors showed a tunable release rate from these nanocapsules depending on the microenvironmental pH. Hence, the release rate of IMI was slowed down, as compared to neutral pH, at pH 10.0, the pH specific to the gut of *Glyphodes pyloalis*, a type of moth.

Garlic (*Allium sativum* L.) essential oil exhibits strong insecticidal activity but it is volatile and water insoluble, which hampers

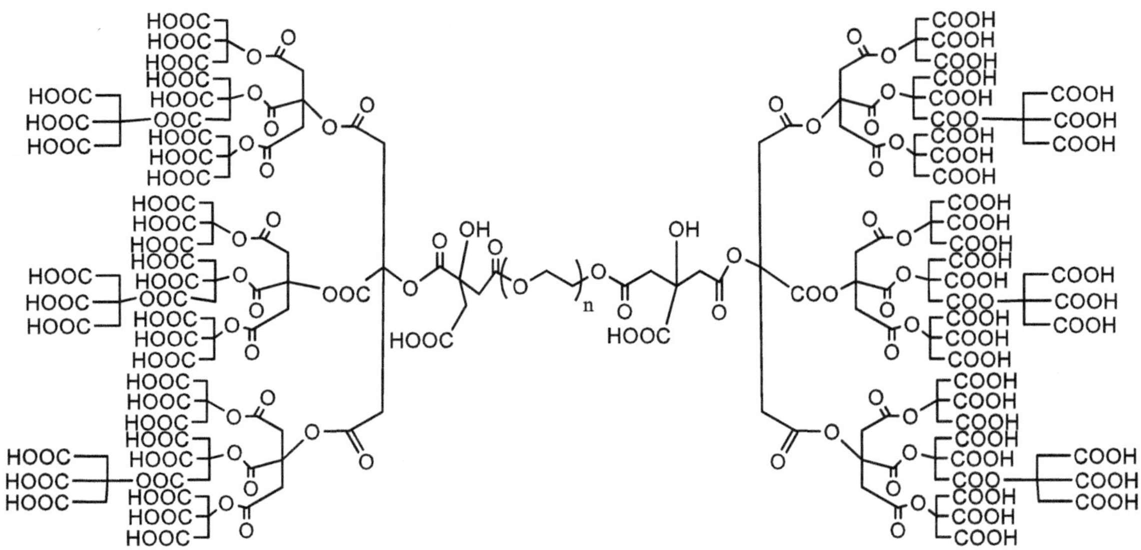

Figure 4.7. The structure of the linear dendritic amphiphilic triblock copolymer PCA–PEG–PCA (Tavakoli Naeini et al., 2010).

its utilization as a natural insecticide. Yang et al. (2009) prepared poly(ethylene glycol) (PEG) nanocapsules loaded with garlic essential oil using the melt-dispersion method. Briefly, PEG 6000 was heated and after being melt, garlic essential oil was added under slight stirring. The mixture was ground in a mortar box, cooled to room temperature, and sieved. A loading efficiency as high as 80% was achieved at the optimal essential oil/PEG ratio. The biological activity of garlic oil-loaded PEG nanocapsules was tested against *Tribolium castaneum*, a worldwide pest of stored products. Briefly, rough rice samples of identical weights and milled rice content have been treated with increasingly doses of free garlic essential oil, and encapsulated garlic essential oil, respectively in 250 mL jars. Then, 60 insects were introduced in each sample. After 5 days, each sample was examined and active, knocked down, and immobile insects were counted. The bioassays were repeated identically at monthly intervals. After five months, pest control efficacy remained over 80% of the initial value in the case of nanoencapsulated garlic essential oil, while free garlic essential oil retained only 11% of its initial pest control efficacy after 5 months. These results obtained at a dose of 8000 mg nanoparticles/kg were ascribed to the controlled-release properties of the nanoformulation.

Other examples of nanoencapsulation of pesticides can be found in Table 4.1 at the end of this section.

Table 4.1 Polymer-Based Nanopesticide Delivery Systems

Type of nanocarrier	Encapsulated pesticide(s)	Polymer(s)	Target organism(s)	Reference(s)
Nanocapsules	LB	Poly(MMA-*co*-St)	Nematodes	Yin et al. (2012)
	Atrazine Ametryn Simazine	PCL	*Brasica* sp.	Pereira et al. (2014) Grillo et al. (2012)
	Neem oil (Aza)	PCL	*P. xylostella*	Forim et al. (2013)
	IMI	ALG	Leafhopper	Kumara et al. (2014)
	Photodegradable nano IMI	CHI–ALG	*M. dermestoides*	Guan et al. (2008)
	Acetamipirid	ALG–CHI	Insects	Kumar et al. (2015)
	Methomyl	Photocrosslinkable CMCS	Armyworm larvae	Sun et al. (2014)
	Onopordopicrin	PEG–PBA–PEG	Fungi and bacteria	Esmaeili and Saremnia (2012)
	IMI	PCA–PEG–PCA	*G. pyloalis*	Memarizadeh et al. (2014)
	Garlic essential oil	PEG	*T. castaneum*	Yang et al. (2009)
	Acephate	PEG	Insects	Choudhury et al. (2012)
Nanospheres	Aza	PCL	Insects	da Costa et al. (2014)
	Bifenthrin	Poly(acrylic acid)-*b*-poly(butyl acrylate) (PAA-*b*-PBA) Poly(styrene)-*b*-poly(ethylene oxide) (PSt-*b*-PEG)		Liu et al. (2008a)
Micelles	IMI	Poly [poly (oxyethylene-300)-oxy glutaroyl] nanopolymer Poly [poly (oxyethylene-600)-oxy glutaroyl] nanopolymer Poly [poly (oxyethylene-1000)-oxy glutaroyl] nanopolymer and similar for the adipic, pimelic, and suberic acids	Insects	Adak et al. (2012)
	Carbofuran	Poly[poly(oxyethylene-18000)-oxy-5-decanyloxyisophthaloyl]	Insects Nematodes	Shakil et al. (2010)

(*Contined*)

Table 4.1 Polymer-Based Nanopesticide Delivery Systems (*cont.*)

Type of nanocarrier	Encapsulated pesticide(s)	Polymer(s)	Target organism(s)	Reference(s)
	β-Cyfluthrin	Poly-[poly-(oxyethylene-600/1000/1500/2000)-oxyisophthaloyl]	Insects	Loha et al. (2011)
	Aza	Ricinoleic acid-grafted CMCS (R-CMCS)	Insects	Feng and Peng (2012)
	Rotenone	*N*-(octadecanol-1-glycidyl ether)-*O*-sulfate chitosan (NOSCS)	Insects	Lao et al. (2010)
	CPF	CS-*co*-PLA-DPPE	Insects	Zhang et al. (2013)
	IMI	CS-*co*-PLA	Insects	Li et al. (2011)
Nanogels	*L. sidoides* oil	CS + cashew gum	Third-instar larvae of *S. aegypti* Ticks Mites	Abreu et al. (2012)
	Cu(II) ions	CS	*F. graminearum*	Brunel et al. (2013)
	Carum copticum (L.) essential oil	Miristic acid–chitosan (MA-CS)	*Sitophilus granarius* (L.)—the granary weevil *Tribolium confusum* Jacquelin du Val—a type of darkling beetle	Ziaee et al. (2014)
Nanofibers	(*Z*)-9-dodecenyl acetate pheromone	Polyamide 6 Cellulose acetate	European grape berry moth	Hellmann et al. (2011)
Polymeric chelate nanoparticles	Cu(II) ions	CS	*A. solani* *F. oxysporum*	Saharan et al. (2013, 2015)

3.2 Nanospheres

Unlike nanocapsules which are heterogenous reservoir type structures, nanospheres are homogenous monolithic system in which the bioactive ingredient is uniformly dispersed throughout the polymer matrix.

da Costa et al. (2014) have prepared Aza-loaded PCL nanospheres both as colloidal suspensions and as powders. The method used was the emulsion-solvent diffusion method which relies on the interfacial deposition of the polymer occurring as a consequence of the diffusion of a water miscible organic solvent from the oily phase into the aqueous phase. Powders were prepared from the colloidal suspension by freeze–drying and provide the best protection against UV light-induced degradation of the limonoid Aza in the neem product (da Costa et al., 2014).

Liu et al. (2008a) used the flash nanoprecipitation technique developed by Johnson and Prud'homme (Liu et al., 2008b) to prepare polymer-stabilized bifenthrin nanoparticles. In order to attain high supersaturation enabling subsequent rapid nucleation and growth of nanoparticles (flash nanoprecipitation), the authors used a multiinlet vortex mixer (MIVM) of a special design.

3.3 Micelles

Amphiphilic block copolymers self-assemble in water to form colloidal particles with a core–shell morphology called micelles. The self-assembly process is driven by the hydrophobic interactions developed on the formation of the hydrophobic micellar core which is surrounded by a hydrophilic shell or corona. However, aggregation occurs only after the concentration of the individual amphipathic molecules in solution exceeds a certain threshold concentration named the critical micellar concentration (CMC) and it is marked by an abrupt change in many physicochemical properties of the aqueous solution of the amphiphile. So, micelles are dynamic structures in the sense that if the amphiphile concentrations drops below CMC, then disassembly takes place.

There is no clean cut division between micelles and nanospheres prepared from amphiphilic block copolymers. That means that as the length of the hydrophobic block increases, the central hydrophobic core of the micelles becomes more dense resembling nanospheres.

Adak et al. (2012) prepared controlled-release formulations of IMI using amphiphilic copolymers, which self-assemble in aqueous media forming nanosized micellar aggregates. The amphiphilic copolymers were prepared reacting PEG of different molecular weights (300, 600, 1000) with various dicarboxylic acids (glutaric, adipic, pimelic, and suberic acids). The low CMC value ensures the stability of the aggregates to dilution which is very important from a practical point of view. As compared to commercial formulation, encapsulation of IMI in the aforementioned nanomicelles slows down pesticide diffusion resulting in slow and sustained

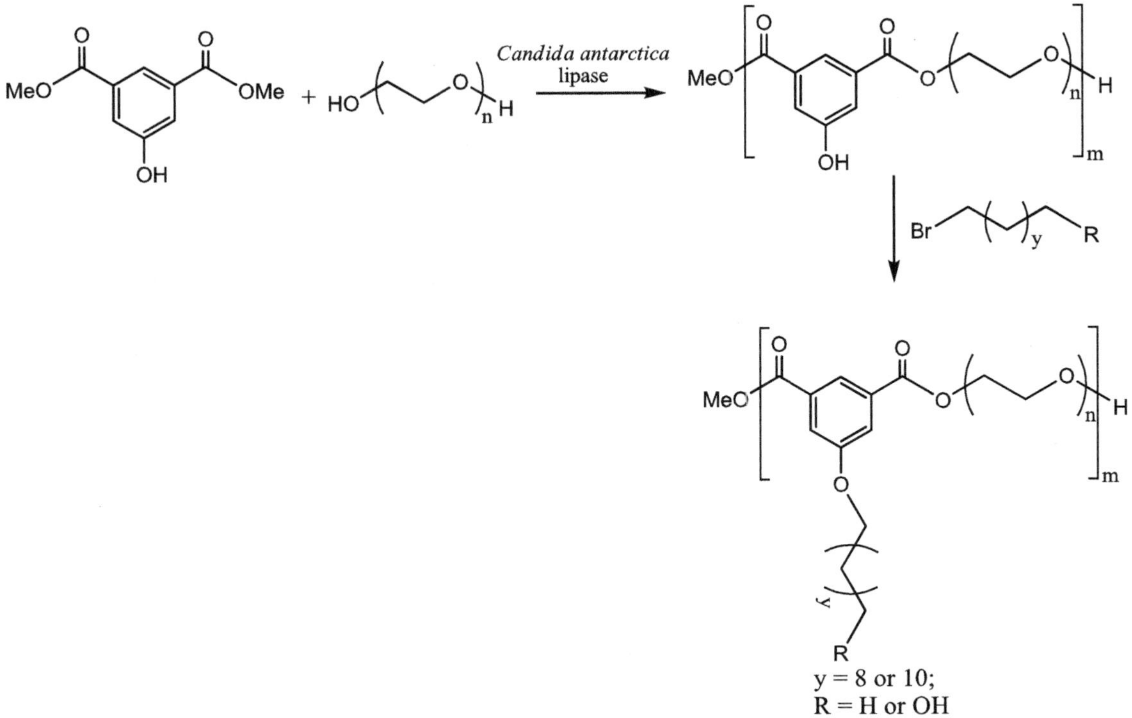

Figure 4.8. Synthesis of amphiphilic polyester copolymers for sustained delivery of carbofuran encapsulated in nano micelles (Shakil et al., 2010).

release. The time taken for 50% of the encapsulated IMI to be released ranged from 2.32 to 9.31 days.

In a similar approach, Shakil et al. (2010) have synthesized a series of amphiphilic polyester copolymers through the enzyme-catalyzed reaction between PEG of various molecular weights and 5-hydroxy-dimethylisophthalate as shown in Fig. 4.8. When placed in water these copolymers formed nanomicelles, which were used to encapsulate the systemic insecticide–nematicide carbofuran. The best results in terms of slow sustained–release performance were obtained for the copolymer prepared from PEG 1800 with $y = 8$, and R = H. Using the same type of nanocarrier, the authors have been able to prepare controlled release formulations of β-cyfluthrin, too (Loha et al., 2011).

Feng and Peng (2012) accomplished micellar solubilization of lipophilic Aza in water using an amphiphilic ricinoleic acid-grafted CMCS. The polymeric nanocarrier (R-CMCS) was prepared by reacting CMCS with ricinoleic anhydride (R). The nanocarrier was dissolved in deionized water of pH 6.8 and blended together with Aza to get the Aza/R-CMCS water dispersion. The loading efficiency was up to 56%. Aza/R-CMCS water dispersions provided better protection against Aza degradation than Aza sodium ricinoleate water/acetone suspensions. This was proved in outdoor tests by the higher residual Aza concentrations in the leaching liqiud of Aza/R-CMCS samples as compared to control groups.

Another type of CHI based polymeric micelles have been obtained by Lao et al. (2010). In order to render amphiphilic properties to CHI, the authors have grafted the hydrophobic octadecanol-1-glycidyl ether and the hydrophilic sulfate groups to the amino, and hydroxyl moieties of CHI, respectively. By the reaction sequence depicted in Fig. 4.9, they synthesized a novel amphipathic CHI derivative, that is, *N*-(octadecanol-1-glycidyl ether)-O-sulfate

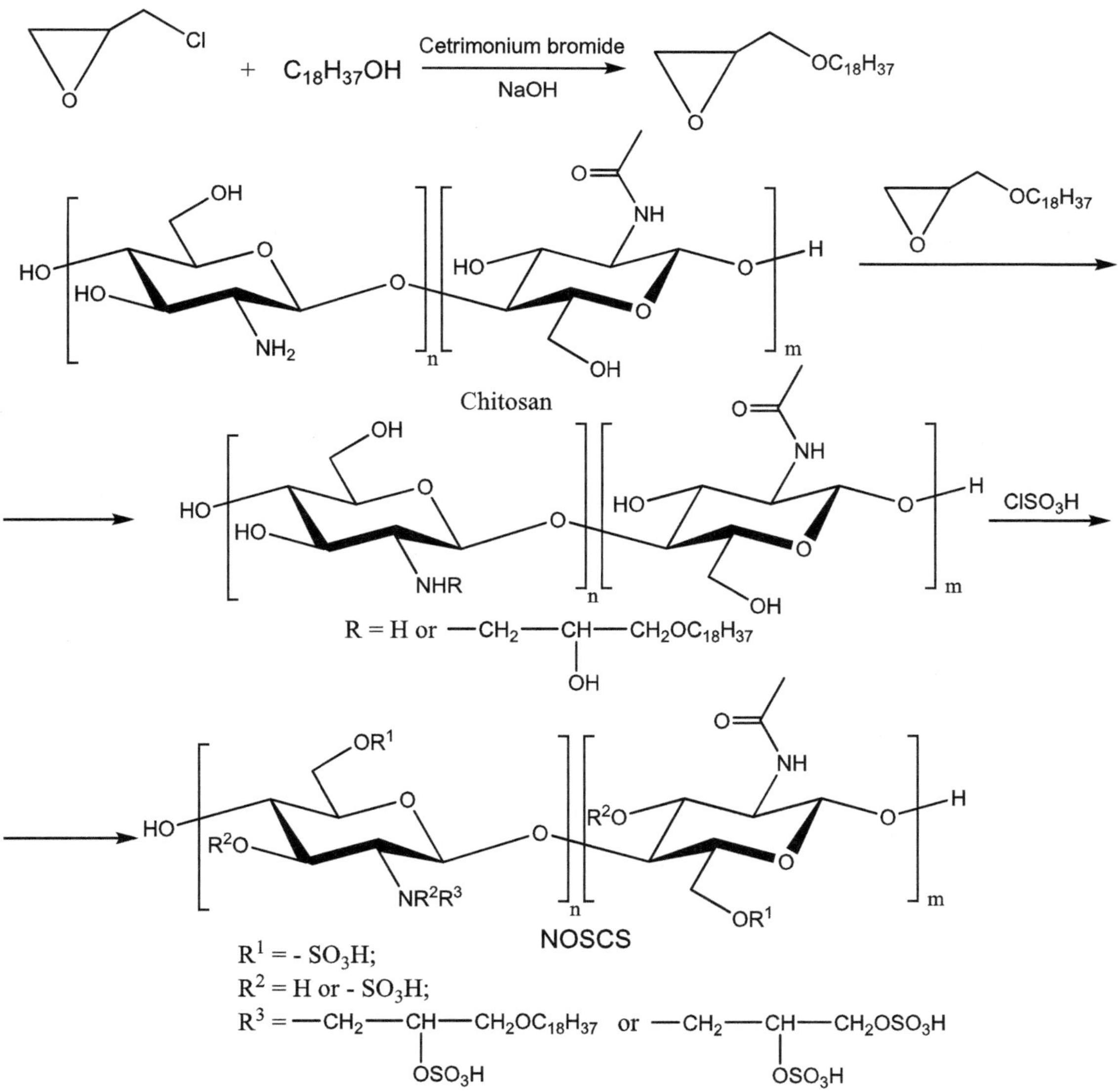

Figure 4.9. Synthesis of *N*-(octadecanol-1-glycidyl ether)-O-sulfate chitosan (NOSCS) (Lao et al., 2010).

chitosan (NOSCS) which underwent self-assembling in aqueous media to form polymeric micelles. The authors used the reverse micelle method to entrap the water insoluble natural insecticide rotenone into NOSCS micelle solutions. Briefly, NOSCS was added into a previously prepared acetone ethanol (1:1 v/v) solution of rotenone. Next, distilled water was added slowly drop by drop to the above solution under stirring. The organic solvents were evaporated at room temperature under stirring and the remaining aqueous solution was lyophilized. Using micellar solubilization, a 13,000-fold increase in the solubility of rotenone in water was obtained.

The group of Zhang et al. (2013) prepared a novel nanocarrier for delivery of the organophosphate insecticide CPF based on an amphiphilic copolymer of CHI with polylactide (PLA) and 1,2-dipalmitoyl-*sn*-glycero-3-phosphoethanolamine (DPPE). CHI oligomers were first prepared by oxidative degradation of CHI with hydrogen peroxide (Wu et al., 2005) and further used to synthesize the CHI–PLA graft copolymer, CS-*co*-PLA (Fig. 4.10). The authors adopted a grafting-from strategy using CS as a macroinitiator for the ring-opening polymerization of D,L-lactide in the presence of triethylamine (Wu et al., 2005). Next, the graft copolymer was activated as the *p*-nitrophenyl carbonate CS-*co*-PLA-pNP by treatment with *p*-nitrophenyl chloroformate (pNP). Eventually, upon treatment with DPPE, displacement of the good leaving group 4-nitrophenoxy by the DPPE moiety occurred yielding the final amphiphilic graft copolymer CS-*co*-PLA-DPPE. The loading of CPF was achieved by the use of two different encapsulation techniques, that is, nanoprecipitation and emulsion-solvent evaporation. In brief, in the nanoprecipitation approach, CPF and the amphiphilic copolymer were dissolved in acetone and the solution was injected dropwise into the aqueous phase under magnetic stirring. The organic solvent was evaporated and the nanoparticles harvested by centrifugation were eventually washed with deionized water (Govender et al., 1999). In the emulsion-solvent evaporation method, a methylene chloride solution of the amphiphilic copolymer and CPF was emulsified by sonication in an aqueous solution (1% w/v) of PVA. The organic solvent was evaporated under vacuum, the nanoparticles were collected by centrifugation, and washed with deionized water. The authors studied the effects of the CPF content and method of preparation on the size and controlled release performances of the fabricated nanocarriers. The size of the nanocarriers ranged from 132.2 to 282.6 nm and generally increased with the increase of the pesticide content. Moreover, nanoparticles prepared by emulsion-solvent evaporation method were generally larger (218.4–282.6 nm) than those obtained by nanoprecipitation (132.2–180.9 nm). The

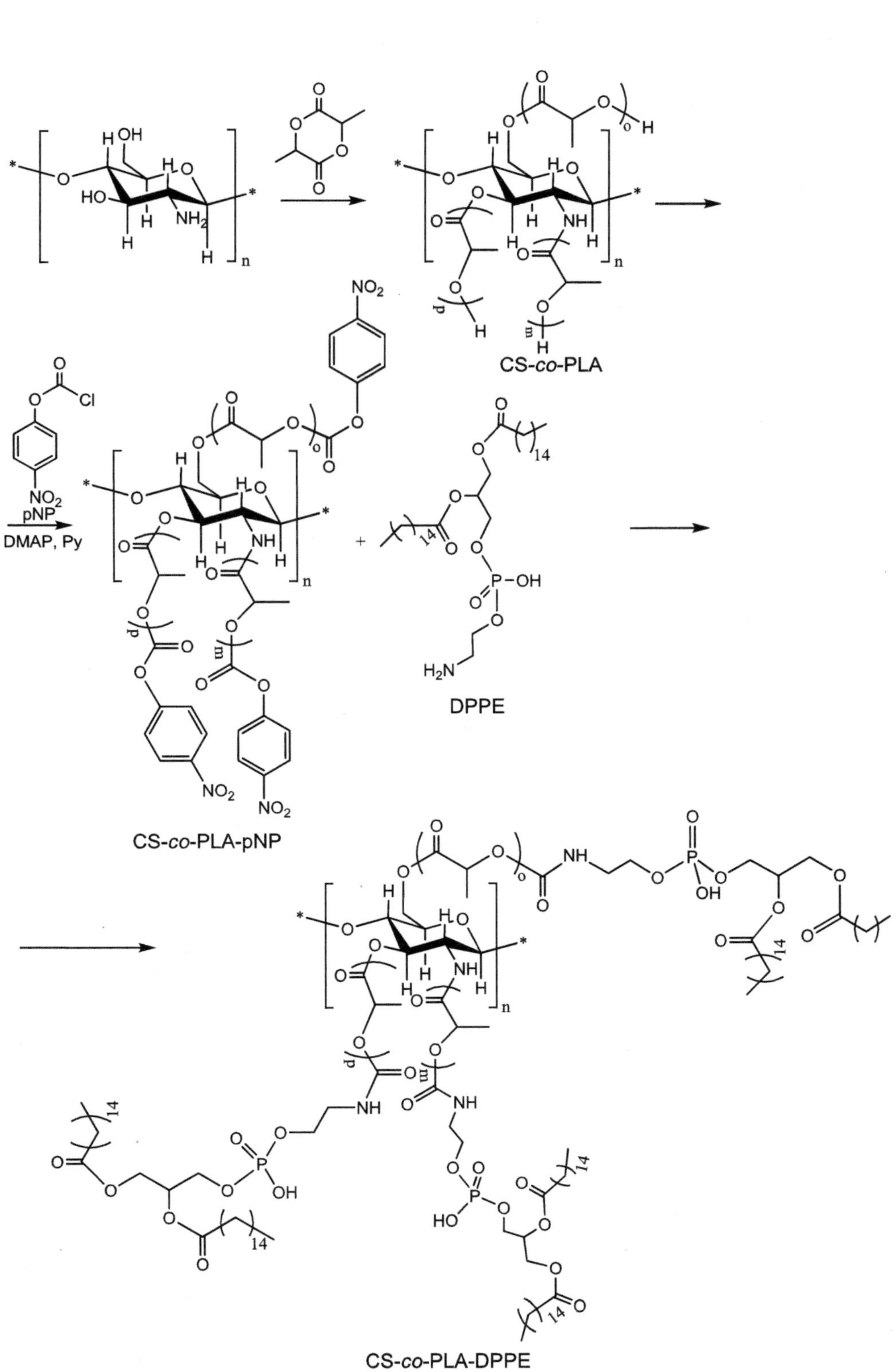

Figure 4.10. Synthetic pathways to the amphiphilic graft copolymers CS-*co*-PLA and CS-*co*-PLA-DPPE.

prepared CS-*co*-PLA-DPPE micelles exhibited good steric stability in vitro and slowed down the pesticide release rate. Controlled release studies carried out at various copolymer/CPF mass ratios (5:1, 10:1, 50:1, and 100:1) revealed that decreasing the pesticide content the release rate increased, that is, the highest release rate was obtained at the copolymer/CPF mass ratio 100:1, while the lowest release ratio at a copolymer/CPF mass ratio of 5:1. The authors gave the following explanation: the highest the content of hydrophobic CPF, the stronger the hydrophobic interactions between the pesticide and the copolymer and the lower the release rate. Controlled release formulations of the neonicotinoid insecticide IMI were developed by the same research group based on the amphiphilic graft copolymer CS-*co*-PLA (Li et al., 2011).

3.4 Nanogels

The term "nanogel" usually defines water-swollen nanosized polymeric networks consisting of either physically or chemically cross-linked hydrophilic or amphiphilic polymer chains that can swell but do not dissolve in water (Kabanov and Vinogradov, 2009).

Abreu et al. (2012) prepared *Lippia sidoides* oil-loaded nanogels based on CHI and cashew gum. Solutions of 1, 5, and 10% (w/v) cashew gum in deionized water were prepared and added to CHI dissolved in 1% aqueous acetic acid by means of a peristaltic pump. Thereby, polymer complexes of gum:CHI were prepared at various gum:CHI ratios, that is, 1:10, 1:2, 1:1, 2:1, and 10:1. Separately, an O/W emulsion of *L. sidoides* oil was prepared using Tween 80 as emulsifier. The latter emulsion was slowly added to the polymer complexes. Two different polymer matrix:oil ratios were used that is, 10:1, and 10:2 (w/w), respectively. Gum:CHI nanogels were eventually obtained by the spray–drying of the turbid solution. The authors studied the effects of gum:CHI composition, the cashew gum concentration and the matrix:oil relative content on various important characteristics of the prepared nanogel particles, such as size, loading capacity, encapsulation efficiency, and sustained-release features. Nanogel nanoparticles prepared exhibited positive zeta potential values and sizes ranging from 335 to 558 nm. Increasing of the CHI content in the polymer matrix resulted in nanoparticles of larger sizes probably due to the increased electrostatic repulsion between the positively charged amino groups in the CHI chains. Nanoparticles prepared from 5% cashew gum solution at a ratio gum:CHI of 1:1 showed the highest loading capacity (11.8%) and an encapsulation efficiency of 70%. In vitro release studies revealed prolonged-release of the encapsulated oil. Bioassays performed with third-instar larvae of

Stegomyia aegypti showed 87% mortality after 48 h, the mortality reaching over 90% after 72 h.

In order to control microbial growth, Brunel et al. (2013) produced pure CHI nanogels which were further loaded with Cu(II) ions to nicely exploit the synergistic effect between CHI and cooper for treating a devastating disease of wheat and cereal grains produced by the pathogenic microorganism *Fusarium graminearum*. CHI nanogels were prepared by an original method previously developed by the same author which is a purely physical gelation process occurring in reverse emulsion characterized by the absence of any cross-linker (Brunel et al., 2008). The formation of physical CHI hydrogel is based on the decreasing of CHI solubility in the medium by enhancing chain–chain interactions at the expense of chain–solvent interactions. CHI solubility can be reduced by decreasing repulsive electrostatic interactions between the polymer chains, or in other words by reducing the charge density of the polyelectrolyte. Another necessary condition for a network to be formed is an initial polymer concentration above the chain entanglement concentration. In brief, CHI oligomers with a degree of acetylation ≤30% were solubilized in water by adding a stoichiometric amount of acetic acid with respect to the free amino moieties. Then, this solution was emulsified by sonication in Miglyol 812N containing the low HLB surfactant Span 80 (sorbitan monooleate). After 5 min of ultrasound treatment, physical gelation was induced by passing of an ammonia stream until the medium pH was increased up to 9. Eventually, nanogel nanoparticles were separated from the supernatant through centrifugation, washed twice with ethanol and twice with water, and redispersed in ammonium acetate buffer. Copper (II) complexation occurred on mixing copper acetate solutions of various concentrations with the CHI nanogel suspension in ammonium acetate/acetic acid solution. The ionization degree of CHI which depends on pH critically influenced the amount of copper (II) ions loaded on CHI nanogels. The maximum adsorption capacity was obtained at pH 5.5. Lowering pH resulted in decomplexation of adsorbed Cu(II) ions due to protonation of free amino groups. To estimate the biological activity, the growth rates of the fungus *F. graminearum* in the presence of these copper-loaded CHI nanogels were evaluated. An interesting synergistic effect was revealed as the minimum inhibitory concentration (MIC) value for Cu (II) ions was reduced by a factor of 3 or 17, in the presence of CHI in dispersion or solution. These copper-based biopesticides exhibit a series of great advantages: (1) high Cu (II)-loading capacity; (2) acidification as produced by a growing pathogen triggers Cu (II) ions release from the nanocarrier; (3) the CHI nanogels is biodegradable by the

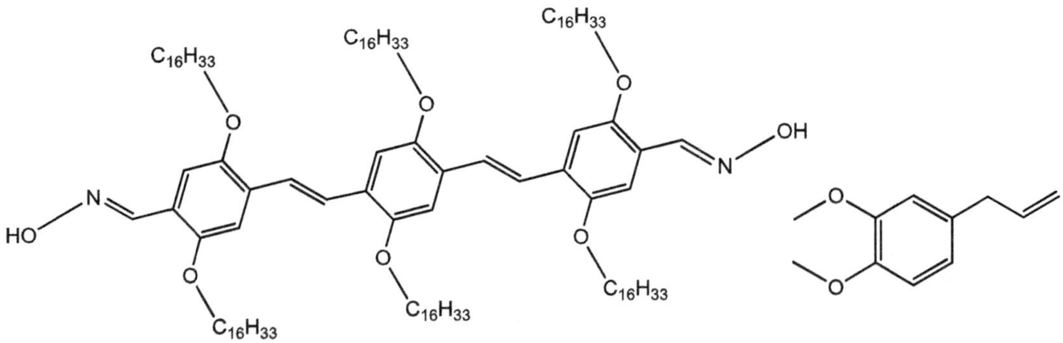

all-*trans*-tri(*p*-phenylenevinylene)bis-aldoxime   Methyl eugenol (ME)

Figure 4.11. Chemical structures of the low molecular mass gelator (LMMG) all-*trans* tri(*p*-phenylenevinylene)bis-aldoxime and of the methyl eugenol (ME) pheromone.

chitosanolytic enzymes of pathogenic fungi resulting in complete release of Cu (II) ions, and (4) synergistic effect of CHI and copper against the phytopathogenic fungus *F. graminearum*.

Bhagat et al. (2013) developed a very simple and environmentally friendly method to control the population of *Bactrocera dorsalis*, a harmful fruits pest. They used a nanogel containing the pheromone methyl eugenol (ME) as a bait trap. Preparation of the pheromone nanogel is quite simple. The authors used a low molecular mass gelator (LMMG) that is all-*trans* tri(*p*-phenylenevinylene)bis-aldoxime (Fig. 4.11) which has the ability to induce gelation of specific solvents through a self-assembly process driven by weak intermolecular noncovalent interactions, such as π–π stacking, van der Waals forces and hydrogen bonding. The pheromone itself was used by the authors as a solvent. All-*trans* tri(*p*-phenylenevinylene)bis-aldoxime was dissolved in warm ME (65°C) at a concentration of 2.5 mg/mL. At this temperature, the pheromone was stable. By simply cooling at room temperature, the initial solution turned into a viscous gel. As one can see, the procedure for ME immobilization in the nanogel is quite simple without any need for organic solvents or cross-linking agents. The gel–sol transition temperature (T_{gel}) increased with the concentration of the gelator and at a concentration of 12 mg/mL it was determined to be as high as 63°C. Hence, the thermal stability of the nanogel makes it suitable for on field application even in hot climates. Moreover, the gel exhibited good rheological properties and mechanical stability. The nanogel protected the immobilized ME against thermal or photochemical decomposition as it has been experimentally proved in a several-weeks-lasting open orchard trial. The authors also proved that through immobilization in the nanogel, the release rate of the volatile ME pheromone significantly decreased thereby prolonging the period over which the pheromone remains effective. For instance, the number of insects that were caught in the control trap containing ME alone steadily decreases over the first week and from the 8th day onward *B. dorsalis* flies were no longer attracted to the trap. However, the trap containing the pheromone immobilized in the nanogel remained active up to 3 weeks. As the nanogel of pheromone ME is water insoluble, it could be utilize also in the rainy season when the pest *B. dorsalis* exhibits maximum activity.

3.5 Nanofibers

Electrospun nanofibers loaded with the pheromone (*Z*)-9-dodecenyl acetate were prepared by Hellmann et al. (2011). The spinning solution contained the pheromone in various concentrations along with the polymer matrix. Taking into account their different biodegradability features and mechanical properties, the authors have chosen polyamide 6 and cellulose acetate, respectively, as polymeric matrices. In one approach, polyamide 6 was used due to its high stiffness which prevents mechanical rupture or chemical decomposition which might result in formation of shorter nanorods that could enter the body for instance through inhalation and cause health problems. Obviously, this advantage comes at the cost of a longer persistence of the polymer in the fields. A pheromone loading of 20% could be achieved for electrospun polyamide 6 nanofibers. The fibers diameters were in the range from 200 to 400 nm. The pheromone was phase separated in the fibers as revealed by transmission electron microscopy (TEM). In the second approach, the bio-based cellulose acetate was used as the polymer matrix. This polymer has the advantage of a higher loading capacity up to 33.3%. Fibers with a large size distribution (100 nm^{-1} μm) were obtained. The disadvantage is the poor mechanical strength. Hence, short nanorods formed by nanofibers disruption could pose some health risks. Thermogravimetric analysis (TGA) experiments were performed on pheromone containing electrospun nanowovens that were stored in containers at room temperature for various predetermined time periods. The results of the previous experiments showed a continuous loss of the pheromone from the both used polymeric matrices meaning that the pheromone is released continuously. However, these "in vitro" studies could not reveal the effect of various environmental factors, such as winds and rains and further on field studies are required. The authors suggested that such electrospun nanofibers could be distributed across the field to be protected very similar to spider webs, thereby ensuring an uniform release of pheromones.

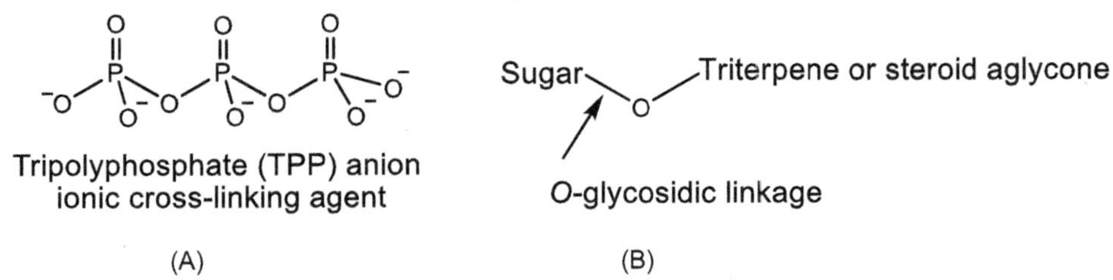

Figure 4.12. (A) Chemical structure of the TPP anion; (B) general structure of saponins.

3.6 Polymeric Chelate Nanoparticles

The group of Saharan used CHI as an effective Cu(II) ionic chelating agent (Saharan et al., 2013, 2015). First, they prepared CHI nanoparticles by ionic gelation using the tripolyphosphate anion (TPP; Fig. 4.12) as cross-linking agent. Briefly, low molecular weight CHI with a degree of deacetylation of 80% was dissolved in 1% acetic acid (w/v) at a concentration of 0.1% and into the above solution an equal volume of an 1% (w/v) solution of TPP in ultrapure water was added under vigorously magnetic stirring. Before complete gelation has occurred, a solution of $CuSO_4$ (0.01%) was introduced into the mixture and stirring was continued. The pellets were separated from the liquid by ultracentrifugation and resuspended in ultrapure water followed by ultrasonication. After three cycles of centrifugation–ultrasonication, the solid nanoformulation was lyophilized (Saharan et al., 2013). The antifungal activity was estimated in earthen pot experiments carried out in a net house under natural conditions of light and temperature (Saharan et al., 2015). Twenty-day old healthy tomato seedlings with four to six true leaves were transferred in pots filled with surface soil. The whole aerial part of the tomato seedlings were sprayed with an aqueous suspension of viable spores of *Alternaria solani*, a fungus that cause the tomato and potato plants disease called early blight. To create the high humidity conditions required for fungal growth, the plants were kept covered with transparent plastic bags for the first two days. At day 4 after inoculation, equal volumes of aqueous suspensions of Cu—CHI nanoparticles of different concentrations (0.08, 0.1, and 0.12%) were uniformly sprayed on the leaves of each plant. Similarly, tomato plants were artificially inoculated with *Fusarium oxysporum* by drenching the soil around the root collar region with an aqueous spore suspension of the fungus. During the first two days after inoculation, the plants were covered with transparent plastic bags to sustain humidity. At day 3, aqueous dispersions of Cu–CHI nanoparticles of various concentrations (0.08, 0.1, and 0.12%) were uniformly applied to the soil near the root zone. The disease extent was evaluated one week after the treatment. In the case of early blight disease, plants treated with Cu–CHI nanoparticles exhibited only isolated black or brown leaf lesions measuring 1–2 mm in size, while in control plants (water treatment) lesions merged covering large portions of the leaves. The disease severity was assessed using the formula given by Chester (1959) and Wheeler (1969) resulting in a calculated disease severity of 55% for the control group as compared with a degree severity of only 6.6% for the plants treated with the aqueous Cu–CHI nanoparticles dispersion at a concentration of 0.12%. These data translate into a percentage of disease control (PEDC) of 87.7%. The control group of plants that were infected with *F. oxysporum* showed obvious signs of the blockage of the plant vascular tissue resulting in yellowing and wilting. The calculated disease severity was 66.6%. By applying the treatment with Cu–CHI nanoparticles, the disease severity was cut down by half. In *Fusarium* wilt, a PEDC of 61.1% was found in plants treated with 0.12% (w/v) aqueous dispersion of Cu–CHI nanoparticles. The authors suggested that the positive zeta potential of Cu–CHI nanoparticles (+22.6 mV) is responsible for both the stability and the higher antifungal activity of the above nanoparticles as a consequence of their enhanced interaction with the negatively charged biological membranes. Relying on the known ability of the CHI biopolymer to effectively elicit plant defense mechanisms, the authors also launched the hypothesis of a synergistic effect between activation of defense enzymes by CHI and release of the incorporated Cu(II) ions. Organic acids secreted by the fungi cause a local pH drop at the place of infection resulting in protonation of the free amino groups in the CHI chains followed by release of Cu^{2+} ions with antifungal properties. Moreover, the Cu–CHI nanoparticles prepared by this group are nontoxic exhibiting no inhibitory effects on the growth of tomato seedlings.

The same authors conducted a research studies aiming to increase the antifungal activity of CHI by incorporation at the nanoscale level of the natural plant defense compounds saponins (Saharan et al., 2013). Using very similar methods to those described above, they prepared CHI-saponin nanoparticles. Saponins are high-molecular-weight glycosides consisting of a hydrophobic triterpene or steroid aglycone attached to a hydrophilic sugar moiety through a glycosidic ether bond (Fig. 4.12). Due to this amphiphilic structure, they are able to disrupt cell membranes and many of them exhibit antifungal properties (Lanzotti et al., 2012a, 2012b). The antifungal activity of the CHI-saponin nanoparticles against *Alternaria alternata* was evaluated by an in vitro bioassay using the spore germination method. The

CHI-saponin nanoparticles at 0.1% concentration showed an inhibitory effect of 82.9% on spore germination of *A. alternata*. However, this result was poorer by comparison to CHI nanoparticles (87.1% inhibition rate) and to Cu–CHI nanoparticles (87.4% inhibition rate) proving that CHI-saponin nanoparticles were less effective against spore germination of *A. alternata*.

The polymer-based nanopesticides are summarized in Table 4.1.

4 Lipid-Based Nanopesticide Delivery Systems

4.1 Nanoliposomes

Nanoliposomes are vesicular structures consisting of a phospolipid bilayer enclosing an internal aqueous cavity at the nanoscale level. When placed in water amphiphilic phospholipids undergo a self-organization process forming a bilayer membrane. During this process, the hydrophobic tails of phospholipid molecules approach each other becoming tightly packed in a parallel alignment within the bilayer and squeezing out water molecules from this region, while the polar heads of the phospholipid molecules are positioned at the margins of the supramolecular aggregate being in contact with the surrounding polar water molecules. With the aid of an energy input, these flat membranes can be converted into nanoparticulate delivery systems with a bilayer vesicular morphology (nanoliposomes). The methods to produce liposomes can be divided in two main categories: mechanical and nonmechanical. Mechanical methods include sonication/ultrasonication, high-pressure homogenization (HPH), extrusion, microfluidization, colloid mill, and others. From the nonmechanical methods, we mention here reversed-phase evaporation and depletion of mixed detergent–lipid micelles (Nuruzzaman et al., 2016). The fluidity of the lipid bilayer can be modulated by incorporation into the phospholipid membrane of cholesterol which prevents crystallization of the acyl chains of phospholipids and enhances the shape stability of nanoliposomes. However, long-term storage of these nanocarriers is problematic because of the physical and chemical instabilities of liposomes in aqueous dispersions. The most used method to prolong shelf-life of nanoliposomes is lyophilization (Chen et al., 2010). In this case, measures have to be taken in order to preserve membrane integrity during lyophilization. The main destabilizing factors are the following ones: the lipid bilayer can be damaged by the ice crystals formed during freezing, dehydrated vesicles are prone to fusion, and phase transition can occur during rehydration. Therefore, one has to use lypoprotectants to protect lipid bilayers during lyophilization. Disaccharides like trehalose are among the most effective lypoprotectants (Chen et al., 2010).

Bang et al. (2009) encapsulated the insecticide etofenprox into liposomes prepared from phosphatidylcholine used as an amphiphilic compound and chlolesterol used as a shape stabilizer. The liposomes were prepared by ultrasonic homogenization (UH). Their size could be reduced up to 150 nm by increasing the lecithin ratio and extending homogenization time (2–6 min). Moreover, the zeta potential could be modulated by further coating of nanoliposomes. When CHI (molecular weight 30.000 Da) was used as a first coating the zeta potential was +10.3 mV and it was changed to a negative value of −21.8 mV by coating with a second layer of ALG. The same authors prepared CHI-coated nanoliposomes by UH technique and a combination of UH and electrospraying (Bang et al., 2011) and studied the effect of the ratio and molecular weight of the coating material on the size of the prepared nanocarrier systems (Hwang et al., 2011).

4.2 Solid Lipid Nanoparticles

SLNs are composed of a high melting point lipid matrix with spherical morphology and size ranging from 40 to 1000 nm, the fat particles being dispersed in an aqueous phase. Surfactants are used to stabilize the dispersion. There are several formulation techniques for the production of SLNs, such as: HPH, emulsification–sonification, microemulsion, solvent emulsification–evaporation, solvent diffusion, solvent injection, and double emulsion W/O/W which is particularly suited for the production of SLNs loaded with hydrophilic pesticides (Das and Chaudhury, 2011).

From the aforementioned preparation techniques, the most used one is HPH which can be accomplished using either hot or cold temperatures. In the hot HPH, the pesticide is dissolved or homogenously dispersed in the melted lipid phase at a temperature 5–10°C higher than the melting point of the lipid(s). Then the aqueous phase containing the surfactant is heated (at the same temperature) and subsequently added to the pesticide-lipid melt. The resulted mixture is homogenized with the aid of a high shear mixing device to obtain a hot preemulsion which is further subjected to a high-pressure homogenizer at the same temperature. The homogenization process is repeated as many times as is deemed necessary until a nanoemulsion of the desired average particle size is eventually obtained. The final nanoemulsion is cooled to room temperature when the lipid droplets recrystallize forming lipid nanoparticles with solid matrix. In the cold HPH, one proceeds similarly by dissolving or dispersing the pesticide in the melted lipid(s). However, the pesticide-lipid melt is suddenly cooled by means of liquid nitrogen or dry ice and subsequently milled using a ball mill or mortar. The resulted microparticles are suspended in the cold aqueous surfactant solution and subjected to HPH below the room temperature to form lipid nanoparticles.

In the solvent emulsification–evaporation technique, the lipid(s) dissolved in a water immiscible organic solvent are emulsified in the aqueous phase containing the surfactant. The organic solvent is subsequently evaporated resulting in lipid precipitation.

Aiming to develop new eco-friendly pesticide products, Lai et al. (2006) have incorporated *Artemisia arborescens* L. essential oil into SLNs. *A. arborescens* L. essential oil was proved to exhibit pesticidal activity against *Aphis gossipy* (a pest of citrus fruits), adult and young *Bemisia tabaci* (sweet potato whitefly), and *Lymantria dispar* L. (pest of *Quercus suber*). The authors adopted the hot HPH method to prepare *A. arborescens* L. essential oil-loaded SLNs. Briefly, the essential oil was dissolved in melted Compritol 888 ATO (a mixture of mono-, di-, and triglycerides) at 85°C and the lipid phase was next dispersed in the hot aqueous phase containing either Poloxamer 188 (SLN 1) or Miranol Ultra C32 (sodium cocoamphoacetate) (SLN 2) as surfactants. The mixture was vigorously stirred for 1 min at 8000 rpm and the preemulsion was homogenized at high pressure (3 cycles, 500 bar). The encapsulation efficiencies were 87% for SLN 1 and 92% for SLN 2, respectively. Both SLN formulations loaded with *A. arborescens* L essential oil showed high physical stability, in particular the average diameters of the SLNs did not change during storing for 2 months at various temperatures and increased only slightly after spraying the SLN dispersions over the plants. In vitro release studies highlighted the capability of SLN formulations to prevent rapid evaporation of the essential oil AI and to release it in a controlled manner. The comparison was made with aqueous emulsion formulations prepared at the same concentrations of the AI and using the same surfactants, that is, Poloxamer 188 for EMU 1 and Miranol Ultra C32 for EMU 2, respectively. Both emulsion formulations exhibited a burst effect, with a loss of 21.6% of the total essential oil for EMU 1, and of 13.52% for EMU 2, respectively, after 1 h. By contrary, both SLN formulations showed no burst effect. After 48 h, the cumulative release was 37.07% and 45.51% for SLN 1 and SLN 2, respectively, as compared to 69.56% for EMU 1 and 80.77% for EMU 2, respectively.

Campos et al. (2015) have prepared SLNs loaded with the fungicides carbendazim (MBC) and tebuconazole (TBZ) using the emulsification-solvent evaporation technique. In brief, glyceryl tripalmitate and equal amounts of the AIs MBC and TBZ were dissolved in the water immiscible organic solvent chloroform. Separately, an aqueous solution of the hydrophilic emulsifier PVA was prepared. The lipid phase was emulsified into the aqueous phase by sonication for 4 min. Then, the resulted preemulsion was further homogenized by vigorous stirring at 1400 rpm for 7 min. By rotary evaporation of the organic solvent, followed by concentration to a final volume of 10 mL, SLNs loaded with MBC and TBZ at a concentration level of 1% (w/v) were obtained. The fungicides-loaded SLNs showed an average hydrodynamic diameter of 317.6 ± 2.7 nm as revealed by the nanoparticle tracking analysis (NTA) and this value remained unchanged over 120 days. Consequently, the SLNs were quite stable with no tendency to aggregation. The polydispersity index (PDI) exceeded 0.2. The encapsulation efficiency was higher than 99%. Release studies were performed in tube systems, by putting the SLNs in contact with deionized water in order to release the fungicide payload. The fastest release rate was observed during the first 5 h; afterward the release rate slowed down. TBZ was released faster as compared to MBC. However, after 6 days only 30% of the MBC, and 51% of the TBZ were released. The slow release is a beneficial feature because futile use of excessive pesticide amounts can be avoided since the concentration of the AI can be adjusted to the minimum effective concentration as a function of time and it can be maintained in the field within the range of biological effectiveness concentrations. Moreover, leaching of the AI that could affect nontarget organism is reduced. For instance, after nine washes only 4.8% of the encapsulated MBC was released from SLN as compared to 17% release from commercial formulation. The cytotoxicity of the nanoformulation was evaluated in vitro through a cell viability assay, that is, the reduction of 3(4–5 dimethylthiazol-2-yl)-2,5-diphenyltetrazolium bromide (MTT). To this end, three different cell types (two normal and one cancerous cell lines) namely preosteoblast (MC3T3-E1), fibroblast (Balb/c 3T3), and, respectively, adenocarcinoma (HeLa) cell lines were used. For normal cells, the MTT assay revealed a significantly lower cytotoxicity of SLN formulations as compared to commercial formulations. In the case of HeLa cells, the cytotoxicity of fungicides-loaded SLNs was higher than that of commercial formulations and this was due to the enhanced cellular uptake of the SLN formulations corroborated with the known ability of MBC to inhibit proliferation of human cancer cells. The authors also tested the effect of the SLN encapsulating fungicides on plant emergence using *Phaseolus vulgaris* seeds. The germination index of seeds was unaffected neither by nanoparticle formulations nor by commercial product. However, in the case of emergence, there was a decrease in the fresh weights of roots and shoots after treatment with nanoformulations of different concentrations. The higher the concentration of the AI, the stronger the effect. The authors concluded that these lipid-based nanoformulations provide new prevention and treatment options for fungal diseases in plants.

5 Noanosized Metals and Metal Oxides

Metal and metal oxides nanoparticles have grown in interest due to their versatility and emerging applications in various domains from medicine (hyperthermia, drug delivery capabilities, biofilm formation prevention) to environmental protection (water treatment, soil treatment) and agricultural applications (nanopesticides, fertilizers). The advantages these particles have to offer are obvious, arising from the huge surface to volume ratio when compared to microparticles or to traditional formulations.

A rather unique and innovative approach was used by the group of Sooresh et al. (2011) to create nanovectors for insect control. The nanomaterial this group chose to use consists of silver core nanoparticles and a deltamethrin shell, the deposition of the deltamethrin on the surface of the silver nanoparticles highly increasing its potency. This type of conjugated system also has another benefit, the fact that it allows tracking of the product in the insect subsystems, such as the hemolymph. The tracking can be achieved via metal detection, thus the deltamethrine content can be traced via the corresponding metal content found. This is an important achievement because it allows a better understanding over the processes that occur in the insect and eventual development of new pest control methods.

The use of silver nanoparticles in order to create a nanoformulation for the agricultural delivery of the pyrethroid insecticide cyhalothrin has been explored by the group of Abouelkassem et al. (2016) in order to increase the potency and the delivery efficiency. The required concentration in order to obtain the desired effect was, as the group reported, decreased by 100 times compared to the pesticide in its native formulation. The main problems solved by the nanoformulation are the hydrophobicity, which limits the effectiveness in water solutions and promotes the use of other harmfull organic solvent for the dispersion and the high dosage required in order for this pesticide to have the desired effect against mosquito larva. The LC_{50} drops from 4.134 to 0.031 mg/L in the case of the nanoformulated pesticide. The issue still remains whether the nanoparticles are more harmfull in the environment than the pesticides, hence the cautious attitude of the scientific community toward the large scale use of nanoparticles or nano-formulated systems based on silver.

In a very similar approach to that already discussed in Section 3.2 (Guan et al., 2008), Guan et al. (2011) applied the layer-by-layer self-assembly of biocompatible polyelectrolytes to prepare novel photodegradable W/TiO_2/Av nanocomposites. This type of delivery system could alleviate the concern caused by the general use of pesticides in any ecosystem, a harmful chemical that undergoes photochemical self-decomposition to inoffensive substances after the usage cycle has completed becoming attractive even for those users that are more preoccupied with traditional agricultural habits which usually yield a lower production.

6 Porous Silica Nanoparticles

Silica nanoparticles are another type of simple, efficient and easy to use delivery system, being widely used in a variety of applications. Sustained release of pesticides aims to enhance efficacy and simultaneously to reduce the dose required to achieve the desired effect.

The group of Wibowo et al. (2014) used biocompatible silica nanocapsules in order to safely deliver fipronil in a sustained release fashion. The authors developed a novel oil-in-water nano-emulsion technique to produce oil-core silica–shell nanocapsules with tailored shell thickness through an eco-friendly, biomimetic dual-templating approach. The group synthesized and tested three different shell thicknesses. The results were very promicing, and the group demonstrated that the increase in shell thickness further restricts the diffusional pathways in the nanocapsule, resulting in a slower release, result which was to be expected considering a diffusional release mechanism. The in vitro release studies showed a 40.7, 24.3, and 15.2% release after 142 h from the nanocapsule with 8, 25, and 44 nm, respectively. The in vivo studies showed 100% termite mortality in 6 days.

Nanosized silica was the main thread followed by the group of Prado et al. (2011) in their attempt to developed a better, nanosized, delivery vector for any type of herbicide. Picloram was the herbicide used by this group as a model, but the results were promising and the group postulated the potential use for other herbicides as well. The novelty of this study is the introduction of suitable functional groups that can act as anchor points for pesticide attachment. A new silylating agent bearing pendant carboxyl groups was synthesized by reacting 3-aminopropyltrimethoxysilane with chloroacetic acid. Next, the new silylating agent and tetraethoxysilane (TEOS) were polymerized in water using *n*-dodecylamine as a template. Eventual extraction of the template by an ethanol reflux resulted in the formation of a hexagonal mesoporous silica network with carboxyl anchoring groups. Controlled release studies revealed that this new carboxyl-modified mesoporous silica nanocarrier has the ability to delay the release of the herbicide. Only 17.31% of the total amount of immobilized picloram was released after 7 days and the slow and sustained release profile was maintained up to 30 days. To conclude, by pesticide anchoring the effectiveness increased and, at the same time, losses by leaching were decreased. Moreover, unlike conventional pesticides, which are easily transported in soil, the mobility of the herbicide anchored on the modified silica surface has to decrease due to the known ability of clay to act as a binder agent for silica.

The same strategy of surface chemical functionalization was used by Qin et al. (2016) to graft a natural proteic biopesticide, that is, the *Bacillus thuringiensis* chitinase (Chi9602) enzyme, onto the surface of the silica nanocarrier. The enzyme was immobilized by means of either electrostatic adsorption or covalent cross-linking through amide bond or base Schiff formation. To this purpose, the authors prepared several types of silica nanoparticles (SNP) modified with amino, carboxyl, and formyl functional groups on the outer surface. They started with unmodified hydroxylated nano SiO_2 (silica nanoparticles SNP1). SNP1 were first functionalized with amino groups by treatment with (3-aminopropyl)triethoxysilane (APTES) when the silica nanoparticles denoted as SNP2 were obtained. SNP2 were further used as a starting material for the preparation of both carboxyl-modified silica nanoparticles (SNP3) and formyl-modified silica nanoparticles (SNP4). The amino surface groups of SNP2 were converted to carboxyl groups by treatment with succinic anhydride, and to formyl groups by reaction with glutaraldehyde, respectively. SNP1, SNP2, and SNP3 were used for electrostatic immobilization of the chitinase, while the enzyme was covalently attached to SNP3 and SNP4 through amide bond, and, respectively, Schiff base formation. The best results were obtained with the chitinase electrostatically adsorbed on the surface of SNP2. These silica nanoparticles exhibited the highest enzyme immobilization rate (80.2%) and, at the same time, the highest residual enzyme activity (94.1%). Bioassays showed that immobilization onto the silica nanocarrier SNP2 resulted in a synergistic enhancement of the nematicidal activity of the chitinase against *Caenorhabditis elegans* N2. Both the LC_{50} and the time required for the dosage to be effective have been significantly reduced.

Wen et al. (2005) fabricated porous hollow silica naoparticles (PHSNs) by a sol–gel process using calcium carbonate nanoparticles as a sacrificial template and sodium silicate as silica source. Briefly, an aqueous solution of sodium silicate was added dropwise under stirring to a heated (80°C) suspension of calcium carbonate containing the surfactant cetyltrimethylammonium bromide (CTAB). The pH was adjusted to 9–10 by addition of hydrochloric acid. After cooling, filtration, rinsing with deionized water and air calcination at 700°C a porous core–shell nanocomposite material with calcium carbonate core and silica shell was obtained. Removal of the calcium carbonate template by treatment with hydrochloric acid eventually yielded PHSNs. The size of the hollow center was about 70 nm, the outer diameter was approximately 100 nm, while the pores in the walls had a diameter of 4–5 nm with a narrow pore-size distribution as determined by TEM and nitrogen adsorption–desorption analyses, respectively. Next, the synthesized PHSNs were immersed into an acetone solution of Av (weight ratio Av:PHSNS = 4:1) at room temperature and normal pressure for a period of 14 days. After removal of the unencapsulated Av by washing with ethanol, the powders were dried. This simple loading technique afforded 58.3 (w/w) percent encapsulation as determined by TGA. The controlled release assays revealed a multistage release behavior, which meets the requirements of a sustained release profile. After an initial burst effect caused by the fast desorption of surface adsorbed Av the release rate slowed down which was ascribed to the slow diffusion of Av from the hollow core and the pores of the nanomaterial. The loading capacity plays an important role in nanocarrier performance and efficiency since a higher loading capacity allows the amount of nanocarrier required to encapsulate a particular amount of AI to be reduced. The loading method used by the authors, that is, simple immersion took 2 weeks to reach the adsorption saturation for Av because of the difficulties the pesticide molecules face in penetrating the tiny nanosized pore channels in the shell of PHSNs. To reduce the loading time without affecting the encapsulated amount, the authors used another loading technique, that is, the supercritical fluids technology, to encapsulate the antifungal antibiotic validamycin into PHSNs (Liu et al., 2006). A supercritical fluid is a substance at a temperature and a pressure that are both above its critical temperature (T_c) and critical pressure (p_c), respectively. Once the T_c and p_c have been reached, the two distinct liquid and gas phases merge into one homogenous phase, the "supercritical fluid". Supercritical fluids combine the properties of gases and liquids in a new unique state of matter. Due to its mild critical conditions, the most employed supercritical fluid is carbon dioxide. Due to their compressibility and low viscosity, which enhance mass transfer properties, supercritical fluids resemble gases, but at the same time, they are characterized by the typical density of a liquid and preserve its solvent properties. Moreover, the lack of surface tension allows full penetration of nanopores (Branch and Bartlett, 2015). Therefore, these remarkable properties, that is, high dissolving power, compressibility, low viscosity, and the absence of surface tension all facilitate the load of pesticides into the PHSNs carriers. Prior to the loading process, the PHSNs were vacuum-dried. Next, validamycin and the PHSNs carriers at a ratio of 2:1 (w/w) were put separately in a supercritical fluid pesticide loading equipment operating at a pressure of 40 MPa and a temperature of 35°C. After completion of the adsorption process and decompression, the powders were collected and dried in a vacuum oven. The loading capacity achieved using this special supercritical fluid encapsulation process (36% w/w) was much higher as compared to simple immersion method in this case.

Mesoporous silica nanoparticles (MSNs) with an average diameter of 162 nm, and an average pore size of 3.2 nm have been prepared by Wanyika (2013) by a sol–gel method using TEOS as the silica source and CTAB as the structure-directing agent. Then, the MSNs were suspended into an aqueous solution of the fungicide metalaxyl and stirred for 12 h at room temperature. Eventually, water was slowly removed under vacuum using a rotary evaporator and nanoparticles were dried. The amount of fungicide encapsulated was estimated by TGA as being about 14 wt.%. The author set up experiments to evaluate the release of encapsulated fungicide in both water and soil. Release kinetics in water was determined in batch experiments by suspending metalaxyl-loaded MSNs in water contained in screw cap closed bottles. At different predetermined time intervals, the bottles were centrifuged and the supernatant filtered and analyzed for the metalaxyl content by high performance liquid chromatography (HPLC). Soil release kinetics studies were performed as follows. Soil columns each having a volume of 25 cm^3 were prepared in glass separatory funnels and settled by the addition of 20 mL of water. Next, equal amounts of metalaxyl-loaded MSNs were added on the top of each soil column. Ten milliliters of pure water was applied to the columns every 3 days for 1 month. The elutes were filtered and analyzed by HPLC. An amount of free fungicide equaling the amount encapsulated in MSNs was applied to each soil column in the control group. The results showed the sustained release of metalaxyl from MSNs. After 30 days, the controlled release system released only 47 and 11.5% of its metalaxyl payload in water, and in soil, respectively. By comparison, about 76% of the free metalaxyl was released in soil within the same period of time.

7 Clay-Based Nanomaterials and Layered Double Hydroxides

7.1 Clay-Based Nanomaterials

Clay based materials have been investigated by some research groups as an innovative approach for an ecofriendly pesticide delivery system.

The group led by Chevillard et al. (2012a,b) investigated the feasibility of using organic modified montmorillonite to enhance the slow release properties of a biopolymer-based nanodelivery system. The authors used a wheat gluten (WG)-based nanocarrier to encapsulate the herbicide ethofumesate as a model pesticide. The organic modified montmorillonite was a nanoclay marketed under the name Cloisite 30B by Southern Clay (Gonzales, TX). Cloisite 30B is an alkyl quaternary ammonium salt bentonite which has both nonpolar and polar groups imparting affinity for both ethofumesate and WG. The biodegradation processes of commercial ethofumesate and of the WG-based ethofumesate nanoformulation in soil have been studied comparatively. Biodegradation was expressed as percentages of CO_2 released in respirometric tests. These tests showed that commercial ethofumesate was not biodegraded after 640 days displaying an ecotoxic effect on soil. By contrary, WG-based nanoformulations containing 0.26% wt. of pesticide were still biodegradable in spite of the presence of nonbiodegradable ethofumesate, although the biodegradation rate was slightly but significantly slowed down as compared to the WG nanocarrier alone. When Cloisite 30B was introduced in the nanoformulation this delaying effect on biodegradation pattern disappeared and at the same time, the slow release properties were improved. The main merit of this study that should be emphasized is the development of a nanopesticide delivery system able to significantly reduce soil pollution. However, the effective bioavailability of the nanoformulated pesticide in soil remains to be determined in further studies.

A set of three clay materials, namely bentonite, kaolinite, and Fuller's earth in combination with carboxymethylcellulose was investigated by the group led by Chouhary et al. (2006) for their possible use in carbofuran delivery nanovectors. The formulations based on kaolinite and bentonite showed a maximum release after 35 days, Fuller's earth showed a maximum release after

28 days. The interesting feature of this type of formulation is that a single application can last for the whole growth span of the crop, allowing efficient nematode control.

Halloysite clays are an important class of clays since they occur naturally in a nanotube shape, this hollow cylindrical morphology giving rise to potential controlled release applications of organic molecules similar in behavior to the more expensive counterpart, the carbon nanotubes. Abdullayev and Lvov (2011) detailed the use of this type of material in comparison with other types of materials, like imogolite, in their paper. The main advantages those materials poses come from their small dimensions (10–20 nm lumen and 50–100 nm external diameter), enabling them to accommodate any number of small molecules and the possibility of capping as well, cap which can act as a trigger releasing the load only when some conditions are met.

7.2 Layered Double Hydroxides

LDHs, also known as anionic or hydrotalcite-like clay (HTs) are brucite-like layered materials with the general formula $[M^{2+}_{1-X}M^{3+}_{X}(OH)_2]^{X+}(A^{n-})_{X/n}\cdot mH_2O$ where M^{2+} and M^{3+} are metal cations ($M^{2+} = Mg^{2+}, Zn^{2+}, Ni^{2+}, Cu^{2+},\ldots; M^{3+} = Al^{3+}, Fe^{3+},\ldots$) and A^{n-} is the interlayer anion ($A^{n-} = CO_3^{2-}, NO_3^{-}, SO_4^{2-}$, and other ionic species; Fig. 4.13). The divalent and trivalent metallic cations occupy octahedral positions in the brucite-like layer, which is positively charged and requires the presence of negative counterions A^{n-} in the interlayer space to assure electrical neutrality of the compound. Taking advantage of the exchangeability of the interlayered anions, bioactive organic anions can be intercalated within the layered structure of LDHs and subsequently released in a

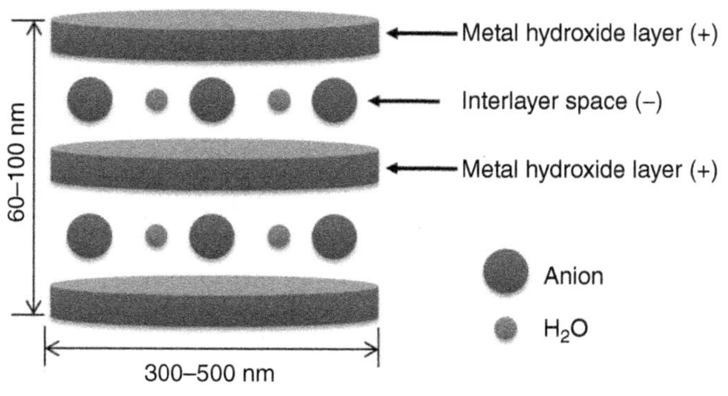

Figure 4.13. The general structure of layered double hydroxides (LDHs) $[M^{2+}_{1-X}M^{3+}_{X}(OH)_2]^{X+}(A^{n-})_{X/n}\cdot mH_2O$.

controlled fashion. Intercalation of organic anions within LDHs can be achieved by several synthetic methods such as: (1) direct synthesis using the coprecipitation method; (2) indirect synthesis using the regeneration method; (3) indirect synthesis using the ion exchange method (Cardoso et al., 2006).

Cardoso et al. (2006) used all the aforementioned three methods to intercalate a Mg/Al LDH with the anionic herbicides 2,4-dichlorophenoxyacetic acid (2,4-D), 4-chloro-2-methylphenoxyacetic acid (MCPA), and picloram. Herein we will briefly describe only the coprecipitation method. An aqueous solution containing $Mg(NO_3)_2$ and $Al(NO_3)_3$ in a molar ratio of 2:1 was added dropwise under stirring to a water solution of the acidic herbicide containing 10-fold molar excess of pesticide relative to the amount of the Al^{3+} salt. The pH was maintained about 10 by addition of sodium hydroxide solution. During the addition, the temperature was kept between 55 and 80°C depending on the nature of the herbicide. The resulting slurries were aged for 3 days at a temperature 10°C higher than the coprecipitation temperature. The resulting nanomaterials were separated by filtration, washed with water, and vacuum dried. In order to estimate the controlled release of the herbicide from the LDH-herbicide complexes, the authors carried out soil column leaching tests. Carbonate and hydroxyl anions from water effectively replace the acidic herbicide anions from the LDH complexes. Breakthrough curves (BTCs) were obtained for both free herbicides (dissolved in water) and LDH-herbicide complexes by plotting the pesticide concentration in the column effluent versus the volume of water added. At pH = 7.9 (the pH of the soil used in the leaching tests), the acidic herbicides are predominantly in the anionic form and, hence, retardation of the free pesticides by the soil columns could be hardly seen, if any. The BTCs showed a sharp peak close to one pore volume (volume of pores in the system filled with water which equals 200 mL in the experimental setup that was used). Application of the LDH-herbicide complexes resulted in dramatic changes in the shape of the BTC plots. The maximum concentration peaks shifted to larger volumes of added water and, at the same time, the heights of the peaks were greatly reduced, hence the BTCs tended to assume a more flattened appearance. These modifications clearly indicate retarded leaching of the herbicides. The maximum concentration was decreased by more than sixfold in the case of 2,4-D (from 5.0 to 0.8 mg/L), by more than fivefold for MCPA (from 6.3 to 1.2 mg/L), and by almost threefold for picloram (from 5.5 to 2.0 mg/L). Moreover, the maxima were shifted to a value of the amount of water added larger with 150 mL than the one corresponding to the free herbicides. To put it otherwise, as compared to free pesticides, in the case of LDH-herbicide complexes it took 3 more days for the leachates to reach the maximum pesticide concentration. An important consequence of this modified release profile was the dramatic decrease of the total amount of 2,4-D accumulated in leachates. When 2,4-D was applied as free herbicide, 82% of the amount applied was accumulated in leachates. This value dropped to only 18% after application of 2,4-D as an LDH complex. The slow release of 2,4-D from the LDH complex prolonged the residence time of the herbicide in the soil column thereby heightening the chances of biodegradation by the microorganisms present in soil. However, this was not the case with MCAP and picloram. After application of these herbicides as LDH complexes, the total herbicide amounts in the leachates were 79% for picloram and 60% for MCPA, respectively. The authors assumed that biodegradation occurred to a lesser extent in the case of these herbicides, their assumption being consistent with the known persistence of these pesticides in soil: picloram > MCPA > 2,4-D. Bioassays performed on garden watercress (*Lepidium sativum*) showed that the activity of herbicides was not affected by the nanoencapsulation. The authors concluded that LDHs could act as effective nanocarriers for the slow release of herbicides that are able to minimize transport losses while maintaining efficient weed control.

Park et al. (2010) synthesized an LDH-cinnamic complex and studied its behavior in soil and its controlled release property. Cinnamic acid is a naturally occurring organic acid with antimicrobial activities (antibacterial and antifungal). The results reported by the authors clearly demonstrate that intercalation of cinnamate within the layered structure of Mg/Al layered double hydroxide rendered complexes with slow release properties and, at the same time, protected the AI against degradation. Antifungal activity against the growth of *Phytophthora capsici*, a plant pathogen that causes blight and fruit rot of peppers and other important commercial crops, was tested comparatively in soils treated with free cinnamic acid (C-soil), and in soils treated with LDH-cinnamate complexes (H-soil). At 6 days after inoculation with the pathogen, the red peppers in the C-soil got infected with root rot and wilted, while the red peppers in the H-soil remained unaffected. These results demonstrate that nanoencapsulation protected the active compound against degradation occurring in soil, while the slow release of the antifungal agent from the LDH-cinnamate complex enhanced its effectiveness in controlling root rot of red pepper.

In a very similar approach, Ghazali et al. (2013) intercalated 3,4-dichlorophenoxyacetic acid (3,4-D) into zinc–aluminum-layered double hydroxide by the coprecipitation method.

We can conclude from these examples that LDHs appear as a promising alternative for green formulation of pesticides.

8 Nanoemulsions

Nanoemulsions are emulsions with droplet size in the nanometer range. They are kinetically stable but not thermodynamically stable. So, one can say that nanoemulsions are metastable systems and their stability depends on the method of preparation (Wang et al., 2007). There are two main types of methods to prepare nanoemulsions: high-energy emulsification methods which make use of high-shear stirring, high-pressure homogenizers, and ultrasonic generators, and low-energy emulsification methods which take advantage of the energy stored in the system to promote the formation of small droplets (Izquierdo et al., 2005).

Balaji et al. (2015) have prepared a new nanovector for the hydrophobic insect repellent *N,N*-diethyl phenylacetamide (DEPA) by a low-energy emulsification method, that is, the so-called phase inversion temperature (PIT) method. The principle of this method introduced by Shinoda and Saito (1969) is briefly explained further. The method is based on the ability of polyethoxylated nonionic emulsifiers to change their hydrophilic–lipophilic balance (HLB) number with temperature. The higher the temperature, the lower the HLB, the drop being caused by the dehydration of the ethoxylate units. Hence, at a fixed composition, the relative affinity of the surfactant for the different phases can be tailored by changing the temperature (Anton et al., 2007). At low temperature, the polyethoxylated surfactant is hydrated, having more affinity with the aqueous phase and thereby promoting the formation of a stable O/W macroemulsion. Increasing the temperature, the stability of the O/W emulsion gradually decreases as the surfactant becomes more lipophilic because of dehydration of the polyoxyethylene chain. At higher temperatures, the surfactant stabilizes W/O emulsions. The PIT or the HLB temperature is the temperature at which the nonionic surfactant has very close affinities for both immiscible phases. At PIT both O/W and W/O macroemulsions are unstable, and the ternary system oil/water/surfactant shows a bicontinuous microemulsion structure and/or a lamellar liquid crystalline structure (Anton et al., 2007). The interfacial tension reaches almost zero, thereby favoring formation of nanosized emulsions. Taking advantage of this behavior, nanoemulsions can be produced. Fabrication of kinetically stable nanoemulsions by a transitional inversion involves preparation of emulsions near the PIT followed by rapid cooling or heating. By quickly cooling an emulsion prepared in the region of the PIT, the W/O emulsion inverts to an O/W emulsion. Rapid heating results in the opposite phase inversion process, the O/W emulsion being inverted to a W/O emulsion. The temperature increase or decrease by about 25–30°C must occur fast in order to obtain kinetically stable W/O, or O/W nanoemulsions, respectively; otherwise, slow temperature change results in coarse emulsions. Following this procedure, Balaji et al. prepared kinetically stable water dispersible nanoformulations of the hydrophobic aromatic amide DEPA and evaluated their larvicidal bioefficacy against *Culex tritaeniorhynchus* (the vector of the Japanese encephalitis). First, the authors prepared an O/W macroemulsion by addition of the aqueous phase consisting of Tween 20 and soy lecithin in 10 mM NaCl to the organic phase containing DEPA, various amounts (0–9% v/v) of PEG and DCM under continuous stirring at 800 rpm for 20 min. Next, the authors determined the PIT by the conductometric method (Allouche et al., 2004). The O/W emulsion conducts electricity since the continuous phase is water with NaCl added in low concentrations. On the other hand, when phase inversion process occurs at PIT, the conductivity approaches zero, since the continuous phase of the inverted W/O emulsion is oil which does not conduct the electricity. The O/W emulsion was heated, passing through the HLB temperature (PIT) being marked by the sudden drop to zero of the conductivity. The heating rate was 5°C/min. Upon PIT emulsification, the W/O emulsion was quickly cooled by diluting it tenfold with ultrapure chilly water (10°C) to eventually get the O/W nanoemulsion of DEPA. Bioassays performed on third instars *C. tritaeniorhynchus* larvae revealed a drop in the median lethal concentration from 0.416 mg/L for bulk DEPA to only 0.052 mg/L for nano DEPA (Balaji et al., 2015).

Another low-energy method to prepare nanoemulsions is the emulsion inversion point (EIP) method (Bouchama et al., 2003; Perazzo et al., 2015). In this case, phase inversion is prompted not by a change in temperature like in the PIT method, but rather by a change in composition. In essence, the method consists in dilution with water of an abnormal W/O emulsion which means a W/O emulsion that is stabilized by a hydrophilic surfactant which has a greater affinity for the discontinuous aqueous phase than for the continuous oil phase. A normal emulsion is an emulsion stabilized by a surfactant with greater affinity for the continuous phase. Initially addition of water leads to nothing else but the formation of more water droplets within the continuous oil phase of the emulsion. However, once a critical amount of water is exceeded, the rate of coalescence of the water droplets overwhelms that of the oil droplets and the abnormal W/O emulsion irreversibly switches to a normal O/W emulsion (Fig. 4.14) (McClements, 2011). This

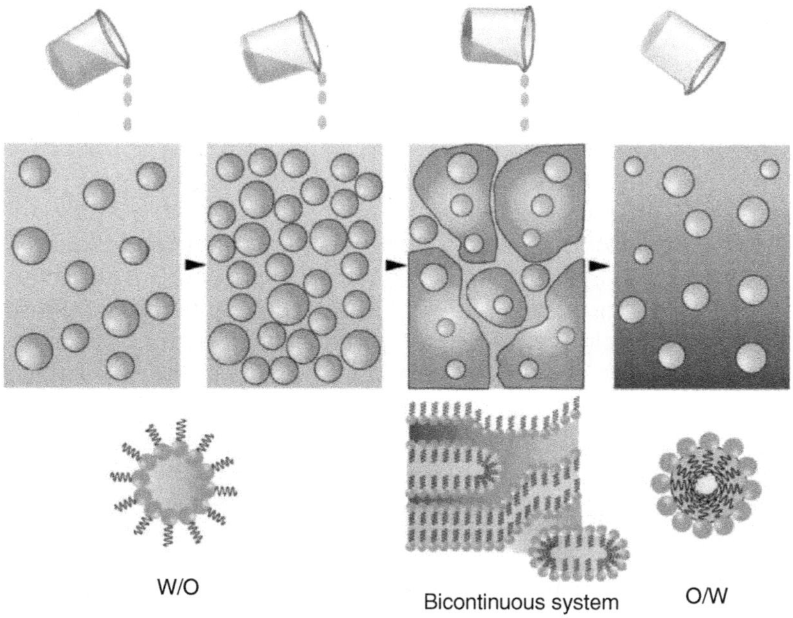

Figure 4.14. Mechanism of low-energy emulsification by the catastrophic phase inversion (CPI) method. Reproduced with permission from reference (McClements, 2011).

phase inversion process is called a catastrophic phase inversion (CPI) to distinguish it from the transitional phase inversion, which occurs between two normal emulsions. The EIP method was applied by Kalaitzaki et al. (2015) to obtain pyrethrin-containing kinetically stable O/W nanoemulsions. The authors reported for the first time the preparation of micro- and nanoemulsions as encapsulation media based exclusively on safe and naturally nontoxic materials. The botanical insecticides pyrethrins were dissolved in lemon essential oil containing 97.5% terpenes and then mixed at 25°C with a high HLB surfactant, that is, either Tween 20 (polyoxyethylene sorbitan monolaureate) or Tween 80 (polyoxyethylene sorbitan monooleate) to get the oily phase. Next, single phase W/O microemulsions were obtained by addition of water and glycerol in a ratio of 2:1. Eventually, O/W nanoemulsions loaded with pyrethrins were obtained after a 100-fold dilution of the W/O microemulsions either with tap water or with a 2:1 mixture of ultrapure water and glycerol. The insecticidal activity of the encapsulated natural pyrethrin was tested on 3–4 days old nymphs of the cotton aphid *Aphis gossypii* Glover and compared with the activity of a commercial suspension concentrate pyrethrum formulation, namely Pyrethro Vioryl 5 SC. Five concentrations were tested for both the commercial product and the pyrethrin nanoemulsions. The bioassays were performed using the leaf-dip method. Stalked leaves containing 15–50 individuals of *A. gossypii* were detached from eggplants and immersed for 10 s into each type of formulations (commercial, and O/W nanoemulsions, respectively). Then, the leaves were transferred for the next 24 h to well ventilated plastic containers placed in a growth chamber kept at a constant temperature of 25 ± 1°C, a relative humidity of 65 ± 2%, and a photoperiod light:dark = 16:8 h. The leaf moisture was maintained with the aid of a wet cotton–wool bandage applied around the edge of the petiole. Dead nymphs were counted after 24 h. Lethal concentrations 50 (LC_{50}) and 95% confidence intervals (CI) were determined from the dose-response curves using probit analysis. The LC_{50} (95% CI) values were decreased from 965.5 (742.0–1186.5) $\times 10^{-6}$ mg/mL for the commercial product to 609.1 (443.2 − 773.3) $\times 10^{-6}$ mg/mL for the pyrethrin nanoemulsion. However, possible adverse effects on beneficial arthropods were not yet assessed and remain to be evaluated in the future.

A slightly modified low-energy emulsification method was applied by Lim et al. (2012a, 2012b) to prepare nanoemulsions containing 41% (w/w) glyphosate isopropylamine salt as herbicide AI. To reduce the environmental harm, the authors used green nonionic surfactants and naturally derived oil phase. A mixture of fatty acid methyl esters (FAMEs) encompassing hexanoate, octanoate, decanoate, and laureate was used as oil phase [methyl hexanoate/octanoate/decanoate/laurate = 3.2/50.8/44.0/2.0 (w/w)]. As ecofriendly nonionic surfactants short-chain alkyl polyglucosides (SAPG), long-chain alkyl polyglucosides (LAPG), and 3-(3-hydroxypropyl)-heptamethyltrisiloxane (organosilicone) were used (Fig. 4.15). Phase diagrams

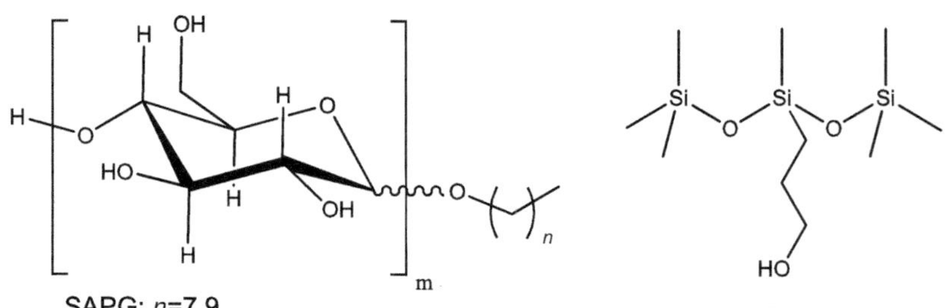

Figure 4.15. Structures of the nonionic surfactants employed in the fabrication of glyphosate-loaded O/W nanoemulsions.

were constructed for pseudoternary systems of FAMEs, water, and surfactants containing 41% (w/w) glyphosate isopropylamine salt in order to study their phase behavior and to select those systems able to form microemulsions. Such phase diagrams were built for each single surfactant and for mixtures of SAPG:organosilicone, and LAPG:organosilicone in different proportions (9:1, 8:2, 7:3, 6:4, and 9:1, 8:2, 7:3, respectively) as well. The outcomes of the aforementioned study were used to prepare microemulsion-based preformulations. By diluting the latter with large amounts of water (1:200) under low-speed stirring (200 rpm for 5 min) O/W nanoemulsion formulations of glyphosate with droplet size less than 200 nm were eventually produced. The performances of the prepared glyphosate-laden nanoemulsions in controlling *Eleusine indica*, a narrow-leaved weed, were estimated by comparison with a commercially available formulation of glyphosate, namely Roundup. The best results were obtained for the following composition of the nanovehicle: 74.58% (w/w) water, 3.27% (w/w) FAMEs oil, and 22.15% (w/w) 8:2 LAPG:organosilicone surfactant. The phytotoxicity study was carried out on 7–8 day old weed. The herbicide was applied by spraying. Nine different glyphosate doses were used. The sigmoidal dose–response curves were constructed and linearized by probit transformation, and the effective dose ED_{50} values of the treatments were determined. The mean weed control rates corresponding to the nanoformulation significantly overcome those of the commercial product at the following doses: 0.25, 0.50., 0.75, and 1.00 kg herbicide/ha. The ED_{50} of the nanoemulsion formulation (0.40 kg herbicide/ha) was lower than that of Roundup (0.48 kg/ha). Moreover, the nanoemulsion formulations exhibited lower surface tensions than the commercial product thereby promoting leaf wettability and facilitating pesticide penetration.

Similarly, Wang et al. (2007) used O/W nanoemulsions to formulate the water insoluble insecticide, β-cypermethrin (CP). Methyl decanoate was used as oil phase and polyoxyethylene (7) lauryl ether as surfactant. A two-step procedure was followed. First, CP was incorporated into a 1:1 (weight ratio) oil/surfactant mixture, and then water was added to obtain a microemulsion concentrate containing 50 wt.% water. Next, the microemulsion concentrate was rapidly injected into a very much larger amount of water under mild stirring to yield the final O/W nanoemulsion ("crash dilution" method). When the amount of CP incorporated was less than 12 wt.%, a nanoemulsion with very small droplet sizes (about 30 nm) and narrow particle size distribution (PDI < 0.2) was obtained. The stabilities of the prepared CP-loaded nanoemulsion and of a commercial CP microemulsion were evaluated by comparing the increase in average droplet size with time and the pesticide solubilizing powers on dilution. Spray solutions were prepared from both the commercial product and the nanoemulsion. After 24 h storage, pesticide precipitation could be observed in the spray solution obtained from the commercial CP-microemulsion, while the spray solution prepared from the CP-nanoemulsion showed no sign of phase separation (precipitation).

Nanoemulsions prepared from natural ingredients poses the ultimate quality of being biodegradable and environmental friendly, and on an economical note, come from a renewable source. The group of Anjali et al. (2012) succeeded to synthesize neem-oil based nanopesticides as O/W nanoemulsions using Tween 20 as hydrophilic surfactant. At an oil:surfactant ratio of 1:3, nanoemulsions with a droplet size as small as 31.03 nm were obtained. The LC_{50} was found to decrease with the decrease in droplet size, being 11.75 mg/L at 31.03 nm droplet size.

9 Microemulsions

Unlike nanoemulsions, microemulsions are thermodynmically stable systems because the free energy of the dispersed system is lower than the separated oil and water phases. Consequently, microemulsions require no energy input during their preparation and are readily obtained using low-energy emulsification methods. Being thermodinamicaly stable, microemulsions allow self-emulsification of the system. However, the emulsification process is reversible, microemulsions becoming unstable at low or high temperatures. Once, the temperature is brought back within the stability range, the microemulsion reforms. Microemulsions are bicontinuous systems containing extended regions of both oil and water separated by surfactant/cosurfactant rich interfacial regions (Beaglehole et al., 1984). Therefore, formation of microemulsions, requires relatively large amount of surfactants to stabilize the large interfacial area. The free energy change of microemulsion formation is given by the following Eq. (4.1) (Ruckenstein and Chi, 1975):

$$\Delta G_{\mathrm{f}} = \gamma \Delta A - T \Delta S \tag{4.1}$$

where, γ is the surface tension at the oil–water interface, ΔA is the change in the interfacial area on microemulsification, T is the absolute temperature, and ΔS is the entropy change accompanying microemulsification. Despite being named microemulsions, the droplet sizes in microemulsions are generally in the range 10–100 nm. Consequently, ΔA, the interfacial area created by the nanodroplets is very large. However, since surfactants are able to produce very low interfacial tensions γ is very small and the first positive term in the right member of Eq. (4.1) is offset by the large entropic change occurring on mixing the two immiscible phases. Hence, due to a negative change in free energy, microemulsification occurs spontaneously if the aqueous phase, the oily phase, and the surfactants are mixed in the appropriate ratios and microemulsions are thermodynamically stable systems. Microemulsions are clear and transparent dispersions with a homogenous appearance on the macroscopic scale but microscopically heterogenous (Vinod et al., 2011). An important advantage provided by the thermodynamic stability of microemulsions is their longer shelf life as compared to nanoemulsions, for instance.

Anjali et al. (2010) prepared highly wettable nanosized particles of the hydrophobic insecticide permethrin using a method previously developed by the same research group (Magdassi et al., 2007, 2008; Margulis-Goshen and Magdassi, 2009; Margulis-Goshen et al., 2009). The preparation method consists of the following operations: (1) solubilization of the water insoluble organic compound in a hydrophobic organic solvent which is more volatile than water; (2) addition of proper surfactants, cosurfactants, and water to the previously prepared organic solution to form a transparent thermodynamically stable microemulsion; and (3) removal of all the solvents (organic and aqueous) through evaporation at reduced pressure or by spray drying yielding a highly wettable nanosized powder which is readily redispersible in water (Margulis-Goshen et al., 2009). The organic solvent used to dissolve permethrin was *n*-butyl acetate (nBuAC). Then, the saponin ammonium glycyrrhizinate (AG), soybean phosphatidylcholine (SbPc), and *sec*-butyl alcohol (secBuOH) were added to the above permethrin solution to form the oily phase. Next, aqueous sucrose (18 wt.%) was added until a transparent, isotropic O/W microemulsion system was formed. The composition of the microemulsion was nBuAC/secBuOH/AG/SbPc/sucrose/water = 4/14/9/9/9/8.5/46.5 wt.%. Eventually, the microemulsion was lyophilized to afford a nonopowder with the following composition: permethrin 13 wt.%, AG 29.5 wt.%, SbPc 29.5%, and sucrose 28 wt.%. The nanopowder was easily water dispersible forming a translucent and stable nanosuspension. The mean particle size after redispersion of powder in water was 131 ± 9 nm (Suresh Kumar et al., 2013). The larvicidal activities of nanopermethrin and bulk permethrin against *Culex quinquefasciatus* were compared. The larval group exposed to a concentration of nanopermethrin of 10 mg/L for 24 h showed 100% mortality, while the bulk pesticide at the same concentration produced about 89% mortality within the same period of time. The LC_{50} was reduced from 0.715 mg/L for bulk permethrin to only 0.117 mg/L for nanopermethrin. The authors also tested the efficiency of formulated nanopermethrin against *Aedes aegypti* (Suresh Kumar et al., 2013). Larvae exposed for only 2 h to a concentration of 26 ppb nanopermethrin showed 100% mortality, while at the same concentration the bulk counterpart gave a mortality of only 60% after 24 h of exposure. For 24 h exposure, the LC_{50} values were found to be 0.0199 mg/L for permethrin, and only 0.0063 mg/L for nanopermethrin. The authors concluded that formulation of permethrin as water dispersible nanopowder makes it a valuable green pesticide since it lengthens the pesticide life and it reduces the administered doses, the nanopesticide eliciting a greater toxic response at lower concentrations as compared to the conventional formulation. Moreover, being freely dispersible in water and giving stable nanosuspensions, this type of nanoformulation offers the opportunity to get rid of toxic and volatile organic solvents. Besides being more toxic toward target organisms, nanopermethrin has been shown to be less toxic than bulk permethrin to nontarget organisms like beneficial bacteria in the soil or useful plant species like grains and vegetables. Antibacterial activity against *Bacillus subtilis* and *Escherichia coli* (ATCC 13534 and 25922) was estimated using the disk diffusion method. Both nano and bulk pesticide showed no antibacterial activity. Comparative phytotoxicity studies were carried out on seeds of *Lycopersicum esculentum* (tomato), *Cucumis sativus* (cucumber), and *Zea. mays* (maize). The roots emerged from seeds exposed to different concentrations of bulk permethrin were significantly shorter than those originating from seeds treated with nanopermethrin. Moreover, seeds treated with nanopermethrin showed 100% germination in all cases, while the germination rate decreased significantly, (up to 70%) when seeds were exposed to bulk permethrin. Genotoxicity tests were performed on root cells of *Allium cepa* (onion). The authors found a decrease in the percentages of cells in various mitotic stages in samples treated with 0.13 mg/L bulk permethrin compared to those exposed to the same concentration of nanopermethrin. The chromosomal aberrations percentage was significantly lower (0.35%) in samples treated with 0.52 mg/L nanopermethrin as compared to samples treated with the same concentration of bulk permethrin (1.2%) (Suresh Kumar et al., 2013).

The same research group prepared nanoparticles of the water insoluble insecticide novaluron using the same method of converting volatile O/W microemulsions into water dispersible powders (Elek et al., 2010). The oil phase consisted of a mixture of a solution of novaluron in isobutyl acetate (IsoBuAc) and isopropanol (IPA). The following surfactants: SDS, sodium linear alkyl benzene sulfonate (LABS), and sodium alkyl naphthalene sulfonate condensate (Morwet D-425) were dispersed in deionized water. An O/W microemulsion with the following composition (% w/w): novaluron (1.2), SDS (6.15), LABS (2.31), Morwet (1.54), IPA (25), IsoBuAc (38.8), and water (25) were prepared by mixing the two phases at room temperature. The composition of the continuous aqueous phase was: 1.6% (v/v) IsoBuAc, 39.6% (v/v) IPA, and 58.8% (v/v) water. A value of 6.2 nm for the diameter of the dispersed novaluron droplets was calculated from the diffusion coefficient of novaluron using the Stokes–Einstein equation. Next, the novaluron-containing O/W microemulsion was spray dried when a nanopowder containing 10.71% (w/w) novaluron, 54.91% (w/w) SDS, 20.63% (w/w) LABS, and 13.75% (w/w) Morwet was obtained. The novaluron particles in the powder were rather amorphous as revealed by the X-ray powder diffraction analysis (XRPD), a feature imparting higher water solubility and improved bioactivity. The powder was dispersed into water (0.1% w/w dispersion). CryoTEM images showed the presence of both small (20–40 nm) and large (90–100 nm) particles in the aqueous dispersion. To evaluate the dispersion stability, the particle size was monitored every 15 min for 4.5 h. Only a slight increase in the particle size could be observed during this time period. The biological activity of the nanoformulation was assessed in vivo against the Egyptian cotton leafworm *Spodoptera littoralis* larvae. The nanoformulation and the commercial formulation exhibited similar toxicities.

Xu et al. (2010) prepared neem oil microemulsions by mixing the neem oil, the emulsifier system, and water at the weight ratio of 1:3.5:5.5. The emulsifier system consisted of a mixture of the surfactant and cosurfactant in a weight ratio surfactant/cosurfactant of 4:1. The surfactant employed was actually a mixture of two surfactants, that is, Tween 80 and dodecyl benzene sulfonate: (SDBS) (the mixing ratio by weight was 4:1 Tween 80:SDBS). As cosurfactants, various compounds (amyl alcohol, hexylalcohol, or heptyl alcohol) have been used. The acaricidal activity against *Sarcoptes scabiei* var. *cuniculi* larvae was assessed in vitro by measuring the speed of kill. The median lethal time value LT_{50} was 81.7463 min.

10 Nanosuspensions

Nanosuspensions, also called nanodispersions are formed by dispersion of crystalline or amorphous nanoparticles of the AI in liquid media (Kah et al., 2013). Nanosuspensions can be prepared from O/W microemulsions as illustrated in Section 9 by the examples of the aqueous dispersions of nanopermethin (Anjali et al., 2010; Suresh Kumar et al., 2013) and of novaluron nanoparticles (Elek et al., 2010). Using the same approach, Zeng et al. (2008) prepared nanosuspensions of beta cypermethrin with narrow size distribution.

Saini et al. (2014) reported the preparation of an aqueous suspension of pyridalyl containing ALG nanocapsules. The authors synthesized pyridalyl-loaded ALG nanocapsules by an ionotropic pregelation method and evaluated in vitro the insecticidal activity of the nanocapsule suspension against larvae of *Helicoverpa armigera*, a worldwide insect pest that has developed resistance toward conventional insecticides causing 20–60% loss in tomato crops. Briefly, sodium ALG was dissolved in distilled water at 50–60°C, and the hydrophilic surfactant Tween 80 was added to this solution within 15 min under continuous stirring. Subsequent dropwise addition of an ethanolic solution of pyridalyl at room temperature afforded an emulsion, which was further sonicated for 15 min. Next, a solution (2 mg/mL) of $CaCl_2$ was dropped into the latter emulsion over a course of 60 min. The stirring was continued for another 60 min and the resulting nanocapsule suspension was allowed to stand overnight. Then, the solvent was evaporated at 45–50°C under reduced pressure for 30 min eventually yielding an aqueous suspension of pyridalyl nanocapsules. The mean size of the dispersed particles and the encapsulation efficiency were dependent on the concentrations of the polymer and the AI at constant concentrations of surfactant and calcium chloride in the resulting nanosuspensions. The minimum particle size was 107 ± 0.8 nm, while the maximum one was 546 ± 2.1 nm. The encapsulation efficiency varied between 23.26% and 32.97%. Two distinct methods, that is, the leaf dip technique and the leaf spray technique, were used to assess the insecticidal activity of the pyridalyl nanosuspension in comparison to a commercial formulation of pyridalyl. As contact poison (leaf spray method), the nanoformulation was 3.125 times more active than the commercial formulation, while as stomach poison (leaf dip method), the nanoformulation was 6.125 times more active than the commercial formulation as resulted from the statistical estimation of the LC_{50} values and of the confidence limits (leaf spray method LC_{50} for the commercial formulation = 250 μg/mL, LC_{50} for the nanoformulation = 80 μg/mL; leaf dip method LC_{50} for the commercial formulation = 250 μg/mL, LC_{50} for the nanoformulation = 40 μg/mL) (Saini et al., 2014).

Strom, Price, and Lubetkin synthesized aqueous stable nanodispersions of a series of compounds with pesticidal activity including atrazine herbicide, epoxiconazole fungicide, natural spynosins (spinosad insceticide), and triazole insecticides (Strom et al., 2001).

11 Conclusions and Future Perspectives

Despite their many advantages like fast action, high availability, and reliability, conventional pesticides as chemical pest control agents also present a series of serious drawbacks and risks, the most important ones being low selective toxicity, low biodegradability, and development of pesticide resistance in target organisms associated with the excessive and improper use of these compounds.

Nanotechnology comes with some new concepts and innovative solutions to the aforementioned problems. Development of nanopesticide delivery systems brings in a series of important advantages over their classical bulk counterparts, the major ones being listed here:

- The water solubility and, hence, the bioavailability of poorly water soluble pesticides is increased.
- Nanoencapsulation protects the AI from being prematurely degraded.
- Nanoencapsulation slows down the rate of pesticide delivery, thereby lengthening the period of time over which the pesticide remains effective.
- Nanopesticide delivery systems enhance pesticide uptake by the target organism.
- Nanopesticide delivery systems can be engineered so they deliver their payload in a well-controlled fashion, the release of the pesticide being triggered by specific features of the local microenvironment, such as the pH value; thereby, one can gain spatial and temporal control over the release process. This major achievement allows the amount of the pesticide actually required for pest control to be significantly reduced and avoids the use of excessive large amounts of pesticides, which is not only futile but often hazardous.
- Nanoencapsulation can improve leaf adhesion and penetration thereby increasing treatment efficacy.
- Nanoencapsulation can reduce pesticide losses through leaching and runoff. Hence, not only the costs of pest control, but also the risks of environmental pollution are greatly reduced.
- Smart nanopesticide delivery systems are also able to improve the selective toxicity and to overcome pesticide resistance.
- The development of novel photodegradable pesticide carriers that once delivery of the AI has been accomplished are able to decompose themselves along with the toxic residuals is another major achievement in the field which should be highlighted.

However, in the field of nanodelivery systems a great deal of attention has been focused on the development of nanocarriers for the transport of pharmaceuticals and nutraceuticals. Relatively few papers deal with the use of nanodelivery systems as carriers of pesticides with potential application in plant protection. So, one can say that the huge potential these new delivery systems could provide for the development of safer and greener pesticides still remains unexploited and a lot of work has to be done in the future.

Nevertheless, we have to notice that the data concerning the environmental fate of these nanoparticles and their possible negative impact are scarce and there is a lack of knowledge in the field. Therefore, many studies have to be designed and conducted in the future until a reliable assessment of the benefits/risks balance of nanopesticides can be made.

References

Abdullayev, E., Lvov, Y., 2011. Halloysite clay nanotubes for controlled release of protective agents. J. Nanosci. Nanotechnol. 11, 10007–10026.

Abouelkassem, S., El-Borady, O.M., Mohamed, M.B., 2016. Remakable enhancement of cyhalothrin upon loading into silver nanoparticles as larvicidal. Int. J. Contemp. Appl. Sci. 3 (1), 252–264.

Abreu, F.O.M.S., Oliveira, E.F., Paula, H.C.B., de Paula, R.C.M., 2012. Chitosan/cashew gum nanogels for essential oil encapsulation. Carbohydr. Polym. 89, 1277–1282.

Adak, T., Kumar, J., Shakil, N.A., Walia, S., 2012. Development of controlled release formulations of imidacloprid employing novel nano-ranged amphiphilic polymers. J. Environ. Sci. Health B-Pestic. 47, 217–225.

Allouche, J., Tyrode, E., Sadtler, V., Choplin, L., Salager, J.-L., 2004. Simultaneous conductivity and viscosity measurements as a technique to track emulsion inversion by the phase-inversion-temperature method. Langmuir 20, 2134–2140.

Anjali, C.H., Khan, S.S., Margulis-Goshen, K., Magdassi, S., Mukherjee, A., Chandrasekaran, N., 2010. Formulation of water-dispersible nanopermethrin for larvicidal applications. Ecotox. Environ. Safe. 73, 1932–1936.

Anjali, C.H., Sharma, Y., Mukherjee, A., Chandrasekaran, N., 2012. Neem oil (*Azadirachta indica*) nanoemulsion—a potent larvicidal agent against *Culex quinquefasciatus*. Pest Manag. Sci. 68 (2), 158–163.

Anton, N., Gayet, P., Benoit, J.-P., Saulnier, P., 2007. Nano-emulsions and nanocapsules by the PIT method: an investigation on the role of the temperature cycling on the emulsion phase inversion. Int. J. Pharm. 344, 44–52.

Balaji, A.P.B., Mishra, P., Suresh Kumar, R.S., Mukherjee, A., Chandrasekaran, N., 2015. Nanoformulation of poly(ethylene glycol) polymerized organic insect repellent by PIT emulsification method and its application for Japanese encephalitis vector control. Colloid Surf. B 128, 370–378.

Balaure, P.C., Grumezescu, A.M., 2014. Methods for synthesizing the macromolecular constituents of smart nanosized carriers for controlled drug delivery. Curr. Med. Chem. 21, 3333–3374.

Bang, S.H., Yu, Y.M., Hwang, I.C., Park, H.J., 2009. Formation of size-controlled nano carrier systems by self-assembly. J. Microencapsul. 26 (8), 722–733.

Bang, S.H., Hwang, I.C., Yu, Y.M., Park, E.H., Kwon, H.R., Park, H.J., 2011. Application of the combined use of ultrasonic homogenization and electro-spraying in the formation of nano carrier systems. J. Microencapsul. 28 (6), 557–567.

Beaglehole, D., Clarkson, M.T., Upton, A., 1984. Structure of the microemulsion/oil/water interfaces. J. Colloid Interface Sci. 101, 330–335.
Bhagat, D., Samanta, S.K., Bhattacharya, S., 2013. Efficient management of fruit pests by pheromone nanogels. Sci. Rep. 3, 1294.
Bouchama, F., van Aken, G.A., Autin, A.J.E., Kope, G.J.M., 2003. On the mechanism of catastrophic phase inversion in emulsions. Colloid Surf. A 231 (1–3), 11–17.
Branch, J.A., Bartlett, P.N., 2015. Electrochemistry in supercritical fluids. Phil. Trans. R. Soc. A 373, 20150007.
Brunel, F., Véron, L., David, L., Domard, A., Delair, T., 2008. A novel synthesis of chitosan nanoparticles in reverse emulsion. Langmuir 24 (20), 11370–11377.
Brunel, F., El Gueddari, N.E., Moerschbacher, B.M., 2013. Complexation of copper(II) with chitosan nanogels: toward control of microbial growth. Carbohydr. Polym. 92, 1348–1356.
Cai, D., Wu, Z., Jiang, J., Ding, K., Tong, L., Chu, P.K., Yu, Z., 2009. A unique technology to transform inorganic nanorods into nano-networks. Nanotechnology 20, 255302.
Campos, E.V.R., de Oliveira, J.L., da Silva, C.M.G., Pascoli, M., Pasquoto, T., Lima, R., Abhilash, P.C., Fraceto, L.F., 2015. Polymeric and solid lipid nanoparticles for sustained release of carbendazim and tebuconazole in agricultural applications. Sci. Rep. 5, 13809.
Cardoso, L.P., Celis, R., Cornejo, J., Valim, J.B., 2006. Layered double hydroxides as supports for the slow release of acid herbicides. J. Agric. Food Chem. 54, 5968–5975.
Carvalho, F.P., 2006. Agriculture, pesticides, food security and food safety. Environ. Sci. Policy 9, 685–692.
Chen, C., Han, D., Cai, C., Tang, X., 2010. An overview of liposome lyophilization and its future potential. J. Control. Release 142, 299–311.
Chen, M., Jensen, S.P., Hill, M.R., Moore, G., He, Z., Sumerlin, B.S., 2015. Synthesis of amphiphilic polysuccinimide star copolymers for responsive delivery in plants. Chem. Commun..
Chester, K.S., 1959. In: Horsfall, J.G., Diamond, A.E. (Eds.), Plant Pathology: An Advances Traits. Academic Press, New York, NY, pp. 199–242.
Chevillard, A., Angellier-Coussy, H., Guillard, V., Gontard, N., Gastaldi, E., 2012a. Investigating the biodegradation pattern of an ecofriendly pesticide delivery system based on wheat gluten and organically modified montmorillonites. Polym. Degrad. Stabil. 97 (10), 2060–2068.
Chevillard, A., Angellier-Coussy, H., Guillard, V., Gontard, N., Gastaldi, E., 2012b. Controlling pesticide release via structuring agropolymer and nanoclays based materials. J. Hazard. Mater. 205–206, 32–39.
Choudhury, S.R., Pradhan, S., Goswami, A., 2012. Preparation and characterisation of acephate nano-encapsulated complex. Nanosci. Methods 1, 9–15.
Chouhary, G., Kumar, J., Walia, S., Parsad, R., Parmar, B.S., 2006. Development of controlled release formulations of carbofuran and evaluation of their efficacy against *Meloidogyne incognita*. J. Agric. Food Chem. 54, 4727–4733.
Cohen, J.E., 2005. Human population grows up. Sci. Am. Special issue, 26–33.
da Costa, J.T., Forim, M.R., Costa, E.S., de Souza, J.R., Mondego, J.M., Boica Junior, A.L., 2014. Effects of different formulations of neem oil-based products on control *Zabrotes subfasciatus* (Boheman, 1833) (Coleoptera: Bruchidae) on beans. J. Stored Prod. Res. 56, 49–53.
Das, S., Chaudhury, A., 2011. Recent advances in lipid nanoparticle formulations with solid matrix for oral drug delivery. AAPS PharmSciTech 12 (1), 62–76.
Department of Economic and Social Affairs, Population Division, 2015. World Population Prospects. The 2015 Revision. Key Findings and Advance Tables. United Nations, New York.

d'Ischia, M., Napolitano, A., Pezzella, A., Meredith, P., Sarna, T., 2009. Chemical and structural diversity in eumelanins: unexplored bio-optoelectronic materials. Angew. Chem. Int. Ed. 48, 3914–3921.

Elek, N., Hoffman, R., Raviv, U., Resh, R., Ishaaya, I., Magdassi, S., 2010. Novaluron nanoparticles: formation and potential use in controlling agricultural insect pests. Colloid Surf. A-Physicochem. Eng. 372, 66–72.

Esmaeili, A., Saremnia, B., 2012. Preparation of extract-loaded nanocapsules from *Onopordon leptolepis* DC. Ind. Crop. Prod. 37, 259–263.

Feng, B.-H., Peng, L.-F., 2012. Synthesis and characterization of carboxymethyl chitosan carrying ricinoleic functions as an emulsifier for azadirachtin. Carbohydr. Polym. 88, 576–582.

Food and Agriculture Organization of the United Nations, International Fund for Agricultural Development, World Food Programme, 2015. The State of Food Insecurity in the World, Meeting the 2015 international hunger targets: taking stock of uneven progress. Rome.

Forim, M.R., Soares Costa, E., das Graças Fernandes da Silva, M.F., Batista, J., Fernandes, Marques Mondego, J., Boiça Junior, A.L., 2013. Development of a new method to prepare nano-/microparticles loaded with extracts of *Azadirachta indica*, their characterization and use in controlling *Plutella xylostella*. J. Agric. Food Chem. 61, 9131–9139.

Funk, C.C., Brown, M.E., 2009. Declining global per capita agricultural production and warming oceans threaten food security. Food Sec. 1, 271–289.

Ghazali, S.A.I.S.M., Hussein, M.Z., Sarijo, S.H., 2013. 3,4-Dichlorophenoxyacetate interleaved into anionic clay for controlled release formulation of a new environmentally friendly agrochemical. Nanoscale Res. Lett. 8, 362.

Ghormade, V., Deshpande, M.V., Paknikar, K.M., 2011. Perspectives for nano-biotechnology enabled protection and nutrition of plants. Biotechnol. Adv. 29, 792–803.

Govender, T., Stolnik, S., Garnett, M.C., Illum, L., Davis, S.S., 1999. PLGA nanoparticles prepared by nanoprecipitation: drug loading and release studies of a water soluble drug. J. Control. Release 57, 171–185.

Grillo, R., dos Santosc, N.Z.P., Maruyama, C.R., Rosa, A.H., de Lima, R., Fraceto, L.F., 2012. Poly(ε-caprolactone)nanocapsules as carrier systems for herbicides: physico-chemical characterization and genotoxicity evaluation. J. Hazard. Mater. 231–232, 1–9.

Guan, H., Chi, D., Yu, J., Li, X., 2008. A novel photodegradable insecticide: preparation, characterization and properties evaluation of nano-Imidacloprid. Pest. Biochem. Physiol. 92, 83–91.

Guan, H.-N., Chi, D.-F., Yu, J., Zhang, S.-Y., 2011. Novel photodegradable insecticide W/TiO_2/Avermectin nanocomposites obtained by polyelectrolytes assembly. Colloid Surf. B-Biointerfaces 83, 148–154.

Hayashi, A., Goto, Y., Nakayama, M., Sato, H., Watanabe, T., Miyata, S., 1992. Novel photoactivatable nonlinear optical polymers: poly[((4-azidophenyl)carboxy) ethyl methacrylate]. Macromolecules 25 (19), 5094–5098.

Hellmann, C., Greiner, A., Wendorff, J.H., 2011. Design of pheromone releasing nanofibers for plant protection. Polym. Adv. Technol. 22, 407–413.

Hwang, I.C., Kim, T.H., Bang, S.H., Kim, K.S., Kwon, H.R., Seo, M.J., Youn, Y.N., Park, H.J., Yasunaga-Aoki, C., Yu, Y.M., 2011. Insecticidal effect of controlled release formulations of etofenprox based on nano-bio technique. J. Fac. Agr., Kyushu Univ. 56 (1), 33–40.

Izquierdo, P., Feng, J., Esquena, J., Tadros, T.F., Dederen, J.C., Garcia, M.J., Azemar, N., Solans, C., 2005. The influence of surfactant mixing ratio on nano-emulsion formation by the pit method. J. Colloid Interface Sci. 285, 388–394.

Jia, X., Sheng, W.-B., Li, W., Tong, Y.-B., Liu, Z.-Y., Zhou, F., 2014. Adhesive polydopamine coated avermectin microcapsules for prolonging foliar pesticide retention. ACS Appl. Mater. Interfaces 6, 19552–19558.

Kabanov, A.V., Vinogradov, S.V., 2009. Nanogels as pharmaceutical carriers: finite networks of infinite capabilities. Angew. Chem. Int. 48, 5418–5429.

Kah, M., Hofmann, T., 2014. Nanopesticide research: current trends and future priorities. Environ. Int. 63, 224–235.

Kah, M., Beulke, S., Tiede, K., Hofmann, T., 2013. Nanopesticides: state of knowledge, environmental fate, and exposure modeling. Crit. Rev. Environ. Sci. Technol. 43, 1823–1867.

Kalaitzaki, A., Papanikolaou, N.E., Karamaouna, F., Dourtoglou, V., Xenakis, A., Papadimitriou, V., 2015. Biocompatible colloidal dispersions as potential formulations of natural pyrethrins: a structural and efficacy study. Langmuir 31, 5722–5730.

Kumar, S., Chauhan, N., Gopal, M., Kumar, R., Dilbaghi, N., 2015. Development and evaluation of alginate–chitosan nanocapsulesfor controlled release of acetamiprid. Int. J. Biol. Macromol. 81, 631–637.

Kumara, S., Bhanjana, G., Sharma, A., Sidhu, M.C., Dilbaghi, N., 2014. Synthesis, characterization and on field evaluation of pesticide loaded sodium alginate nanoparticles. Carbohydr. Polym. 101, 1061–1067.

Lai, F., Wissing, S.A., Müller, R.H., Fadda, A.M., 2006. *Artemisia arborescens* L essential oil-loaded solid lipid nanoparticles for potential agricultural application: preparation and characterization. AAPS PharmSciTech 7 (1), E1–E9.

Lanzotti, V., Romano, A., Lanzuise, S., Bonanomi, G., Scala, F., 2012a. Antifungal saponins from bulbs of white onion, *Allium cepa* L. Phytochemistry 74, 133–139.

Lanzotti, V., Barile, E., Antignani, V., Bonanomi, G., Scala, F., 2012b. Antifungal saponins from bulbs of garlic, *Allium sativum* L. var. Voghiera. Phytochemistry 78, 126–134.

Lao, S.-B., Zhang, Z.-X., Xu, H.-H., Jiang, G.-B., 2010. Novel amphiphilic chitosan derivatives: synthesis, characterization and micellar solubilization of rotenone. Carbohydr. Polym. 82, 1136–1142.

Li, M., Huang, Q., Wu, Y., 2011. A novel chitosan-poly(lactide) copolymer and its submicron particles as imidacloprid carriers. Pest Manag. Sci. 67, 831–836.

Lim, C.J., Mahiran, B., Dzolkhifli, O., Mohd Basyaruddin, A.R., Abu Bakar, S., Raja Noor Zaliha Raja, A.R., Ahmad, S., 2012a. Green nano-emulsion intervention for water-soluble glyphosate isopropylamine (IPA) formulations in controlling *Eleusine indica* (*E. indica*). Pest. Biochem. Physiol. 102, 19–29.

Lim, C.J., Mahiran, B., Dzolkhifli, O., Mohd Basyaruddin, A.R., Abu Bakar, S., Raja Noor Zaliha Raja, A.R., 2012b. Physicochemical characterization and formulation of glyphosate-laden nano-emulsion for herbicide formulation. Ind. Crop. Prod. 36, 607–613.

Liu, F., Wen, L.X., Li, Z.Z., Yu, W., Sun, H.Y., Chen, J.F., 2006. Porous hollow silica nanoparticles as controlled delivery system for water-soluble pesticide. Mater. Res. Bull. 41, 2268–2275.

Liu, Y., Tong, Z., Prud'homme, R.K., 2008a. Stabilized polymeric nanoparticles for controlled and efficient release of bifenthrin. Pest Manag. Sci. 64, 808–812.

Liu, Y., Cheng, C., Liu, Y., Prud'hommea, R.K., Fox, R.O., 2008b. Mixing in a multi-inlet vortex mixer (MIVM) for flash nano-precipitation. Chem. Eng. Sci. 63, 2829–2842.

Loha, K.M., Shakil, N.A., Kumar, J., Singh, M.K., Adak, T., Jain, S., 2011. Release kinetics of β-Cyfluthrin from its encapsulated formulations in water. J. Environ. Sci. Health B 46, 201–206.

Magdassi S, Netivi H, Margulis-Goshen K., 2007. Patent number: WO2008032327 (A2). Organic nanoparticles obtained from microemulsions by solvent evaporation.

Magdassi S, Dayan B, Levy-Ruso G., 2008. Patent number: US2,010,015,236 (A1). Pesticide nanoparticles obtained from microemulsions and nanoemulsions.

Margulis-Goshen, K., Magdassi, S., 2009. Formation of simvastatin nanoparticles from microemulsion. Nanomed. Nanotechnol. Biol. Med. 5 (3), 274–281.

Margulis-Goshen, K., Netivi, H.D., Major, D.T., Gradzielski, M., Raviv, U., Magdassi, S., 2009. Formation of organic nanoparticles from volatile microemulsions. J. Colloid Interface Sci. 2, 283–292.

McClements, D.J., 2011. Edible nanoemulsions: fabrication, properties, and functional performance. Soft Matter 7, 2297–2316.

Memarizadeh, N., Ghadamyari, M., Adeli, M., Talebi, K., 2014. Preparation,characterization and efficiency of nanoencapsulated imidacloprid under laboratory conditions. Ecotox. Environ. Safe. 107, 77–83.

Nuruzzaman, M., Rahman, M.M., Liu, Y., Naidu, R., 2016. Nanoencapsulation, nano-guard for pesticides: a new window for safe application. J. Agric. Food Chem. 64 (7), 1447–1483.

Organization for Economic Co-operation and Development, 2010. Challenges for agricultural research. OECD Publishing. Available from: http://dx.doi.org./10.1787/9789264090101-en

Park, M., Lee, C.-I., Seo, Y.J., Woo, S.R., Shin, D., Choi, J., 2010. Hybridization of the natural antibiotic, cinnamic acid, with layered double hydroxides (LDH) as green pesticide. Environ. Sci. Pollut. Res. 17, 203–209.

Perazzo, A., Preziosi, V., Guido, S., 2015. Phase inversion emulsification: current understanding and applications. Adv. Colloid Interface Sci. 222, 581–599.

Pereira, A.E.S., Grillo, R., Mello, N.F.S., Rosa, A.H., Fraceto, L.F., 2014. Application of poly(epsilon-caprolactone) nanoparticles containing atrazine herbicide as an alternative technique to control weeds and reduce damage to the environment. J. Hazard. Mater. 268, 207–215.

Postma, A., Yan, Y., Wang, Y., Zelikin, A.N., Tjipto, E., Caruso, F., 2009. Self-polymerization of dopamine as a versatile and robust technique to prepare polymer capsules. Chem. Mater. 21, 3042–3044.

Prado, A.G.S., Moura, A.O., Nunes, A.R., 2011. Nanosized silica modified with carboxylic acid as support for controlled release of herbicides. J. Agric. Food Chem. 59, 8847–8852.

Preston, G.W., Wilson, A.J., 2013. Photo-induced covalent cross-linking for the analysis of biomolecular interactions. Chem. Soc. Rev. 42, 3289–3301.

Qin, X., Xiang, X., Sun, X., Sun, H., Ni, H., Li, L., 2016. Preparation of nanoscale *Bacillus thuringiensis* chitinases using silica nanoparticles for nematicide delivery. Int. J. Biol. Macromol. 82, 13–21.

Ruckenstein, E., Chi, J.C., 1975. Stability of microemulsions. J. Chem. Soc., Faraday Trans. 2, 1690–1707, 71.

Saharan, V., Mehrotra, A., Khatik, R., Rawal, P., Sharma, S.S., Pal, A., 2013. Synthesis of chitosan based nanoparticles and their in vitro evaluation against phytopathogenic fungi. Int. J. Biol. Macromol. 62, 677–683.

Saharan, V., Sharma, G., Yadav, M., Choudhary, M.K., Sharmab, S.S., Pal, A., Raliya, R., Biswas, P., 2015. Synthesis and in vitro antifungal efficacy of Cu-chitosan nanoparticles against pathogenic fungi of tomato. Int. J. Biol. Macromol. 75, 346–353.

Saini, P., Gopal, M., Kumar, R., Srivastava, C., 2014. Development of pyridalyl nanocapsule suspension for efficient management of tomato fruit and shoot borer (*Helicoverpa armigera*). J. Environ. Sci. Health B 49, 344–351.

Shakil, N.A., Singh, M.K., Pandey, A., Kumar, J., Pankaj, Parmar, V.S., Singh, M.K., Pandey, R.P., Watterson, A.C., 2010. Development of poly(ethylene glycol) based amphiphilic copolymers for controlled release delivery of carbofuran. J. Macromol. Sci. Part A-Pure Appl. Chem. 47, 241–247.

Shinoda, K., Saito, H., 1969. The stability of O/W type emulsions as functions of temperature and the HLB of emulsifiers: the emulsification by PIT method. J. Colloid Interface Sci. 30 (2), 258–263.

Sooresh, A., Kwon, H., Taylor, R., Pietrantonio, P., Pine, M., Sayes, C.M., 2011. Surface functionalization of silver nanoparticles: novel applications for insect vector control. ACS Appl. Mater. Interfaces 3, 3779–3787.

Soppimath, K.S., Aminabhavi, T.M., Kulkarni, A.R., Rudzinski, W.E., 2001. Biodegradable polymeric nanoparticles as drug delivery devices. J. Control. Release 70, 1–20.

Storm, R.M., Price, D.C., Lubetkin, S.D., 2001. Aqueous dispersion of agricultural chemicals. US Patent 20,010,051,175.

Strom, R.M., Price, D.C., Lubetkin, S.D., 2001. Aqueous dispersions of agricultural chemicals. Patent number: US 0,051,175 (A1).

Sun, C., Shu, K., Wang, W., Ye, Z., Liu, T., Gao, Y., Zheng, H., He, G., Yin, Y., 2014. Encapsulation and controlled release of hydrophilic pesticide in shell cross-linked nanocapsules containing aqueous core. Int. J. Pharm. 463, 108–114.

Suresh Kumar, R.S., Shiny, P.J., Anjali, C.H., Jerobin, J., Margulis Goshen, K., Magdassi, S., Mukherjee, A., Chandrasekaran, N., 2013. Distinctive effects of nano-sized permethrin in the environment. Environ. Sci. Pollut. Res. 20, 2593–2602.

Tavakoli Naeini, A., Adeli, M., Vossoughi, M., 2010. Poly(citric acid)-block-poly(ethylene glycol) copolymers—new biocompatible hybrid materials for nanomedicine. Nanomed. Nanotechnol. Biol. Med. 6, 556–562.

UNICEF, World Health Organization, World Bank Group, 2016. Levels and trends in child malnutrition. Key findings of the 2015 edition. Available from: http://www.unicef.org/media/files/JME_2015_edition_Sept_2015.pdf.

Vinod, S., Bushettii, S.S., Appala Raju, S., Rizwan, A., Mamta, S., Anupam, B., 2011. Microemulsions as promising delivery systems: a review. Indian J. Pharm. Educ. Res. 45 (4), 392–401.

Wang, L., Li, X., Zhang, G., Dong, J., Eastoe, J., 2007. Oil-in-water nanoemulsions for pesticide formulations. J. Colloid Interface Sci. 314, 230–235.

Wanyika, H., 2013. Sustained release of fungicide metalaxyl by mesoporous silica nanospheres. J. Nanopart. Res. 15, 1831.

Wen, L.X., Li, Z.Z., Zou, H.K., Liu, A.Q., Chen, J.F., 2005. Controlled release of avermectin from porous hollow silica nanoparticles. Pest. Manag. Sci. 61, 583–590.

Wheeler, B.E.J., 1969. An Introduction to Plant Disease. John Wiley and Sons Limited, London, pp. 301.

Wibowo, D., Zhao, C.X., Peters, B.C., Middleberg, A.P.J., 2014. Sustained release of fipronil insecticide in vitro and in vivo from biocompatible silica nanocapsules. J. Agric. Food Chem. 62, 12504–12511.

Wu, Y., Zheng, Y., Yang, W., Wang, C., Hu, J., Fu, S., 2005. Synthesis and characterization of a novel amphiphilic chitosan-polylactide graft copolymer. Carbohydr. Polym. 59, 165–171.

Xiang, Y., Wang, M., Sun, X., Cai, D., Wu, Z., 2014. Controlling pesticide loss through nanonetworks. ACS Sustain. Chem. Eng. 2, 918–924.

Xu, J., Fan, Q.J., Yin, Z.Q., Li, X.T., Du, Y.H., Jia, R.Y., Wang, K.Y., Lv, C., Ye, G., Geng, Y., Su, G., Zhao, L., Hu, T.X., Shi, F., Zhang, L., Wu, C.L., Tao, C., Zhang, Y.X., Shi, D.X., 2010. The preparation of neem oil microemulsion (*Azadirachta indica*) and the comparison of acaricidal time between neem oil microemulsion and other formulations in vitro. Vet. Parasitol. 169, 399–403.

Yang, F.-L., Li, X.-G., Zhu, F., Lei, C.-L., 2009. Structural characterization of nanoparticles loaded with garlic essential oil and their insecticidal activity against *Tribolium castaneum* (Herbst) (Coleoptera: Tenebrionidae). J. Agric. Food Chem. 57, 10156–10162.

Yin, Y., Xu, S., Chang, D., Zheng, H., Li, J., Liu, X., Xu, P., Xiong, F., 2010. One-pot synthesis of biopolymeric hollow nanospheres by photocrosslinking. Chem. Commun. 46, 8222–8224.

Yin, Y.-H., Guo, Q.-M., Han, Y., Wang, L.-J., Wan, S.-Q., 2012. Preparation, characterization and nematicidal activity of lansiumamide B nano-capsules. J. Integr. Agric. 11 (7), 1151–1158.

Zeng, H., Li, X., Zhang, G., Dong, J., 2008. Preparation and characterization of beta cypermethrin nanosuspensions by diluting O/W microemulsions. J. Dispersion Sci. Technol. 29 (3), 358–361.

Zhang, J., Li, M., Fan, T., Xu, Q., Wu, Y., Chen, C., Huang, Q., 2013. Construction of novel amphiphilic chitosan copolymer nanoparticles for chlorpyrifos delivery. J. Polym. Res. 20 (3), 107.

Zhou, Z., Ye, J., Chen, L., Ma, A., Zou, F., 2010. Simultaneous determination of ropivacaine, bupivacaine and dexamethasone in biodegradable PLGA microspheres by high performance liquid chromatography. Yakugaku Zasshi-J. Pharm. Soc. 130 (8), 1061–1068.

Ziaee, M., Moharramipour, S., Mohsenifar, A., 2014. Toxicity of Carum copticum essential oil-loaded nanogel against *Sitophilus granarius* and *Tribolium confusum*. J. Appl. Entomol. 138 (10), 763–771.

5

NANOPESTICIDES: A REVIEW OF CURRENT RESEARCH AND PERSPECTIVES

John Hayles, Lucas Johnson, Clare Worthley, Dusan Losic
The University of Adelaide, School of Chemical Engineering, Adelaide, SA, Australia

1 Introduction

Contemporary agricultural pest and pathogen control methods result in ~90 % of the applied pesticides being lost to the air and as run-off, adversely affecting both farmers financially and the environment (Stephenson, 2003). Additionally, the indiscriminate use of pesticides intensifies pest and disease resistance, lessens nitrogen fixation, reduces soil biodiversity, and increases the bioaccumulation of pesticides (Tilman et al., 2002). These are significant issues, which require considerable focus; in order to reduce costs to stakeholders, increase productivity, improve efficiency, and reduce environmental impact. The application of new pesticide concepts based on nanotechnology, which are collectively referred to as "nanopesticides" is anticipated to address these issues by increasing pesticide efficacy, reducing dose required, improve stability of payloads delivered from the environment (i.e., UV degradation); subsequently diminishing run-off and alleviating environmental concerns. This new research field compromises a broad research aspect including study for fundamental understanding of interaction of nanoscale materials and insects, formulation of the active ingredients into nanoemulsions and dispersions using existing pesticides, development of new nanopesticide formulations using nanomaterials as active pesticide agents (silicia, titania, silver, etc.) or using these nanomaterials as nanocarriers for their delivery (polymer nanoparticles). There is confidence that nanopesticides will address the main limitations of existing pest control strategies and provide new advanced nano

New Pesticides and Soil Sensors. http://dx.doi.org/10.1016/B978-0-12-804299-1.00006-0

based formulation that remain stable and active in the spray environment (sun, heat, rain), penetrate the organism (fungus, insect), can be delivered to the target, resist defense of the pest/pathogen, remain benign to plants and mammals, be cost effective to formulate and manufacture and preferably possess a new mode of action (Smith et al., 2008). The following chapters will present an overview of recent advancements in this research field describing these concepts their advantages and limitations followed with conclusions and future perspectives.

2 Nanoscale Particles for Agriculture: Definition, Concepts and Perspectives

Nanoscale particles can be defined as a subclass of ultrafine particle with characteristic dimensions from 1 to 100 nm and have properties that are not shared by nonnanoscale particles with the same chemical composition (Auffan et al., 2009). The basis of the 100-nm limit is the fact that unique properties that differentiate particles from the bulk material typically develop at a critical length scale of under 100 nm. However, because other phenomena (transparency or turbidity, ultrafiltration, stable dispersion, etc.) that extend the upper limit are occasionally considered, the use of the prefix "nano" is accepted for dimensions smaller than 500 nm (Alemán et al., 2007). The size, shape (spherical, rods, tubes, irregular), surface-to-volume ratio, crystal phase (crystalline, amorphous), chemical composition (metallic, carbon, inorganic, organic, polymeric, etc.) are key parameters which define many outstanding properties of these materials relevant for their pesticide application including toxicity. A broad variety of materials have been synthesized or used from natural materials to make NPs, in different forms and chemical composition including emulsions, dispersions of metal, metal oxides, semiconductor quantum dots (QDs), carbon, ceramics, silicates, lipids, polymers, proteins, dendrimers, and so on (Niemeyer et al., 2001; Oskam, 2006; Puoci et al., 2008). Some common benefits of nanoparticles based pesticide formulations include the increased solubility of water insoluble active ingredients, increased stability of formulation, elimination of toxic organic solvents in comparison to conventionally used pesticides, providing capability to slow release of active ingredients, improve stability and prevent their early degradation, improve their mobility and higher insecticidal activity due to smaller particle size and higher surface area, extend their longevity (Sasson et al., 2007).

The mode of action against target pests is expected to be enhanced with nanoparticles, as opposed to bulk materials. Increased mobility of nanoparticles enables superior insecticidal activity through contact with the insect's cuticle or ingestion into the digestive tract (Sasson et al., 2007). Additionally, nanoparticles observed penetration into plants (Boehm et al., 2003), uniform leaf coverage, and improved diffusion properties to soil (Cameron and Mitchell, 2007) further promote their beneficial use in agriculture.

3 Pesticides as Nanoemulsions and Nanodispersions

3.1 Common Issues With Conventional Pesticide Formulations

The fundamental limitation with the use of current agroherbicides and pesticides is that they are generally comprised of virtually insoluble compounds (Whitehouse and Rannard, 2010). This lack of solubility requires the addition of large amounts of organic solvents to dissolve them, for suitable efficacy and uniform application in the field. The necessity to use solvents increases costs, environmental pollutants, and increased user exposure (Stackelberg et al., 2001). In many applications, it is necessary to disperse the active ingredients (a.i.'s) of chemical pesticides in a liquid phase, as this facilitates spraying application. By far the most convenient liquid for applying pesticides is water, owing to its low cost, availability, and environmental compatibility (Lawrence and Warisnoicharoen, 2006; Pratap and Bhowmick, 2008). However, one of the main problems associated with many pesticides is that they are poorly soluble, or even insoluble in water. This is most often due to:

1. The pesticide being highly lipophilic (nonpolar), which makes mixing these pesticides into water thermodynamically unfavorable (increasing the contact surface area between the two incompatible phases increases the interfacial free energy).
2. In some instances, the pesticide having strong intermolecular bonding and a high lattice energy in the solid state (represented by a melting point above 200°C) (Yadollahi et al., 2009).

Consequently, droplets or particles of these pesticides are driven to demix from water, which occurs by coalescence, flocculation, sedimentation, creaming, and Ostwald ripening processes (Fig. 5.1) unless continuous vigorous agitation is carried out. As a result of this separation, it is much more difficult to apply the

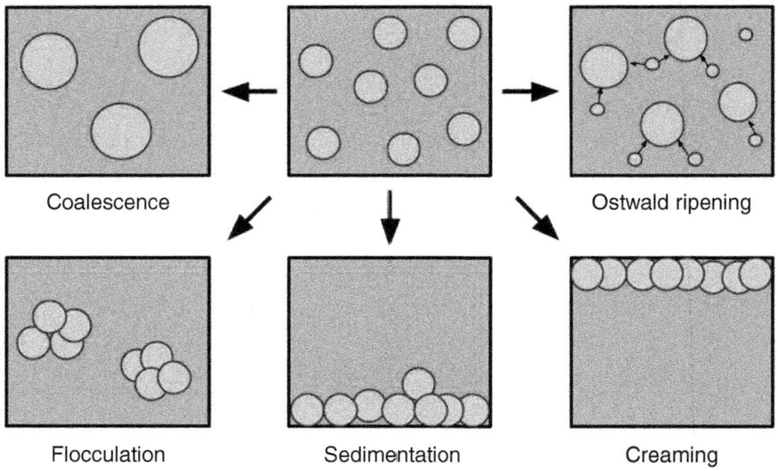

Figure 5.1. Depiction of the mechanisms by which dispersed droplets of nonpolar pesticides demix from water, which include droplet coalescence, flocculation, sedimentation, creaming, and Ostwald ripening.

pesticide uniformly on treated surfaces, thereby requiring much higher quantities to be applied to ensure that a sufficient dose is present in all areas to control the target pest. Not only does this increase costs, but it also increases the negative environmental and health impacts of the pesticide. These significant problems can be addressed by using nanotechnology to reduce particle size of pesticide materials to nano or colloidal scale, which substantially increases their water solubility, dissolution rate, and uniform dispersion when applied. Furthermore, the production of nanosized particles results in partially or fully amorphous products that are distinctly more soluble than their crystalline equivalents (Hancock and Parks, 2000; Yu, 2001).

One way by which solubility problem is commonly solved in commercial formulations is to combine the pesticide with surfactants; a type of molecule that is comprised of both a polar head group and a nonpolar group (such as an alkyl chain). When mixed with water, the surfactant molecules localize at the pesticide-water interface due to the thermodynamically unfavorable contact between the surfactants nonpolar groups and water (the hydrophobic effect), which causes the surfactant molecules to be arranged with the polar portions extending into the aqueous solution, and the nonpolar portions facing inward toward the pesticide (Fig. 5.2A). In doing so, they help to lower the interfacial surface energy, thereby facilitating dispersal of the pesticide in the form of small particles. In the case of liquid pesticides, these formulations are called emulsifiable concentrates (or coarse emulsions), while solid pesticides are referred to as wettable powders. Typically, particle sizes for these formulations are in the micron range (1–20 μm in diameter).

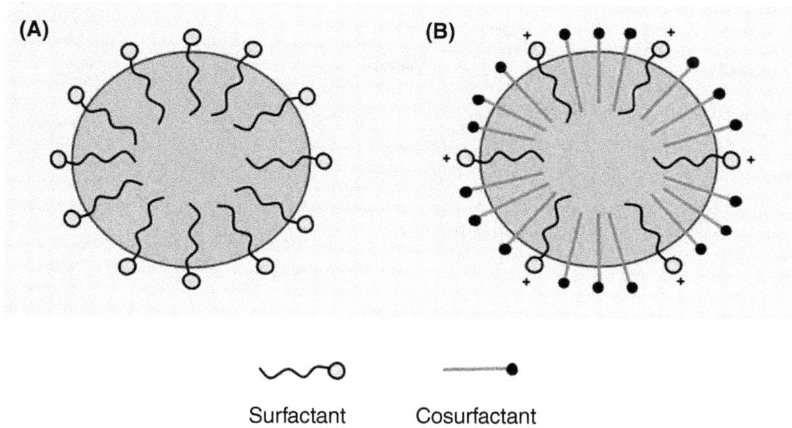

Figure 5.2. (A) Diagram showing the arrangement of surfactant molecules at the interface of a nonpolar pesticide droplet and water, with the nonpolar tail of the surfactant oriented inward into the droplet, and the hydrophilic head group facing the aqueous solution, (B) in the case of highly repelling surfactants (such as ionic surfactant), cosurfactant molecules are also added, which act as spacers that reduce repulsion between ionic surfactants on the droplet surface.

While this type of formulation has improved stability, they still tend to demix after a relatively short period of time unless constant agitation is applied. A more recent approach to further improve this stability involves dispersing the pesticide a.i. in water as a colloid, where the pesticide is in the form of nanosized droplets or solid particles (diameter <250 nm) that are stabilized with the aid of surfactants (McClements, 2012). The formation of a pesticide colloid helps prevent demixing of the pesticide from water in several ways. Firstly, preparing a colloid where the vast majority of particles are <200 nm in diameter effectively prevents creaming and sedimentation, as Brownian motion overcomes forces due to buoyancy and gravity respectively (McClements, 2012). Secondly, surfactants can generate a strong repulsive force between the droplets/particles (such as by electrostatic repulsion or steric hindrance), which helps prevent flocculation and coalescence, by establishing a large energy barrier that needs to be overcome in order for these processes to occur (McClements, 2012). Note that in the case of strongly repelling surfactants, a cosurfactant is often added (typically an aliphatic alcohol) which acts as a spacer between the surfactant molecules (Fig. 5.2B). This helps limit unwanted repulsion between surfactant molecules on a given colloidal particle, which would otherwise lower the density of surfactant at the interface and give a lower stability. Additionally, the preference for surfactants is toward the use of nonionic surfactants, in order to optimize the inertness between the surfactant and the pesticide, and to minimize the effect of varying water hardness (which can dramatically reduce the effectiveness of ionic surfactants as emulsion stabilizers) (Pratap and Bhowmick, 2008).

In the case of liquid a.i.'s (or solids that are dissolved in a small amount of organic solvent), these colloids are referred to as nanoemulsions. In the case of solid particles (comprised either of solid pesticides or liquid pesticides entrained within an inert nonpolar matrix), they are referred to as nanodispersions (Green and Beestman, 2007). These categories are each discussed in the following sections.

3.2 Nanoemulsions

A pesticide nanoemulsion [more generally referred to as an oil-in-water (O/W) emulsion] is where the pesticide is dispersed as nanosized droplets in water, with surfactant molecules localized at the pesticide-water interface. Depending upon the quantity and type of surfactant used, nanoemulsions can be classified as either being thermodynamically stable or kinetically stable.

3.2.1 Thermodynamically Stable Nanoemulsions

This type of nanoemulsion forms when (1) the nonpolar pesticide is at least partially soluble in the aqueous phase and (2) a strongly repelling surfactant is present in the aqueous phase at concentrations higher than the so called critical micelle concentration (CMC). Under these conditions, the surfactant molecules greatly prefer to assemble into spherical aggregates called micelles, which are arranged with the polar portions of the molecules extending outward into the aqueous solution, and the nonpolar portions of the molecules facing inward and associating with each other, creating a hydrophobic core (Fig. 5.3A). When the nonpolar pesticide is added to this aqueous solution, the pesticide molecules are driven to diffuse into the micelle interiors in order to minimize the free energy, there by swelling the micelles to form small droplets (Fig 5.3B). The size of these droplets is primarily determined by the chemical nature and quantity of the surfactant and pesticide (Green and Beestman, 2007; Lawrence and Warisnoicharoen, 2006; Knowles, 2005).

This type of nanoemulsion is considered to be thermodynamically stable (under a particular range of temperatures and concentrations), as the swollen micelle state has the lowest free energy.

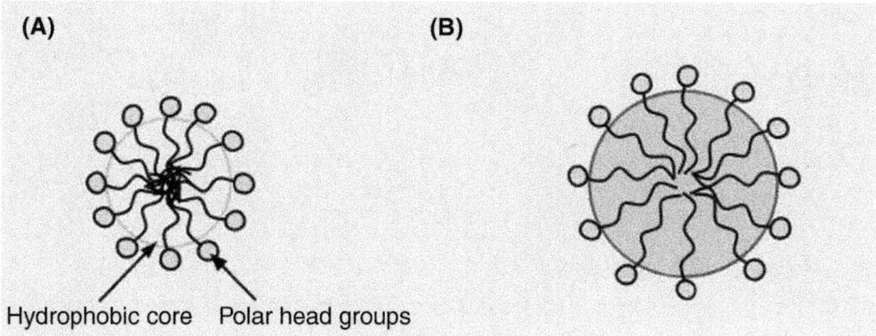

Figure 5.3. (A) Depiction of a micelle, which is an aggregate of surfactant molecules that forms in solution at concentrations greater than the critical micelle concentration (CMC). In aqueous solution, the surfactant molecules orient with the nonpolar portions aggregating to form a hydrophobic core and the polar portion facing out toward the aqueous solution, (B) a micelle that has been swollen with nonpolar pesticide to form a nanosized droplet. Pesticide migrates into the micelles via diffusion in order to minimize free energy.

Consequently, these nanoemulsions remains stable indefinitely, provided the initial conditions are not altered. This also means that these emulsions form spontaneously when the surfactant, pesticide, and water components are brought together, although in practice, the presence of kinetic energy barriers and/or slow mass transport processes may make it necessary to mechanically agitate or heat the system in order to prepare the nanoemulsion (Green and Beestman, 2007; Lawrence and Warisnoicharoen, 2006).

The high stability and simple preparation to form these nanoemulsions makes them highly advantageous for pesticide formulations, and as such, there are many commercial formulations currently available on the market (Tomlin, 2009; Green and Beestman, 2007; Knowles, 2005). However, this type of nanoemulsion also comes with several disadvantages. For example, the substantial quantities of surfactant required (typically about 20% of the formulation by weight) make them costly, and only limited quantities of pesticide can be incorporated into the micelles (less than 30% by weight of the total formulation) (Tadros et al., 2004; Lawrence and Warisnoicharoen, 2006). The high quantity of surfactant is also undesirable with respect to unintended phytotoxicity to exposed plants (Katagi, 2008).

Additionally, only highly repelling surfactant systems are suitable, as they have a greater tendency to form micelles. The optimum combination of surfactants and cosurfactants will also vary depending upon the pesticide that is to be emulsified, making formulation development a time consuming process (McClements, 2012).

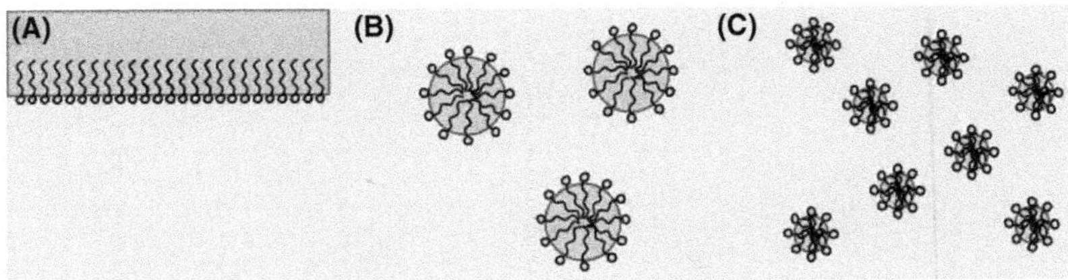

Figure 5.4. (A) Two-phase system of nonpolar pesticide and water, with surfactant molecules arranged at the interface, (B) large droplets of pesticide formed from shearing the two-phase system, which are stabilized by surfactant, (C) further shear reduces the droplet size further, until nanosized droplets stabilized by surfactant are formed.

3.2.2 Kinetically Stable Nanoemulsions

In contrast to thermodynamically stable nanoemulsions, kinetically stable nanoemulsions are formed under conditions where it is much less energetically favorable for the surfactant molecules to aggregate into micelles (such as at lower concentrations or with weakly repelling surfactants), and the pesticide is almost completely insoluble in the aqueous phase. In this case, the mixture of water, pesticide and surfactant initially forms a two-phase system, with the surfactant molecules preferentially assembling at the pesticide-water interface (Fig. 5.4A). If shear is then applied to the system (such as by stirring), the pesticide phase breaks up into droplets that are coated with surfactant and are inhibited from demixing due to interfacial repulsion (Fig. 5.4B). As this emulsion is sheared further, larger pesticide droplets are stretched, undergo a capillary instability, and rupture into smaller droplets. This process is continued until nanosized droplets of pesticide are formed (Fig. 5.4C) (Lawrence and Warisnoicharoen, 2006; Mason et al., 2006; Anton et al., 2008; Song et al., 2009).

Nanoemulsions of this type are thermodynamically unstable, as the nanoemulsion has a higher free energy than the demixed state. As a result, the droplets will eventually separate from the aqueous phase, primarily by Ostwald ripening. However, the presence of surfactant at the droplet surfaces provides an energy barrier that opposes demixing, thereby slowing the rate of these processes. In this case, the pesticides droplets in the nanoemulsion will remain dispersed for an extended period of time, and so are considered to be kinetically stable. This stability can be as high as several years for large energy barriers (>20 kT), which is sufficient for most practical applications (McClements, 2005; Lawrence and Warisnoicharoen, 2006; Gutierrez et al., 2008).

As micelles are not required, kinetically stable nanoemulsions may be formed using substantially less surfactant than a thermodynamically stable nanoemulsion (5–10% of the formulation by weight). Furthermore, a wider range of surfactant systems can be utilized (McClements, 2012). However, as stated previously, one of the key requirements to prepare this type of nanoemulsion is that the pesticide phase needs to be broken up into nanosized droplets before the surfactant molecules can coat and stabilize them. Some methods used to achieve this dispersal involve intensively mixing the pesticide and water using high–energy processes involving extreme shear, which is necessary to disperse the pesticide as nanosized droplets as the vast majority of the energy input is lost to viscous dissipation. This makes these approaches inefficient, difficult to scale up for commercial agrochemical production, and impractical for on-site preparation (Anton et al., 2008). The principal examples of these high-energy mixing methods are:

Ultrasonication: In this method, a vibrating solid surface agitates the coarse emulsion at ultrasonic frequencies (typically greater than 20 kHz) and high power. This leads to cavitations, where small liquid-free bubbles are produced and then implode, causing intensive shock waves and high velocity jets of liquid that act to break up emulsion droplets. Since the emitted sound field is typically inhomogeneous, it is often necessary to recirculate the emulsion so that all droplets experience the highest shear rate (Mason, 1992; Lauterborn and Ohl, 1997; Mason et al., 2006). While this method is often performed at laboratory scale, it is hard to scale up to produce commercially relevant quantities of pesticide nanoemulsions (Wang et al., 2007).

High Pressure Homogenization: This method uses a high-pressure positive displacement pump (up to 2000 atmospheres) to force a premade coarse emulsion of pesticide, water, and surfactant (<10 μm in diameter) through rigid microchannels (about 100-μm wide), which direct the resulting fluid flows into an interaction chamber. This subjects the emulsion droplets to extreme hydraulic shear, intense turbulence, collisions, and cavitations, which result in the production of very fine droplets in the submicron range. The coarse emulsion may be passed through the microchannels repeatedly until the desired particle size is obtained. The bulk emulsion is then filtered to remove large droplets, resulting in a uniform nanoemulsion. To enhance the efficiency of the emulsification, the emulsion is preferably prepared at high volume fractions of pesticide, and then diluted afterwards. Although this may result in coalescence, more surfactant can be added to prevent this (Jafari et al., 2007; Lovelyn and Attama, 2011). This method can be used for the preparation of nanoemulsions at both laboratory and industrial scales (Graves et al., 2005; Mason et al., 2006).

Given the disadvantages of extreme shear mixing, more recent research has focused on developing a variety of low-energy emulsification methods to disperse nonpolar liquids as nanosized droplets. These methods take advantage of the phase behavior properties of the emulsion constituents to promote the formation of nanosized droplets, chiefly by changing the parameters which would affect the solubility, or hydrophilic–lipophilic balance (HLB) of the surfactants (such as temperature and composition). These methods are usually more cost-effective to employ than high-energy methods, but are much more difficult to formulate (Rang and Miller, 1999; Anton et al., 2008).

The main low energy methods (reviewed in Lovelyn and Attama, 2011) include:

Phase Inversion Temperature: This approach takes advantage of the temperature-dependent solubility of nonionic surfactants (in particular polyethoxylated surfactants) to modulate the size of pesticide droplets in an emulsion. The first step of this method involves preparing a coarse O/W emulsion using the nonionic surfactant. The emulsion is then heated, which causes the nonionic surfactant to become more soluble in the pesticide phase and less soluble in the aqueous phase (decreases the HLB). This is accompanied by a concurrent decrease in the size of the pesticide droplets (to create more surface area to accommodate the surfactant). Eventually, a critical temperature is reached (the phase inversion temperature or PIT), where the surfactant starts to become preferentially solubilized in the pesticide phase and the initial O/W emulsion undergoes phase inversion to water-in-oil (W/O) emulsion (Fig. 5.5). Further increases in temperature lead to an increase in the size of the water droplets.

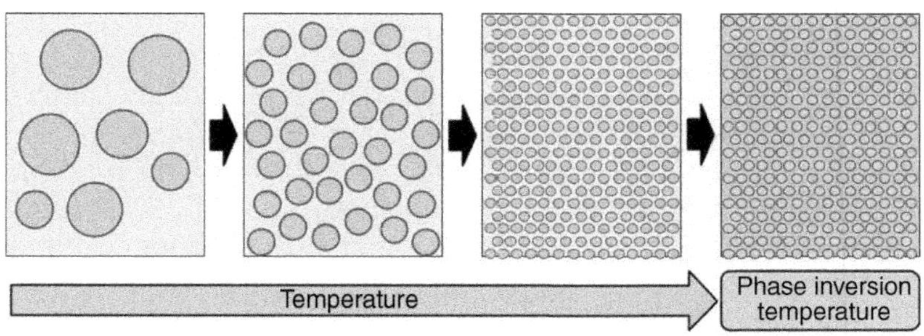

Figure 5.5. Heating an oil-in-water (O/W) emulsion results in a decrease in droplet size to accommodate the surfactant (increase surface area) as it becomes more soluble in the pesticide phase. This size reduction continues until a critical temperature is reached, whereupon a phase inversion to a water-in-oil (W/O) emulsion occurs.

At temperatures just below the PIT, the droplet size reaches a minimum. However, these small droplets are unstable and coalesce very rapidly. In order to stabilize the resulting nanoemulsion, it is rapidly cooled (at least 20°C below the PIT), which slows coalescence and Ostwald ripening by increasing the fluid viscosity and slowing the pesticide diffusion rate through the water (Shinoda and Saito, 1968; Forster et al., 1995; Izquierdo et al., 2002, 2004, 2005; Morales et al., 2003).

Phase Transition: As with the PIT method, this approach involves modifying the conditions so that the temperature is just below the PIT, in order to promote the formation of nanosized droplets of pesticide. In this case, however, the temperature is kept fixed and the composition is gradually changed in a stepwise fashion, which modifies the PIT for the emulsion. This may be achieved by starting with a mixture of surfactant and pesticide, and then gradually adding water (which decreases the surfactant concentration and the pesticide to water ratio) (Fig. 5.6) (Forgiarini et al., 2000, 2001a,b).

Self-Emulsification: This method involves a mixture of pesticide, surfactant and a cosolvent (chemical that is mutually soluble in the pesticide and water) first being prepared, which is then added to a large quantity of water. This contact with the water then results in the spontaneous formation of an O/W nanoemulsion (Lopez-Montilla et al., 2002). While the precise mechanisms by which these nanoemulsions form remains the subject of intensive

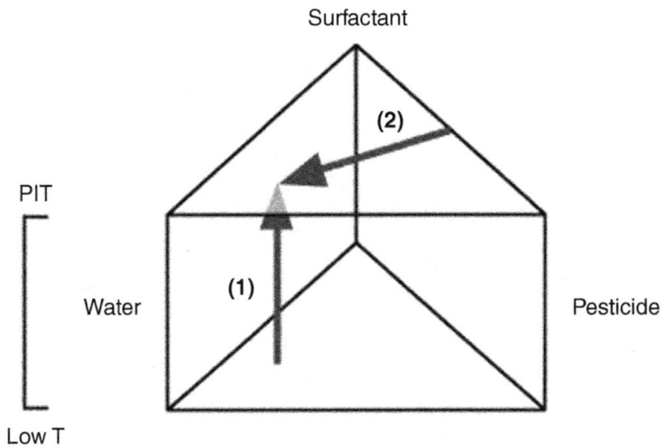

Figure 5.6. Three-dimensional phase diagram for a mixture comprising nonpolar pesticide, water, and surfactant, with the different levels corresponding to different temperatures. (1) Corresponds to heating an emulsion to near the phase inversion temperature in order to reduce the droplet size. (2) Corresponds to approaching this phase transition by gradually diluting the mixture with water.

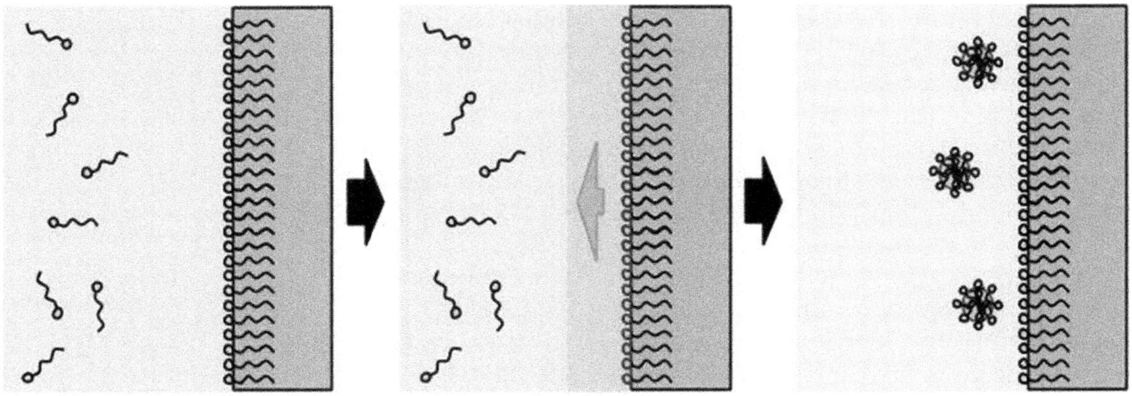

Figure 5.7. Depiction of the interface of a bulk pesticide phase in an aqueous solution of surfactant, where the pesticide phase also contains a cosolvent that is soluble in both pesticide and water. This cosolvent gradually diffuses out of the pesticide phase, creating a region at the surface that contains a mixture of water, cosolvent and dissolved pesticide. As the cosolvent diffuses further into the aqueous phase, the dissolved pesticide suddenly becomes insoluble and demixes from the water. This demixed pesticide is stabilized in the form of nanosized droplets due to the presence of nearby surfactant molecules, which rapidly assemble at the droplet surface.

basic research, the predominant mechanism that is currently accepted for self-emulsification is the "diffusion and stranding" mechanism (Pouton, 1997; Miller, 2005). In this mechanism, the cosolvent begins to diffuse into the aqueous phase when mixing takes place, taking some of the pesticide with it (forming a three component phase near the interface). As the cosolvent diffuses further into the aqueous phase and dilutes, it is unable to keep the pesticide dissolved in the three component phase, causing it to separate from the water in the form of nanosized droplets (super saturation) which are rapidly stabilized by the assembly of surfactant at the interface (Fig. 5.7) (Pons et al., 2003; Bataller et al., 2004; Lamaallam et al., 2005; Dicharrya et al., 2003).

3.3 Nanodispersions

In nanodispersions the pesticide is dispersed as solid nanosized particles in water. In the same manner as for nanoemulsions, nanodispersions are stabilized against demixing from the water by their small size and the presence of surfactant molecules localized at the particle surface, which are similarly arranged with the polar portions extending into the aqueous solution and the nonpolar portions associating with the solid pesticide (Acosta, 2009; Muller and Junghanns, 2006; Muller et al., 1995). While nanodispersions with long-term stability may be prepared with particles as large as 200 nm in diameter, smaller particles (diameter less than 50 nm) are preferred, as they yield the greatest improvement in pesticide solubility. In contrast to nanoemulsions, only kinetically stable nanodispersions can be prepared (Muller and Junghanns, 2006).

A variety of well-established methods for preparing nanodispersions are currently available, which were originally developed for the food industry (to allow the incorporation of bioactive compounds), and have been more recently utilized in the pharmaceutical sector. The main preparation methods are dry/wet milling, extraction precipitation, solvent evaporation from nanoemulsions, and high-pressure homogenization (which has been discussed in the section on nanoemulsions) (Muller and Junghanns, 2006).

3.3.1 Milling

In this method, high-shear ball mills (also known as pearl mills) are used to break down solid pesticides either into a nanoparticle powder (dry milling) or directly into a nanodispersion (wet milling). These mills are comprised of a milling chamber, which contains small balls made from aluminum oxide ceramic or highly cross-linked polystyrene resin (Hu et al., 2004; Liverside et al., 1992; Peters and Muller, 1996). This method is easy to scale up and gives reproducible results, but erosion of the balls can lead to contamination of the final product (Chingunpituk, 2007).

3.3.2 Extraction/Precipitation

This method involves dissolving the pesticide into a suitable nonpolar solvent, then carefully adding this solution to a polar liquid containing surfactant that is miscible with the nonpolar solvent. The resulting shift in pesticide solubility causes precipitation to occur, which is restricted to small particle sizes due to the stabilization effects of the surfactant. Particle size can be preserved until use by lyophilisation (freeze drying) or spray drying the resulting nanodispersion. While simple to carry out, the limitation of this technique is the requirement for the drug to be soluble in at least one solvent, which also needs to be miscible with a nonsolvent (Gassmann et al., 1994).

3.3.3 Solvent Evaporation From Nanoemulsions

In this approach, the pesticide is first dissolved in a volatile organic solvent that is partially miscible in water, such as butyl lactate, benzyl alcohol, or ethyl acetate. A nanoemulsion of the dissolved pesticide with water is then formed by high-pressure homogenization or other techniques. Dilution with water leads to the formation of nanosuspensions, through a combination of diffusion of the organic solvent into the aqueous phase and evaporation of the organic solvent, which converts the droplets into solid particles. The size of the emulsion droplets determines the final particle size (Kocbek et al., 2006; Trotta et al., 2001). As with the extraction/precipitation method, the resulting nanoparticles may be isolated by lyophilization of spray drying for long-term storage. The main disadvantage of this approach is presence of residual organic solvents in the final products (Kocbek et al., 2006; Zhang et al., 2008).

3.4 Advantages of Nanoemulsions and Nanodispersions

While the main objective of preparing colloids of chemical pesticides is to improve water solubility, and hence delivery of the active ingredients, recent research has shown that reformulation of chemical pesticides as a colloid can also influence other important properties of the pesticide.

3.4.1 Bioavailability

The majority of this research concerns evaluation of the bioavailability, and hence efficacy, of the formulations. In many cases, a significant increase in bioavailability is observed, due to a combination of greater surface area for exposure (smaller particle sizes in addition to enhanced wetting and spreading of the pesticide on treated surfaces) and enhanced penetration through waxy plant and insect cuticles (Tadros et al., 2004; Katagi, 2008; Abribat et al., 2004). For example, studies by Anjali et al. (2012) on neem oil nanoemulsions showed that the median lethal concentration (LC_{50}) against southern house mosquitoes (*Culex quinquefasciatus*) was highly dependent on the emulsion droplet size, with smaller droplets (11.75 mg/L at 31 nm diameter) being substantially more effective than larger droplets (62.89 mg/L at 251 nm diameter). This was hypothesized to be due to an increase in the surface area of the droplets, which increases the rate of accumulation by the larvae of the insecticidal components of the oil. Likewise, studies by Xu et al. (2010) demonstrated that 10% neem oil nanoemulsions yielded a quicker median lethal response time (LT_{50}: 81.7 min) against itch mites(*Sarcoptes scabiei*) than coarse neem oil emulsions (95.6 min), neem oil solutions in liquid paraffin (156.7 min) and control treatments (1576.2 min). Other research by Kalaitzaki et al. (2015) showed that O/W nanoemulsions of pyrethrins (36–37 nm in diameter) are also more effective than commercially available coarse emulsions against nymphs of the cotton aphid (*Aphis gossypii*), with an LC_{50} of 0.609 mg/L compared with 0.966 mg/L. The herbicide Glyophosate has also been shown to have improved, efficacy when it is formulated as a colloid. Lim et al. prepared glyphosphate nanoemulsions (200 nm diameter) with various proportions of fatty acid methyl esters, organo-silicones, and alkyl glucosides, and compared their efficacy with commercially available formulation Roundup against a variety of plant pests. In these studies, they found that these nanoemulsions yielded improved efficacy against cowsfoot grass (*Eleusine indica*) (ED_{50} of 0.40 vs. 0.48 kg a.i./ha), and had a similar efficacy against creeping foxglove (*Asystasia gangetica*), slender buttonweed (*Diodia ocimifolia*), and buffalo grass (*Paspalum conjugatum*), despite having significantly lower spray deposition on the leaf surface. This increased efficacy was ascribed to enhance penetration of the pesticide active ingredients through the plants cuticles (Lim et al., 2012, 2013).

Nanodispersions of permethrin were also found to be more effective than permethrin microparticles. Kumar et al. (2013) demonstrated that permethrin nanodispersions had greater efficacy against yellow fever mosquito larvae (*Aedes aegypti*), with a 24 h LC_{50} of 6.3 μg/L compared with 20 μg/L for microparticles. Similarly, Anjali et al. (2010) showed that permethrin nanodispersions (151 ± 27 nm diameter) gave enhanced efficacy compared with microparticles (LC_{50} of 117 μg/L vs. 715 μg/L) against southern house mosquito (*C. quinquefasciatus*). One last example is provided by Fan et al., who reported that nanoemulsions of Emamectin-benzoate were significantly more effective against Asian rice borer (*Chilo suppressalis*) compared to commercially available coarse emulsions. They found that nanoemulsions yielded less borer damaged rice seedlings (6.25%) compared to the commercial formulations (12.62%) at a dose of 4 mg/L. By comparison, 47.95% of untreated rice seedlings were damaged by the insects. This improvement was ascribed to the much lower surface tension of these formulations, which leads to improved retention of the pesticide on the treated leaf surfaces (Fan et al., 2010).

Importantly, it should also be mentioned that some reports show no improvement in efficacy when formulating a pesticide as a colloid. For example, Huang et al. investigated the efficacy of O/W nanoemulsions of Chlorpyrifos (51.8 nm diameter) against the cotton bollworm (*Helicoverpa armigera*). Laboratory assays gave no statistically significant difference in LC_{50} values for the nanoemulsion (500 mg/L) and a commercially available coarse emulsion (561 mg/L). Field tests also showed no improvement in efficacy (Huang et al., 2006). In another study by Elek et al. (2010), nanodispersions of novaluron (200 ± 50 nm diameter) were found to offer no statistically significant improvement in efficacy compared to equivalent doses of commercial pesticides with the same active ingredients.

3.4.2 Enhanced Stability

Another area of research concerns the stability of the pesticides prepared as colloids. Many chemical pesticides are known to be susceptible to degradation, which can occur through a variety of mechanisms. One of the most important degradation processes of a pesticide in water is abiotichydrolysis, where the pesticide reacts with H_3O^+ and OH^- species in water, converting it into a molecule with greatly reduced biological activity. Incorporation of chemical pesticides into an O/W nanoemulsion may restrict degradation by hydrolysis, as the pesticide experiences a different surrounding environment from the bulk water phase (Katagi, 2002). For example, Song et al. prepared O/W nanoemulsions of Triazophos, and compared the decomposition rates with a coarse emulsion of Triazophos (over a 48 hour period) under a range of temperatures and pH conditions. They reported that decomposition rates were lower in the nanoemulsions over the temperature range 25–45°C (1.45 vs. 2.02% at 25°C, 8.23 vs. 12.56% at 45°C), and over a pH range of 5–9 (1.19 vs. 1.59% at pH 5, 1.64 vs. 2.86% at pH 9). This was ascribed to limited diffusion of the $H3O^+$ and OH^- species from the aqueous phase into the nonpolar micelle cores (Song et al., 2009).

However, it should be noted that the selection of an appropriate surfactant to protect the pesticide from hydrolysis is critical. For example, Balakrishnan et al. studied the stability of nanoemulsions of fenitrothion prepared using the cationic surfactant cetyltrimethylammonium hydroxide (CTA^+OH^-). This was ascribed to the orientation of the pesticide in the micelle core, with the aromatic ring and aliphatic side chains oriented toward the micelle interior and the vulnerable P = S group associating with the polar surfactant head groups, which acted to electrostatically attract OH^- ions, thereby increasing the local concentration (Fig. 5.8) (Balakrishnan et al., 2004, 2005; Han et al., 2006).

Colloidal formulations have also been used to stabilize pesticides against photodegradation from exposure to UV light. For instance, work by Nguyen et al. (2012a,b) showed that by combining deltamethrin with lipids (such as corn oil and beeswax) and then converting into a colloid, a moderate level of photo-protection can be achieved, with an up to 1.8-fold increase in photo-stability after a 12 h exposure to UV light.

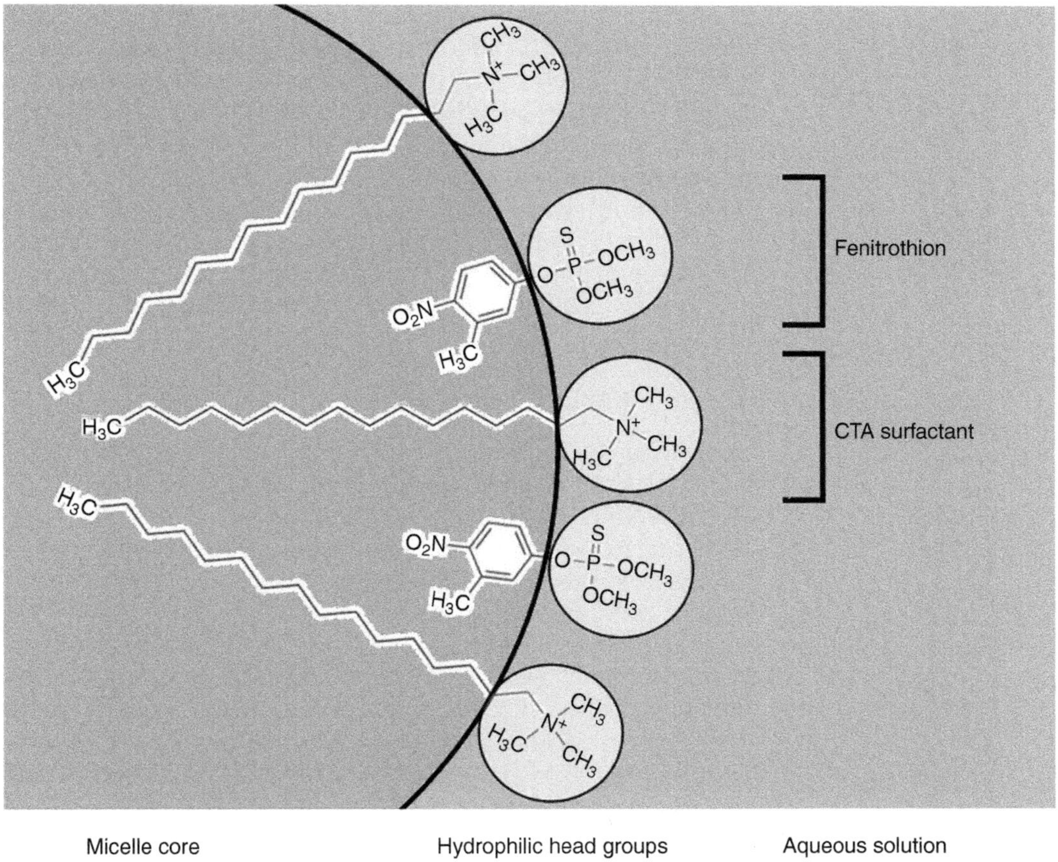

Figure 5.8. Nanoemulsions of fenitrothion prepared using cetyltrimethylammonium (CTA) surfactant arrange with the pesticide molecules orienting at the micelle interface to present the hydrolytically vulnerable P = S group to the aqueous solution. This results in an increase in the degradation rate compared with nanoemulsions of other nonpolar pesticides, which typically lie in the core of the micelle rather than at the surface.

3.4.3 Controlled Release

Previous studies showed that the release kinetics of pesticide active ingredients from colloidal formulations, can be used to slow the release process, resulting in more sustained exposure and longer term efficacy (Zeng et al., 2008). One example of this is given by Lai et al., who demonstrated that incorporation of tree wormwood (*Artemisia arborescens* L.) essential oil into lipid nanodispersions (200–300 nm diameter) yielded substantially slower evaporation of the essential oil compared to coarse emulsions. Both burst release rates (1 h, 3.0 vs. 21.6% w/w) and longer-term release rates (48 h, 37.07 vs. 69.56% w/w) were decreased. Different release rates for different surfactants were also observed (Lai et al., 2006).

In another example, Yang et al. investigated the long term insecticidal activity of lipid nanodispersions (<240 nm diameter) loaded with garlic (*Allium sativum*) essential oil against adult red flour beetle (*Tribolium castaneum*). They found that the nanodispersion efficacy against adult *T. castaneum* remained over 80% after 5 months (at a dose of 640 mg/kg total formulation), which was hypothesised to be due to the slow and persistent release of the essential oils from the nanoparticles. In contrast, the efficacy of free garlic essential oil at the same concentration was only 11% (Yang et al., 2009).

4 Polymer-Based Nanopesticides

As with nanoemulsions, polymer-based pesticide nanocarriers serve to increase dispersion in aqueous media, act as a protective reservoir, and facilitate diffusion-controlled release of pesticides. Controlled and slow release of the active molecules can be achieved based on degradation properties of the nanocarrier, bonding of the active ingredients to the material and the environmental conditions. Controlled release formulations avoid temporal overdose, and improved stability via protection increases effectiveness and minimizes input and waste—this helps address chemical runoff and alleviate environmental concerns associated with traditional pesticides (Chen and Yada, 2011). Their attractiveness is also based on flexibility to design complex drug delivery systems including incorporating multiple pesticides with different modes of action, scalable preparation, biocompatibility and biodegradability.

Many techniques exist for the formation of polymer-based nanopesticides, including: meltdispersion, spray drying, complex coacervation, interfacial polymerization, and emulsion diffusion (Goncalves et al., 2010). Regardless of the preparation method employed, four main architectures for association of pesticide active ingredients with the nanocarrier arise: absorption onto the nanoparticle surface, covalent attachment via polymeric linkers, encapsulation within a micelle core, or entrapment within the polymeric matrix (Fig. 5.9).

4.1 Absorption on Nanoparticle Surface

In one example the absorption onto the nanoparticle surface, mesoporous silica nanoparticles (MSNs) were employed as nanoscale carriers for the fungicide metalaxyl. The metalaxyl was first dissolved in water via sonication, the MSNs were then added to the solution, and the solvent evaporated under reduced

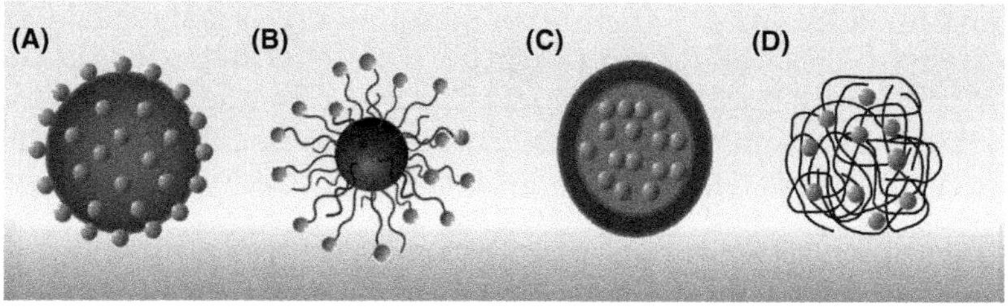

Figure 5.9. Schematic representation of different polymer nanoparticles for delivery of pesticides, (A) adsorption on nanoparticle; (B) attachment on nanoparticle by different linkers; (C) encapsulation inside polymeric hydrophobic or hydrophilic core (polymer micelles); and (D) entrapment inside polymeric nanoparticle.

pressure. Characterization of the loaded MSNs indicated reversible, noncovalent entrapment of metalaxyl within the MSN pores at 14 wt.%. Fungicide release studies showed 47% release in water and 11.5% release in soil within 30 days. Release for free metalaxyl in soil was 76%, showing a 7× delay for loaded MSNs, facilitating longer periods of soil protection without increased amounts of fungicide (Wanyika, 2013).

4.2 Covalent Attachment via Polymeric Linkers

In order to target its release, antibacterial active ingredient kasugamycin was covalently attached to silica nanospheres via an amide bond. These bonds are normally relatively stable and only hydrolyzed slowly in water environments. Plants and many pathogens produce amidase, which enzymatically breaks the bond in the conjugate, resulting in the release of the active ingredient. Free kasugamycin was completely degraded by UV irradiation after 56 h, while conjugated kasugamycin was protected against photo-degradation and showed just 25% degradation after 72 h. Conjugated and free kasugamycin showed the same initial inhibition of *Escherichia coli*, however, after 24 h inhibition by conjugated kasugamycin had dropped to 63.46%, while inhibition by free kasugamycin had dropped to 18.26%, demonstrating sustained bactericidal efficacy of the conjugate (Ding, 2014). Using a different approach, Sarlak modified multiwalled carbon nanotubes (CNTs) with hyperbranchedpolycitric acid (PCA), and then encapsulated the fungicides mancozeb and zineb in the PCA shell, using ultrasonication and stirring in aqueous solution. The CNT-g-PCA encapsulated pesticide had superior toxicity to the bulk pesticide against the fungi *Alternaria alternate*. This effect was attributed to increase contact area between the encapsulated fungicide and fungi (Sarlak, 2014). Another group modified magnetic Fe_3O_4 nanoparticles with carboxymethyl-B-cyclodextrin to act as an inclusion complex for the pesticide diuron. The diminished toxic effect on soil microbial activity compared to free diuron was attributed to slow release of the diuron from the complex (Liu, 2014).

4.2.1 Encapsulation Within Polymer Micelle Core

For targeted release, the insecticide imidacloprid was encapsulated within an ABA-type copolymer of poly(citric acid) and poly(ethylene glycol). This copolymer self assembles into nanoparticles, capable of encapsulating a guest molecule (Naeini et al., 2010). Characterization of the product demonstrated that the imidacloprid became part of the self-assembly via the formation of hydrogen bonds with the PCA blocks of the copolymers, at a loading rate of 14 wt.%. Encapsulated imidacloprid showed increased release rate at optimum pH for *Glyphodes pyloalis's* gut (pH = 10) compared to pH 7. After 5 days the required dose of nanoimidacloprid for 50% mortality was lower than for bulk imidacloprid, indicating better performance (Memarizadeh, 2014).

4.3 Entrapment Within Polymeric Matrix

Polymeric nanogels (also known as hydrogel nanoparticles) are small cross-linked polymeric particles that absorb large quantities of water due to the presence of hydrophilic groups (Goncalves et al., 2010). The properties of nanogels can be controlled via the functional monomers, degree of crosslinking, and preparation method, to enhance responsiveness to the surrounding environment (Kettel, 2014). For example, pure chitosan nanogels were produced with neutralized amino groups able to complex large amounts of copper (II). Maximum copper (II) loading of 300 mg/g was achieved at pH 5.5, and corresponded to approximately 80% of the chitosan amino groups having associated copper. The active ingredient, copper (II), could be released by protonation of amino groups by acidification caused by a growing pathogen, or by chitosanolytic enzymes present in many phytopathogenic fungi. The enzyme also breaks the nanogel into chitosan oligomers, which have plant-strengthening activity. A synergistic effect was observed between the chitosan and the copper against *F. graminearum* (Brunel, 2013). Bhagat et al. prepared a nanogel of the pheromone methyl eugenol (ME), which acted to protect the pheromone from volatilization via exposure to air, water, and sunshine. Pheromones are highly specific, naturally occurring disruptors of mating and sexual communication in insect pests. Due to their volatile nature, they are susceptible to decomposition under ambient conditions.

The nanogel also facilitated the controlled release of ME over a sustained period and showed prolonged shelf life. At 50°C, ME alone completely evaporated in 3 weeks, compared to 30 weeks for evaporation of ME for the nanogel (Bhagat, 2013).

In another study, the natural pesticide essential oil *Cuminum cyminum* was loaded into myristic acid-chitosan nanogel. Tests were performed against two pest species, *Sitophilus garnarius* and *Tribolium confusum*, the oil-loaded nanogels showed increased toxicity of 97% after 24 h, relative to 18% for the free oil. The oil-loaded nanogels also showed improved persistence, with 54% mortality after storage for 10 days, while the free oil dropped to 9% mortality after storage for only 4 days (Ziaee et al., 2014). The broad-range insecticide permethrin was complexed into a β-cyclodextrin nanogel to coat textiles for protection against insects. Compared to the noncomplexed a.i., irreversible photo degradation was decreased for the complexed permethrin, and biological effectiveness was not affected (Kettel, 2014).

4.3.1 Other Nanopesticide Composites

Layered double hydroxides (LDHs) consist of double metal cation hydroxides, with interlayer charge-balancing cations. Their unique properties allow biomolecules to be intercalated between the layers, for protection from degradation and facilitated release in soils. Hybridization of natural antibiotic, cinnamic acid, with LDH led to the protection of cinnamate against degradation, as well as controlled release in soils (Park et al., 2010).

The antibiotic amphotericin B (AMB) has been shown to self-assemble with phospholipids and scaffold proteins, into nanoscale ternary complexes called nanodisks (NDs), resulting in increased water solubility and protection against environmental damage. AMB-NDs were shown to be effective against phytopathogenic fungi in chickpeas and wheat (Perez-de-leque, 2012).

5 Solid Nanoparticles as Nanopesticides

Many nanoparticles are known to have intrinsic antibacterial/pesticidal properties and have therefore naturally been suggested as potential candidates not only as nanocarriers, but also as active pesticide agents or biopesticides.

5.1 Inert Dusts as Insecticides

The mode of action of inert dusts, such as silica, alumina, and clays is through damage to the wax coating on the insect cuticle through both sorption and abrasion. The damage causes the insects to lose water and die due to desiccation. Since the mode of action is physical, it is considered unlikely that insects will develop resistance (Shah and Khan, 2014).

5.1.1 Silica

Due to silicon's ability to help increase plant's tolerance to abiotic and biotic stresses, the use of silica nanoparticles (SNPs) for agricultural pest control has been logically suggested. (Barik et al., 2008). Debnath (2011) investigated the toxicity of amorphous hydrophilic, hydrophobic, and lipophilic SNPs against the rice weevil *Sitophilus oryzae*, and found it to be highly effective, and more effective than bulk silica. No fresh infestation was found after 2 months of storage. The silica NPs were physio-sorbed by the cuticular lipids disrupting the protective epidermis layer and thereby causing death of insects purely by physical means with similar mode of action observed on diatoms particles used for protection of stored grain (Barik et al., 2008; Korunic, 1998; Arthur, 1996). Furthermore, surface charged modified hydrophobic silica NPs (3–5 nm) were successfully used to control a range of agricultural insect pests and animal ectoparasites of veterinary importance (Ulrichs et al., 2006). It was successfully applied as a thin film on seeds to decrease fungal growth and boost cereal germination (Robinson and Salejova-Zadrazilova, 2010). Application of NPs on the leaf and stem surface did not alter either photosynthesis or respiration in several groups of horticultural and crop plants. They did not cause alteration of gene expression in insect trachea and were, thus, qualified for approval as the nanobiopesticide. Additionally, the use of amorphous silica as a nanobiopesticide is considered safe for humans by World Health Organization (WHO).

SNPs have also been explored as carriers for traditional pesticides. Song et al. (2012) loaded dispersible SNPs with insecticide chlorfenapyr and found increased biological efficacy compare to microsized chlorfenapyr. They attributed this to both the nanosize, and the intrinsic pesticidal action of the SNPs themselves. Additionally, porous hollow SNPs have been reported to protect the short half-life pesticide avermectim from UV degradation and enable its slow release. The SNP carriers were observed to facilitate the slow release of avermectim for ~30 days (Li et al., 2007).

5.1.2 Diatomaceous Earth (DE)

DE is composed mainly of amorphous silica derived from fossilized phytoplankton. DE is commonly used to protect stored grain from pest insects. The main drawback of DEs is the need to apply at high dosages, having adverse effect on grain properties, primarily bulk density. Recent research has focused on enhanced DEs with other insecticides to allow control at low doses. For example, a mixture of DE with the plant extract bitterbarkomycin was evaluated against grain pest *Rhyzopertha dominica*, and found to be effective at dose rates as low as 150 ppm (Athanassiou et al., 2008).

5.1.3 Alumina

Stadler et al. (2010) presented the discovery of nanostructured alumina (NSA) as an effective insecticide against two grain pests, *S. oryzae* and *R. dominica*. Stadler et al. (2012) also compared his NSA formulations against a leading commercial DE product and found their formulation was more effective. More recent research using NSA dusts synthesized using a modified glycine-nitrate combustion process revealed that their use was more effective against *S. oryzae* than *R. dominica*. With results demonstrating that particle size, surface area, and morphology are key factors, which determine insecticidal efficacy. However, the authors suggested that these are not the sole factors, and modifying the synthesis route will achieve better results for targeted species (Buteler, 2015).

5.1.4 Clays

Nanoclays are thin sheets of silicate materials in the order of 1 nm thick and 70–150 nm wide. They are produced from montmorillonite clays commonly found in volcanic ash, and their size is reduced and surface modified to form nanoclays that are biocompatible and have low toxicity. The group from these organic materials which is seen to have the most potential is LDHs, also referred to as anionic clays. They have already been successfully used as carriers for the plant growth regulator α-naphthalene acetate and for the controlled release of the herbicide 2, 4-dichlorophenoxyacetate (Bin Hussein et al., 2005). Their use was further investigated by Park et al. (2010) who successfully layered double hydroxide as a carrier for the antibiotic cinnamate, which is used for pest control. This natural antibiotic is prone to rapid degradation in soil and requires high doses. Park et al. (2010) successfully demonstrated slow release of the antibiotic and extended retention in the soil. This indicates excellent promise of nanoclays to be used for slow/targeted delivery of pesticides and fungicides.

5.2 Metal Nanoparticles

There are three hypothesized modes of biocidal action by metal particles; (1) antimicrobial activity via photocatalysis—absorbed photons lead to the release of superoxide radicals, which cause the death of bacterial, fungal, and viral organisms by oxidation of critical molecular structures; (2) accumulation and dissipation in the cell membrane, leading to membrane damage and release of cell contents; (3) uptake of metallic ions into cells followed by disruption of DNA replication (Chatterjee et al., 2014). Nanometals show enhanced activity due to the increased surface area (Paret et al., 2013).

5.2.1 Silver

Silver nanoparticles (AgNPs) have been largely considered the most favorable, attributed to their: bactericidal and viricidal efficacy, low toxicity, charge capacity, high surface area, crystallographic structure, and adaptability to various substrates (Nangmenyi and Economy, 2009). Silver nanoparticles were investigated against fungal phytopathogen *Raffaelea*, which causes the destructive disease oak wilt. Fungal growth was inhibited in a dose-dependent manner, and cell wall damage was observed (Kim et al., 2009). The most recent nanosilver study by Kim et al. (2012) demonstrated the in vitro activity of AgNPs against 18 plant pathogens. The use of AgNPs over synthetic fungicides is suggested: reduced human toxicity, pest resistance, plant protection costs, and environmental pollution (Jo et al., 2009; Jung et al., 2010). However, none of these potential advantages have to be realized. Additionally, the open field use of AgNPs is optimistic due to its production cost and regulatory obstacles.

5.2.2 Titanium Dioxide

The application of titanium dioxide to crops has demonstrated effective antimicrobial activity, with suppression of bacterial and fungal pathogens (Norman and Chen, 2011). More recently, Paret et al. (2013) investigated the effect of TiO_2, and TiO_2 doped with zinc and silver against bacterial spot disease of tomato. Protection was comparable to the grower standard (copper + mancozeb) without adverse effects on tomato yield. Repeated use of the formulation did induce increased leaf phytotoxicity (5–10%); however, this can be mitigated by the use of electrostatic sprayers instead of conventional ones (Paret et al., 2013). The main enhancement of the titanium dioxide/zinc formulation presented, is its potential to lower ecological and toxicological risks, compared with current grower standard.

5.2.3 Copper

Nanocopper was investigated against pomegranate bacterial blight, and was found to be effective at very low concentrations. Cell wall damage was observed in nanocopper treated bacterial cells (Mondal and Mani, 2012). There is scarce peer reviewed literature on the efficacy on nanocopper formulations other than (a patent in Gogos et al., 2012), which demonstrated an 8% increase in efficiency compared to a formulation of copper hydroxides salts currently in use. The Mondal and Mani (2012) study was limited to in vitro studies and did not reveal formulation details. As noted by Kah and Hofmann (2014) in order to comprehensively evaluate the efficacy of nanocopper formulations more in depth investigations need to be undertaken.

6 Toxicity and Environmental Impacts

There is a concern about toxicity and environmental impact of nanoscale-based formulations, which requires more investigation and research. Little is yet known about the predicted environmental concentration of nanoformulations in soil, surface water, and ground water, and potential impacts on nontarget organisms. Apart from the characteristics of the nanoformulations discussed later, environmental fate also depends on environmental factors, such as pH, ionic strength and dissolved molecules in the media (Kookana, 2014). Some of key issues are highlighted in the following sections.

6.1 Direct toxicity on Humans and Environment

The toxicity of the most of pesticides used in nanoscale formulation is proved by authority however, their nanoscale formulation due possible impact of nanodimension should be also taken into account with possible negative impact. More research is required to confirm toxicity of these nanoscale formulation and influence of size, charge, shape, and chemistry of these nanoparticles on toxicity.

6.2 Durability and Persistence

A key criterion for risk assessment purposes is the durability of the nanoformulation following application of the nanopesticide.

Delayed release could continue or even increase over a long time period, possibly affecting nontarget species exposure (Kah et al., 2013).

6.3 Bioavailability

One possible deleterious effect of nanocarriers is the facilitated transport of active ingredients that would otherwise be considered immobile (Kah and Hofmann, 2014). A number of nanoformulations have been shown to increase uptake by the target organism. It is important that this occurs without increasing the risk to nontarget organisms.

6.4 Release Profile/Degradation

Release of the active ingredient depends on the type of nanocarrier, and the dispersion of the active ingredient within the matrix. Research indicates that release of the active ingredient will be through a combination of desorption from the surface, diffusion through the polymer matrix, and degradation of the polymer which all could influence their environmental impact and toxicity (Kah and Hofmann, 2014).

6.5 Fate of the Carrier

Much recent research focuses on carriers that are based on natural biodegradable polymers, polysaccharides, or lipids, which degrade into products that are of little concern (Kah and Hofmann, 2014).

7 Conclusions

Numerous publications and reports showed very strong research in this field and considerable confidence that nanopesticide based formulation, such as nanoemulsions, nanodispesions, nanoparticles, and so on have a bright future and potential for developing safer and more effective chemical pesticide formulations for pest control which potentially could make revolutionary change in this field. This confidence is recently confirmed by pesticide companies who have recently released their first nanopesticide products on the market. The approaches involving encapsulation of pesticide active ingredients within nanoparticles with three major concepts including the improvement of conventional pesticide formulations, development of new delivery systems using nanoparticle as nanocarriers and solid nanoparticles used as active pesticide agents are promising strategy for the development of novel nanopesticide based formulations. However, due potential toxicity concerns of nanomaterials, which are not standardized yet, not well understood and not explored, this development will likely go through a strong scrutiny from international and national safety regulations with request for more research on environmental and humans impact of these materials.

Acknowledgments

Authors acknowledge the support provided by the Grain Research and Development Corporation (GRDC) through the grants numbers UA 000134 and UA 000151 and School of Chemical Engineering, the University of Adelaide.

References

Abribat, B., Lachut, F., Anderson, T., Pompeo, M., Michail, D., 2004. Microemulsions as adjuvants for agricultural chemicals. WO Patent 2004080177.

Acosta, E., 2009. Bioavailability of nanoparticles in nutrient and nutraceutical delivery. Curr. Opin. Colloid Interface Sci. 14, 3–15.

Alemán, J., Chadwick, A.V., He, J., Hess, M., Horie, K., Jones, R.G., Kratochvil, P., Meisel, I., Mita, I., Moad, G., Penczek, S., Stepto, R.F.T., 2007. IUPAC Recommendations. 2007. Pure Appl. Chem. 79, 1801.

Anjali, C.H., Sudheer Khan, S., Margulis-Goshen, K., Magdassi, S., Mukherjee, A., Chandrasekaran, N., 2010. Formulation of water-dispersablenanopermethrin for larvicidal applications. Ecotoxicol. Environ. Saf. 73, 1932–1936.

Anjali, C.H., Sharma, Y., Mukherjee, A., Chandrasekaran, N., 2012. Neem oil (*Azadirachta indica*) nanoemulsion as potent larvicidal agent against *Culex quinquefasciatus*. Pest Manag. Sci. 68 (2), 158–163.

Anton, N., Benoit, J.P., Saulnier, P., 2008. Design and production of nanoparticles formulated from nano-emulsion templates: a review. J. Control. Release 128, 185–199.

Arthur, F.H., 1996. Grain protectants: current status and prospects for the future. J. Stored Prod. Res. 32, 293–302.

Athanassiou, C.K., Kavallieratos, N.G., Vayias, B.J., Vassiliki, K.S., 2008. Evaluation of a new enhanced diatomaceous earth formulation for use against the stored products pest *Rhyzopertha dominica* (Coleoptera: Bostrychidae). Int. J. Pest Manag. 54 (1), 43–49.

Auffan, M., Rose, J., Bottero, J.-Y., Lowry, G.V., Jolivet, J.-P., Wiesner, M.R., 2009. Towards a definition of inorganic nanoparticles from an environmental, health and safety perspective. Nat. Nanotechnol. 4, 634–641.

Balakrishnan, V.K., Han, X., VanLoon, G.W., Dust, J.M., Toullec, J., Buncel, E., 2004. Acceleration of nucleophilic attack on an organophosphorothioate neurotoxin, fenitrothion, by reactive counterion cationic micelles. Regioselectivity as a probe of substrate orientation within the micelle. Langmuir 20, 6586–6593.

Balakrishnan, V.K., Buncel, E., VanLoon, G.W., 2005. Micellar catalyzed degradation of fenitrothion, an organophosphorus pesticide, in solutions and soils. Environ. Sci. Technol. 39, 5824–5830.

Barik, T.K., Sahu, B., Swain, V., 2008. Nanosilica—from medicine to pest control. Parasitol. Res. 103 (2), 253–258.

Bataller, H., Lamaallam, S., Lachaise, J., Graciaa, A., Dicharry, C., 2004. Cutting fluid emulsions produced by dilution of a cutting fluid concentrate containing a cationic/nonionic surfactant mixture. J. Mater. Process. Technol. 152, 215–220.

Bhagat, D.S., 2013. Efficient management of fruit pests by pheromone nanogels. Nat. Sci. Rep. 3, 1294.

Bin Hussein, M.Z., Yahaya, A.H., Zainal, Z., Kian, L.H., 2005. Nanocomposite-based controlled release formulation of an herbicide, 2,4-dichlorophenoxyacetate incapsulated in zinc–aluminium-layered double hydroxide. Sci. Technol. Adv. Mater. 6 (8), 956–962.

Boehm, A.L., Martinon, I., Zerrouk, R., et al., 2003. Nanoprecipitation technique for the encapsulation of agrochemical active ingredients. J. Microencapsul. 20 (4), 433–444.

Brunel, F.E., 2013. Complexation of copper (II) with chitosan gels: toward control of microbial growth. Carbohydr. Polym. 92, 1348–1356.

Buteler, M.S., 2015. Development of nanoalumina dust as insecticide against *Sitophilus oryzae* and *Rhyzopertha dominica*. Int. J. Pest Manag. 61 (1), 80–89.

Cameron, N.M.S., Mitchell, M.E., 2007. Nanoscale: issues and perspectives for the nano century. In: Kimbrell, G.A. (Ed.), The potential environmental hazards of nanotechnology and the applicability of the existing low. first edn. Wiley, Hoboken.

Chatterjee, A., Chakraborty, R., Basu, T., 2014. Mechanism of antibacterial activity of copper nanoparticles. Nanotechnology 25, 135101.

Chen, H., Yada, R, 2011. Nanotechnologies in agriculture: new tools for sustainable development (Review). Trends Food Sci. Technol. 22, 585–594.

Chingunpituk, J., 2007. Nanosuspension technology for drug delivery. Walailak J. Sci. Technol. 4 (2), 139–153.

Debnath, N.D., 2011. Entomotoxic effect of silica nanoparticles against *Sitophilus oryzae* (L). J Pest Sci. 84, 99–105.

Dicharrya, C., Batallera, H., Lamaallama, S., Lachaisea, J., Graciaa, A., 2003. Microemulsions as cutting fluid concentrates: structure and dispersion into hard water. J. Dispersion Sci. Technol. 24 (2), 237–248.

Ding, G.L., 2014. Preparation and characterisation of kasuga-silica-conjugated nanospheres for sustained microbial activity. J. Nanopart. Res. 16, 2671.

Elek, N., Hoffman, R., Raviv, U., Resh, R., Ishaaya, I., Magdassi, S., 2010. Formation and potential use in controlling agricultural insect pests. Colloids Surf. A 372, 66–72.

Fan, P., Gu, Z.Y., Xu, D.J., Xu, X.L., Xu, G.C., 2010. Action analysis of drops of emamection-benzoate microemulsion on rice leaf. Chin. J. Rice Sci. 24, 503–508.

Forgiarini, A., Esquena, J., Gonzalez, C., Solans, C., 2000. Studies of the relation between phase behavior and emulsification methods with nanoemulsion formation. Prog. Colloid Polym. Sci. 115, 36–39.

Forgiarini, A., Esquena, J., Gonzalez, C., Solans, C., 2001a. Formation and stability of nano-emulsions in mixed nonionic surfactant systems. Prog. Colloid Polym. Sci. 118, 184–189.

Forgiarini, A., Esquena, J., Gonzalez, C., Solans, C., 2001b. Formation of nano-emulsions by low-energy emulsification methods at constant temperature. Langmuir 17 (7), 2076–2083.

Forster, T., Rybinski, W.V., Wadle, A., 1995. Influence of microemulsion phases on the preparation of fine-disperse emulsions. Adv. Colloid Interface Sci. 58 (2–3), 119–149.

Gassmann, P., List, M., Schweitzer, A., Sucker, H., 1994. Hydrosols-alternatives for the parenteral application of poorly water soluble drugs. Eur. J. Pharm. Biopharm. 40 (2), 64–72.
Gogos, A., Knauer, K., Bucheli, T.D., 2012. Nanomaterials in plant protection and fertilization: current state, foreseen applications, and research priorities. J. Agric. Food Chem. 60, 9781–9792.
Goncalves, C., Pereira, P., Gama, M., 2010. Self-assembled hydrogel nanoparticles for drug delivery applications. Materials 3 (2), 1420–1460.
Graves, S., Meleson, K., Wilking, J., 2005. Structure of concentrated nanoemulsions. J. Chem. Phys. 122 (13), 134703.
Green, J.M., Beestman, G.B., 2007. Recently patented and commercialized formulation and adjuvant technology. Crop Prot. 26 (3), 320–327.
Gutierrez, J.M., Gonzalez, C., Maestro, A., Sole, I., Pey, C.M., Nolla, J., 2008. Nano-emulsions: new applications and optimisation of their preparation. Curr. Opin. Colloid Interface Sci. 13, 245–251.
Han, X., Balakrishnan, V.K., VanLoon, G.W., Buncel, E., 2006. Degradation of the pesticide fenitrothion as mediated by cationic surfactants and α-nucleophilic reagents. Langmuir 22, 9009–9017.
Hancock, B.C., Parks, M., 2000. What is the true solubility advantage for amorphous pharmaceuticals? Pharm. Res. 17 (4), 397–404.
Hu, J., Johnson, K.P., Williams, III, R.O., 2004. Nanoparticle engineering processes for enhancing the dissolution rates of poorly water soluble drugs. Drug Dev. Ind. Pharm. 30 (3), 233–245.
Huang, Q.L., Zhang, W.J., Li, F.M., She, D.M., Zhang, C.H., Bu, X.L., 2006. Solubilization of chlorpyrifos in the mixed system of surfactants and the bioactivity evaluation. Chin. J. Pest. Sci. 8, 71–76.
Izquierdo, P., Esquena, J., Tadros, Th.F., Dederen, J.C., Garcia, M.J., Azemar, N., Solans, C., 2002. Formation and stability of nano-emulsions prepared using the phase inversion temperature method. Langmuir 18 (1), 26–30.
Izquierdo, P., Esquena, J., Tadros, Th.F., Dederen, J.C., Feng, J., Garcia-Celma, M.J., Azemar, N., Solans, C., 2004. Phase behavior and nano-emulsion formation by the phase inversion temperature method. Langmuir 20 (16), 6594–6598.
Izquierdo, P., Feng, J., Esquena, J., Tadros, Th.F., Dederen, J.C., Garcia, M.J., Azemar, N., Solans, C., 2005. The influence of surfactant mixing ratio on nano-emulsion formation by the pit method. J. Colloid Interface Sci. 285 (1), 388–394.
Jafari, S.M., He, Y., Bhandari, B., 2007. Optimisation of nanoemulsion production by microfluidization. Eur. Food Res. Technol. 225 (5–6), 733–741.
Jo, Y.K., Kim, B.H., Jung, G., 2009. Antifungal activity of silver ions and nanoparticles on phytopathogenic fungi. Plant Disease 93, 1037–1043.
Jung, J.-H., Kim, S.-W., Min, J.-S., Kim, Y.-J., Lamsal, K., Kim, K.S., Lee, Y.S., 2010. The effect of nano-silver liquid against the white rot of the green onion caused by *Sclerotium cepivorum*. Mycobiology 38, 39–45.
Kah, M., Beulke, S., Tiede, K., Hofmann, T., 2013. Nanopesticides: state of knowledge, environmental fate, and exposure modelling. Crit. Rev. Env. Sci. Technol. 43 (16), 1823–1867.
Kah, M., Hofmann, T., 2014. Nanopesticide research: current trends and future priorities. Environ. Int. 63, 224–235.
Kalaitzaki, A., Papanikolaou, N.E., Karamaouna, F., Dourtoglou, V., Xanakis, A., Papadimitriou, V., 2015. Biocompatible colloidal dispersions as potential formulations of natural pyrethrins: a structural and efficacy study. Langmuir 31 (21), 5722–5730.
Katagi, T., 2002. Abiotic hydrolysis of pesticides in the aquatic environment. Rev. Environ. Contam. Toxicol. 175, 79–261.

Katagi, T., 2008. Surfactant effects on environmental behaviour of pesticides. Rev. Environ. Contam. Toxicol 194, 71–177.

Kettel, M.S., 2014. Nanogels with high active B-cyclodextrin content as physical coating system with sustained release properties. Appl. Mater. Inter. 6, 2300–2311.

Kim, S., Kim, K., Lamsal, K., Kim, Y., Kim, S., Jung, M., Sim, S., Kim, H., Chang, S., Kim, J., Lee, Y., 2009. An in vitro study of the antifungal effect of silver nanoparticles on oak wilt pathogen *Raffaelea* sp. J. Microbiol.Biotechnol. 19 (8), 760–764.

Kim, S.W., Jung, J.H., Lamasal, K., Kim, Y.S., Min, J.S., Lee, Y.S., 2012. Antifungal effects of silver nanoparticles (AgNPs) against various plant pathogenic fungi. Mycobiology 40, 53–58.

Knowles, A., 2005. New developments in crop protection product formulation. Agrow Reports. T & F Informa. UK Ltd., UK.

Kocbek, P., Baumgartner, S., Kristl, J., 2006. Preparation and evaluation of nanosuspensions for enhancing the dissolution of poorly soluble drugs. Int. J. Pharm. 312 (1-2), 179–186.

Korunic, Z., 1998. Diatomaceous earths, a group of natural insecticides. J. Stored Prod. Res. 34, 87–97.

Kookana, R.B., 2014. Nanopesticides: guiding principles for regulatory evaluation of environmental risks. J. Agric. Food Chem. 64, 4227–4240.

Kumar, R.S.S., Shiny, P.J., Anjali, C.H., Jerobin, J., Goshen, K.M., Magdassi, S., Mukherjee, A., Chandrasekaran, N., 2013. Distinctive effects of nano-sized permethrin in the environment. Environ. Sci. Pollut. R. 20 (4), 2593–2602.

Lai, F., Wissing, S.A., Muller, R.H., Fadda, A.M., 2006. *Artemisia arborescens* L essential oil-loaded solid lipid nanoparticles for potential agricultural application: preparation and characterization. AAPS PharmaSciTech 7 (1), E1–E9.

Lamaallam, S., Bataller, H., Dicharry, C., Lachaise, J., 2005. Formation and stability of miniemulsions produced by dispersion of water/oil/surfactants concentrates in a large amount of water. Colloids Surf. A 270–271, 44–51.

Lauterborn, W., Ohl, C.D., 1997. Cavitation bubble dynamics. Ultrason. Sonochem. 4, 65–75.

Lawrence, M.J., Warisnoicharoen, W., 2006. Recent advances in microemulsions as drug delivery vehicles. In: Torchilin, V.P. (Ed.), Nanoparticles as drug carriers. Imperial College Press, London.

Li, Z.Z., Chen, J.F., Liu, F., Liu, A.Q., Wang, Q., Sun, H.Y., Wen, L.X., 2007. Study of UV-shielding properties of novel porous hollow silica nanoparticle carriers for avermectin. Pest Manag. Sci. 63, 241–246.

Lim, C.J., Basri, M., Omar, D., Rahman, M.B.A., Salleh, A.B., Rahman, R.N.Z.A., 2012. Physicochemical characterization and formation of glyphosate-laden nano-emulsion for herbicide formulation. Ind. Crop Prod. 36 (1), 607–613.

Lim, C.J., Basri, M., Omar, D., Rahman, M.B.A., Salleh, A.B., Rahman, R.N.Z.A., 2013. Green nanoemulsion-laden glyphosate isopropylamine formulation in suppressing creeping foxglove (*A. gangetica*), slender button weed (*D. ocimifolia*) and buffalo grass (*P. conjugatum*). Pest Manag. Sci. 69 (1), 104–111.

Liu, W.Y., 2014. Synthesis of a novel nanopesticide and its potential toxic effect on soil microbial activity. J. Nanopart. Res. 16, 2677.

Liverside, G.G., Cundy, K.C., Bishop, J.F., Czekai, D.A., 1992. USA Patent 5,145,689. Surface modified drug nanoparticles.

Lopez-Montilla, J.C., Hererra-Morales, P.E., Pandley, S., Shah, D.O., 2002. Spontaneous emulsification: mechanisms, physicochemical aspects, modelling, and applications. J. Dispersion Sci. Technol. 23 (1–3), 219–268.

Lovelyn, C., Attama, A.A., 2011. Current state of nanoemulsions in drug delivery. J. Biomater. Nanobiotechnol. 2, 626–639.

Mason, T.G., Wilking, J.N., Meleson, K., Chang, C.B., Graves, S.M., 2006. Nanoemulsions: formation, structure, and physical properties. J. Phys.: Condens. Matter 18, R635–R666.

Mason, T.J., 1992. Industrial sonochemistry: potential and practicality. Ultrasonics 30 (3), 192–196.

McClements, D.J., 2005. Food Emulsions: Principles, Practice, and Techniques. CRC Press, Boca Raton.

McClements, D.J., 2012. Nanoemulsions versus microemulsions: terminology, differences, and similarities. Soft Matter 8, 1719–1729.

Memarizadeh, N.G., 2014. Preparation, characterisation and efficiency of nanoencapsulated imidacloprid under laboratory conditions. Ecotoxicol. Environ. Saf. 107, 77–83.

Miller, C.A., 2005. Spontaneous emulsification: recent developments with emphasis on self-emulsification. In: Sjoblom, J. (Ed.), Emulsions and Emulsion Stability. CRC Press, NY, USA.

Mondal, K., Mani, C., 2012. Investigation of the antibacterial properties of nanocopper against *Xanthomonas axonapodis* pv. *punicae*, the incitant of pomegranate bacterial blight. Ann. Microbiol. 62, 889–893.

Morales, D., Gutierrez, J.M., Garcia-Celma, J.M., Solans, C., 2003. A study of the relation between bicontinuous microemulsions and oil/water nano-emulsion formation. Langmuir 19 (18), 7196–7200.

Muller, R.H., Peters, K., Becker, R., Kruss, B., 1995. Nanosuspensions for the i.v. administration of poorly soluble drugs: stability during sterilization and long-term storage. P. Control. Release Soc. 22, 574–575.

Muller, R.H., Junghanns, J.U., 2006. Drug nanocrystals/nanosuspensions for the delivery of poorly soluble drugs. In: Torchilin, V.P. (Ed.), Nanoparticles as drug carriers. Imperial College Press, London, pp. 307–328.

Naeini, A.T., Adeli, M., Vossoughi, M., 2010. Poly(citric acid)-*block*-poly(ethylene glycol) copolymers—new biocompatible hybrid materials for nanomedicine. Nanomedicine: NBM 6 (4), 556–562.

Nangmenyi, G., Economy, J., 2009. Nonmetallic particles for oligodynamic microbial disinfection. In: Savage et al., (Ed.), Nanotechnology Applications for Clean Water. William Andrew, Norwich, NY, pp. 3–15.

Nguyen, H.M., Hwang, I.C., Park, J.W., Park, H.J., 2012a. Enhanced payload and photo-protection for pesticides using nanostructured lipid carriers with corn oil as liquid lipid. J. Microencapsul. 29 (6), 596–604.

Nguyen, H.M., Hwang, I.C., Park, J.W., Park, H.J., 2012b. Photoprotection for deltamethrin using chitosan-coated beeswax solid lipid nanoparticles. Pest Manag. Sci. 68 (7), 1062–1068.

Niemeyer, B.A., Bergs, C., Wissenbach, U., Flockerzi, V., Trost, C., 2001. Competitive regulation of CaT-like-mediated Ca^{2+}entry by protein kinase C and calmodulin. Proc. Natl. Acad. Sci. U S A 98, 3600–3605.

Norman, D.J., Chen, J., 2011. Effect of foliar application of titanium dioxide on bacterial blight of geranium and xanthomonas leaf spot of poinsettia. Hortscience 46, 426–428.

Oskam, G., 2006. Met oxide nanoparticles: synthesis, characterization and application. J. Sol. Gel. Sci. Technol. 37, 161–164.

Paret, M., Vallad, G., Averett, D., Jones, J., Olson, S., 2013. Photocatalysis: effect of light-activated nanoscale formulations of TiO_2 on *Xanthomonas perforans* and control of bacterial spot of tomato. Phytopathology 103 (3), 228–236.

Park, M., Lee, C., Seo, Y., Woo, S., Shin, D., Choi, J., 2010. Hybridization of the natural antibiotic, cinnamic acid, with layered double hydroxides as green pesticide. Environ. Sci. Pollut. Res. 17, 203–209.

Perez-de-leque, A.C., 2012. Effect of amphotericin B nanodisks on plant fungal diseases. Pest Manag. Sci. 68, 67–74.

Peters, K., Muller, R.H., 1996. Nanosuspensions for the oral application of poorly-soluble drugs. Proceedings of the European Symposium for the Formulation of Poorly-Available Drugs for Oral Administration, Paris.

Pons, R., Carrera, I., Caelles, J., Rouch, J., Panizza, P., 2003. Formation and properties of miniemulsions formed by microemulsions dilution. Adv. Colloid Interface Sci. 106, 129–146.

Pouton, C.W., 1997. Formulation of self-emulsifying drug delivery systems. Adv. Drug Deliver. Rev. 25, 47–58.

Pratap, A.P., Bhowmick, D.N., 2008. Pesticides as microemulsion formulations. J. Dispersion Sci. Technol. 29, 1325–1330.

Puoci, F., Iemma, F., Spizzirri, U.G., Cirillo, G., Curcio, M., Picci, N., 2008. Polymer in agriculture: a review. American J. Agric. Biol. Sci. 3, 299–314.

Rang, M.J., Miller, C.A., 1999. Spontaneous emulsification of oils containing hydrocarbon, nonionic surfactant, and oleyl alcohol. J. Colloid Interface Sci. 209, 179–192.

Robinson, D., Salejova-Zadrazilova, G., 2010. Nanotechnologies for nutrient and biocide delivery in agricultural production. Observatory NANO.

Sarlak, N.T., 2014. Synthesis of nanopesticides by encapsulating pesticide nanoparticles using functionalised carbon nanotubes and application of new nanocomposite for plant disease treatment. J. Agr. Food Chem. 62, 4833–4838.

Sasson, Y., Levy-Ruso, G., Toledano, O., Ishaaya, I., 2007. Nanosuspensions: emerging Novel agrochemical formulations. In: Ishaaya, I., Nauen, R., Horowitz, A.R. (Eds.), Insecticides Design Using Advanced Technologies. first edn. Springer, Berlin/Heidelberg.

Shah, M.A., Khan, A.A., 2014. Use of diatomaceous earth for the management of stored-product pests. Int. J. Pest Manag. 60 (2), 100–113.

Shinoda, K., Saito, H., 1968. The effect of temperature on the phase equilibria and the types of dispersions of the ternary system composed of water, cyclohexane, and nonionic surfactant. J. Colloid Interface Sci. 26 (1), 70–74.

Smith, K., Evans, D.A., El-Hiti, G.A., 2008. Role of modern chemistry in sustainable arable crop protection. Phil. Trans. R. Soc. B. 363, 623–637.

Song, M.C., Cui, S., Gao, F., Liu, Y., Fan, C., Lei, T., Liu, D., 2012. Dispersible silica nanoparticles as carrier for enhanced bioactivity of chlorfenapyr. J. Pestic. Sci. 37 (3), 258–260.

Song, S.L., Liu, X.H., Jiang, J.H., Qian, Y.H., Zhang, N., Wu, Q.H., 2009. Stability of triazophos in self-emulsifying pesticide delivery system. Colloids Surf. A 350, 57–62.

Stackelberg, P.E., Kauffman, L.J., Ayers, M.A., Baehr, A.L., 2001. Frequently co-occurring pesticides and volatile organic compounds in public supply and monitoring wells, southern New Jersey, USA. Environ. Toxicol. Chem. 20 (4), 853–865.

Stadler, T.B., Buteler, M., Weaver, D., 2010. Novel use of nanostructured alumina as an insecticide. Pest Manag. Sci. 66, 577–579.

Stadler, T., Buteler, M., Weaver, D.K., Sofie, S., 2012. Novel Comparative toxicity of nanostructured alumina and a commercial inert dust for Sitophilus oryzae (L.) and Rhyzopertha dominica (F.) at varying ambient humidity levels. J. Stored Prod. Res. 48, 81–90.

Stephenson G. R., 2003 Pesticide use and world food production: risks and benefits. In: Coats, J.R., Yamamoto, H., (Eds.), Environmental Fate and Effects of Pesticides. ACS Symposium Series, Washington, vol. 853. pp. 261–270.

Tadros, T., Izquierdo, R., Esquena, J., Solans, C., 2004. Formation and stability of nanoemulsions. Adv. Colloid Interface Sci. 108, 303–318.

Tilman, D., Cassman, K.G., Matson, P.A., Naylor, R., Polasky, S., 2002. Agricultural sustainability and intensive production practices. Nature 418, 671–677.

Tomlin, C.D.S., 2009. The pesticide manual, 15th edn British Crop Protection Council, Surrey.

Trotta, M., Gallarate, M., Pattarino, F., Morel, S., 2001. Emulsions containing partially water-miscible solvents for the preparation of drug nanosuspensions. J. Control. Release 76 (1–2), 119–128.

Ulrichs, C., Krause, F., Rocksch, T., Goswami, A., Mewis, I., 2006. Electrostatic application of inert silica dust based insecticides onto plant surfaces. Commun. Agric. Appl. Biol. Sci. 71, 171–178.

Wang, L., Li, X., Zhang, G., Dong, J., Eastoe, J., 2007. Oil-in-water nanoemulsions for pesticide formulations. J. Colloid Interface Sci. 314, 230–235.

Wanyika, H., 2013. Sustained release of fungicide metalaxyl by mesoporous silica nanospheres. J Nanopart. Res. 15, 1831.

Whitehouse, P., Rannard, S., 2010. The application of nanodispersions to agriculture. Outlook Pest Manag. 21 (4), 190–192.

Xu, J., Fan, Q.J., Yin, Z.Q., Li, X.T., Du, Y.H., Jia, R.Y., Wang, K.Y., Lv, C., Ye, G., Geng, Y., Su, G., Zhao, L., Hu, T.X., Shi, F., Zhang, L., Wu, L.C.L., Tao, C., Zhang, Y.X., Shi, D.X., 2010. The preparation of neem oil microemulsion (*Azadirachta indica*) and the comparison of acaricidaltime between neem oil microemulsion and other formulations in vitro. Vet. Parasitol. 169, 399–403.

Yadollahi, R., Vasilev, K., Simovic, S., 2009. Nanosuspension technologies for delivery of poorly soluble drugs. J. Nanomater. 2015, 216375.

Yang, F.L., Li, X.G., Zhu, F., Lei, C.L., 2009. Structural characterization of nanoparticles loaded with garlic essential oil and their insecticidal activity against *Tribolium castaneum* (Herbst) (Coleoptera: Tenebrionidae). J. Agr. Food Chem. 57, 10156–10162.

Yu, L., 2001. Amorphous pharmaceutical solids: preparation, characterization and stabilization. Adv. Drug Deliv. Rev. 48 (1), 27–42.

Zeng, H., Li, X.F., Zhang, G.Y., Dong, J.F., 2008. Preparation and characterization of beta cypermethrin nanosuspensions by diluting O/W microemulsions. J. Dispersion Sci. Technol. 29, 358–361.

Zhang, H.F., Wang, D., Butler, R., Campbell, N.L., Long, J., Tan, B.E., Duncalf, D.J., Foster, A.J., Hopkinson, A., Taylor, D., Angus, D., Cooper, A.I., Rannard, S.P., 2008. Formation and enhanced biocidal activity of water-dispersable organic nanoparticles. Nat. Nanotechnol. 3, 506–511.

Ziaee, M., Moharramipour, S., Mohsenifar, A., 2014. MA-chitosan nanogel loaded with *Cuminum cyminum* essential oil for efficient management of two stored product beetle pests. J. Pest Sci. 87, 691–699.

6

AN OVERVIEW OF NANOPESTICIDES IN THE FRAMEWORK OF EUROPEAN LEGISLATION

Juan José Villaverde, Beatriz Sevilla-Morán, Carmen López-Goti, Pilar Sandín-España, José Luis Alonso-Prados
National Institute for Agricultural and Food Research and Technology (INIA), DTEVPF, Plant Protection Products Unit, Madrid, Spain

1 Introduction

Agriculture is one of the most important food sources worldwide. Pesticides play a key role in the protection of crops against weeds, pests, and diseases, improving crop yields and reducing costs. According to the European Commission (European Commission, 2015), a pesticide is defined as "something that prevents, destroys, or controls a harmful organism (pest) or disease, or protects plants or plant products during production, storage and transport." The term pesticide is also defined by the US EPA (2015) as "any substance or mixture of substances intended for preventing, destroying, repelling, or mitigating any pest."

Since 1940s, the use of synthetic pesticides has spread around the world and, nowadays, it is one of the most commonly used methods in agriculture for pest control. Indeed, the global pesticide trade (expressed as the sum of imports and exports) is constantly growing and it reached a value of nearly $60,000 million in 2012 (Fig. 6.1) (FAOSTAT, 2012). In this scenario, the largest contributor to the global pesticide trade is by far Europe (including Russia) and more concretely the European Union, accounting for about 49.2 and 44.0% of the total world, respectively (FAOSTAT, 2012).

Pesticides show a large variety of chemical structures with a wide spectrum of physicochemical and toxicological properties. Although pesticides seem a heterogeneous set of chemicals, there are different ways of classifying them. The most common

New Pesticides and Soil Sensors. http://dx.doi.org/10.1016/B978-0-12-804299-1.00007-2

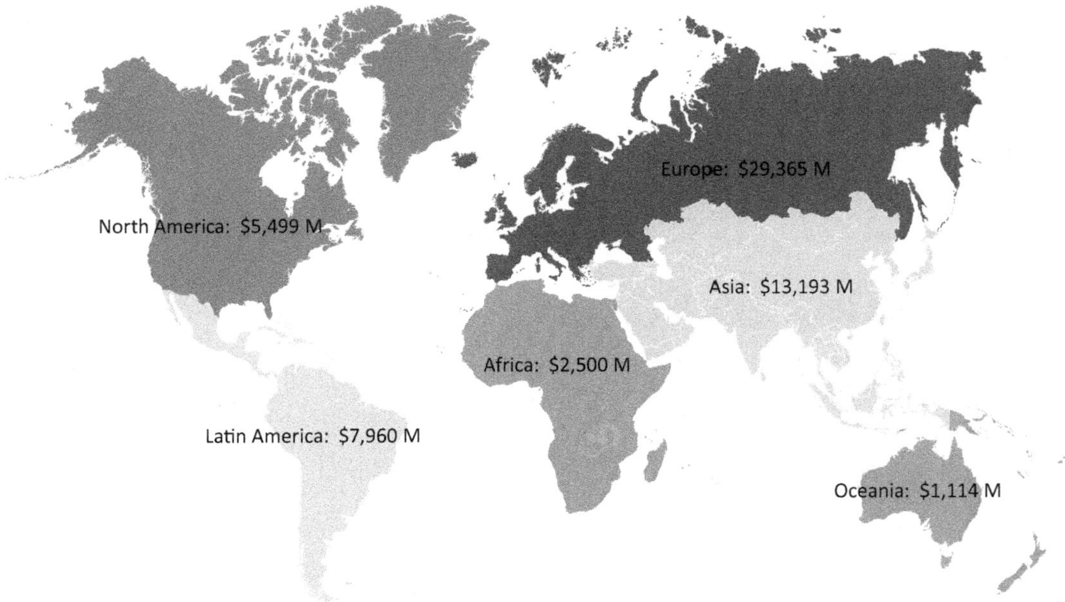
Europe: $29,365 M
North America: $5,499 M
Asia: $13,193 M
Africa: $2,500 M
Latin America: $7,960 M
Oceania: $1,114 M

Figure 6.1. Global distribution of pesticide trade (expressed as the sum of imports and exports) in 2012 (FAOSTAT, 2012). (For statistical purpose, FAOSTAT includes Russia and Turkey in Europe and Asia, respectively.)

classifications are based on the target pest and the pesticide chemical structure. According to the target pest, it can be distinguished mainly insecticides (control insects and other arthropods), herbicides (control weeds), fungicides (control fungi), acaricides (control mites), nematicide (control nematodes), and other pesticides (control rodents, mollusks, algae, etc.). According to their chemical structures, pesticides are grouped into different chemical classes or families, divided in turn into several subclasses. Pesticides belonging to the same family often show similarities in their chemical behavior and usually share a common mode of action. The Table 6.1 lists some of the most common pesticide families.

Despite their initial success, it was soon reported that synthetic pesticides had serious adverse effects on nontarget organisms and on the environment. The main adverse effects include the appearance of pesticide resistances, loss of biodiversity, bioaccumulation, and biomagnification of pesticide residues through the food chain and contamination of different environmental compartments. In this context, government authorities of several countries are continuously working to develop different regulatory frameworks that allow protecting human and animal health and the environment from the use of pesticides.

Table 6.1 Selected Pesticides, Families According to Their Chemical Structures (Tomlin, 2006)

Chemical Family	Examples
Amide	Alachlor, boscalid
Azole	Amitrole, hexaconazole
Aryloxyalkanoic acid	2,4-D; MCPA
Bipyridylium salts	Paraquat, diquat
Carbamate	Carbaryl, methiocarb
Neonicotinoid	Imidacloprid, acetamiprid
Organochlorine	DDT, lindane
Organophosphorus	Glyphosate, parathion
Pyrethroid	Cypermethrin, cyhalothrin
Triazine	Atrazine, terbutryn
Urea	Diuron, linuron

The "first generation" of synthetic pesticides was characterized by its broad-spectrum toxicity, persistence, and insolubility (e.g., DDT, aldrin, lindane). Then, pesticide industry has tended to research and develop more selective compounds with minimal nontarget organism toxicity, effective at low application rates and with polar character and easily degradable to prevent their persistence in the environment (second and third pesticide generations). Some of the most recent synthetic pesticides dealing with these goals include insecticides (e.g., spinosyns, neonicotinoids), herbicides (e.g., imidazolines, cyclohexanediones), or fungicides (e.g., strobirulins, phenylpyrroles), just to name a few (Fig. 6.2). However, these new compounds are not exempt of risk since some of their physicochemical properties, such as the polar and nonvolatile character and water solubility make them highly mobile in the environment (Hernández et al., 2012; Marín et al., 2006; Parham and Rahbar, 2010; Sevilla-Morán et al., 2008, 2014). Likewise, these pesticides can be susceptible to degradation due to the action of biotic and abiotic processes in order to reduce their persistence. However, these transformations frequently conduct to the formation of new chemical entities known as metabolites or degradation/transformation products. Often, the lack of knowledge about transformation products of pesticides conducts

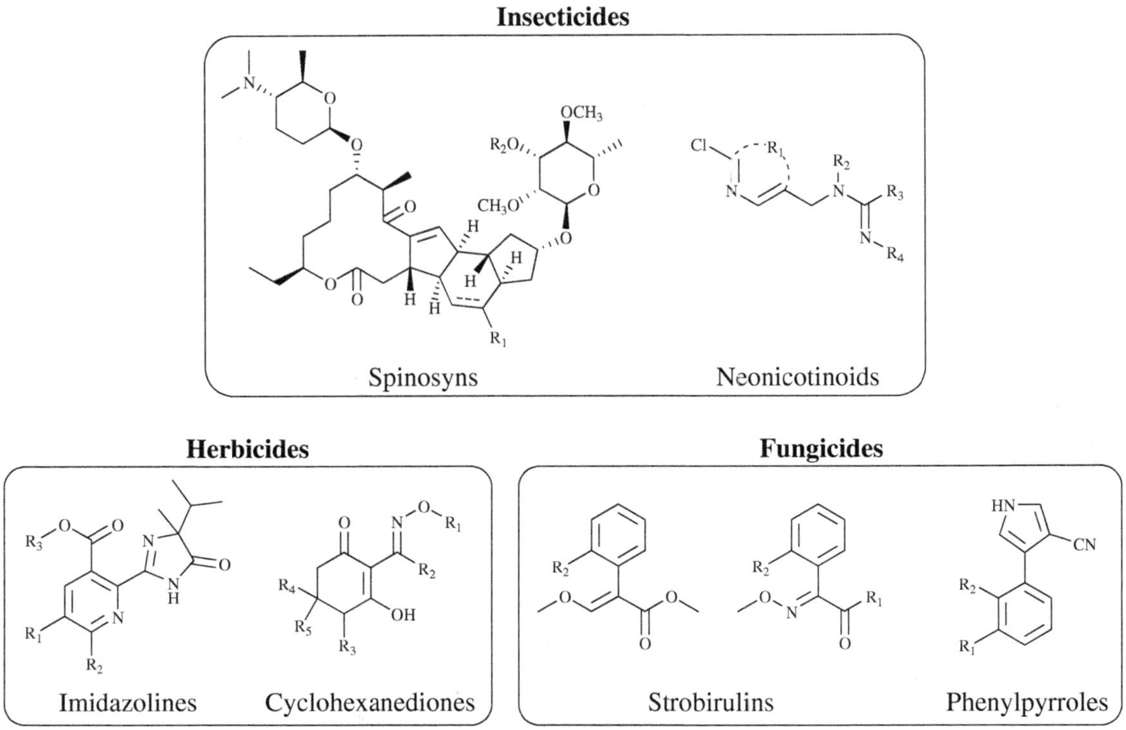

Figure 6.2. Chemical structures of some recent families of synthetic pesticides.

to underestimate the real impact of pesticides usage. Thus, many researches have pointed out that transformation products of pesticides in the environment may greatly differ from their parent compounds since they can display very different physicochemical and toxicological properties (Hildebrandt et al., 2008; Kruawala et al., 2005; Rosenbom et al., 2010; Sandín-España et al., 2015).

Nowadays, the efforts of agrochemical industry to avoid the deleterious effects of pesticides, are not only focused on the development of new active substances, but also in new pesticide formulations. In this sense, nanotechnology has recently become a promising option to improve the pest control in agriculture.

Although some nanomaterials have been unconsciously used by humans for hundreds of years (e.g., nanogold), the concept of nanotechnology was not introduced till 1959 by Richard P. Feynman, who spoke about the ability to manipulate matter at the atomic level (Feynman, 1960). Later, K. Eric Drexler (1986, 1992) provided the scientific and technological foundations to develop the manufacturing components and systems of nanotechnology. Over the past few years, there have been major advances in the field of nanoscience and nanotechnology and, nowadays, its applications have great impact in different disciplines, such as medicine, electronics, material science, energy, or environment, among many others. However, the application of nanotechnology in agriculture is still in the early stages and there is limited information on the impact of this technology to humans, animals, and the environment. Therefore, it is a challenge for scientists and government officials to improve the knowledge about this field.

Recently, INIA (National Agronomic Research and Technology Institute) has been authorized by the Spanish Ministry of Agriculture, as Independent Organism for the Evaluation of the required documentation for the approval of active substances and authorization of plant protection products (active substance/s + formulant/s) under the Regulation (EC) No. 1107/2009 (European Commission, 2009b). This review analyses the recent state of knowledge on nanopesticides, focusing the attention in the problems that should overcome in order to allow their authorization in Europe. In this sense, it will be reviewed the current legislative situation at European level concerning the placing of plant protection products on the market, focusing on nanopesticides. In order to achieve this issue, a review of regulatory needs that arose in the last 25 years and that first led to the Directive 91/414/EEC (European Commission, 1991) and later to the current Regulation (EC) No. 1107/2009 (European Commission, 2009b) will be carried out. The new opportunities that the Directive 2009/128/EC of sustainable use (European Commission, 2009a) provide to nanopesticides will also be analyzed.

2 Nanopesticides

According to Rai and Ingle (2012) the prefix *nano* is developed from the Greek word, meaning dwarf. In technical terms, *nano* means 10^{-9} or one billionth part of something. The European Commission (EC) also accepts these definitions and uses the nanotechnology term to refer to "science and technology at the nanoscale of atoms and molecules, and to the scientific principles and new properties that can be understood and mastered when operating in this domain. Such properties can then be observed and exploited at the micro- or macroscale, for example, for the development of materials and devices with novel functions and performance" (Commission of the European Communities, 2008). For regulatory purposes, a definition of nanomaterial should fulfill the next four main requirements (Lövestam et al., 2010): (1) to be a single definition broadly applicable in EU legislation and policies; (2) to be legally clear and unambiguous; (3) to be enforceable through agreed measurement techniques and procedures; (4) to be in line with other approaches worldwide. However, there is not an international agreement about definition for the term nanomaterials. In fact, the efforts of several national and international standardization bodies, organizations, and authorities to establish a definition for this term have conducted to incompatible definitions.

The International Organization for Standardization (ISO), the European Standardization Committee (CEN) and the Organization for Economic Cooperation and Development (OECD), among others, refer the term nanomaterial to materials, with internal structures or external dimensions, which are on a nanoscale (size range typically between 1 and 100 nm) (House of Lords, 2010; Lövestam et al., 2010). In this sense, they have focused on the quantitative measure of these materials. However, some other definitions assume that nanomaterials should show novel properties and behavior, regarding those of bulk materials with similar chemical composition, as a result of their small (nanoscale) size (Barlow et al., 2009; Daniel and Astruc 2004). Scientific literature on nanopesticides also includes particles in the whole nanoscale (1–1000 nm) as long as they display different properties or behavior from their macrosized counterparts (Bhagat et al., 2013; McClements, 2011, 2012; Porras et al., 2008). Regarding the agencies and authorities focused on the management of plant protection products, the United States Environmental Protection Agency (US EPA), defines engineered (manufactured) nanoscale material as any particle, substance, or material that has been engineered to have one or more dimensions in the nanoscale (US EPA, 2007). However, there is not an official established definition of nanomaterial proposed by the European Food Safety Authority (EFSA). The EC recommends define nanomaterial as "natural, incidental, or manufactured material containing particles, in an unbound state or as an aggregate or as an agglomerate and where, for 50% or more of the particles in the number size distribution, one or more external dimensions is in the size range 1–100 nm. In specific cases and where warranted by concerns for the environment, health, safety, or competitiveness the number size distribution threshold of 50% may be replaced by a threshold between 1% and 50%" (European Commission, 2011a). Alternatively, "fullerenes, graphene flakes, and single wall carbon nanotubes with one or more external dimensions below 1 nm" and materials "where the specific surface area by volume of the material is greater than 60 m^2/cm^3" should also be considered as nanomaterials (European Commission, 2011a). Therefore, the EC recommendation contains a rather broad description of the term nanomaterial. However, again, this definition only takes into account morphology considerations, mainly size. Few days after this EC recommendation, Regulation (EU) No. 1169/2011 (European Commission, 2011c) defined engineered nanomaterial as "any intentionally produced material that has one or more dimensions of the order of 100 nm or less or that is composed of discrete functional parts, either internally or at the surface, many of which have one or more dimensions of the order of 100 nm or less, including structures, agglomerates, or aggregates, which may have a size above the order of 100 nm but retain properties that are characteristic of the nanoscale. Properties that are characteristic of the nanoscale include: (1) those related to the large specific surface area of the materials considered; and/or (2) specific physico-chemical properties that are different from those of the nonnanoform of the same material." Therefore, this new definition includes some changes in the properties derived from the nanoform. In conclusion, nanoparticles form nanomaterials and only should be considered as such those particles that show features according to the posture adopted (i.e., size in the nanoscale range and/or novel properties derived from a smaller size).

An unequivocal official definition of nanomaterial would be desirable in order to provide consumers sufficient information to choose a product, either with or without nanomaterial ingredients. This definition might also be useful to select which materials need a closer control concerning the small size and/or altered features. In this context, pesticide nanoformulations (nanomaterials with properties against pests by themselves or thanks to the presence of an active ingredient) commonly known as nanopesticides could fall or not within the nanomaterials according to definition selected. For instance, it is well-known that microemulsions have particle sizes typically smaller than 100 nm (De et al., 2014; Kah et al., 2013; McClements, 2011) and, hence, pesticides formulations based on microemulsions should be considered as nanopesticide formulations according to the morphology criterion proposed by EC (mainly particle size) (European Commission, 2011a). Conversely, other promising formulations, such as pesticide nanoemulsions [20–200–500 nm (McClements, 2011, 2012; Porras et al., 2008)] could be excluded from EC recommendation (European Commission, 2011a) despite of displaying additional advantages over their microemulsion and/or bulk material counterparts, despising their novel properties. This undefined situation is favoring an incorrect use of the prefix *nano*, that is, (1) companies do not reference their formulations as *nano* due to the association that is currently done with possible undesirable effects, or (2) formulations are referenced as *nano* only due to its connotation with novelty or enhanced activity, without cover both or one of the definitions of nanomaterials.

In general, the main objectives of pesticide nanoformulations are to improve the solubility of insoluble or poorly soluble pesticides, a more precise and controlled release of pesticides and the protection of pesticide against premature degradation under biotic or abiotic conditions (Pérez-de-Luque and Rubiales, 2009; Kah et al., 2013; Nair et al., 2010). Therefore, it is expected that such improvements offer some advantages over the conventional formulations, including a better pest control without multiple treatments, reduction of pesticide doses, an increase of bioavailability (better penetration through tissues and increased uptake) or less pesticide lost by volatilization.

However, the use of pesticide nanoformulations is not exempt of risk since new chemical entities with poorly understood physicochemical and toxicological properties would be introduced in the environment (Kah et al., 2013; Kah and Hofmann, 2014). For instance, increasing solubility of nanopesticide can lead to enhanced mobility of the active substance in the environment, being potential contaminants of water bodies. Moreover, the protection of pesticide against early degradation can lead to a longer persistence of biologically active compounds, being potentially harmful to nontarget organisms. Besides, the incorporation of pesticides into nanoparticles can conduct to unexpected toxicity against nontarget organisms due to synergic effects.

With regard to the classification, EFSA proposes three types of nanomaterials devoted to agricultural sector based on its chemical nature: organic nanomaterials, inorganic nanomaterials, and combinations of organic and inorganic nanomaterials (or hybrids) (Peters et al., 2014). In this context, this review reports some current advances in nanopesticide formulations covering these three categories.

2.1 Organic Nanopesticide Formulations

The organic nanopesticide formulations refer to nanostructures of organic nature that retain or "encapsulate" existing pesticides. Often these structures are so-called nanodelivery systems, controlled release systems or nanoencapsulates (Peters et al., 2014). The release mechanisms of the pesticide can be controlled by diffusion, dissolution, and/or degradation, depending of encapsulated composition, pesticide properties, and pesticide distribution.

Regarding to the morphology, scientific literature describe different geometric forms to retain pesticides (Fig. 6.3). Nanospheres and nanocapsules are the most common shapes reported in nanopesticide formulations (Fig. 6.3) (Perlatti et al., 2013; Ragaei

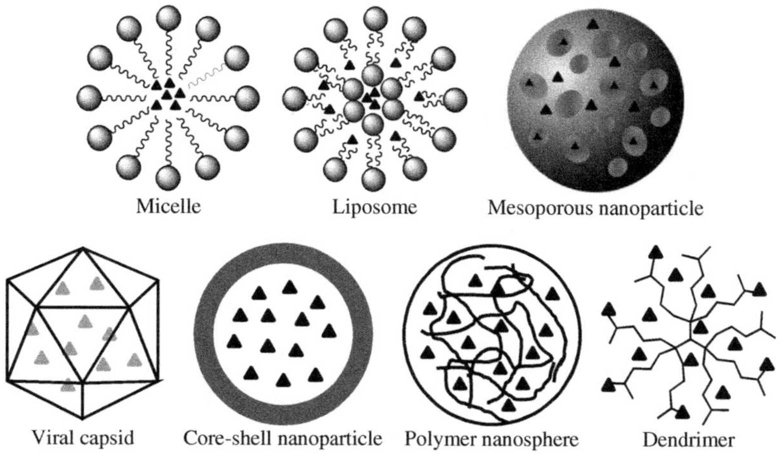

Figure 6.3. Selection of nanoparticle shapes used to design nanopesticides formulations (▲ symbolize the active ingredient of nanopesticide).

and Sabry, 2014; Ramos Campos et al., 2015). Nanospheres are monolithic systems where the pesticide is dissolved or dispersed in a matrix, while nanocapsules or (core–shell nanoparticles) are reservoir systems where a shell encloses the dissolved pesticide. Moreover, it can be found other nanostructures that retain pesticides, such as dendrimers (i.e., polymers composed of highly branched monomers that emerge from a central core) or hydrogels (i.e., hydrophilic polymeric networks) (Göller et al., 2001; Liu et al., 2015; Ramos Campos et al., 2015).

Regarding to the composition, the most frequent types of organic nanopesticides are formulated from lipids, proteins, and polymers.

2.1.1 Lipid-Based Nanopesticide Formulations

Emulsions are one of the most common lipid-based formulations used in agriculture applications. In recent years, nanoemulsions have attracted interest of many researchers due to their potential advantages as delivery systems of pesticides over conventional emulsions.

Nanoemulsions consist of a complex mixture of the pesticide, water, water immiscible oil, surfactants, and cosurfactants. These systems typically are oil-in-water (O/W) emulsions, where nanoparticles or "nanodroplets" of oil (with the previously dissolved pesticide) are dispersed inside the continuous aqueous phase. Although nanoemulsions are thermodynamically unstable, they show high stability for a long time with a droplet size ranging from 20 to 500 nm (De et al., 2014; Forgiarini et al., 2001; Solans et al., 2003).

The main aim of nanoemulsions is to enhance solubility of insoluble or poorly water-soluble pesticides with lower surfactant concentrations than microemulsions (McClements, 2012). Thus, the use of nanoemulsions is highly attractive for preparing formulations containing essential oils (or their components) since the preparation of conventional formulations has several limitations related to their hydrophobic character, reactivity and volatility of these antimicrobial substances. For instance, nanoemulsions of lemongrass oil (56–88 nm) and oregano oil (148 nm) showed a good antimicrobial activity against *Salmonella typhimurium* and *Escherichia coli* during the storage of grape berries (Kim et al., 2014) and lettuce (Bhargava et al., 2015). In the same way, promising results with nanoemulsions containing glyphosate (water soluble herbicide) (Jiang et al., 2012) and β-cypermethrin (poorly water soluble insecticide) (Zhu et al., 2009) have been reported. However, some authors have pointed out that the use of nanoemulsions for solubilizing pesticides is not the best application but a commercial one (Gutiérrez et al., 2008).

It is worth to mention that other types of nanoemulsions are recently described, namely water-in-oil (W/O) emulsions and multiple emulsions [oil-in-water-in-oil (O/W/O) and water-in-oil-in-water (W/O/W)] in which the dispersed droplets are themselves emulsions (Choi et al., 2011; ElShafei et al., 2010; Landfester et al., 2000; McClements, 2010, Usón et al., 2004).

Other types of lipid-based formulations are those based on liposomes. Unlike lipid-based nanoemulsions, liposomes are vesicles of rather uniform particle size distribution (50–500 nm) (Sopeña et al., 2009) formed by (phospho)lipid bilayers that enclose an aqueous compartment. Due to their amphiphilic character, this system is able to solubilize a wide range of compounds, that is, retaining hydrophobic pesticides in their bilayer and hydrophilic pesticides in their aqueous cavity.

Although the major application of liposomes in agriculture field is related to the detection of pesticides (nanobiosensors), they can be use as delivery systems of pesticides with a wide range of solubilities (Quinn and Perrett, 1996; Sopeña et al., 2009; Taylor et al., 2005). For instance, Milne and Shelby (1999) have reported a method to prepare pesticide formulations containing boron compounds (e.g., borates, boric acids, and boric oxides) by means of the encapsulation of the active ingredient in liposomes (mixture of lecithin and organic solvent).

2.1.2 Protein-Based Nanopesticide Formulations

Nowadays, protein-based nanopesticides are being investigated in order to reduce pesticide use and to develop more environmental friendly formulations. In this regard, viruses have received considerable interest since they can carry pesticides inside their capsids (Coulibaly et al., 2007; Chang et al., 2003). Virus capsids are coat or shell structures in the nanometer range composed of protein subunits (Pérez-de-Luque and Rubiales, 2009; Manchester and Steinmetz, 2009).

Coulibaly et al. (2007) described the structure of two viruses (i.e., cypoviruses and baculoviruses) as polyhedral shells able to entrap active substances, such as pesticides. It was found that these structures have good stability under dehydration and freezing conditions, and enzymatic degradation, whereas they can release their load when exposed to basic pH. In a recent work, Cao et al. (2015) have developed a delivery system for the biopesticide abamectin by encapsulating it into capsids of red clover necrotic mosaic virus (<100 nm). This nanopesticide improved the stability and bioavailability of abamectin, enlarged the zone of protection in the soil and increased the control of root knot nematode *Meloidogyne hapla* infection of tomato seedlings.

Scientists of Louisiana State University AgCenter are working on developing protein-based nanopesticides from nanoparticles made of zein, a biodegradable corn-derived protein (Blanchard, 2015). The particles were designed to entrap the insecticide methoxyfenozide for a better control of soybean looper.

2.1.3 Polymer-Based Nanopesticide Formulations

Different polymers can be used to retain pesticides at nanoscale level, including naturally occurring polymers (e.g., cellulose, chitosan, alginate) or synthetic polymers (e.g., cellulose derivatives, polyethers, polyamides) (Masuda, 2011; Perlatti et al., 2013; Ramos Campos et al., 2015). For instance, Oliveira et al. (2015) reported a good control of mustard (*Brassica juncea*) during the postemergence treatment with nanocapsules, of poly(epsilon-caprolactone) (polyester compound) containing atrazine. The authors showed that the polymeric nanocapsules of atrazine not only provided a gradual released of the herbicide, but also nanoencapsulation enhanced the herbicidal activity in comparison with a commercial atrazine formulation, which allowed to reduce the atrazine dosage up to 10-fold without comprising the effectiveness (Oliveira et al., 2015). Similarly, it was proved that the gradual release of other encapsulated pesticides, such as azadirachtin-A, carbofuran, azoxystrobin, or β-cyfluthrin in amphiphilic polymers formulations pesticides provide an efficient control of different pests with a significantly reduction of dosage (Kumar et al., 2010; Kumari et al., 2015; Loha et al., 2011; Shakil et al., 2010).

Kaushik et al. (2013) observed that the quality of soybean seeds during the storage could be improved by means of coatings with polymeric nanoformulations containing the pesticide thiram. The quality improvement not only was due to the antifungal activity of thiram and its controlled release, but also to the action of the polymeric coatings as barriers to moisture, which reduce the rate of seed deterioration.

Photoinactivation is also an issue of concern since the effectiveness of pesticides can be reduced during field applications as a consequence of photodegradation processes. Boehm et al. (2003, 2000) prepared a stable formulation of the photolabile pesticide ethiprole from polymeric nanospheres. Although the formulations are not as good as the classical suspension of ethiprole in terms of controlled release, the nanospheres improved the penetration of the pesticide through the plant and protected it against photoinactivation.

Volatilization of pesticides is an important transport route of pesticides from the initial application site to nontarget locations, which leads to the contamination of different compartments. In this regard, some authors proposed micro- and nanoencapsulation as a potential option to reduce the volatilization and increased its effectiveness, avoiding reapplications (Bhagat et al., 2013; Hellmann et al., 2011). For instance, the nanoencapsulation of garlic oil in nanoparticles of poly(ethylene glycol) allow improving efficacy of this essential oil against the insect *Tribolium castaneum* over a 80%, while the control efficacy of free garlic essential oil was only 11% (Yang et al., 2009).

2.2 Inorganic Nanopesticide Formulations

The inorganic pesticide nanoformulations refer to those nanosized compounds of inorganic nature that display pesticide activity. There are diverse inorganic compounds used to formulate inorganic nanopesticides, including metals (e.g., Ag, Cu), metal oxides (e.g., SiO_2, TiO_2, ZnO, Al_2O_3), carbon nanotubes, or combinations thereof.

Historically, silver is one of the most extensively studied inorganic compounds due to high effectiveness as antimicrobial agent against bacteria, viruses, and fungi (Liu and Jiang, 2015; Morrill et al., 2013). Different formulations containing nanoparticles of silver are currently on the market although its usage is limited to health care or biocide applications (European Commission, 2014b; Nowack et al., 2011). However, the application of nanosilver as nanopesticide in the agriculture sector is still under development. Different authors have instigated the use of nanosilver as alternative to conventional organosynthetic fungicides. For instance, Krishnaraj et al. (2012) have biosynthesized silver nanoparticles (10–50 nm) showing an excellent activity against a variety of fungal plant pathogens (i.e., *Alternaria alternata, Sclerotinia sclerotiorum, Macrophomina phaseolina, Rhizoctonia solani, Botrytis cinerea*, and *Curvularia lunata*). Similarly, Jo et al. (2009) showed that the preventive application of silver nanoparticles (20–30 nm) significantly inhibited colony formation of two plant-pathogenic fungi, *Bipolaris sorokiniana* and *Magnaporthe grisea*, within 3 h.

Nanoparticles of silica (SiO_2) are also extensively studied to control insects in agriculture. This compound is absorbed into cuticular lipids of insects, damaging their protective wax layer, which led to death of insects by desiccation (Aslani et al., 2014). Debnath et al. (2011) and Goswami et al. (2010) obtained a successful control of different insects and pathogens after the treatment with nanoparticles of silica with a mortality rate nearly 90–100%.

Nanoparticles of silica are also used as carrier and delivery systems of other inorganic compounds (Oh et al., 2006; Zielecka, 2011). For instance, nanoparticles of Ag–SiO_2 have a strong antifungal effect against *B. cinerea* by the presence of silver (Oh et al., 2006). Similarly, Zheng et al. (2012) described a core–shell nanoparticle of Ag–SiO_2 (118 nm) with antifungal activity against a phytopathogenic fungi. These authors reported that the antifungal effect was not just due to dissolved Ag^+ released from the nanoparticles, but also was probably due to the appearance of reactive oxygen species that inhibit fungi growth (Zheng et al., 2012).

Other metal oxides, such as TiO_2, ZnO, CuO, Al_2O_3, and so on, also can display activity against different pests. Thus, nanoparticles of Al_2O_3 provided a better control of the insects *Sitophilus oryzae* and *Rhyzopertha dominica* than commercial formulations of SiO_2 (Buteler et al., 2015; Stadler et al., 2010). Goswami et al. (2010) demonstrated that nanoparticles of ZnO and TiO_2 inhibit the growth of the two bacterial strains of *Klebsellia*. Likewise, nanoparticles of TiO_2 have potential for controlling *Xanthomonas* bacterial blight in geranium and leaf spot on poinsettia (Norman and Chen, 2011).

However, some of these inorganic nanopesticides can show carcinogenic effects related with the low size, what difficult their commercialization in the European Union. For example crystalline silica, also known as quartz sand (SiO_2, CAS No. 14808-60-7), is classified as carcinogen category 1A (C1A) when it contains >0.1% (w/w) of particles of a diameter below 50 μm (European Commission, 2012a). Classification of quartz sand as C1A impedes its commercialization in the European Union (see Section 4). Diatomaceous earth, also known as amorphous silicon dioxide [$(SiO_2)_n$, CAS No. 61790-53-2], is other good example. This active substance also shows a maximum limit of 0.1% of particles of crystalline silica with a diameter below 50 μm (European Commission, 2013c).

2.3 Organic/Inorganic Nanopesticide Formulations

Organic/inorganic nanopesticide formulations entail those compounds formed by a mixture of nanomaterials of organic and inorganic nature. The main function of these formulations is to protect the active compound against premature degradation, as well as providing a slow release of them.

As mentioned before, silica-based nanoparticles has been used to load and release inorganic compounds, such as silver or cupper (Oh et al., 2006; Zielecka, 2011). Likewise, different studies pointed that silica nanoparticles are also promising carriers in applications requiring sustained release of organosynthetic pesticides. Porous hollow nanoparticles of silica (Fig. 6.3) seem a suitable shape to carry pesticides since it has high loading capacity into its hollow and a porous shell that controls the release. In this sense, Tan et al. (2012) obtained good controlled-release of uniconazole using porous hollow nanoparticles of silica with a shell thickness of ~15 nm and a particle size of 80–100 nm. Moreover, compared with free uniconazole, the application of porous hollow nanoparticles of silica improved retardation effects on rice growth (Tan et al., 2012). The encapsulation of pesticides into porous hollow silica also provides UV protection due to UV-shielding properties of these nanoparticles. For example, the photostability of avermectin was significantly improved after its encapsulation into hollow core of the nanoparticle, which can lead to a major efficiency against pests (Li et al., 2007).

Nanospheres and nanocapsules of silica also provide good results regarding to control release of pesticides. In this regards, Ao et al. (2013) described the preparation of nanospheres of silica conjugated with a growth regulator. The nanoconjugate SiO_2-regulator displayed a better efficacy in promoting root formation than free regulator and a long-duration sustained-release performance. Similarly, core–shell nanoparticles of silica have been synthetized, which are formed by a shell of silica surrounded an oil core of fipronil (insecticide) (Wibowo et al., 2014) Fig. 6.3. The release rate of fipronil decreased with increasing the shell thickness, which allowed a sustained control of subterranean termites for longer time.

Clay minerals are appropriate materials to be used in controlled release formulations, since they are able to absorb and desorb pesticides at a slow rate (Rashidzadeh et al., 2014). The main clay minerals used in agriculture sector entail both cationic clays (e.g., bentonite, montmorillonite) and anionic clays [e.g., layered double hydroxides (LDHs)]. Cationic clays are negatively charged layers that contain hydrated cations in the interlayer region, while anionic clays are positively charged layers that contain hydrated anions in the interlayer region (Zhang et al., 2004). The ions in the interlayer region can easily be replaced. This fact allows the direct intercalation of hydrophilic compounds. In the same way, the substitution of inorganic ions by organic ions in the interlayer region allows the adsorption of hydrophobic compounds (Gámiz et al., 2015; Singla et al., 2012).

Ionic pesticides, such as the herbicide 2,4-D (Hussein et al., 2009) or the growth regulator β-naphthoxyacetic acid (Li et al., 2015) have been successfully prepared by intercalation into LDHs formulations, providing a good controlled release of the pesticides. On the other hand, the modification of LDH surface by addition of surfactants allowed to intercalate nonionic pesticide into LDHs structures (Zhenlan et al., 2009).

Scientific literature also report nanopesticide formulations based on clay minerals containing biopesticides, such as essential oils or living organism or their derived product. Thus, the encapsulation of Neemazal® was successfully performed using a polymer-montmorillonite nanocomposite as controlled release system (Rashidzadeh et al., 2014). Ghormade et al. (2011) have developed chitosan/kaolin nanoparticles (350 nm) loaded with the *Myrothrecium verrucaria* enzyme complex as active ingredient. The encapsulation allowed to stabilize the enzyme complex, increasing its biological activity against the cotton mealy bug (*Psudococcus gossypiphilous*). Moreover, the presence of chitosan in this nanoformulation provided an additional control of the soil borne pathogen *Fusarium* (Ghormade et al., 2011).

3 Pesticide Legislation at European Level

With the Maastricht Treaty in the early 1990s (European Commission, 1992b), the real need to harmonize national laws on marketing about pesticides arose. In July 1991, the European Directive 91/414/EEC was adopted in order to harmonize the criteria for the assessment and registration of plant protection products intended for marketing within the European Economic Community [and later within the European Union (EU)] (European Commission, 1991). This Directive failed to introduce an unique registration system at European level, although two agreements of great importance were reached: (1) to create a single positive list of active substances approved at European level and included in the Annex I of this Directive; (2) to establish common principles in the Member States (MSs) for assessment and decision making for the registration of plant protection products. In this sense, only those products whose active substances were incorporated in Annex I could achieve an authorization to be commercialized as plant protection products. The unique market was accomplished by setting that all authorization granted by a MS has to being recognized by the others (mutual recognition), providing that the agro-environmental conditions of MSs are comparable. Thus, a review program for the existing active substances in the EU market before 1993 was developed to determine their inclusion or not in Annex I following the new uniform principles and requirements established by the Directive 91/414/EC (European Commission, 1991). This review program was divided into four stages (European Commission, 1992a, 2000b, 2002). The active substances were approved by inclusion Directives in Annex I and plant protection products containing them were subjected to a review program, called reregistration, for authorization in the MSs (European Commission, 2011d).

In June 2011 the Regulation (EC) No. 1107/2009 (European Commission, 2009b) replaced the Directive 91/414/EEC (European Commission, 1991). The main purpose of the Regulation is to ensure a high level of protection of both human and animal health and the environment and at the same time to safeguard the competitiveness of Community agriculture. Furthermore, with this Regulation the most recent scientific and technical developments and the experience gained with the Directive 91/414/EC were adopted (European Commission, 1991). The application of the Regulation remove as far as possible obstacles to trade and speed up the approval of active substances and authorization of plant protection products with the establishment of strict deadlines. This Regulation, currently in force, grouped EU MSs according to their agroclimatic conditions (northern, central, and south) (Table 6.2) [Annex I of Regulation (EC) No. 1107/2009]. These groups were performed to share the workload between the various MSs. In addition, the mutual recognition of authorizations is improved and tight deadlines are set to carry out the review process. These mechanisms are accelerating the arrival of new solutions for plant protection into the market, such as new nanopesticides.

However, criteria to address and to assess the risk of these solutions based on scientific data (risk assessment) still need more harmonization among MSs. While active substances are approved at EU level, agreeing a common pesticide risk assessment through

Table 6.2 Northern, Central and Southern Zones Established in the EU Regulation (EC) 1107/2009 (European Commission, 2009b)

Zone	Country	Abbreviations
Northern	Denmark	DK
	Estonia	EE
	Finland	FI
	Latvia	LV
	Lithuania	LT
	Sweden	SE
Central	Austria	AT
	Belgium	BE
	Czech Republic	CZ
	Germany	DE
	Hungary	HU
	Ireland	IE
	Luxembourg	LU
	Netherlands	NL
	Poland	PL
	Romania	RO
	Slovakia	SK
	Slovenia	SI
	United Kingdom	UK
Southern	Bulgaria	BG
	Cyprus	CY
	France	FR
	Greece	EL
	Italy	IT
	Malta	MT
	Portugal	PT
	Spain	ES

the conclusion of the EFSA, formulated products are evaluated at zonal level and authorized at national level. In this sense, the efforts for risk-mitigation of one MS can be contrary to a divergent approach taken by another neighboring MS. The Regulation (EU) No. 546/2011 (European Commission, 2011b) establishes the uniform principles in order to harmonize the risk assessment for formulated products, trying to avoid those situations. Guidance documents on the risk assessment of plant protection products are also developed to provide guidance for agrochemical companies and authorities (Antunović et al., 2011). Nevertheless, these guidance documents do not include the evaluation of the risk produced by the application of a plant protection product formulated as nanopesticides. All these guidance documents should be reviewed to include the assessment of this new technology. Risk mitigation measures also need additional harmonization because each MS in a given territory is responsible for participating in risk management surrounding the use of pesticides (Guidance Document, 2011).

4 Nanopesticides Within the Regulation (EC) No. 1107/2009

The communication "Toward a European Strategy for Nanotechnology" (Commission of the European Communities, 2008) was assumed by the EC on May 12, 2004. This document fixes the basis of an integrated and responsible strategy for the development of nanotechnology. The most important issue of this strategy is that nanotechnology should not generate damage despite of its benefits. Development together with the technological progress need to complement the scientific investigation and assessment of possible health or environmental risks associated with nanotechnology. It is also addressed the environmental, health, safety, and social concerns. In this context, the main needs on nanotechnology identified in the previous cited communication (Commission of the European Communities, 2008) are shown in Table 6.3. These considerations still continue today as part of an integrated approach to maintain and strengthen the European research and development on nanotechnology. The objective is the exploitation of the knowledge generated by this contemporary technology for the benefit of society.

In 2008, the EC published a communication to the European Parliament, the Council and the European Economic and Social Committee regarding regulatory aspects of nanomaterials (Commission of the European Communities, 2008), where it was

Table 6.3 The Main Needs on Nanotechnology Identified in the Communication "Toward a European Strategy for Nanotechnology" (Commission of the European Communities, 2008)

Needs on Nanotechnology
To increase the investment and coordination in research and development
To create research institutions of excellence
To encourage the interdisciplinary education and training of research personnel
To ensure favorable conditions for technology transfer and innovation
To integrate the social considerations
To address public health, safety, environmental, and consumer risks of nanotechnology-based products
To encourage the cooperation and initiatives at the international level

stated that current European legislation covers in principle the potential health, safety and environmental risk in relation to nanomaterials. Nanomaterials as substances are covered by the Regulation (EC) No 1907/2006 concerning Registration, Evaluation, Authorization, and Restriction of Chemicals (REACH) (European Commission, 2006). REACH does not explicitly reference nanomaterials. However, they are covered by its substance definition, which addresses chemicals in whatever size, shape, or physical state (European Commission, 2008). The European Chemicals Agency (ECHA) has recently published a guidance on information requirements and chemical safety assessment (ECHA, 2015), with recommendations for nanomaterials applicable to physicochemical properties. Additionally, various actions are ongoing to further improve the regulatory framework for nanomaterials (e.g., revision of REACH annexes and EC nanomaterial definition and working groups at the ECHA), in order to introduce safer nanomaterials into the market (Peters et al., 2014).

In this context, public health, safety, environmental, and consumer protection require to address any potential risk of nanotechnology-based products. Moreover, research results should be made available as soon as possible to all stakeholders, such as public authorities, regulatory bodies, and industry. Engineering a substance with nanotechnology can be compared to producing a new chemical, because of the unpredictable change of its properties as a consequence of classical physics and quantum mechanical effects. Therefore, nanotechnology-based products require evaluate the possible use of previous data considered valid and generate new data on their physicochemical properties, environmental fate, toxicology, and ecotoxicology, including exposure data and dose response. Therefore, specific and easy-to-use instruments for analysis and measurement and analytical methods with high specificity, accuracy, and precision are needed. If required, risk assessment methods should also be adjusted.

Currently, the approval and authorization procedure for active substances and plant protection products, respectively, takes place at Community level under the Regulation (EC) No. 1107/2009 (European Commission, 2009b). According to this Regulation, the term active substance (also known as active ingredient in the open literature) is applied to chemical substances and microorganisms, with general or specific action against harmful organisms or on plants, parts of plants, or plant products. Substances are defined as those chemical elements and their compounds that occur naturally or by manufacture. Plant protection products are formulations consisting of or containing active substances, safeners, or synergists, and intended for protecting crops or desirable or useful plants (Articles 2 and 3 of Regulation (EC) No. 1107/2009). Therefore, pesticide active ingredients and formulations on a nanoscale are covered by this Regulation (European Commission, 2009b). The stages of risk analysis are the follows: hazard identification, exposure characterization, risk assessment, risk management, and communication of risk. The risk assessment of an active substance or plant protection product involves first the identification of the risk factor, followed by quantification of exposure and finally the risk assessment, taking into account the safety factor for humans, including vulnerable groups, consumers, operators, workers, bystanders, environment, and nontarget organisms resulting from its use. In addition, the rules of this authorization procedure should be updated from time to time as a result of new scientific knowledge and lessons learned. The principle that governs the current European food law is not to market unsafe food. In fact, this principle is a worldwide trend, mainly in those countries with important trading partners, as a consequence of the globalization of markets. Therefore, in Europe, plant protection products cannot be commercialized without demonstrate in a rigorous and scientific way that they do not have negative effects on human and animal health and the environment, that they are sufficiently effective and show low capacity to contaminate water (surface and groundwater). The main challenge for the industry dedicated to the development and marketing of active substances and plant protection products is to find new tools to maintain or increase food production, while safeguarding protection of all stakeholders (consumer, animals, and environment) and diversity of crops without increase the land dedicated to them.

On February 2, 2000, the EC adopted the precautionary principle (Commission of the European Communities, 2000), which is particularly important for risk management. The principle of prior approval through a positive list of active substances (Annex I), before placing plant protection products on the market, is an approach of applying the precautionary principle, by shifting responsibility for producing scientific evidence. The safety level is increased with the Regulation (EC) No. 1107/2009 by introducing the nonapproval (cut-off) criteria (Table 6.4) (European Commission, 2009b). In this sense, the active substances will be simply banned because of their classification within a toxicological, environmental, and ecotoxicological classification cut-off criteria shown in Table 6.4, which involves a perceptible and an unacceptable risk (Commission of the European Communities, 2000). Only if the exposure of humans to an active substance that fails in the cut-off criteria is (1) negligible under realistic proposed conditions of use (Annex II, Point 3 of Regulation (EC) No. 1107/2009) and (2) necessary to control a serious danger to plant health which cannot be contained by other available means including non-chemical methods (Article 4, Point 7 of Regulation (EC) No. 1107/2009), it could be possible to approve the active substance. Therefore, the cut-off criteria push to an eventual loss of active substances and plant protection products despite being proved their safety.

First, in the year 2006, the EC and the European Crop Protection Association (ECPA, 2006) and later, in the year 2008, the Pesticides Safety Directorate (PSD) of the United Kingdom (PSD, 2008; Theodoris, 2008) and the Kemikalieinspektionen Swedish Chemicals Agency (KEMI) (KEMI, 2008; Theodoris, 2008) presented their analysis of the likely percentage of active substances affected by the nonapproval criteria (Table 6.5). Their conclusions varied significantly and a comparison of the main differences between analyses is needed to understand the variances (ECPA, 2006; PSD, 2008; KEMI, 2008; Theodoris, 2008): The Commission evaluation was based on those substances that were included in the Annex I of Directive 91/414/EEC (European Commission, 1991). Therefore, Commission did not analyze substances under EU review and pending an Annex I decision at that moment. The ECPA analysis was based on substances that remain on the market as of October 2006 and presented by the ECPA full member companies, but excluding the substances of

Table 6.4 Categories of Active Substances Recognized by the Regulation (EC) No. 1107/2009, Together With Their Maximum Period of Authorization and Main Requirements for Their Classification (European Commission, 2009b)

	Maximum Validity		
Classification	**1st approval**	**Renewal**	**Requirements**
Nonapproved substances with cut-off criteria	n/a	n/a	Environmental cut-off criteria: • Persistent organic pollutant (POP) • Persistent, bioaccumulative, and toxic (PBT) • Very persistent, very bioaccumulative (vPvB) Ecotoxicological cut-off criteria: • Adverse endocrine effects to non-target organisms and honeybees Toxicological cut-off criteria: • Carcinogens (C1A and C1B) • Mutagens (M1A and M1B) • Toxic for reproduction (R1A and R1B)
Candidates for substitution	7 years	7 years	Toxicological criteria: • Low acceptable daily intake (ADI), acute reference dose (ARfD), or acceptable operator exposure level (AOEL) • Exceptions to classification as C1A or C1B • Exceptions to classification as R1A or R1B Environmental criteria: • Two criteria of PBT substances Ecotoxicological criteria: • Exceptions to adverse endocrine effects Further criteria: • Concerned situations of use • Significant proportion of nonactive isomers
Standard substances	10 years	15 years	Approval criteria: • The obligatory complete dossier shall contain information to establish, where relevant, ADI, ARfD, and AOEL, to carry out a risk assessment and for enforcement purposes • Take into account efficacy, relevance of metabolites, composition of the active substance, methods of analysis, impact on human health, fate and behavior in the environment, ecotoxicology, residue definition and fate and behavior concerning groundwater

Table 6.4 Categories of Active Substances Recognized by the Regulation (EC) No. 1107/2009, Together With Their Maximum Period of Authorization and Main Requirements for Their Classification (European Commission, 2009b) (*cont.*)

Classification	Maximum Validity 1st approval	Maximum Validity Renewal	Requirements
			• Considering the above criteria for the active substance, at least one formulation (and its residues) with this substance for at least one representative use in at least one MS: (1) shall not have hazardous effects on human and animal health and on the environment, on plants/plant products, or on ground water; (2) shall be sufficiently effective; (3) shall not cause unnecessary suffering to vertebrates to be controlled • There shall be methods for measuring residues
Low risk substances	15 years	15 years	Toxicological criteria: • Not classified as carcinogenic, mutagenic, toxic to reproduction, sensitizing chemicals, very toxic or toxic, explosive or corrosive Further criteria: • Not persistent or endocrine disrupter • Bioconcentration factor not higher than 100 • Not have neurotoxic or immunotoxic effects
Basic substances	Unlimited	Unlimited	Approval criteria: • Without concern • Without inherent capacity to cause endocrine disrupting, neurotoxic, or immunotoxic effects • Not predominantly used for plant protection purposes • Not placed on the market as a plant protection product Further criteria: • Fulfil the criteria of a foodstuff

the List 4 of the fourth stage of the EC review program (European Commission, 2002) mainly formed by unconventional chemicals (e.g., biopesticides) (Villaverde et al., 2014b, 2016a). Moreover, the methodology for measuring active substances differed between the Commission and the ECPA. In this sense, while the Commission evaluation was based only on substances already classified,

Table 6.5 Predicted Impact of the Regulation (EC) No. 1107/2009 in the Classification of Active Substances, According to the European Commission (EC), the European Crop Protection Association (ECPA), the PSD of the United Kingdom and the Kemikalieinspektionen Swedish Chemicals Agency (KEMI) (ECPA, 2006; Commission of the European Communities, 2006a; KEMI, 2008; Theodoris, 2008)

			PSD		
	EC	ECPA	Commission Criteria	Parliament Criteria	KEMI
Cut-off criteria (%)	5	30	16	41	8
Candidates for substitution (%)[a]	10–15	Up to 50	20	43	—
Total affected (%)[b]	20	60	36	84	8

[a]Percentages on those active substances that do not fall within the cut-off criteria.
[b]Active substances that could be impacted by either rejection or substitution candidate criteria.

the ECPA also considered the possibility that substances may be (re)classified in future. The study of PSD (now CRD) was based on those substances included in the Annex I of Directive 91/414/EEC (European Commission, 1991), including the substances of the List 3 under review as part of the third stage of the EC review program (European Commission, 2000b). Furthermore, the PSD analysis took into account both the Commission and also the European Parliament criteria. Finally, the KEMI proposal was based on the substances included in the Annex I of Directive 91/414/EEC (European Commission, 1991) and pending on third stage of the EC review program (European Commission, 2000b), taking into account the national criteria and principles.

With this background, it is clear that several active substances will have difficulties to renew their approval, most probably those included in the first, second and third stage of the EC review program and the new substances included in the Annex I after 1992 (Villaverde et al., 2014a,b). In fact, most of these substances will have to be reassessed for renewal of their approval between 2016 and 2021 (Villaverde et al., 2014a). A withdrawal of plant protection products from the market could involve an increase in the pests incidence and an increase of cases of resistance, causing a drastic yield reduction while increase the price of food products. Therefore, one of the main challenges of the Regulation (EC) No. 1107/2009 involves the application of cut-off criteria for pesticides without losing tools for future agriculture (especially for minor uses) (European Commission, 2009b).

The higher safety level of the Regulation (EC) No. 1107/2009 (European Commission, 2009b) in comparison with the Directive 91/414/EEC (European Commission, 1991) is also observed through the establishment of the following new four categories of approved substances recognized by the Regulation: candidates for substitution [Article 24 of Regulation (EC) No. 1107/2009], standard [Article 4 of Regulation (EC) No. 1107/2009], low risk [Article 22 of Regulation (EC) No. 1107/2009], and basic substances [Article 23 of Regulation (EC) No. 1107/2009]. The criteria for their classification are summarized in Table 6.4, where basic and low risk substances (especially the first) show the strictest ones. Depending on their classification, the substances have an associated period of validity and renewal of approval (Table 6.4), being inversely proportional to their level of risk. These periods clearly denote an additional difficulty for those substances classified as candidates for substitution. The criteria show in Table 6.4 to identify substances candidates for substitution leave more margins for interpretation than criteria established for basic and low-risk substances.

In July 2015, the Commission draft list of substances candidates for substitution contained 77 proposals. This quantity represents 17% of all approved substances (474 substances in total) after discounting those that fall within the nonapproval criteria (5%). Moreover, it is a value very close to that predicted ten years ago (Table 6.5). To include the substances in the provisional list, MSs and stakeholders were consulted and an analysis was conducted by comparing the agreed and peer reviewed endpoints, against the requirements specified in Table 6.4. The information was grouped in a comprehensive database that is updated on a regular basis (European Commission, 2015). The previous worst-case evaluations carried out by the ECPA (ECPA, 2006) and PSD (PSD, 2008; Theodoris, 2008) showed that up to 50% of the active substances would fall in the category of candidate for substitution (Table 6.5). The substances considered in the analyses, which lead to the differences were already listed previously. Meanwhile, KEMI did not make a detailed impact assessment with regards to the adopted candidate criteria (KEMI, 2008). Therefore, between 8% and

84% of substances would be impacted by at least the rejection or substitution candidate criteria (Table 6.5).

Classification of substances as candidates for substitution, based on very restrictive conditions of use (i.e., exceptions to the cut-off criteria in Table 6.4), should not be misled. This is not an easily renewable status that delays or slows their disappearance. Nothing could be further from the truth. In fact, the MSs will perform a comparative risk assessment of the applications for authorization of plant protection products containing these active substances [Article 50 of Regulation (EC) No. 1107/2009], taking into account the availability of adequate solutions for plant protection (chemical and nonchemical) and of sufficient active substances in the market with other modes of action to prevent appearance of resistances. In this situation, it seems evident that nanoformulations with standard and low risk substances, with better features for crop protection in comparison with basic substances (Table 6.4), can play an important role in the imminent decline of active substances. The reason is found in the ability of nanoformulations to increase the availability of tools using both groups of active substances (i.e., standard and low risk substances), providing them novel physicochemical and toxicological properties against pests. Examples of active substances that could suffer a reemerging interest due to their use in nanoformulations are those naturally occurring and known to exhibit pesticidal properties [e.g., monoterpenes (Jalali et al., 2012; Peixoto et al., 2015), sesquiterpenes (Jalali et al., 2013; Ma et al., 2014), phenolic compounds (Cespedes et al., 2014; Santos et al., 2012, 2013)], especially those obtained from biomass residues in agroforest and pulping industries for the integrated exploitation of biomass within the biorefinery concept (Domingues et al., 2011; Villaverde et al., 2016a). In fact, several recent research works have already tested some of these substances (Feng and Peng, 2012; Gonzalez et al., 2014; Hellmann et al., 2011; Lao et al., 2010; Yang et al., 2009).

It is worth noting that Article 29 of Regulation (EC) No. 1107/2009 requires that the technical formulation of the plant protection product to be registered is such that user exposure or other risks are limited as much as possible without compromising the functioning of the product (European Commission, 2009b). This means that nanoformulation could be an opportunity to reduce the exposure, and reduce the risk, maintaining or increasing the efficiency against the harmful organisms. This fact will allow to maintain active substances in the market and a sufficient battery of modes of action to manage the risk of appearance of resistances.

Information, tests, and analysis that the agrochemical companies must submit (data requirements) are established by the Regulations (EU) No. 283/2013 (European Commission, 2013a) and 284/2013 (European Commission, 2013b) for active substances and formulated products, respectively. Part B of both Regulations covers requirements relating to microorganisms, including viruses. In the case of low-risk substances, a reduced dossier for their registration is accepted, what also encourages the development of nanoformulations with this kind of substances. It should be highlighted that active substances are approved at EU level. Meanwhile, plant protection products are authorized at national level after assessment under "uniform principles" throughout the zone, which are set out in the Annex of Commission Regulation (EU) No. 546/2011 (European Commission, 2011b). The uniform principles guarantee the application by all MSs of the Article 29, Point 1 of Regulation (EC) No. 1107/2009 (European Commission, 2009b). Therefore, toxicity to target organisms and efficacy for each intended use are assessed with the same requirements regardless of the MS, reaching a high level of protection of human and animal health and the environment.

5 Physicochemical Considerations for Analytical Instruments With Nanopesticides

It should be taken into account that, according to the Article 36 of Regulation (EC) No. (European Commission, 2009b), assessment of a plant protection product should be carried out in the light of current scientific and technical knowledge. The MS that examines an application shall make an independent, objective, and transparent assessment, taking into account the cited Article. In this sense, all MSs in the same zone will also have the opportunity to participate in the assessment procedure by submitting comments and may suggest any novel analytical instrument to be considered which maybe provides better results in the risk assessment. Therefore, the European pesticide legislative framework will evolve over time, in response to challenges posed by the new nanotechnologies for pest control. The working groups, the concerns shown by MSs during assessments and/or comments and the new identified needs, which cannot be satisfied using the accepted science-based approaches, guidance documents, and/or data requirements, are the engines that lead this evolution.

The traceability of an analytical result is based on both identity and quantity (mass or number of particles) (Koeber et al., 2010). Today, there is an open discussion concerning the suitability of the analytical instruments to monitor nanomaterials (Antunović et al., 2011; Barlow et al., 2009; Blasco and Picó, 2011; Bleeker et al., 2013; Linsinger et al., 2013; von der Kammer et al., 2011), which includes nanopesticides. The underlying problem could be found in that determination of nanoparticles shows difficult challenges to overcome today. According to the nanoparticle concept, their unequivocal identification seems imply two kinds of information, namely morphology and chemical composition. Powerful instruments, capable of measure simultaneously both requirements for each particle will be required. Henceforth, in order to provide a clearer approximation to the real problem, the discussion will be limited only to the size aspect of particle morphology. Regarding quantification, it is essential to note that particles of the same chemical composition maybe differ in their physical properties (i.e., mass, size, and density). Therefore, unless the nanoparticles are perfectly spherical and pose uniform and known physical properties, no suitable conversion exists between, mass and amount of nanoparticles and intensity of the signal.

In the following discussion, the problem is briefly reviewed, with special attention on the major challenges for analytical instruments and validation scope.

According to the EC recommendation about nanomaterial (European Commission, 2011a), information about size is important to know whether a particle is in its nanoform. However, the size of a nanoparticle is a blurred property as a consequence of the numerous sizes that nonspherical particles show (even measuring the same material repeatedly), or due to the differences observed in multiple circumstances between nanoparticles in the dried or dispersed state. Moreover, the different instruments employed for the particle size analysis, measure different parameters, although the output is always called size. Therefore, talks about size of a particle without identify the size measured and the method for its determination does not have sense. Both issues (i.e., unclear size of nanoparticles and differences between the analytical measurement principles) seem to generate a challenge intractable today. In this sense, a preferred technique for all situations does not exist, being necessary a combination of them. The ideal case would be the one in which the particles are perfectly spherical. In this situation, measurements from different methods could be comparable. However, this situation is rarely observed.

Mahl et al. (2011) made a comparative study of several measurement techniques [i.e., scanning electron microscopy (SEM), transmission electron microscopy (TEM), dynamic light scattering (DLS), analytical disc centrifugation, and nanoparticle tracking analysis (Brownian motion analysis)] used for the characterization of pure dispersions of gold and silver nanoparticles almost spherical with diameters around 15 and 70 nm, respectively, and their 50:50 mixture (w:w) stabilized with poly(vinylpyrrolidone). This study, in agreement with other studies of different authors (Bootz et al., 2004; Fissan et al., 2014; Hole et al., 2013; Hussain et al., 2009; Landsiedel et al., 2010; Lange 1995), showed that the compared techniques for particle size analysis gave different results even for the same well-defined ensemble of particles. The difference was attributed to the fact that all these methods are based on different physical principles and/or detection methods. For example, SEM and TEM are usual electron microscopy techniques that measure the lateral dimensions of an ultrathin sampling projection. Electron microscopy gives a direct image of a part of a particle population, providing the diameter of the nanoparticles and its data can be quantified by counting individual particle sizes (Bootz et al., 2004; Fissan et al., 2014; Hussain et al., 2009; Landsiedel et al., 2010; Lange, 1995; Mahl et al., 2011). DLS is one of the most frequently used techniques. It involves the measurement of the intensity of the light scattered from a solution. Opposed to direct imaging techniques, such as SEM or TEM, the samples can be measured in its natural state, what requires small particle concentrations to avoid multiple scattering effects. DLS is an instrument technique used to determine the Stokes radius of particles [similar to the hydrodynamic radius in the case in which the particles are nonspherical or flexible (Pecora, 2000)] and is a rough measure of the average particle size (Bootz et al., 2004; Fissan et al., 2014; Hussain et al., 2009; Landsiedel et al., 2010; Lange 1995; Mahl et al., 2011). This size is the radius of a hypothetical hard sphere that diffuses with the same speed as the particle under examination (Cecere et al., 2003; Pecora, 2000).

According to the guidance for risk assessment of nanomaterials published by EFSA (Antunović et al., 2011), at least electron microscopy and other independent method should be used to measure the size parameter because the results obtained from different measurement techniques differ as a consequence of the physical principles of the measurement method (Antunović et al., 2011; Domingos et al., 2009). The requirement of use two or more methods is also established by the OECD preliminary guidance notes on sample preparation and dosimetry for the safety testing of manufactured nanomaterials (OCDE, 2010). In summary, the confirmatory methods can in the whole meaning of the word not confirm the result of the primary methods.

Other issue to have especially into account, related with the nanoparticle size discussed previously, is that sizes of nanoparticles frequently show broad distributions. Determination of this range is also essential (Antunović et al., 2011; Barlow et al., 2009; Bowen, 2002; Cumberland and Lead 2009; Dieckmann et al., 2009; Planken et al., 2008). However, currently there are not accurate and precise methods available for the determination of number based size distributions with some trustworthiness. For example, electron microscopy techniques, such as SEM and TEM provide number based distributions. However, broad particle size distributions need to measure a vast number of particles to ensure representative results, which implies a huge time consuming (Dieckmann et al., 2009). Sample preparation is critical and can affect the real particle size distribution (Dieckmann et al., 2009). Mixtures with particles of very different sizes are complicate to obtain accurate size distribution data because the resolution is not sufficient (for the small particles) or the number of visible particles is too small (for the large particles) (Mahl et al., 2011). On the other hand, for the determination of particle size distribution using analytical ultracentrifugation (AUC) technique, the separation is based on the size and density differences of particles (Dieckmann et al., 2009), and the detectors are able to measure the migration of particles obtaining their sedimentation coefficient distributions (Colfen and Pauck, 1997). However, conversion factors from mass or intensity weighted distributions to number based distributions are not suitable, although occasionally are used for comparison reasons without a greater purpose (Dieckmann et al., 2009). In addition, AUC results may suffer artefacts like particle charge (Dieckmann et al., 2009).

There are other physicochemical parameters (e.g., pH, viscosity, dustiness) that determine the properties and probable biological effects of a nanomaterial, in addition to the size and size distribution. The selection of these parameters together with the characterization methods depends on the nature and planned uses of the nanomaterial. Choices of parameters and methods need to be made case by case. EFSA, in its document on the risk assessment of the application of nanoscience and nanotechnologies in the food and feed chain (Antunović et al., 2011), establishes 15 essential physicochemical parameters for characterization and identification of nanomaterials, from which 6 are required for all nanomaterials (i.e., chemical composition, particle size and size distribution, physical state, surface charge, solubility and partition properties, and chemical reactivity). Moreover, EFSA also lists some of the currently available methods to determine the previous parameters, such as TEM, SEM, DLS, AUC, liquid chromatography, mass spectrometry (MS), and nuclear magnetic resonance spectroscopy (Antunović et al., 2011). However, these methods show drawbacks to accurate detection and characterization, some of which were already highlighted by Montaño et al. (2014). For example, information on chemical composition of the nanomaterial can be determined by inductive couples plasma (ICP)-MS, X-ray absorption spectroscopy (XAS), and so on. Specifically, these methods are not able to distinguish the origin of the particles (i.e., natural or engineered) and sample preparation may modify sample representativeness, they may involve acidification destroying the particle integrity (e.g., ICP-MS) and concentration of nanomaterial in sample may be too low (e.g., XAS) (Antunović et al., 2011; Montaño et al., 2014).

In line with the aforementioned, there are also other challenges that the analytical methods and protocols should overcome, in order to achieve an accurate and precise determination of nanoparticles. For example, morphologies of the particles can change between producers and even in the same producer. Coformulants may also be changed between nanoformulations and producers. Therefore, methods should respond in the same way to nanoparticles from different suppliers and production processes. Otherwise, it would be required a detailed identification of the source before carry out the quantitative analysis, something impossible for monitoring environmental samples without traceability. On the other hand, classical steps in sample preparation could significantly alter the properties of nanoparticles. Extraction, digestion and/or concentration of sample might cause aggregation or dissolution of particles, which result in analytical mistakes. However, the final analytical instrument should be able to distinguish, for example, between the free and encapsulated form of the active substance. In this sense, validation of the analytical method should prove the integrity of the particles by direct or nondirect way (von der Kammer et al., 2011). Other issue that requires attention is that related with the especial characteristics of the analyte, which impede a suitable approximation by a normal distribution of particles without collecting a huge quantity. This is a problem during the quantification step, where only a small fraction is studied. Therefore, numerous analyses are required in order to account a large number of particles.

Finally, European research projects, such as the NanoLyse project, funded by the European Commission under the 7th Framework Program (European Commission, 2010), are being implemented to follow established validation approaches while making necessary adjustments for the specificities of the measurement of nanomaterials (Linsinger et al., 2013).

6 Opportunities of Nanopesticides Within the Directive 2009/128/EC of Sustainable Use

Before beginning to develop this section, it might be useful to define the integrated pest management (IPM) concept. This is not an easy task. In fact, Bajwa and Kogan (2002) carried out a compendium of IPM definitions, collecting them from more than 65 recognized sources. The difficult lies in that IPM is an approach, a strategy to pest control. Therefore, there is not a defined methodology. The idea behind IPM is that combining different practices (e.g., cultural, chemical, biological, and/or technical measures appropriate to an individual situation); it could be possible to overcome their individual limitations. Its main advantage is the adaptability to all pest problems. Nevertheless, the European legislation has fixed one definition in order to establish rules that allow the IPM implementation in the management of plant protection products and measure their progress (see below).

The Regulation (EC) No. 1107/2009 addresses the authorization process by fixing the conditions for the placing of plant protection products on the market (European Commission, 2009b). However, this Regulation does not impede to find undesirable amounts of residues in agricultural products and in the environmental media (Reemtsma et al., 2013; Sánchez-Ávila et al., 2011; Sevilla-Morán and Sandín-España, 2012; Sevilla-Morán et al., 2016; Villaverde et al., 2016b), as long as it was demonstrated that they do not represent a risk for humans, animals, and environment and compile with the approval and authorization criteria established in the articles 4 and 29 of Regulation (EC) No. 1107/2009 (European Commission, 2009b). Neither the Regulation (EC) 396/2005/EC on maximum residue levels of pesticides in or on food and feed of plant and animal origin (European Commission, 2005) nor the European Water Framework Directive (WFD) 2000/60/EC (European Commission, 2000a), complemented by other more specific EU laws (European Commission, 2014a), are enough to avoid these situations. However, it is worth noting the maximum residue levels of pesticides established under the Regulation (EC) 396/2005 are safe for consumer taking into account the chronic and the acute exposure.

The shortcoming is solved by the "Thematic Strategy on the Sustainable Use of Pesticides" (Commission of the European Communities, 2006b,c), published by the European Commission in June 2006, which complements the existing legislative framework. The thematic strategy guides the use phase of plant protection products and was approved by the European Parliament on January 13, 2009 (European Commission, 2012b). Later, in October 2009, the Directive 2009/128/EC was approved, establishing a framework for Community action to achieve the sustainable use of pesticides (European Commission, 2009a). This Directive, which will enter into force in stages from 2011 to 2020 (Villaverde et al., 2014a), provides clear references on how to manage pesticides to achieve their sustainable use, by promoting the use of IPM practices and of alternative approaches or techniques. Both, the Directive 2009/128/EC (European Commission, 2009a) together with the Regulation (EC) No. 1107/2009 (European Commission, 2009b), are the main legislative instruments containing the measures proposed in the Thematic Strategy on the sustainable use of pesticides (Commission of the European Communities, 2006b,c).

The main objective of the thematic strategy and of the Directive 2009/128/EC (European Commission, 2009a) is focused on the promotion of IPM policies within the National Action Plans (NAPs), in order to reduce the risks and impacts of pesticide use on human and animal health and the environment. NAPs should be adopted by MSs to set up their quantitative objectives, targets, measures, and timetables (Article 4 of Directive 2009/128/EC).

According to the Article 3 of Directive 2009/128/EC, IPM "means careful consideration of all available plant protection methods and subsequent integration of appropriate measures that discourage the development of populations of harmful organisms and keep the use of plant protection products and other forms of intervention to levels that are economically and ecologically justified and reduce or minimize risks to human health and the environment. 'Integrated pest management' emphasizes the growth of a healthy crop with the least possible disruption to agro-ecosystems and encourages natural pest control mechanisms" (European Commission, 2009a). This definition includes the three pillars of sustainable development (i.e., economic, environmental, and social) (United Nations, 2002) through the incorporation of the notions included in the next sentence "economically and ecologically justified and reduce or minimize risks to human health and the environment."

Prokopy (1993) proposed four levels of IPM according to their degree of development. The lower level combines diverse strategies against one pest on one crop. The highest level covers all pests and crops within an overall system that implicates all stakeholders (e.g., consumers, authorities, regulatory bodies, and industry), taking into account of the social, cultural, and ecological context. The IPM promoted by the European Union through the Thematic Strategy (Commission of the European Communities, 2006b,c) and the Directive 2009/128/EC (European Commission, 2009a) aspires to reach the requirements established to be classified in the fourth level. To achieve it, their IPM approach highlights between its principles the necessity of prevent and/or suppress harmful organisms together with their motorization, the responsibility of the professional user to apply measures based on scientific data, at the necessary levels and to check the success of the measures adopted, the preference for nonchemical methods, the requirement of specific pesticides for the target with the least side effects and the implementation of antiresistance strategies (Annex III of Directive 2009/128/EC).

In order to achieve a full development of the IPM practices in Europe, it would be suitable to encourage nanopesticides and other friendly environmental technologies in agriculture. Recent published works focused on the IPM programs show how correcting pest management practices can reduce the pesticide use without negative consequences (Hassanali et al., 2008; Pretty, 2008; Resosudarmo, 2012; Sharma et al., 2015). Pretty (2008) analyzed the impact of an important number of IPM initiatives through their classification in four groups according to the effects observed in pesticide use and yield increase, namely, A (pesticide use and yields increase), B (pesticide use increases, but yields decline), C (both pesticide use and yields fall), and D (pesticide use declines, but yields increase). Over 60% of the projects fall into the category D. The European Union shows curiously several cases, mainly cereal-framing systems, where the IPM projects are in category C. However, in these cases, the yields fall slightly while pesticide use falls dramatically (Pretty, 2008). Therefore, it should be bet for the development of new technologies, such as the nanopesticides, and its suitable use within IPM programs. They could help to correct this little diversion regarding the best class D, with the ambitious objective to place all European IPM programs within this category. Furthermore, to achieve it, the Thematic Strategy on the sustainable use of pesticides (Commission of the European Communities, 2006b,c) and the Directive 2009/128/EC (European Commission, 2009a) also include between their aims the training and awareness of end users, the inspection of application equipments, the prohibition of aerial spraying, the application of specific actions to protect aquatic environments, the solicitation of specific measures to appropriate handling of pesticides, the measuring of the progress of risk reduction by appropriate indicators, and the exchange of information and best practice.

There is no doubt that nanopesticides represent an attractive technology from the standpoint of improving the European IPM programs. The success of nanopesticides will lie in the integration of their usage with traditional plant protection products due to their major advantages such as high efficacy at lower doses, easier pest control, fewer volatilization, and higher bioavailability. However, their way will not be easy. The environmental fate and behavior of nanopesticides may differ from traditional formulations. Therefore, new or refined risk assessment approaches maybe needed for implementation of these new nanoformulations within IPM programs. Furthermore, with everything said so far, the use of nanopesticides still requires considerable knowledge by all stakeholders, especially the farmers who use them, in order to avoid risks on human and animal health and on the environment. It seems that compliance with the aforementioned objectives is essential to the establishment of this new technology. Additionally, new legislative requirements for nanomaterials/nanopesticides, still in elaboration, may cause problems for some of them.

7 Conclusions

The Regulation (EC) No. 1107/2009 constitutes the basis of the European pesticide legislative framework. This Regulation is showing a great capacity to maintain a sustainable, viable, and safe agriculture. This capacity safeguards the competitiveness of the European agriculture, regarding those developed in other countries with less stringent legislations, ensuring agricultural products with own characteristics. Therefore, the European agricultural products show a strategic advantage towards consumers each day more concerned about their diet.

An official definition of nanomaterial is being discussed. In this context, there is an unquestionable and clear willingness by the EC and all stakeholders to achieve an effective system to approve active substances and register nanoformulations. The current European legislation covers the potential health, safety, and environmental risk in relation to nanomaterials. Recent studies and communications seem to indicate future troubles to regularize the marketing of nanopesticides. However, the actual Regulation is versatile enough to provide response to the new challenges.

Most health, safety, and environmental concerns about nanopesticides are related with their mobility, novel toxicological effects, and potential of nanoparticles to cross biological barriers. Therefore, reliable methods for characterizing nanopesticides, as well as methods for detection and quantification of nanoparticles in plants, plant products, foodstuff (of plant and animal origin), and feeding stuff (of plant origin) are required. Validation of methods for nanoparticles shall mainly cover morphology, chemical composition, and mass or number fraction, as a consequence of the nanoparticle concept. Nowadays, the adequacy of current validation requirements to the specificities of each analytical technique for nanoparticles is the best approach.

It would be suitable to encourage the use of nanopesticides, in order to achieve a full development of the European IPM practices. Nanoformulations could represent a good technology to reduce the risk for humans, animals, and environments, maintaining or increasing the effectiveness against the harmful organism. However, it is necessary to check that current data requirements are sufficient to characterize the risk and the exposure produced during the application of a nanopesticide.

References

Antunović, B., Barlow, S., Chesson, A., Flynn, A., Hardy, A., Jany, K.-D., Jeger, M.-J., Knaap, A., Kuiper, H., Larsen, J.-C., Lovell, D., Noerrung, B., Schlatter, J., Silano, V., Smulders, F.P.V., 2011. Scientific opinion. Guidance on the risk assessment of the application of nanoscience and nanotechnologies in the food and feed chain. EFSA J. 9, 1–36.

Ao, M., Zhu, Y., He, S., Li, D., Li, P., Li, J., Cao, Y., 2013. Preparation and characterization of 1-naphthylacetic acid-silica conjugated nanospheres for enhancement of controlled-release performance. Nanotechnology 24, 24.

Aslani, F., Bagheri, S., Muhd Julkapli, N., Juraimi, A.S., Hashemi, F.S.G., Baghdadi, A., 2014. Effects of engineered nanomaterials on plants growth: an overview. Sci. World J. 2014, 1–28.

Bajwa, W.I., Kogan, M., 2002. Compendium of IPM definitions (CID)—what is IPM and how is it defined in the worldwide literature? IPPC Publication 998, 1–19.

Barlow, S., Chesson, A., Collins, J.D., Flynn, A., Hardy, A., Jany, K.-D., Knaap, A., Kuiper, H., Larsen, J.C., Le Neindre, P., Schans, J., Schlatter, J., Silano, V., Skerfving, S., Vannier, P., 2009. The potential risks arising from nanoscience and nanotechnologies on food and feed safety. EFSA J. 958, 1–39.

Bhagat, D., Samanta, S.K., Bhattacharya, S., 2013. Efficient management of fruit pests by pheromone nanogels. Sci. Rep. 3, 1–8.

Bhargava, K., Conti, D.S., da Rocha, S.R.P., Zhang, Y., 2015. Application of an oregano oil nanoemulsion to the control of foodborne bacteria on fresh lettuce. Food Microbiol. 47, 69–73.

Blanchard, 2015. Researchers look to nanoparticles to reduce pesticide use in agriculture. LSU AgCenter Communications. Available from: www.lsuagcenter.com/news_archive/2015/July/headline_news/Researchers-look-to-nanoparticles-to-reduce-pesticide-use-in-agriculture.htm

Blasco, C., Picó, Y., 2011. Determining nanomaterials in food. Trends Anal. Chem. 30, 84–99.

Bleeker, E.A.J., de Jong, W.H., Geertsma, R.E., Groenewold, M., Heugens, E.H.W., Koers-Jacquemijns, M., van de Meent, D., Popma, J.R., Rietveld, A.G., Wijnhoven, S.W.P., Cassee, F.R., Oomen, A.G., 2013. Considerations on the EU definition of a nanomaterial: science to support policy making. Regul. Toxicol. Pharmacol. 65, 119–125.

Boehm, A.L.L.R., Martinon, I., Zerrouk, R., Rump, E., Fessi, H., 2003. Nanoprecipitation technique for the encapsulation of agrochemical active ingredients. J. Microencapsul. 20, 433–441.

Boehm, A.L.L.R., Zerrouk, R., Fessi, H., 2000. Poly epsilon-caprolactone nanoparticles containing a poorly soluble pesticide: formulation and stability study. J. Microencapsul. 17, 195–205.

Bootz, A., Vogel, V., Schubert, D., Kreuter, J., 2004. Comparison of scanning electron microscopy, dynamic light scattering and analytical ultracentrifugation for the sizing of poly(butyl cyanoacrylate) nanoparticles. Eur. J. Pharm. Biopharm. 57, 369–375.

Bowen, P., 2002. Particle size distribution measurement from millimeters to nanometers, and from rods to platelets. J. Dispersion Sci. Technol. 23, 631–662.

Buteler, M., Sofie, S.W., Weaver, D.K., Driscoll, D., Muretta, J., Stadler, T., 2015. Development of nanoalumina dust as insecticide against *Sitophilus oryzae* and *Rhyzopertha dominica*. Int. J. Pest Manag. 61, 80–89.

Cao, J., Guenther, R.H., Sit, T.L., Lommel, S.A., Opperman, C.H., Willoughby, J.A., 2015. Development of abamectin loaded plant virus nanoparticles for efficacious plant parasitic nematode control. ACS Appl. Mater. Interfaces. 7, 9546–9553.

Cecere, D., Bruno, A., Minutolo, P., D'Alessio, A., 2003. DLS measurements on nanoparticles produced in laminar premixed flames. Synth. Met. 139, 653–656.

Cespedes, C.L., Salazar, J.R., Ariza-Castolo, A., Yamaguchi, L., Avila, J.G., Aqueveque, P., Kubo, I., Alarcon, J., 2014. Biopesticides from plants: *Calceolaria integrifolia* s.l. Environ. Res. 132, 391–406.

Chang, J.H., Choi, J.Y., Jin, B.R., Roh, J.Y., Olszewski, J.A., Seo, S.J., O'Reilly, D.R., Je, Y.H., 2003. An improved baculovirus insecticide producing occlusion bodies that contain Bacillus thuringiensis insect toxin. J. Invertebr. Pathol. 84, 30–37.

Choi, A.-J., Kim, C.-J., Cho, Y.-J., Hwang, J.-K., Kim, C.-T., 2011. Characterization of capsaicin-loaded nanoemulsions stabilized with alginate and chitosan by self-assembly. Food Bioprocess. Technol. 4, 1119–1126.

Colfen, H., Pauck, T., 1997. Determination of particle size distributions with angstrom resolution. Colloid Polym. Sci. 275, 175–180.

Commission of the European Communities, 2000. Communication from the Commission of the precautionary principle. COM(2000) 1, pp. 1–29.

Commission of the European Communities, 2006a. Proposal for a regulation of the European Parliament and of the Council concerning the placing of plant protection products on the market. COM(2006) 388 final. pp. 1–91.

Commission of the European Communities, 2006b. A thematic strategy on the sustainable use of pesticides. pp. 1–13.

Commission of the European Communities, 2006c. A thematic strategy on the sustainable use of pesticides—Technical annex. pp. 1–22.

Commission of the European Communities, 2008. Communication from the Commission to the European Parliament, the Council and the European Economic and Social Committee. Regulatory aspects of nanomaterials. SEC(2008) 2036. pp. 1–11.

Coulibaly, F., Chiu, E., Ikeda, K., Gutmann, S., Haebel, P.W., Schulze-Briese, C., Mori, H., Metcalf, P., 2007. The molecular organization of cypovirus polyhedra. Nature 446, 97–101.

Cumberland, S.A., Lead, J.R., 2009. Particle size distributions of silver nanoparticles at environmentally relevant conditions. J. Chromatogr. A 1216, 9099–9105.

Daniel, M.C., Astruc, D., 2004. Gold nanoparticles: assembly, supramolecular chemistry, quantum-size-related properties, and applications toward biology, catalysis, and nanotechnology. Chem. Rev. 104, 293–346.

De, A., Bose, R., Kumar, A., Mozumdar, S., 2014. Targeted Delivery of Pesticides Using Biodegradable Polymeric Nanoparticles. Springer, New Delhi.

Debnath, N., Das, S., Seth, D., Chandra, R., Bhattacharya, S.C., Goswami, A., 2011. Entomotoxic effect of silica nanoparticles against *Sitophilus oryzae* (L.). J. Pest. Sci. 84, 99–105.

Dieckmann, Y., Colfen, H., Hofmann, H., Petri-Fink, A., 2009. Particle size distribution measurements of manganese-doped ZnS nanoparticles. Anal. Chem. 81, 3889–3895.

Domingos, R.F., Baalousha, M.A., Ju-Nam, Y., Reid, M.M., Tufenkji, N., Lead, J.R., Leppard, G.G., Wilkinson, K.J., 2009. Characterizing manufactured nanoparticles in the environment: multimethod determination of particle sizes. Environ. Sci. Technol. 43, 7277–7284.

Domingues, R.M.A., Patinha, D.J.S., Sousa, G.D.A., Villaverde, J.J., Silva, C.M., Freire, C.S.R., Silvestre, A.J.D., Pascoal Neto, C., 2011. Eucalyptus biomass residues from agro-forest and pulping industries as sources of high-value triterpenic compounds. Cellulose Chem. Technol. 45, 475–481.

Drexler, K.E., 1986. Engines of Creation: The Coming Era of Nanotechnology. Anchor Press/Doubleday, New York.

Drexler, K.E., 1992. Nanosystems: Molecular Machinery, Manufacturing and Computation. Wiley-Interscience, New York.

ECHA, 2015. Endpoint specific guidance. In: Guidance on information requirements and chemical safety assessment. ECHA, pp. 1–494 (Chapter R.7a).

ECPA, 2006. ECPA evaluation. Proposal for a regulation concerning the placing on the market of plant protection products—Impact of the criteria for "non-approval" and "candidates for substitution". PP/06/EJ/15809, pp. 1–6.

ElShafei, G.M.S., El-Said, M.M., Attia, H.A.E., Mohammed, T.G.M., 2010. Environmentally friendly pesticides: essential oil-based w/o/w multiple emulsions for anti-fungal formulations. Ind. Crops. Prod. 31, 99–106.

European Commission, 1991. Directive 91/414/EEC. L 230, pp. 1–290.

European Commission, 1992a. Regulation (EEC) No. 3600/92. L 366, pp. 1–14.

European Commission, 1992b. Treaty on European Union 92/C 191/01. C 191, pp. 1–112.

European Commission, 2000a. Directive 2000/60/EC. L 327, pp. 1–72.

European Commission, 2000b. Regulation (EC) No. 451/2000. L 55, pp. 25–52.

European Commission, 2002. Regulation (EC) No. 1112/2002. L 168, pp. 14–30.

European Commission, 2005. Regulation (EC) No 396/2005. L 70, pp.1–16.

European Commission, 2006. Regulation (EC) No 1907/2006 of the European Parliament and of the Council. L 396,pp. 1–101.

European Commission, 2008. CA/59/2008 rev. 1. Follow-up to the 6th meeting of the REACH competent authorities for the implementation of Regulation (EC) 1907/2006 (REACH). pp. 1–21.

European Commission, 2009a. Directive 2009/128/EC. L 309, pp. 71–86.

European Commission, 2009b. Regulation (EC) No 1107/2009. L 309, pp. 1–50.

European Commission, 2010. EU NanoLyse Project. Available from: www.nanolyse.eu

European Commission, 2011a. Commission recommendation on the definition of nanomaterial. L 275, pp. 38–40.

European Commission, 2011b. Regulation (EU) No 546/2011. L 155, pp. 127–175.

European Commission, 2011c. Regulation (EU) No 1169/2011 of the European Parliament and of the Council. L 304, pp. 18–63.

European Commission, 2011d. Guidance document SANCO/10796/2003 rev. 12.2, 1–15.
European Commission, 2012a. Regulation (EU) No 369/2012. L 116, pp. 19–24.
European Commission, 2012b. Thematic strategy on sustainable use of plant protection products - Prospects and requirements for transferring proposals for plant protection products to biocides. pp. 1–304.
European Commission, 2013a. Commission Regulation (EU) No 283/2013. L 93, pp. 1–84.
European Commission, 2013b. Commission Regulation (EU) No 284/2013. L 93, pp. 85–152.
European Commission, 2013c. Regulation (EU) No 293/2013. L 293, pp. 31–33.
European Commission, 2014a. The EU Water Framework Directive. Available from: http://bookshop.europa.eu/en/the-eu-water-framework-directive-pbKH0414216/
European Commission, 2014b. Opinion on Nanosilver: safety, health and environmental effects and role in antimicrobial resistance. 1–103.
European Commission, 2015. Pesticides. Available from: http://ec.europa.eu/food/plant/pesticides/index_en.htm
FAOSTAT, 2012. Food and Agriculture Organization of the United Nations. Statistics Division. Available from: http://faostat3.fao.org/
Feng, B.H., Peng, L.F., 2012. Synthesis and characterization of carboxymethyl chitosan carrying ricinoleic functions as an emulsifier for azadirachtin. Carbohydr. Polym. 88, 576–582.
Feynman, R.P., 1960. There's plenty of room at the bottom. Eng. Sci. 23, 22–36.
Fissan, H., Ristig, S., Kaminski, H., Asbach, C., Epple, M., 2014. Comparison of different characterization methods for nanoparticle dispersions before and after aerosolization. Anal. Methods 6, 7324–7334.
Forgiarini, A., Esquena, J., González, C., Solans, C., 2001. Formation of nano-emulsions by low-energy emulsification methods at constant temperature. Langmuir 17, 2076–2083.
Gámiz, B., Hermosín, M.C., Cornejo, J., Celis, R., 2015. Hexadimethrine-montmorillonite nanocomposite: characterization and application as a pesticide adsorbent. Appl. Surf. Sci. 332, 606–613.
Ghormade, V., Dugam, S., Oke, A., Sable, A., Shahapurkar, G., Deshpande, M.V., Paknikar, K.M., 2011. Development of environmentally benign nanomaterial-based enzyme formulations for biocontrol of plant pathogens and pests. ISCB International Symposium, March, 10–11, 2011 New Delhi. pp. 29–30.
Göller, R., Vors, J.-P., Caminade, A.-M., Majoral, J.-P., 2001. Phosphorus dendrimers as new tools to deliver active substances. Tetrahedron Lett. 42, 3587–3590.
Gonzalez, J.O.W., Stefanazzi, N., Murray, A.P., Ferrero, A.A., Band, B.F., 2014. Novel nanoinsecticides based on essential oils to control the German cockroach. J. Pest Sci. 88, 393–404.
Goswami, A., Roy, I., Sengupta, S., Debnath, N., 2010. Novel applications of solid and liquid formulations of nanoparticles against insect pests and pathogens. Thin Solid Films 519, 1252–1257.
Gutiérrez, J.M., González, C., Maestro, A., Solè, I., Pey, C.M., Nolla, J., 2008. Nano-emulsions: new applications and optimization of their preparation. Curr. Opin. Colloid Interface Sci. 13, 245–251.
Hassanali, A., Herren, H., Khan, Z.R., Pickett, J.A., Woodcock, C.M., 2008. Integrated pest management: the push–pull approach for controlling insect pests and weeds of cereals, and its potential for other agricultural systems including animal husbandry. Philos. Trans. R. Soc. B 363, 611–621.
Hellmann, C., Greiner, A., Wendorff, J.H., 2011. Design of pheromone releasing nanofibers for plant protection. Polym. Adv. Technol. 22, 407–413.

Hernández, F., Portolés, T., López, M.C.B., Díaz, R., Botero-Coy, A.M., Fuentes, C.L., Peñuela, G., 2012. Use of time-of-flight mass spectrometry for large screening of organic pollutants in surface waters and solid from a rice production area in Colombia. Sci Total Environ. 439, 249–259.

Hildebrandt, A., Guillamon, M., Lacorte, S., Tauler, R., Barceló, D., 2008. Impact of pesticides used in agriculture and vineyards to surface and groundwater quality (North Spain). Water Res. 42, 3315–3326.

Hole, P., Sillence, K., Hannell, C., Maguire, C.M., Roesslein, M., Suarez, G., Capracotta, S., Magdolenova, Z., Horev-Azaria, L., Dybowska, A., Cooke, L., Haase, A., Contal, S., Mano, S., Vennemann, A., Sauvain, J.J., Staunton, K.C., Anguissola, S., Luch, A., Dusinska, M., Korenstein, R., Gutleb, A.C., Wiemann, M., Prina-Mello, A., Riediker, M., Wick, P., 2013. Interlaboratory comparison of size measurements on nanoparticles using nanoparticle tracking analysis (NTA). J. Nanopart. Res. 15, 12.

House of Lords, 2010. First Report of session 2009–2010: nanotechnologies and food. House of Lords, vol. 1, pp. 1–112.

Hussain, S.M., Braydich-Stolle, L.K., Schrand, A.M., Murdock, R.C., Yu, K.O., Mattie, D.M., Schlager, J.J., Terrones, M., 2009. Toxicity evaluation for safe use of nanomaterials: recent achievements and technical challenges. Adv. Mater. 21, 1549–1559.

Hussein, M.Z., Jaafar, A., Yahaya, A., Zainal, Z., 2009. The effect of single, binary and ternary anions of chloride, carbonate and phosphate on the release of 2,4-dichlorophenoxyacetate intercalated into the Zn–Al-layered double hydroxide nanohybrid. Nanoscale Res. Lett. 4, 1351–1357.

Jalali, H.T., Petronilho, S., Villaverde, J.J., Coimbra, M.A., Domingues, M.R.M., Ebrahimian, Z.J., Silvestre, A.J.D., Rocha, S.M., 2012. Deeper insight into the monoterpenic composition of *Ferula gummosa* oleo-gum-resin from Iran. Ind. Crops Prod. 36, 500–507.

Jalali, H.T., Petronilho, S., Villaverde, J.J., Coimbra, M.A., Domingues, M.R.M., Ebrahimian, Z.J., Silvestre, A.J.D., Rocha, S.M., 2013. Assessment of the sesquiterpenic profile of *Ferula gummosa* oleo-gum-resin (galbanum) from Iran. Contributes to its valuation as a potential source of sesquiterpenic compounds. Ind. Crops Prod. 44, 185–191.

Jiang, L.C., Basri, M., Omar, D., Rahman, M.B.A., Salleh, A.B., Rahman, R.N.Z.R.A., Selamat, A., 2012. Green nano-emulsion intervention for water-soluble glyphosate isopropylamine (IPA) formulations in controlling *Eleusine indica* (*E-indica*). Pest. Biochem. Physiol. 102, 19–29.

Jo, Y.-K., Kim, B.H., Jung, G., 2009. Antifungal activity of silver ions and nanoparticles on phytopathogenic fungi. Plant Dis. 93, 1037–1043.

Kah, M., Beulke, S., Tiede, K., Hofmann, T., 2013. Nanopesticides: state of knowledge, environmental fate, and exposure modeling. Crit. Rev. Environ. Sci. Technol. 43, 1823–1867.

Kah, M., Hofmann, T., 2014. Nanopesticide research: current trends and future priorities. Environ. Int. 63, 224–235.

Kaushik, P., Shakil, N.A., Kumar, J., Singh, M.K., Singh, M.K., Yadav, S.K., 2013. Development of controlled release formulations of thiram employing amphiphilic polymers and their bioefficacy evaluation in seed quality enhancement studies. J. Environ. Sci. Health B 48, 677–685.

KEMI, 2008. Interpretation in Sweden of the impact of the "cut-off" criteria adopted in the common position of the Council concerning the Regulation of placing plant protection products on the market (document 11119/08). 1–14.

Kim, I.-H., Oh, Y.A., Lee, H., Song, K.B., Min, S.C., 2014. Grape berry coatings of lemongrass oil-incorporating nanoemulsion. LWT Food Sci. Technol. 58, 1–10.

Koeber, R., Linsinger, T.P.J., Emons, H., 2010. An approach for more precise statements of metrological traceability on reference material certificates. Accred. Qual. Assur. 15, 255–262.

Krishnaraj, C., Ramachandran, R., Mohan, K., Kalaichelvan, P.T., 2012. Optimization for rapid synthesis of silver nanoparticles and its effect on phytopathogenic fungi. Spectrochim. Acta A 93, 95–99.

Kruawala, K., Sacherb, F., Wernerc, A., Muller, J., Knepperc, T.P., 2005. Chemical water quality in Thailand and its impacts on the drinking water production in Thailand. Sci. Total Environ. 340, 57–70.

Kumar, J., Shakil, N.A., Singh, M.K., Pankaj, Singh, M.K., Pandey, A., Pandey, R.P., 2010. Development of controlled release formulations of azadirachtin-A employing poly(ethylene glycol) based amphiphilic copolymers. J. Environ. Sci. Health B 45, 310–314.

Kumari, A., Kumar, J., Shakil, N.A., Kamil, D., 2015. Bio-efficacy evaluation of CR formulations of azoxystrobin against *Rhizoctonia solani*. Ann. Pl. Protec. Sci. 23, 124–126.

Landfester, K., Willert, M., Antonietti, M., 2000. Preparation of polymer particles in nonaqueous direct and inverse miniemulsions. Macromolecules 33, 2370–2376.

Landsiedel, R., Ma-Hock, L., Kroll, A., Hahn, D., Schnekenburger, J., Wiench, K., Wohlleben, W., 2010. Testing metal-oxide nanomaterials for human safety. Adv. Mater. 22, 2601–2627.

Lange, H., 1995. Comparative test of methods to determine particle size and particle size distribution in the submicron range. Part. Syst. Char. 12, 148–157.

Lao, S.B., Zhang, Z.X., Xu, H.H., Jiang, G.B., 2010. Novel amphiphilic chitosan derivatives: Synthesis, characterization and micellar solubilization of rotenone. Carbohydr. Polym. 82, 1136–1142.

Li, S., Shen, Y., Xiao, M., Liu, D., Fan, L., 2015. Synthesis and controlled release properties of β-naphthoxyacetic acid intercalated Mg–Al layered double hydroxides nanohybrids. Arabian J. Chem.

Li, Z.-Z., Chen, J.-F., Liu, F., Liu, A.-Q., Wang, Q., Sun, H.-Y., Wen, L.-X., 2007. Study of UV-shielding properties of novel porous hollow silica nanoparticle carriers for avermectin. Pest Manag. Sci. 63, 241–246.

Linsinger, T.P.J., Chaudhry, Q., Dehalu, V., Delahaut, P., Dudkiewicz, A., Grombe, R., von der Kammer, F., Larsen, E.H., Legros, S., Loeschner, K., Peters, R., Ramsch, R., Roebben, G., Tiede, K., Weigel, S., 2013. Validation of methods for the detection and quantification of engineered nanoparticles in food. Food Chem. 138, 1959–1966.

Liu, J., Jiang, G., 2015. Silver Nanoparticles in the Environment. Springer, Heidelberg.

Liu, X., He, B., Xu, Z., Yin, M., Yang, W., Zhang, H., Cao, J., Shen, J., 2015. A functionalized fluorescent dendrimer as a pesticide nanocarrier: application in pest control. Nanoscale 7, 445–449.

Loha, K.M., Shakil, N.A., Kumar, J., Singh, M.K., Adak, T., Jain, S., 2011. Release kinetics of β-cyfluthrin from its encapsulated formulations in water. J. Environ. Sci. Health B 46, 201–206.

Lövestam, G., Rauscher, H., Roebben, G., Sokull Klüttgen, B., Gibson, N., Putaud, J.-P., Stamm, H., 2010. Considerations on a definition of nanomaterial for regulatory purposes. JRC-Reference Reports, Luxembourg.

Ma, Z.Q., Li, Y.J., Wu, L.P., Zhang, X., 2014. Isolation and insecticidal activity of sesquiterpenes alkaloids from *Tripterygium wilfordii* Hook f. Ind. Crop. Prod. 52, 642–648.

Mahl, D., Diendorf, J., Meyer-Zaika, W., Epple, M., 2011. Possibilities and limitations of different analytical methods for the size determination of a bimodal dispersion of metallic nanoparticles. Colloid Surf. A 377, 386–392.

Manchester, M., Steinmetz, N.F., 2009. Viruses and Nanotechnology. Springer-Verlag, Berlin.

Marín, J.M., Sancho, J.V., Pozo, O.J., López, F.J., Hernández, F., 2006. Quantification and confirmation of anionic, cationic and neutral pesticides and transformation products in water by on-line solid phase extraction–liquid chromatography–tandem mass spectrometry. J. Chromatogr. A 1133, 204–214.

Masuda, M., 2011. Microencapsulation of Pesticides for Controlling Release from Coatings. Department of Chemical and Biological Engineering, Chalmers University of Technology, Göteborg.

McClements, D.J., 2010. Emulsion design to improve the delivery of functional lipophilic components. Annu. Rev. Food Sci. Technol. 1, 241–269.

McClements, D.J., 2011. Edible nanoemulsions: fabrication, properties, and functional performance. Soft Matter 7, 2297–2316.

McClements, D.J., 2012. Nanoemulsions versus microemulsions: terminology, differences, and similarities. Soft Matter 8, 1719–1729.

Milne, C.G., Shelby, P.P., 1999. United States Patent: US 5,958,463 A. Agricultural pesticide formulations.

Montaño, M.D., Lowry, G.V., von der Kammer, F., Blue, J., Ranville, J.F., 2014. Current status and future direction for examining engineered nanoparticles in natural systems. Environ. Chem. 11, 351–366.

Morrill, K., May, K., Leek, D., Langland, N., Jeane, L.D., Ventura, J., Skubisz, C., Scherer, S., Lopez, E., Crocker, E., Peters, R., Oertle, J., Nguyen, K., Just, S., Orian, M., Humphrey, M., Payne, D., Jacobs, B., Waters, R., Langland, J., 2013. Spectrum of antimicrobial activity associated with ionic colloidal silver. J. Altern. Complement. Med. 19, 224–231.

Nair, R., Varghese, S.H., Nair, B.G., Maekawa, T., Yoshida, Y., Kumar, D.S., 2010. Nanoparticulate material delivery to plants. Plant Sci. 179, 154–163.

Norman, D.J., Chen, J., 2011. Effect of foliar application of titanium dioxide on bacterial blight of geranium and xanthomonas leaf spot of poinsettia. HortScience. 46, 426–428.

Nowack, B., Krug, H.F., Height, M., 2011. 120 Years of nanosilver history: implications for policy makers. Environ. Sci. Technol. 45, 1177–1183.

OCDE, 2010. Preliminary guidance notes on sample preparation and dosimetry for the safety testing of manufactured nanomaterials. ENV/JM/MONO(2010)25, pp. 1–58.

Oh, S.-D., Lee, S., Choi, S.-H., Lee, I.-S., Lee, Y.-M., Chun, J.-H., Park, H.-J., 2006. Synthesis of Ag and Ag-SiO_2 nanoparticles by γ-irradiation and their antibacterial and antifungal efficiency against *Salmonella enterica* serovar *Typhimurium* and *Botrytis cinerea*. Colloids Surf. A 275, 228–233.

Oliveira, H.C., Stolf-Moreira, R., Bueno Reis Martinez, C., Grillo, R., Bispo de Jesus, M., Fernandes Fraceto, L., 2015. Nanoencapsulation enhances the post-emergence herbicidal activity of atrazine against mustard plants. PLoS One 10, 1–12.

Parham, H., Rahbar, N., 2010. Square wave voltammetric determination of methyl parathion using ZrO_2-nanoparticles modified carbon paste electrode. J. Hazard. Mater. 177, 1077–1084.

Pecora, R., 2000. Dynamic light scattering measurement of nanometer particles in liquids. J. Nanopart. Res. 2, 123–131.

Peixoto, M.G., Bacci, L., Blank, A.F., Araujo, A.P.A., Alves, P.B., Silva, J.H.S., Santos, A.A., Oliveira, A.P., da Costa, A.S., Arrigoni-Blank, M.D., 2015. Toxicity and

repellency of essential oils of *Lippia alba* chemotypes and their major monoterpenes against stored grain insects. Ind. Crop. Prod. 71, 31–36.
Pérez-de-Luque, A., Rubiales, D., 2009. Nanotechnology for parasitic plant control. Pest Manag. Sci. 65, 540–545.
Perlatti, B., de Souza Bergo, P.L., Fernandes da Silva, M.F.D.G., Batista Fernandes, J., Rossi Forim, M., 2013. Polymeric nanoparticle-based insecticides: A controlled release purpose for agrochemicals. In: Trdan, S. (Ed.), Insecticides—Development of Safer and More Effective Technologies. Intech, Rijeka, pp. 523–550.
Peters, R., Brandhoff, P., Weigel, S., Marvin, H., Bouwmeester, H., Aschberger, K., Rauscher, H., Amenda, V., Arena, M., Moniz, F.B., Gottardo, S., Mech, A., 2014. External scientific report. Inventory of nanotechnology applications in the agricultural, feed and food sector. EFSA supporting publications. EN-621, 1–125.
Planken, K.L., Kuipers, B.W.M., Philipse, A.P., 2008. Model independent determination of colloidal silica size distributions via analytical ultracentrifugation. Anal. Chem. 80, 8871–8879.
Porras, M., Solans, C., González, C., Gutiérrez, J.M., 2008. Properties of water-in-oil (W/O) nano-emulsions prepared by a low-energy emulsification method. Colloids Surf. A 324, 181–188.
Pretty, J., 2008. Agricultural sustainability: concepts, principles and evidence. Philos. Trans. R. Soc. B 363, 447–465.
Prokopy, R.J., 1993. Stepwise progress toward IPM and sustainable agriculture. IPM Practitioner 15, 1–4.
PSD, 2008. Assessment of the impact on crop protection in the UK of the 'cut-off criteria' and substitution provisions in the proposed Regulation of the European Parliament and of the Council concerning the placing of plant protection products in the market, 1–37.
Quinn, P.J., Perrett, S.F., 1996. Liposomal formulations of agrichemical pesticides. In: Lasic, D.D., Barenholz, Y. (Eds.), Handbook of Nonmedical Applications of Liposomes, Vol IV From Gene Delivery and Diagnosis to Ecology. CRC Press, Boca Raton, pp. 127–152.
Ragaei, M., Sabry, A.-K.H., 2014. Nanotechnology for insect pest control. Int. J. Sci. Environ. Technol. 3, 528–545.
Rai, M., Ingle, A., 2012. Role of nanotechnology in agriculture with special reference to management of insect pests. Appl. Microbiol. Biotechnol. 94, 287–293.
Ramos Campos, E.V., de Oliveira, J.L., Fraceto, L.F., Singh, B., 2015. Polysaccharides as safer release systems for agrochemicals. Agron. Sustain. Dev. 35, 47–66.
Rashidzadeh, A., Olad, A., Salari, D., Jalil Hejazi, M., 2014. On the encapsulation of natural pesticide using polyvinyl alcohol/alginate–montmorillonite nanocomposite for controlled release application. Polym. Eng. Sci. 54, 2707–2714.
Reemtsma, T., Alder, L., Banasiak, U., 2013. Emerging pesticide metabolites in groundwater and surface water as determined by the application of a multimethod for 150 pesticide metabolites. Water Res. 47, 5535–5545.
Resosudarmo, B.P., 2012. Implementing a national environmental policy: understanding the 'success' of the 1989–1999 integrated pest management programme in Indonesia. Singap. J. Trop. Geogr. 33, 365–380.
Rosenbom, A.E., Kjaer, J., Olsen, P., 2010. Long-term leaching of rimsulfuron degradation products through sandy agricultural soils. Chemosphere 79, 830–838.
Sánchez-Ávila, J., Fernández-Sanjuan, M., Vicente, J., Lacorte, S., 2011. Development of a multi-residue method for the determination of organic

micropollutants in water, sediment and mussels using gas chromatography-tandem mass spectrometry. J. Chromatogr. A 1218, 6799–6811.

Sandín-España, P., Sevilla-Morán, B., Villarroya-Ferruz, M., Alonso-Prados, J.L., Santín-Montanyá, M.I., 2015. Comparative phytotoxicity assays of the herbicide alloxydim and its main identified photoproduct in cereal and broadleaves crops. Weed Sci. (In press), doi: 10.1614/WS-D-14-00122.1.

Santos, S.A.O., Villaverde, J.J., Freire, C.S.R., Domingues, M.R.M., Neto, C.P., Silvestre, A.J.D., 2012. Phenolic composition and antioxidant activity of *Eucalyptus grandis, E. urograndis* (*E. grandis* × *E. urophylla*) and *E. maidenii* bark extracts. Ind. Crops Prod. 39, 120–127.

Santos, S.A.O., Villaverde, J.J., Sousa, A.F., Coelho, J.F.J., Neto, C.P., Silvestre, A.J.D., 2013. Phenolic composition and antioxidant activity of industrial cork by-products. Ind. Crops Prod. 47, 262–269.

Sevilla-Morán, B., López-Goti, C., Alonso-Prados, J.L., Sandín-España, P., 2014. Aqueous photodegradation of sethoxydim herbicide: Qtof elucidation of its by-products, mechanism and degradation pathway. Sci. Tot. Environ. 472, 842–850.

Sevilla-Morán, B., Sandín-España, P., 2012. Pesticide degradation in water. In: Rathore, H.S., Nollet, L.M.L. (Eds.), Pesticides. Evaluation of Environmental Pollution. CRC Press Taylor & Francis, Boca Raton, pp. 79–130.

Sevilla-Morán, B., Sandín-España, P., Vicente-Arana, M.J., Alonso-Prados, J.L., García-Baudín, J.M., 2008. Study of alloxydim photodegradation in the presence of natural substances: elucidation of transformation products. J. Photochem. Photobiol. A 198, 162–168.

Sevilla-Morán, B., Villaverde, J.J., Mateo-Miranda, M.M., Alonso-Prados, J.L., Sandín-España, P., 2016. Pesticide transformation products as contaminants of water compartments. In: Chandra, R., Gurjar, B.R., Govil, J.N. (Eds.), Environmental Science & Engineering. Estudium Press LLC, USA.

Shakil, N.A., Singh, M.K., Pandey, A., Kumar, J., Pankaj, Parmar, V.S., Singh, M.K., Pandey, R.P., Watterson, A.C., 2010. Development of poly(ethylene glycol) based amphiphilic copolymers for controlled release delivery of carbofuran. J. Macromol. Sci. A 47, 241–247.

Sharma, R., Peshin, R., Shankar, U., Kaul, V., Sharma, S., 2015. Impact evaluation indicators of an Integrated Pest Management program in vegetable crops in the subtropical region of Jammu and Kashmir. India. Crop Prot. 67, 191–199.

Singla, P., Mehta, R., Upadhyay, S., 2012. Clay modification by the use of organic cations. Green Sust. Chem. 2, 21–25.

Solans, S., Esquena, J., Forigianini, A., Uson, N., Morales, D., Izquierds, P., Azemar, N., Garcla-Celma, M.J., 2003. Nano-emulsion: formation properties and applications. In: Mittal, K.L., Dinesh, O.S. (Eds.), Absorption and Aggregation of Surfactants in Solution. Marcel Dekker Inc., New York (USA), pp. 525–554.

Sopeña, F., Maqueda, C., Morillo, E., 2009. Controlled release formulations of herbicides based on micro-encapsulation. Cien. Inv. Agr. 35, 27–42.

Stadler, T., Buteler, M., Weaver, D.K., 2010. Novel use of nanostructured alumina as an insecticide. Pest Manag. Sci. 66, 577–579.

Tan, W.-M., Hou, N., Pang, S., Zhu, X.-F., Li, Z.-H., Wen, L.-X., Duan, L.-S., 2012. Improved biological effects of uniconazole using porous hollow silica nanoparticles as carriers. Pest Manag. Sci. 68, 437–443.

Taylor, T.M., Weiss, J., Davidson, P.M., Bruce, B.D., 2005. Liposomal nanocapsules in food science and agriculture. Crit. Rev. Food Sci. Nutr. 45, 587–605.

Theodoris, P., 2008. The consequences of the "cut off" criteria for pesticides: agronomic and financial aspects. European Parliament. PE 408.963, pp. 1–36.

Tomlin, C.D.S., 2006. The Pesticide Manual: a World Compendium, fourteenth ed. BCPC Publications, Hampshire.

United Nations, 2002. Report of the world summit on sustainable development A/CONF.199/20*, pp. 1–173.
US EPA, 2007. Concept paper for the nanoscale materials stewardship program under TSCA. Available from: www.epa.gov
US EPA, 2015. Pesticides. Available from: www.epa.gov/pesticides
Usón, N., Garcia, M.J., Solans, C., 2004. Formation of water-in-oil (W/O) nano-emulsions in a water/mixed non-ionic surfactant/oil systems prepared by a low-energy emulsification method. Colloids Surf. A 250, 415–421.
Villaverde, J.J., Sandín-España, P., Sevilla-Morán, B., López-Goti, C., Alonso-Prados, J.L., 2016a. Biopesticides from natural products: current development, legislative framework, and future trends. BioRes. 11, 5618–5640.
Villaverde, J.J., Sevilla-Morán, B., López-Goti, C., Alonso-Prados, J.L., Sandín-España, P., 2016b. Trends in analysis of pesticide residues to fulfil the European Regulation (EC) No. 1107/2009. Trends Anal. Chem. 80, 568–580.
Villaverde, J.J., Sevilla-Morán, B., Sandín-España, P., López-Goti, C., Alonso-Prados, J.L., 2014a. Biopesticides in the framework of the European Pesticide Regulation (EC) No. 1107/2009. Pest Manag. Sci. 70, 2–5.
Villaverde, J.J., Sevilla-Morán, B., Sandín-España, P., López-Goti, C., Alonso-Prados, J.L., 2014b. Challenges of biopesticides under the European regulation (EC) No. 1107/2009: an overview of new trends in residue analysis. In: Atta-ur-Rahman, F. (Ed.), Studies in Natural Products Chemistry. Elsevier, Oxford, pp. 437–482.
von der Kammer, F., Legros, S., Hofmann, T., Larsen, E.H., Loeschner, K., 2011. Separation and characterization of nanoparticles in complex food and environmental samples by field-flow fractionation. Trends Anal. Chem. 30, 425–436.
Wibowo, D., Zhao, C.-X., Peters, B.C., Middelberg, A.P.J., 2014. Sustained release of fipronil insecticide in vitro and in vivo from biocompatible silica nanocapsules. J. Agric. Food Chem. 62, 12504–12511.
Yang, F.L., Li, X.G., Zhu, F., Lei, C.L., 2009. Structural characterization of nanoparticles loaded with garlic essential oil and their insecticidal activity against *Tribolium castaneum* (Herbst) (Coleoptera: Tenebrionidae). J. Agric. Food Chem. 57, 10156–10162.
Zhang, J., Zhang, F., Ren, L., Evans, D.G., Duan, X., 2004. Synthesis of layered double hydroxide anionic clays intercalated by carboxylate anions. Mater. Chem. Phys. 85, 207–214.
Zheng, L.P., Zhang, Z., Zhang, B., Wang, J.W., 2012. Antifungal properties of Ag-SiO_2 core–shell nanoparticles against phytopathogenic fungi. Adv. Mater. Res. 476–478, 814–818.
Zhenlan, Q., Heng, Y., Bin, Z., Wanguo, H., 2009. Synthesis and release behavior of bactericides intercalated Mg–Al layered double hydroxides. Colloids Surf. A 348, 164–169.
Zhu, Y., An, X., Li, S., Yu, S., 2009. Nanoencapsulation of β-cypermethrin by complex coacervation in a microemulsion. J. Surfact. Deterg. 12, 305–311.
Zielecka, M., 2011. Characteristics of silica nanopowders and sol containing immobilized nanoparticles of copper or silver. Polimery 10, 765–768.

7

IS NANOTECHNOLOGY A PROMISING FIELD FOR INSECT PEST CONTROL IN IPM PROGRAMS?

Nabil El Wakeil*,, Saad Alkahtani*, Nawal Gaafar****

**King Faisal University, College of Agriculture and Food Sciences, Arid Land Agriculture Department, Al-Ahsa, Kingdom of Saudi Arabia; **National Research Centre, Pests and Plant Protection Department, Dokki, Cairo, Egypt*

1 Introduction

1.1 Definition of Nanotechnology

Nanotechnology is a new field that has been come in various applied sciences, such as physic, biology, medical sections, chemistry, and engineering divisions. The purposeful research and development to recognize influence and measure at the resources with atomic, molecular, and great molecules sizes is known nanotechnology. Nanotechnology has been in the short term identified as relating to resources, processes, which drive at a scale of 100 nm. Overall nano refers to a dimension scale between 1 and 100 nm. Nanotechnology has numerous uses and applications in many stages: production, storing, processing, packaging, and shipping of various agricultural products (Predicala, 2009; Mousavi and Rezaei, 2011).

The nanoscience and nanoengineering, sometimes called nanomodification, of concrete are terms that have come into common usage and describe two main avenues of application of nanotechnology in concrete research (Scrivener and Kirkpatrick, 2008; Garboczi, 2009). Nanoscience deals with the measurement and characterization of the nano and microscale structure of cement-based materials to better understand how this structure affects macroscale properties and performance through the use of advanced characterization techniques and atomistic or molecular level modeling. Nanoengineering encompasses the techniques of

New Pesticides and Soil Sensors. http://dx.doi.org/10.1016/B978-0-12-804299-1.00008-4

manipulation of the structure at the nanometer scale to develop a new generation of tailored, multifunctional, cementitious composites with superior mechanical performance and durability potentially having a range of novel properties, such as low electrical resistivity, self-sensing capabilities, self-cleaning, self healing, high ductility, and self-control of cracks. Concrete can be nanoengineered by the integration of nanosized building blocks or substances (e.g., nanoparticles and nanotubes) to control material behavior and add novel properties, or by the grafting of molecules onto cement particles, cement phases, aggregates, and additives (including nanosized additives) to provide surface professionally, which can be accustomed to endorse specific interfacial interactions (Sanchez and Sobolev, 2010).

1.2 The Promise of Nanotechnology

Nanotechnology is the improvement and utilize of techniques to study physical fact and create configurations in the physical size range of 1–100 nm, as well as the establishment of these structures into applications. In spite of size is a suitable way of defining the area, it alone is not enough to make a division the nanoscale material from microscopic material. In practice, nanotechnology has more to operate with the examination of novel properties that manifest themselves at that size level, and of the ability to affect and synthetically build structures at that scale. Experiments and computer recreation have been targeted at very small scales for many years. The advances in high speed and high safe capacity computers, as well as precise instruments for measuring and operating at the nanoscale, have accelerated the development of nanoscale structures and devices into authenticity (Kostoff et al., 2006).

The science that underlies nanotechnology can be returned back to the early days of the 19th century. Kostoff et al. (2007) used the citation-assisted background (CAB) approach of Kostoff and Shlesinger (2005) to trace the rich scientific inheritance of nanotechnology back to its earliest roots. The interested reader is strongly advised to access this ~1500 page reference. Predictions about the promise of nanotechnology can be traced back to Feynman's classic 1959 talk (Feynman, 1960), where he stated: "The principles of physics, as far as I can see, do not speak against the possibility of maneuvering things atom by atom." Feynman proceeded to describe building with atomic precision, and outlined a pathway involving a series of increasingly smaller machines (Ragaei and Sabry, 2014). Presently, much effort is devoted to forecasting the role that nanotechnology could play in modern society, and outlining proficient nanotechnology accomplishment strategies and trajectories. Nanotechnology is envisioned in a dual role of both an enabling technology and a disruptive technology. Complicated roadmaps are used to link the end targets of nanotechnology implementation with the development approaches and portfolios necessary to speed up the implementation process.

Criteria for successful science and technology roadmaps are presented by Kostoff and Schaller (2001). A follow-on outline of technology road mapping (Phaal et al., 2004) includes a novel fast-start variant, and illustrates use of the fast-start method in the context of troublesome technological trends from multiple perspectives. Roadmaps geared to bringing potentially disruptive technologies from the concept stage to market products are described generically by Kostoff et al. (2004) and specifically for the nanotechnology case by Walsh (2004). The improvement of production processes through integration of macro-, micro-, and nanotechnologies provides a broad picture of available nanotechnology roadmaps and surveys (Almansa et al., 2006). Additionally, forecasting market size and demand for an early-stage emerging process technology (illustrated through a microsystems example) is mentioned by Linton (2004), and evaluating commercial importance of nanolithographic patenting trends is explained by Eijkel et al. (2006). There are many roadmaps and other forecasting tools that serve to accelerate nanotechnology improvement and deployment.

2 Nanotechnology in Agriculture

Communities, governments, and nations have been stressed with the issue since long. Last years have seen even bigger challenges on this obverse. The future looks even bleaker with food shortage issue threatening large. The challenge is how to feed the growing people by producing more even if landscape is reduced; with less input costs and with lesser dangers to the ecosystem (Anonymous, 2009). In between, nanotechnology has proved its position in agricultural sectors and related industries, as a corrective technology and a pioneer in solve many problems.

Nanotechnology as a new powerful technology has the ability to create massive changes in agricultural systems. The use of nanotechnology in agriculture will likely have ecological earnings (Froggett, 2009). Farm applications of nanotechnology are also powerful awareness. Nanomaterials are being developed that offer the chance to more proficient, safe, and sound direct pesticides, herbicides, and fertilizers by controlling precisely when and where they are released (Kuzma and VerHage, 2006). Nanotechnology is able to introduce new apparatus for use in molecular biology and new materials to identify plant disease microorganisms (Mousavi and Rezaei, 2011). Use of nanotechnology in agriculture can revolutionize this section with new tools for disease detection, targeted treatment, enhancing the ability of plants to absorb nutrients, fight pests, and withstand ecological pressures. Nanotechnology has provided new way outs to problems in plants (postharvest products) and offers new approaches to the rational selection of raw materials, or the processing of such materials to develop the quality of plant products (Sharon et al., 2010).

2.1 Applications of Nanobiotechnology in Plant Protection and Nutrition

Prospective applications of nanotechnology in agriculture are: delivery of nanocides–insecticides encapsulated in nanomaterials for controlled release; establishment of biopesticides with nanomaterials as reported by Debnath et al. (2012); Sahayaraj (2014); slow release of nanomaterial assisted biofertilizers and micronutrients for proficient use; and field applications of agrochemicals, nanomaterials assisted delivery of genetic material for crop development (Ghormade et al., 2011). Nanosensors for plant pathogen and pesticide detection, and NPs for soil protection are other areas in agriculture that can benefit from nanotechnology (Fig. 7.1). Enzyme immobilization for nanobiosensor using nanomaterials involves the high value low volume application of enzymes (Kim et al., 2006). Usually costly, large enzyme volumes are required for biocontrol in agricultural fields that would be practical if spray applications combined high volume with low value. Cost-usefulness of such biocontrol planning can be achieved by immobilization of enzyme/inhibitors on nanostructures, providing large surface areas, to increase the effective concentration of the preparation. In this chapter, we focus on nanomaterial-based technologies and their existing and potential applications in plant protection and nutrition.

2.2 Nanotechnology in Branches of Pests and Plant Diseases Management

Traditionally, managing the pathogens and pests need annually ~2 million metric tons pesticides worldwide (worth US $35 billion), a major part of which are lost to the air during application and as run-off, affecting both the atmosphere and application expenses to the farmers (Stephenson, 2003). Resistance of pests

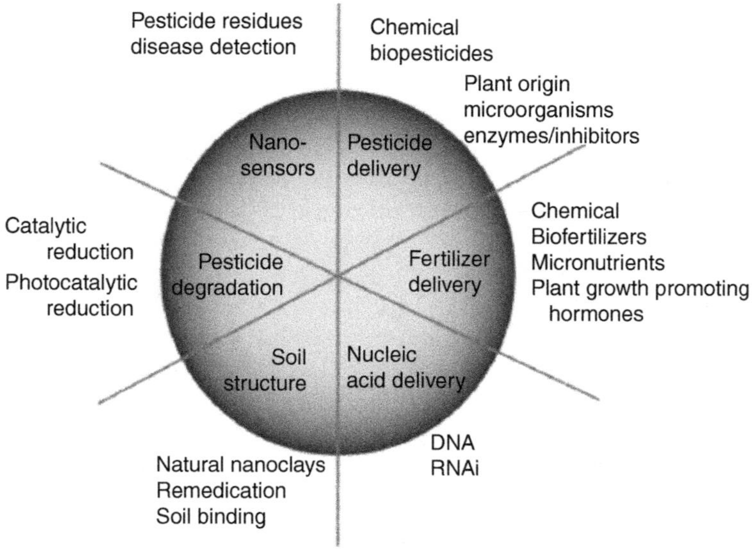

Figure 7.1. Applications of nanobiotechnology in plant protection and nutrition.
Cited from Ghormade et al. (2011).

increase resulting from high pesticide usage, which reduces soil bioassortment, diminishes nitrogen (N) addiction; supplies to bioaccretion of insecticides and pesticides, which affected birds and animals habitats (Tilman et al., 2002). So, there is a vital needing to begin the extreme pesticide uses and fertilizers by (1) rapidly and locally detecting presence of various insects, pesticides, as well as nutrient intensities, (2) finding substitutes the existing chemical fertilizer or pesticide, and (3) upward methods for either agrochemical deletion or degradation to support soil physical or chemical conditions (Ghormade et al., 2011).

Using the nanoparticles and nanocapsules with the ability to control or delayed release are brilliant way to help agricultural scientists to decrease environmental pollution by production of chemical pesticides and fertilizers, absorption and more effective and environmentally friendly; and production of nanocrystals to increase the pesticide effectiveness for applying lower dose insecticides. In near future, nanoparticles for delivery of active components will be at its helm for healing of all pathological sufferings of plants (Mousavi and Rezaei, 2011).

Polymeric nanoparticles, iron oxide nanoparticles, and gold nanoparticles are myriad of nanomaterials, which can be easily synthesized and exploited as pesticide. They could be used to modify the kinetic shapes of remedy material release, leading to more continuous release of therapy materials with a concentrated requirement for recurrent dosing (Sharon et al., 2010). Crop productivity is shackled by many organisms, one of them are plant diseases. The problem with the disease management lies with the detection of the exact stage of avoidance. The viruses' diseases are not easy to control, as one has to stop the spread of the disease by the vectors. However, pesticide application would not be of much use, once it starts showing its signs. For that cause, the key to the success of control of diseases mainly viral diseases, that is recognition of exact stage, such as stage of viral DNA duplication or the production of preliminary viral protein (Mousavi and Rezaei, 2011).

Detection and usages of biomarkers that precisely indicate pest stages is also a new area of research. Measuring differential protein production in both unhealthy and healthy states leads to the identification of the enlargement of several proteins during the infection rotation. These nanobased diagnostic kits not only increase the speed of detection but also increase the power of the detection (Rai and Ingle, 2012). Nanobased viral diagnostics, including multiplexed diagnostic kit development, have taken momentum to detect the exact strain of virus and stage of application of some therapeutic to stop the disease. In the future, nanoscale devices with these properties should be used to create the agricultural systems, which can be described as "smart". Those devices might be able to respond to various situations by taking the suitable action. If not, they will change to act the farmer to the problem. In this way, such devices will act as both a precautionary and warning structures.

3 Nanotech Sensor

Smart delivery systems, as well as smart sensors will help the agricultural production business fight viruses and other crop pathogens. In the next years, nanostructured materials will be accessible which will raise the insecticides effectiveness, allowing lower doses to be used. Smart sensors are the dominant tools for track detect and control with animal and plant pests. Detection of very small amounts of virus or bacteria contaminant in agricultural is envisioned from the integration of chemical, physical, and biological devices working together as an incorporated sensor at the nanoscale (Scott and Chen, 2003). A tiny sensor had been produced at the University of Manitoba, in both microelectronics and nanotechnology departments, which can help farm owners in the early detection of grain spoilage during storeroom.

Correspondingly, if fungus infests the grain, it produces different chemicals. The sensor has seven fragments in it and will identify which fungus is causing the spoilage. "The sensor also measures changes in carbon dioxide to detect incipient and ongoing deterioration of stored grains (Mousavi and Rezaei, 2011). A specific treatment can be used to correct the problem directly when the cause of spoilage is identified." The researchers are also looking at construction the sensor to be wireless, says Neethirajan et al. (2009). Who envisions that various sensors would be distributed throughout the grain to pinpoint problem areas and would communicate with a central hub. The central hub would routinely update a household computer, website, or personal mobile device, such as a cellphone so that a farmer could monitor the grain on a daily basis without having to visit the grain bin. By catching and treating spoilage, before it becomes severe, additional benefits might include reduced chemical usage and better grain quality (Hager, 2011).

The nano sensors could be distributed throughout the field where they can monitor soil conditions and crop growth. One of the most functions for nanotechnology-enabled devices will be the increased use of self-directed sensors linked into a GPS system for real-time observing. Finally, accuracy farming, which using the smart sensors, will allow improved productivity in agriculture by provided that a accurate information, thus will help the farmers to make the best decisions (Joseph and Morrison, 2006). Nanosmart dust and gas sensors are used in determining the amount of pollutants and dust in the air. In a few minutes, it is possible estimating the presence of pollutants in the atmosphere by sensors (Scott and Chen, 2003).

3.1 Nanosensors in Agriculture

Nanotechnology based sensor systems for applications in agriculture are still at the basic research level. Development of sensors and diagnostic devices for on-site monitoring will allow farmers to closely monitor environmental conditions, for plant growth and protection. These detection systems can contribute to increased productivity and decreased the use of agrochemicals (e.g., pesticides, nutrients) by early intervention (Ghormade et al., 2011).

3.2 Nanobiosensors for Pesticide Detection

Several studies were conducted for development of analytical tools for pesticide residue determination. In parallel with typical chromatography, immunochemical assays based on biomolecules were employed as an alternative for pesticide measurement by virtue of its high selectivity, sensitivity, and reliability, as well as its rapidity (Gabaldon et al., 1999). Traditional immunoassay is performed as discrete tests, that is, one assay for one analyte and several detecting runs for all of the components in a complex system. Application of nanomaterials adds further advantages to such systems, such as: further miniaturization, measurement of more variables, greater sensitivity, less sample material required, faster detection rates, read-outs in real time, and application of novel detection methodologies (e.g., electronic, colorimetric, fluorometric, and mass changes).

Currently unimolecular and array type of nanomaterial based biosensors are being developed for detection of pesticides (Table 7.1). However, the format of biosensors varies, from free biomolecules to those conjugated to a substrate, such as NPs, nanowires, nanotubes, and thin-films. Interaction of the target with the biosensor can be measured either directly or indirectly by recording the changes in color, fluorescence or electrical potential. In array technologies, multiple biomolecules are fixed to a substrate allowing multiple analytes to be measured simultaneously.

The unimolecular array systems a gold NPs (30 nm) based dipstick competitive immunoassay with sensitivity of 27 ng/mL was developed to obtain a detector to insecticides like DDT (Table 7.1, Lisa et al., 2009). Gold NPs have the property of agglomeration associated with color production that was used for pesticide detection. Development of a color signal aided easy visual detected when gold NPs labeled antibodies bound to the pesticide residues. The gold NP based dipstick technique was suitable for the detection of several toxins in food and environmental samples and can be applied for rapid on-site testing of pesticides (Lisa et al., 2009). Vinayaka et al. (2009) used cadmium telluride quantum dots (CdTeQDs), semiconductor fluorescent NPs, in a fluoroimmuno assay to detect 2,4-dichlorophenoxyacetic acid (2,4-D), herbicide. It was possible to detect 2,4-D up to 250 pg/L. Wang et al. (2004, 2009) developed a zirconium oxide NPs (~50 nm) based immunoassay for sensitive detection (0.02 nM) of organophosphate pesticides using phosphorylated enzyme acetylcholinesterase as a potential biomarker (Table 7.1). Joshi et al. (2005) developed a disposable, sensitive biosensor for organophosphorus pesticides (0.5 nM) based on acetylcholinesterase binding on multiwall carbon nanotubes modified thick film strip electrode (Table 7.1). The biosensor reproducibly detected low paraoxon at parts per billion (0.145) levels. Gan et al. (2010) also developed an acetylcholinesterase coated iron oxide magnetic NPs (30 nm) bound carbon nanotubes and zirconium oxide NPs (31.5 nm) composite on the

Table 7.1 Applications of Nanotechnology in Agriculture

Application	Nanoparticles	References
Pesticide delivery Chemical Avermectin	Porous hollow silica (15 nm)	Li et al. (2007)
Ethiprole or phenylpyrazole	Poly-caprolactone (135 nm)	Boehm et al. (2003)
Gamma cyhalothrin	Solid lipid (300 nm)	Frederiksen et al. (2003)
Tebucanazole/chlorothalonil	Polyvinylpyridine and polyvinylpyridine-*co*-styrene (100 nm)	Liu et al. (2001)
Biopesticides plant origin: nanosilica for insect control *Artemisia arborescens*	Nanosilica (3–5 nm)	Barik et al. (2008)
Essential oil encapsulation	Solid lipid (200–294 nm)	Lai et al. (2006)
Microganisms: *Lagenidium giganteum* cells in emulsion	Silica (7–14 nm)	Vandergheynst et al. (2007)
Microbial product: absorption of *Myrothrecium verrucaria* enzyme complex	Chitosan/kaolin (250–350 nm)	Ghormade et al. (2015)
Fertilizer delivery NPK controlled delivery	Nanocoating of sulfur (100 nm layer)	Wilson et al. (2008)
	Chitosan (78 nm)	Corradini et al. (2010)
Genetic material delivery DNA	Gold (10–15 nm) Gold (5–25 nm)	Torney et al. (2007) Vijayakumar et al. (2010)
Double stranded RNA	Starch (50–100 nm)	Liu et al. (2008)
	Chitosan (100–200 nm)	Zhang et al. (2010)
Pesticide sensor Carbofuran/triazophos	Gold (40 nm)	Guo et al. (2009)
DDT	Gold (30 nm)	Lisa et al. (2009)
Dimethoate	Iron oxide (30 nm)	Gan et al. (2010)
Organophosphate	Zirconium oxide (31.5 nm)	Wang et al. (2009)
	Zirconium oxide (50 nm)	Wang et al. (2009)
Paraoxon	Silica (100–500 nm)	Ramanathan et al. (2009)
	Carbon nanotubes	Joshi et al. (2005)
Pyrethroid	Iron oxide (22 nm)	Kaushik et al. (2009)
Pesticide degradation Lindane	Iron sulfide (200 nm)	Paknikar et al. (2005)
Imidacloprid	Titanium oxide (30 nm)	Guan et al. (2008)

screen-printed electrode surface for detection of dimethoate, an organophosphorus pesticide (Table 7.1).

The sensitivity of the biosensor was at 50 pg/L. An enzyme based organophosphate array biosensor was developed by Ramanathan et al. (2009). Organophosphate hydrolase (OPH) was conjugated to a pH-responsive fluorophore encapsulated in silica NPs (100–500 nm) and patterned to a waveguide surface (Table 7.1). Silica NP sencapsulated OPH was stable for nearly 60 days and retained a detection limit (34 μM) of parts per million for paraoxon. The ability to integrate enzymes for catalytic detection with the capability to detect chemical agents may potentially extend the versatility of the array nanobiosensor to both biological and chemical contaminants. Kaushik et al. (2009) fabricated a nucleic acid sensor via immobilization of single standard calf thymus deoxyribose nucleic acid onto a chitosan nanobiocomposite film containing iron oxide NPs (Fe_3O_4, 22 nm), deposited onto indium–tin oxide coated glass surface for pyrethroid, cypermethrin, and permethrin, detection (Table 7.1).

This disposable nanobiocomposite bioelectrode was stable for about 2 months under refrigerated conditions and detected cypermethrin and permethrin rapidly (N50 s) at 0.0025 ppm (Kaushik et al., 2009). The widespread use of various pesticides and their mixtures in the agricultural fields causes the multiresidue retention problem in the environment. Thus, it is necessary to simultaneously identify several pesticides in a complex sample. By comparison, multianalyte immunoassay that can simultaneously discriminate at least two analytes in a single run displays noticeable advantages, such as high sample throughput, attractive assay efficiency, and low consumption of reagent, labor, and time (Fu et al., 2007; Kricka, 1992). Guo et al. (2009) developed a gold NPs (40 nm) based portable one-step strip assay allowing simultaneous screening for two pesticides carbofuran and triazophos within a short time (8–10 min) without any equipment (Table 7.1). A bispecific monoclonal antibody (McAb), against both carbofuran and triazophos, was labeled with nanogold in comparison to the nanogold labeled anticarbofuran McAb and antitriazophos McAb as detector reagents. Analysis of spiked water samples, by visual comparison of pesticide standard tests between the two formats, indicated that the detection limit was at parts per million for carbofuran (32 μg/L) and triazophos (4 μg/L) (Guo et al., 2009).

The scope for application of nanotechnology for the development of sensors that are specific, fast, handy, and inexpensive is vast and the key challenge would be the commercialization of biosensors. Furthermore, combining nanotechnology with microfluidic devices, that allow flow of microvolumes of liquid through channels, will promote further miniaturization and rapid sampling. Cantilever nanomechanical devices, with springboard like-mechanism, are interesting as they detect the presence of specific target molecules, when the target binds a reporter molecule attached to the cantilever. Cantilever arrays can give rise to a sensitive nanosensor electronic "nose" or "tongue". The future would see the development of multianalyte array sensors, microfluidic devices, and cantilever arrays to make environmental monitoring easy.

3.3 Nanobiosensors for Plant Pathogen Detection

Currently, several methods of microbial identification and typing are available for most plant pathogens. Traditional culture based methods are time consuming (Fletcher et al., 2006). Techniques based on biochemical profiles for identification are limited by the population of characterized strains in the databases. Sensitive and specific serological techniques, such as ELISA and indirect fluorescent antibody staining depend on the titer and specificity of the antibody either monoclonal or polyclonal (Lister, 1978; Yuen et al., 1998; Uddin et al., 2003). Cross-reactivity among closely related strains prevents their clear identification (Cho and Goodman, 1979: Jain et al., 1992). Costly, nucleic acid based polymerase chain reaction methods, such as restriction fragment length polymorphism, DNA fingerprinting and amplification of the internal transcribed spacer region from rRNA gene increase specificity of identification (Bariana et al., 1994; Schaad et al., 2002; Gao et al., 2004; Doorn et al., 2007).

A novel microbial detection technology based on NPs is being developed. Silica-based NPs (60 nm) were filled with a fluorescent dye and conjugated to an antibody specific to a surface antigen of the microbe of interest (Zhao et al., 2004). Detection of a single bacterial cell was possible using that technique (Zhao et al., 2004). It has potential for sensitive detection of plant pathogens.

4 Application of Nanotechnology in Agricultural Production

4.1 Literature and Functional Points

All living organisms either tiny or huge depend on nanometer-shaped protein machines that perform everything from whipping of flagella to flexing of muscles. Nanometer-sized carbon that develops the mechanical traits of tires, nanometer silver particles that initiate photographic film improvement, and nanometer particles that are the basis of catalysts critical to the petrochemical industry have contributed to commercial products for several years (Huck, 2008; Fiorito, 2008; Bhattacharyya et al., 2010). Nanostructured materials are regularly manufactured using chemical methods. It is very vital to identify the target nanoparticles through the scanning tunneling microscope (STM) and atomic force microscope (AFM). Great prospective for application in ecological protection has been already shown by Nanotechnology researchers (Nowack, 2009; Ying, 2009).

Application of nanoparticles or other nanostructured materials for pollution prevention through environmentally benign synthesis and manufacturing are also being discovered (Duebendorf, 2008; Bhattacharyya et al., 2010). The potential of nanotechnology to renovate the healthiness caring, agriculture, textile, information, and communication technology has been well documented. In fact, numerous products enabled by nanotechnology are formerly in the market and they include antibacterial dressings, strain-resistant plant cultivars, and nanoparticles in ecofriendly insecticides (Sukul et al. 2009; Barik et al., 2008; Gha-Young et al., 2008; Bhattacharyya, 2009).

Generally, preciseness agriculture is a new approach in farm administration. By using nanosensors, we will be informed for each small part of farm, how much needs to fertilizer and chemical insecticides? Consequently, use of inputs will be most positive and safe products and economic effectiveness is increased. Nanosensors help to farmers in maintaining farm with precise control and report timely needs of plants. Nanosensors and nanobased smart delivery systems could help in the efficient use of agricultural natural resources, such as chemicals and nutrients through this farming. Farm managers could remotely detect crop insect pests or evidence of stress, such as drought throughout using nanomaterials and global positioning systems with satellite imaging of fields (Kumar, 2009).

In case we could detect insect, pest, disease, or drought, there would be automatic adjustment of pesticide applications or irrigation levels. Detecting presence of viruses damaged the plant or soil nutrient materials could be prepared by nanosensors dispersed. Nanofertilizers will be rapid absorption by plants. Nanoencapsulated leisurely release fertilizers have also become a trend to save fertilizer utilization as well to minimize ecological pollution. An alternative fuels and reduce environmental pollution could be produced by using nanotechnology tools. Nanotechnology has also exposed that it can modify the genetic creation of the crop plants thereby helping in further improvement of crop plant productivity (Jones, 2006; DeRosa et al., 2010).

4.2 Nanoparticles Based Delivery Systems: Formulations and Applications

Delivery systems in agriculture are important for application of pesticides and fertilizers, as well as during genetic material mediated plant improvement. Application systems for pesticides need to focus on efficacy enhancement and spray drift management while fertilizers face problems of bioavailability due to soil chelating, overapplication and run-offs. A viable alternative for these problems is provided by controlled delivery systems for the pesticide and fertilizer application. Controlled delivery technique aims toward measured release of necessary and sufficient amounts of agrochemicals over a period of time, to obtain the fullest biological efficacy and to minimize the harmful effects (Tsuji, 2001). For this purpose, micronic and submicronic particles were explored as agrochemical delivery vehicles. In comparison to micronic particles ($\geq$1000 nm), nanoparticles ($<$1000 nm) offered the advantage of effective loading due to the larger surface area, easy attachment and fast mass transfer. As depicted in Fig. 7.2, the active ingredient is adsorbed, attached, encapsulated, or entrapped unto or into the nanomatrix (Fig. 7.2). Controlled release of the active ingredient is achieved due to the slow release characteristics of the nanomaterial, bonding of the ingredients to the material and the environmental conditions. In case of genetic material, delivery systems face challenges, such as limited host range, transportation across cell membrane and trafficking to the nucleus. Nevertheless, the use of NPs assisted delivery for genetic material to develop insect resistant plant varieties is being studied. For instance, DNA-coated gold NPs are used as bullets in "gene gun" system, for bombardment of plant cells and tissues to achieve gene transfer (Torney et al., 2007; Vijayakumar et al., 2010).

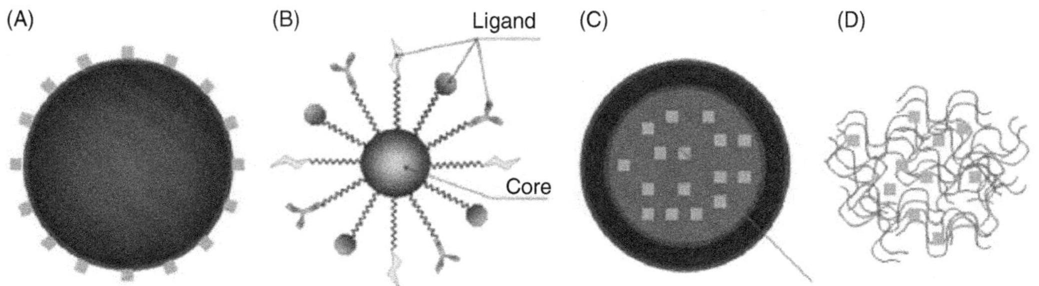

Figure 7.2. Schematic representation of different nanodevices for delivery of pesticides, fertilizers or nucleic acids (A) adsorption on nanoparticle; (B) attachment on nanoparticle mediated by different ligands; (C) encapsulation in nanoparticulate polymeric shell; (D) entrapment in polymeric nanoparticles. Cited from Ghormade et al. (2011).

4.3 The Applied Theories of Management of Insect–pests Using Nanotechnology

The less efficiency of traditional methods leads to the development of modern approaches for insect pest control strategies, which are the need of hour. Keeping in our thinking the nanotechnology applications in agriculture, it should be suggested that nanomaterials uses would give the development of efficient approaches for pest management. Recently studies confirmed that metal nanoparticles are effective against plants pathogens and insect pests. Nanoparticles could be used in the new formulations of pesticides preparation and insect repellants (Barik et al., 2008; Owolade et al., 2008; Gajbhiye et al., 2009; Stadler et al., 2010; Goswami et al., 2010). Torney (2009) mentioned that nanotechnology has talented applications in nanoparticles gene transfer. Deliver DNA and other preferred chemicals into plant-tissue for protection of host plants against insects could be done by using nanotechnology.

Porous hollow silica nanoparticles (PHSNs) encumbered with validamycin (it is pesticide) might be a promising carrier in agriculture, especially for pesticide controlled delivery whose immediate, as well as prolonged release is needed for plants (Liu et al., 2006). Depending on results of Wang et al. (2007), oil in water (nanoemulsions) was practical for the pesticide formulations and these could be efficient against many insects. In the same way, essential oil-loaded solid lipid nanoparticles were also functional for the formulations of nanoinsecticides (Liu et al., 2006). Nanosilica, a type of unique nanomaterial, is prepared from silica. It has many applications in medicine and drug development as catalyst and most importantly, is that it can be used as nanopesticide, as described by Barik et al. (2008) in using nanosilica for producing nanopesticide. This mechanism is depending on that insects used a diversity of cuticular lipids for keeping their water barrier and thereby avoid death from waterlessness. However, nanosilica gets absorbed into the cuticular lipids by physiosorption and thereby causes death of insects purely by physical resources, if it is applied on surfaces of leaves and stem.

4.4 Role of Natural Nanoparticles in Controlling Some Insects

Nanostructures are a probability rich source of products that meet certain specifications (Watson and Watson, 2004). Here, it is an example, where the ordered hexagonal crammed array of constructions in the cicada wings for instance, *Psaltoda claripennis*

Ashton and termite for example, family *Rhinotermitidae* (Zhang and Liu, 2006). The structures tend to have a rounded shape at the apex and protrude some 150–350 nm out from the surface plane. These wing nanoparticles help in the aerodynamic effectiveness of the insect. The emerging industries based on nanotechnology have so far made little use of "free" technology accessible in nature (Bhattacharyya and Debnath, 2008; Ehrlich et al., 2008).

It is known that the performance of a great variety of higher animals is affected by changes in the local magnetic field within their environment. Insects possess ferromagnetic resonance, which is temperature dependent. This material is found in the different insect body parts; abdomen, thorax, and head of insects like *Solenopsis substitute* (Fabricius). These magnetic nanoparticles act as geomagnetic sensors especially in social insects (Esquivel, 2007). Yang et al. (2009) demonstrated activity of insecticidal of polyethylene glycol-covered nanoparticles loaded integrated with garlic essential oil against *Tribolium castaneum* adult in the storage. It has been noticed that mortality percents for adult *T. castaneum* was 80%, most probably due to the sluggish and constant release of the dynamic components from the nanoparticles as well stated by Abduz Zahir et al. (2012) in their studies on *Sitophilus oryzae*.

Recently, a novel photodegradable insecticide involving nanoparticles has been prepared (Guan et al., 2008). Nanostructure components are also present in insect eyes. Wings of butterflies possess bright color components and these color components are nothing but nanoparticles. Naturally, nanoparticles of insects and volatile phytochemicals are solely responsible for plant-insect interaction (Gorb and Gorb, 2009). Furthermore, in the case of silkworm, electrospun silk fibroin-based fibers with average diameter of 700 nm were prepared from aqueous regenerated silkworm silk solutions (Jin et al., 2004; Zhang et al., 2007). The electrospun nanocomposite of silkworm silk helps in producing single wall carbon nanotubes (SWNT) for drug delivery system (Ayutsede et al., 2008).

4.5 Effects of Nanotechnology Materials on Silk Worm, Ants, and Honey Bee

An applications of different type of nanoparticles, namely silver nanoparticles (SNP), titanium dioxide, zinc oxide, and aluminium oxide (ANP) in controlling rice weevil and grasserie disease in *Bombyx mori*, which caused by baculovirus BmNPV (*B. mori* nuclear polyhedrosis virus) and *S. oryzae* have been studied by Goswami et al. (2010). In their study they conducted a practice bioassay, in which they prepared the liquid and solid formulations of the nanoparticles; later, they applied these formulations to control *S. oryzae* on rice and kept in a plastic box with 20 insect-adults and their effects were recorded for one week (7 days). Hydrophilic SNP was most efficient on the 1st day. On the 2nd day, more than 90% mortality was noticed with SNP and ANP. After seven days of introduction this treatment, 95 and 86% mortality were stated with SNP either hydrophilic or hydrophobic and most 70% of treated insects were damaged while lipophilic SNP treated on the rice. However, in case of ANP, 100% mortality was recorded. Correspondingly, in other bioassay conducted for grasserie disease in silkworm, a considerable decrease in viral load was affirmed when leaves of *B. mori* were treated with ethanolic suspension of hydrophobic alumino-silicate nanoparticles as mentioned by Goswami et al. (2010).

Honey bees use geomagnetic field information for direction, homing and foraging (Binhi, 2004). On the other hand, the process that animals use to detect the geomagnetic field is still not known. Many interpretations indicate that intracellular biomineralized magnetite could interact with the geomagnetic field monitoring information on its intensity and direction. Identifying the presence of magnetite particles in various insects and thus showing that insects' behavior is affected by the geomagnetic field is a first try for representative that biogenic magnetite is implicated in geomagnetic field detection (Ishay et al., 2008). Also, the ant *Formica rufa* Linnaeus uses information from the geomagnetic field to find the right direction during their behavior process. The same examination has been done in respect of the ant *Solenopsis invicta* Buren (Slowik et al. 1998). The presence of ferric iron in the abdomen of *S. invicta* workers was also observed (Abracado et al., 2005). The examination which was completed through electron microscope system clearly established that several ant species differentiate magnetic signals with the help of magnetite nanoparticles (Abracado et al., 2005). Isolated nanoparticles of insects have diameters of about 12 and 11 nm in abdomen with petiole and head with antennae, respectively. In the stingless bee *Schwarziana quadripunctata* Lepeletier was observed finding magnetite particles in its head, antennae, thorax and abdomen (Lucano et al., 2006; Esquivel et al., 2007). The magneto sensor is found in *Pachycondyla marginata* Roger and termite species *Neocapritermes opacus* Hagen (Acosta-Avalos et al., 1999; Wajnberg et al., 2004; de Oliveira et al., 2008). Also, ferromagnetic material has been discovered in *Apis mellife*ra Linnaeus abdomens and known as suitable for magnetic reception (Desoil et al., 2005). Magnetic nanoparticles in the *A. mellifera* abdomens are well accepted as involved in their magneto reception mechanism

(El-Jaick et al., 2001). The biogenic magnetic properties of *A. mellifera* were inspected with a view to accepting the bee's physiological response to a magnetic field (Billen, 2006; Hsu et al., 2007; Chambarelli et al., 2008). The magnetizations of bee abdomens on one hand, and heads and thoraxes on the second hand were evaluated separately as functions of temperature and field (Esquivel et al., 2002; Desoil et al., 2005). Both the anti-ferromagnetic responses of the ferrihydrite cores of the iron storage protein ferritin, and the ferromagnetic responses of nanoscale magnetite (Fe_3O_4) particles were observed (Dawson, 2008; Tai Kai, 2008). Using magnetic resonance imaging (MRI) for detecting the natural magnetism in fire ant (*S. invicta*) workers, queens and alates were studied. All ferromagnetic materials are magnetic nanoparticles, which are solely responsible for localization of specific direction for food and insect hosts. In other insects such as cicada wings have been found by atomic force microscopy (AFM) used for observing nanoparticles. The structures consist of hexagonal close-packed protrusions with a lateral spacing of 200 nm and may have multiple functionalities (Bhattacharyya et al., 2010).

4.6 Potential Usage in Controlling Weeds

The nanoencapsulation applications in agriculture have been started. Many paths are now open, and other possibilities remain still unknown. Controlling parasitic plants, nanoencapsulation could be applied to solve problems concerning phytotoxicity on the plant of the herbicides used against the parasitic plants (Goldwasser et al., 2003). For example, it is recognized that broomrape (*Orobanche* spp.) tubercles be active as strong sinks for water and nutrients (Joel, 2000). If nanoencapsulated as herbicides are sprayed, they will enlarge systemically in the plants to avoid such phytotoxicity troubles and/or detoxification. Once the nanocapsules attain the weeds, the herbicide will be discharged. This indicates that minor doses of herbicides such as glyphosate or imidazolinones will be needed.

Encapsulation of another herbicide can also supply enhancements in its treatment. Sulfonylurea is applied throughout the soil to control *Orobanche* spp., but several applications are needed to get efficient control (Joel et al., 2007). If the herbicide are encapsulated and gradually released into the soil during the crop season, an enhanced control might be achieved with sloe treatment and with lower doses. On the other hand, applying encapsulated herbicides as coatings of seed before the sowing, to prevent the several treatments needed with nonencapsulated ones (Jurado-Expósito et al., 1996, 1997). It is probable to link different molecules, some of them valuable for movement through nonpolar substances (cuticle waxes, cell membranes), and others for movement through polar substances (water) (Pérez-de-Luque and Rubiales, 2009).

It may be possible to develop an agrochemical containing diverse substances for different purposes (pest management, fertilization, hormones, etc.) and encapsulated independently to evade interactions between them and degradation. Thus, several stuffs might be treated with the same management to the crop, and the nanocapsules could be synchronized to release their load according to the traits of every loaded substance.

Different active materials (various herbicides) with a harmony effect may be applied individually with the similar treatment and released inside the weed tubercles, so acting more efficiently without harming the plant. Glyphosate, sulfonylureas and imidazolinones should be encapsulated alone within a polymeric shell. The shell will be utilized with surfactants to develop the penetration through the weed cuticle, and treated systemically throughout the leaves (Pérez-de-Luque and Rubiales, 2009).

Therefore, 3 herbicides with 2 different modes of action could be used with the same dealing. Additionally, a remaining effect in the soil should be evaded. Nanoencapsulation may make it potential to fight the weeds with herbicides that regularly cannot be treated systemically (contact herbicides), improving the effectiveness of each treatment and reducing the lethal dose to be distributed (Pérez-de-Luque and Rubiales, 2009).

The same principles applied for nanoencapsulation of herbicides can be applied for other materials developed against weeds. Germination stimulants as mentioned by López-Ráez et al. (2009) may be transported into the soil inside nanocapsules defending about them against herbicide degradation. Natural metabolites, such as mycotoxins (Vurro et al., 2009), could also be applied systemically inside nanocapsules. A different approach might be to use nanocapsules delivered into the rhizosphere for the absorption of chemical signals released by the host, such as germination stimulants or haustorial inducing factors (Palmer et al., 2009). In this case, nanocapsules would absorb the host released substances responsible for triggering specific processes in the parasitic weed cycle (Pérez-de-Luque and Rubiales, 2009).

5 Nanoparticles for Ecological Remediation

Nanoscience and nanotechnology have the potential to produce major impacts on the environment. Nanoscale particles represent a new generation of environmental remediation technologies that could provide cost-effective solution to some of the most challenging environmental cleanup problems. Nanoscale iron particles have large surface areas and high surface reactivity. Equally important, they provide enormous flexibility for in situ applications. Research has shown that nanoscale iron particles are very effective for the transformation and detoxification of a diversity of common ecological contaminants, such as chlorinated organic solvents, organochlorine pesticides, and PCBs. Modified iron nanoparticles, such as catalyzed and supported nanoparticles have been synthesized to improve the speed and effectiveness of remediation (Chinnamuthu and Boopathi, 2009).

The environmental chemistry of metallic or zero-valent iron has been extensively documented. Recent research has suggested that as a remediation technique, nanoscale iron particles have several advantages: (1) effective for transformation of a large variety of environmental contaminants, (2) inexpensive, and (3) nontoxic. Recent laboratory research has largely established nanoscale iron particles as effective reductants and catalysts for a wide variety of common environmental contaminants including chlorinated organic compounds and metal ions (Chinnamuthu and Boopathi, 2009).

Rapid and complete dechlorination of all chlorinated contaminants can be achieved within the water and soil-water slurries. For example, with a nanoscale Pd/Fe particle dose at 6.25 g/L, all chlorinated compounds were reduced to below detectable limits. Ethane was the major product in all tests. Greater than 99% removal was achieved with nanoscale iron particle in 24 h. Some pesticides that are persistent in aerobic environments are more readily degraded under reducing conditions. One application of this technique uses zerovalent iron (ZVI) as a chemical reductant. Under aerobic conditions, oxygen is the usual electron acceptor, while in anaerobic environment, electron release from the reaction of ZVI with water can be coupled to the reaction of chlorinated and nitroaromatic compounds.

Utilization of "magnetic" bacteria seems useful for metallic ion and heavy metal removal from aqueous solutions (e.g. Ag, Hg, Pb, Cu, Zn, Sb, Mn, Fe, As, Ni, Al, Pt, Pd, and Ru). In the presence of magnetic ions such as iron sulphide, heavy metal precipitates onto bacterial cell walls, making the bacteria sufficiently magnetized for removal from suspension by magnetic separation procedure. Research has shown that certain bacteria could produce iron sulfonide, which would act as an adsorbent for several metallic ions. A novel concept was proposed to synthesize mesoporous magnetic nanocomposite particles. These particles could be used for the removal of harmful agents present in the environment. This method employs molecular templates to coat nanoparticles of magnetite with mesoporous silica (Chinnamuthu and Boopathi, 2009).

5.1 Pesticide Degradation

Pesticide-contaminated soil and water treatment ranges from conventional methods such as incineration, phyto-remediation, and photochemical processes to innovative methods such as ultrasound-promoted remediation and other advanced oxidation processes (Hoffmann et al., 1995; Bhatkhande et al., 2001; Chaudhry et al., 2002; Farre et al., 2007). Degradation of bio-recalcitrant pollutants using NPs is another promising approach (Hee Joo and Cheng, 2006; Zhang, 2003). Recent studies showed that pesticides such as atrazine, molinate, and chlorpyrifos are susceptible to degradation with nanosized ZVI (1–100 nm). Cyclodiene insecticides such as endosulfan, however, were generally resistant (Hee Joo and Cheng, 2006).

Nanosized ZVI had a greater reactivity than granular ZVI, and their direct injection into the groundwater plume to minimize installation costs, was suggested (Zhang, 2003). Applications of ZVI structures and iron oxide NPs may be for removal of humic material and toxins (Waychunas et al., 2005; Giasuddin et al., 2007). However, little is known about the long-term performance of these nanoparticles/colloidal systems. The application of NPs such as biopolymer stabilized FeS (200 nm), are in scavenging and degradation of lindane, a persistent organic pollutant found in drinking water as well as in food (Table 7.1, Paknikar et al., 2005).

Other approaches such as photocatalytic decomposition of pesticide residues using titania doped with Fe_2O_3 or other metals sprayed directly on crops or even incorporated into the pesticide formulation are promising (Sasson et al., 2007). Layer-by-layer surface (LbL) nanoengineering is a novel strategy for direct surface modification of colloidal entities, which utilizes sequential adsorption of oppositely charged polyelectrolytes to form a complex assembly via electrostatic interactions. Guan et al. (2008) directly encapsulated microcrystals of the insecticide imidacloprid (IMI) by LbL assembly using polysaccharides chitosan and sodium alginate followed by addition of addition of photocatalytic NPs (Table 7.1). Photocatalytic degradation and mineralization of the IMI by TiO_2 NPs (~30 nm) and silver and sodium dodecyl sulfate modified TiO_2 NPs were reported.

5.2 Soil Structure and Remediation

Clays are sub-micrometric soil particles. Common clays are layered phyllosilicate materials, with a polymeric silicate base, which are nanodimensional in one plane. Transmission electron (TEM) and high resolution transmission electron (HRTEM) microscopy showed that clays are composed of stacked tetrahedral and octahedral sheets (Wilson et al., 2008). Other inorganic nanomaterials such as the tubular aluminosilicate imogolite and its non-tubular precursor called protoimogolite are soil components (Farmer et al., 1983). NPs such as iron and silica originate from natural weathering of bedrocks. Other naturally occurring NPs are iron oxides (2–5 nm length), as colloidal phases of ferrihydrite, associated with organic matter in river-borne material (Allard et al., 2004). However, Yang and Watts (2005) showed that alumina NPs (aluminum oxide) is detrimental to plant root growth.

Remediation is another aspect of the role of NPs in soil structure. In 2003, a nanotechnology based soil binder, a type of quick-setting organic and biodegradable mulch, was developed by a US based company (ETC Group, 2004). The reaction caused silicates in the soil and silicates in the product to self-assemble into a kind of crust that remained up to a year. The crust was claimed to prevent soil runoff and allowed seeds blended into the product to germinate. It was sprayed over 1400 acres of in New Mexico to prevent erosion following forest fires.

Bioremediation of toxic metals is an important aspect that affects plant growth. Copper, as a free ion catalyzes the production of damaging radicals. Thus, all life forms attempt to prevent copper toxicity. Plants diminish excess copper in two structural regions: in sub-aerial tissues by rare hyperaccumulators, that bind cationic copper to organic ligands; and in roots by metal tolerant plants that segregate copper by similar mechanisms. Biomolecular responses to oxidative stress were responsible for the NP formation. Peat cultivation can contribute to copper biorecycling and rhizosphere containment to prevent copper biomagnification.

5.3 Detoxification of Herbicide Residues

Excessive use of herbicides leave residue in soil and cause damage to the succeeding crops. Continuous use of single herbicide leads to evolution of herbicide resistant weed species and shift in weed flora. Atrazine, an s-triazine-ring herbicide, is used globally for the control of preand post-emergence broadleaf and grassy weeds, which has high persistence (half life-125 days) and mobility in some types of soils. Residual problems due to the application of atrazine herbicide pose a threat towards widespread use of herbicide and limit the choice of crops in rotation. Recent finding from Tamil Nadu Agricultural University raises hope to remediate the atrazine residue from soil within a short span of time (Chinnamuthu and Boopathi, 2009).

Using of nanotechnology have a significant effect in the main areas of agriculture, one of these areas is remediation of herbicide and pesticide residues from plant and soil (Moraru et al., 2003). Application of silver modified with nanoparticles of magnetite stabilized with carboxy methyl cellulose (CMC) nanoparticles recorded 88% degradation of herbicide atrazine residue under controlled environment (Susha et al., 2009).

6 Nanotechnology Risks and Regulation

6.1 Some Concerns

The novel characteristics of nanoparticles and other nanomaterials that offer new and desirable traits for a range of industrial applications may also be the source of new forms of hazards to environments and people, such as new forms of toxicity and new forms of pollution (Wilkinson, 2002; Colvin, 2003; Weiss et al., 2006; Scrinis, 2006a). There is little known about the health effects of eating foods that contain nanoparticles, or of workers handling nanomaterials. A report by the British Royal Society has warned of the serious risks of nanotoxicity (Royal Society and the Royal Academy of Engineering, 2004). A key concern regarding human exposure to nanoscale particles is that they have many pathways for entering the body, such as through inhalation, digestion and through the skin. From there they may be able to pass into the bloodstream, penetrate cells, by-pass immune responses, lodge in the lungs, and cross the blood-brain barrier (Scrinis, 2006b).

Proponents of nanofood applications argue that they offer the capacity to bring on-going improvements to agriculture and food systems: they argue it will improve the productivity and efficiency of crop and livestock production, as well as increasing the safety, nutritional value, and shelf-life of food, and helping to increase food production to meet future population growth trends (Joseph and Morrison, 2006; Sanguansri and Augustin, 2006). This chapter was tried to identify and evaluate some of the specific applications and implications of nanotechnology within the various sectors of the agriculture system in the same frame of results obtained by Scrinis and Lyons (2007).

6.2 Safety/Toxicity of Nanoscale Materials

Many current researches that assessed the effects of nanoscale materials on biological organisms have provided very useful data for considerate the human health implications from exposure to these materials and have helped to identify precedence points for further research. While most of the obtainable studies on manufactured nanoscale resources have focused on a very limited range of materials, including quantum dots, carbon nanotubes and fullerenes, the data derived from these studies provides useful information for evaluating the prospective human health and ecological effects that could result from exposure to nanoscale materials (Thomas and Sayre, 2005). The increased reactivity of nanoscale stuffs that arises as a consequence of their larger surface area has created extensive interest in development of a better understanding of the effects of nanoscale materials on biological systems. Nanoscale materials have been assessed in both in vitro and in vivo systems to explore effects from dermal and inhalation exposure. In a broad sense, these experimental studies were designed to characterize the extent to which these materials interact with organ systems and cellular organelles, the biological effects of those interactions, and the potential health effects from acute and chronic contact to nanoscale materials (Oberdorster et al., 2004).

Further studies are needed to find out the reversibility of the observed translocation, and to determine whether similar effects would be seen in humankind. Another significant consideration for evaluating the biological effects of nanoscale materials is the existence and type of surface coating on the material. Although uncoated material was used for the largemouth bass study, a significant amount of the material that will be used in commerce is likely to be coated with one of a variety of materials that have varying levels of biological availability and determination. The traits of the underlying nanoscale material therefore must be understood in combining with the relevant surface coating or treatment (Thomas and Sayre, 2005). Respiratory exposure to nanoscale materials such as carbon nanotubes has also received a considerable amount of interest. Because of the difficulties related with generating aerosols of carbon nanotubes to assist an evaluation of inhaled material, and the high cost of harmonized well-characterized material, several in vivo pulmonary studies have employed intratracheal instillation as the exposure methodology (Rao et al., 2003). Single walled carbon nanotubes (SWCNTs) have been estimated in rodents using this technique. SWCNTs instilled into the lungs of mice produced granulomas in the pulmonary interstitium of the lungs (Lam et al., 2004). Rats exposed to SWCNTs developed multifocal granulomas in the nonappearance of any pulmonary inflammation or cellular proliferation (Warheit et al., 2004) which suggests that SWCNTs may act via a different mechanism of toxicity than other inhaled toxicants such as crystalline silica.

These studies highlight the need for further testing experiments to fully elucidate the mechanisms that are responsible for the behavior of carbon fullerenes and nanotubes. Specifically, to develop a comprehensive evaluation of the human health implications from exposure to nanoscale materials, more data are needed on the adsorption, distribution, metabolism, and excretion of these materials in biological systems. In addition, more data are needed to assess the extent to which the original properties of these materials, such as particle size and size distribution, affect the distribution and elimination of these materials in the body. More studies are also needed to characterize the toxicity of a broader range of commercial nanoscale materials as a function of chemical composition, shape, surface characteristics, and method of production (Thomas and Sayre, 2005).

Several of these characteristics, particularly surface coating, could have a substantial effect on the biological activity of these materials. While only a few studies have been noted here, other recently published review articles capture a broader range of studies that have been performed to assess the human health implications of exposure to nanoscale materials (Oberdorster et al., 2005; Royal Society and the Royal Academy of Engineering, 2004).

7 Nanoparticles—A Green Revolution in Future

There are enormous uses and benefits for nanotechnology. These include agricultural yield improvement relating nanoporous zeolites for leisurely release of nanocapsules for herbicide or pesticides relief and pest control and nanosensors for pest recognition as shown in Table 7.2 (Liu and Du, 2004; Joseph and Morrison, 2006; Scrinis and Lyons, 2007; Scott, 2007). Nanoparticles help to produce new pesticides, insecticides and insect repellants (Owolade et al., 2008). Nanoencapsulation is a procedure throughout which an insecticide is slowly but capably of released to a particular plant for pest management. Nanoencapsulation with nanoparticles in structure of insecticides allows for an appropriate absorption of the chemicals inside the plants unlike the case of larger particles (Scrinis and Lyons, 2007). This process may distribute DNA and other preferred chemicals into tissues of plant for plants protection against various pests (Torney, 2009).

Liberate mechanisms of nanoencapsulation is including the following steps: diffusion, biodegradation, dissolution and osmotic pressure with an exact pH (Vidhyalakshmi et al., 2009; Ding and Shah, 2009). Also, it is known that aluminosilicate filled nanotube can stick to plant surfaces while nano ingredients of nanotube have the ability to stick to the surface hair of insect pests and ultimately

Table 7.2 Nanotechnology Applications in Different Fields of Agriculture

General Term	Different Agriculture Fields	Nanotechnology Applications
Nanotechnology	Food packaging	
	Gene transfer	Crop improvement
	Nanobased products	Nanopesticides Nanofungicide Nanofertilizers
	Precision farming	Remove sensing devices
	Nanofood	

enters the body and influences certain physiological functions (Patil, 2009). Sukul et al. (2009) have reported that potentized drugs significantly increased plant growth, chlorophyll, protein and water content in the leaves as compared to the control. *CCC* 30 (nano) was found to be more effective than *CCC* 30. Potentized drugs are thought to initiate their action on the integral membrane proteins of leaves and modulate cell physiology towards growth. Barik et al. (2008) opined that more ambitious uses of nanoparticles are bio-remediation of contaminated environments, biocides and antifungals on textiles. Research on silkworm, *B. mori* L. race Nistari clearly demonstrates that nanoparticle could stimulate more production of fibroin protein which can help in producing carbon nanotube in future (Bhattacharyya et al., 2008; Bhattacharyya, 2009). The previous highlights the putative effects of nanoparticles on insects, as these small particles are present in their entire body parts. Research on nanoparticles as well their roles in insect control should be geared toward introduction of faster and ecofriendly pesticides in the next decade (Bhattacharyya et al., 2007). It is high time therefore that leading chemical companies to focus on formulation of nanoscale pesticides for delivery into the target host tissue through nanoencapsulation. At present, the toxicological and ecotoxicological risks linked to this expanding technology (emerging technology) cannot be assessed yet. While nanotechnology is increasingly moving into the center of public attention, it is currently not yet linked to any great degree to concerns about health and the environment.

8 Is Nanobio-Farming? A Future of Farming

8.1 Question and Answer

It is important to note that nanomaterials, owing to their increased contact surface area, might have toxic effects that are not apparent in the bulk materials especially in open agricultural ecosystems (Nel et al., 2006). The selection of nanomaterial for application in the field may be critical as materials which are nontoxic, biocompatible, and biodegradable are desirable. Few food and nutrition products that contain nanoscale additives already in the market, such as iron in nutritional drink mixes, micelles that carry vitamins, minerals, and phytochemicals in oil and zinc oxide in breakfast cereals (Hoyt and Mason, 2008).

The future if foreseen would allow the advancements in agricultural nanotechnology to promote "accurate or precision farming" allowing optimum use of the natural resources with judicious farming practices. Different sensor and controlled delivery technologies would change the face of farming. The use of a network of sensors, global positioning system, global information system, and actuators throughout an agricultural area could measure (data and statistics) and report on a number of different environmental, crop, and pest variables. These reports would support the experience of the farmer and permit choices for intervention during irrigation, fertilization, pest control, and even harvesting. Although costly, this would be largely offset by the rising cost of food, the need for higher quality, and increasing legislation. The technology already exists to measure each of these variables. However, measurement requires technical expertise, is labor-intensive and can take days, by which time the opportunity for optimal intervention could be missed. By providing robust, portable, or remote in situ nanotechnology based sensing and monitoring, backed up with analytical software, farmers can begin to make their own informed choices, in real-time, and apply agrochemicals or engage expert help only when necessary.

8.2 Nanosilica—a Novel Nanobiopesticide

In the current context, amorphous nanosilica is a promising new venture. Biodiversity ensures discovery and extraction of new drugs not only for use as human or animal medicines but also as biopesticides for agricultural and domestic use. Those nanosilicas will be absorbed into the cuticular lipid stuffs by physiosorption and thus causing insect death solely by physical resources. Application of nanoparticles on the leaf and stem surface does not alter either photosynthesis or respiration in several groups of horticultural and crop plants (Ragaei and Sabry, 2014). They do not cause alteration of gene expression in insect trachea and are, thus, qualified for approval as the nano-biopesticide in this particular category. To control a range of agricultural insect pests and animal ectoparasites of veterinary importance could use successfully surface charged modified hydrophobic nanosilica (~3–5 nm) for humankind safety (Ulrichs et al., 2005, 2006a,b,c).

Nanoparticles offer a greater surface part and circulate easily and in lepidopteran insects, therefore they are considered special harness stuffs, as well as they will be removed during 24 h from the insect body (Ulrichs et al., 2006c). Lawry (2001) assumed that particles considerably slighter than micron order would be less injurious in the insect hemocoel. In addition, Hui-Peng et al. (2006) confirmed that lipase handling, the only practical option to control BmNPV, interferes in hormonal steadiness and cannot be treated to premolting phase. Plant–stem-derived nanosilica is able to reduce certain classes of lipoproteins found in the hemolymph of silkworm larval. Here, too, infection by nuclear polyhedrosis virus (BmNPV), a scourge in silkworm industry, enhances the level of certain lipids, part of which is reduced by nanosilica. The silkworm model for drug development might be used successfully for controlling other insect and human diseases. In particular, controlling human malaria parasite growth both in vitro and in vivo might be possible (Sharma et al., 1996; Panteghini et al., 2001; Majumder et al., 2006; Ulrichs et al., 2007; Barik et al., 2008; Popat et al., 2012).

9 Conclusions

In this century, rising technologies will face a more skeptical and challenging public—not only must their profits to the public be clear, but scientists must also anticipate and distinguish potential risks related with their accomplishment. In the present case (nanotechnology), those risks surround the possible environmental insinuations of the extensive using of nanomaterials. At the present, nanometerial exposures and health effects are unlikely to pretense any substantial danger to health of the community given the most common contact routes and the partial scope of their use. On the other hand, as the quantity and nanomaterial kinds used in society amplify, the prospective for unintended ecological penalty will also increase. Although it is challenging to evaluate the hazards of engineered nanomaterials before saleable products could be well defined, proactive research is serious to ensure a sustainable nanotechnology production.

In the current agricultural scenario, the extensive use of agrochemicals to boost agricultural production has polluted not only the top soil, but also groundwater. Increasing agricultural productivity is necessary, but keeping in mind the damage to the ecosystem new approaches need to be considered. Nanotechnology is becoming increasingly important for the agricultural sector. Promising results and applications are already being developed in the areas of delivery of pesticides, biopesticides, fertilizers, and genetic material for plant transformation. The use of nanomaterials for delivery of pesticides and fertilizers is expected to reduce the dosage and ensure controlled slow delivery. A main contribution anticipated, is the application of nanoparticles to stabilize biocontrol preparations that will go a long way in reducing the environmental hazard. A major difficulty in the removal of hurtful contaminants from soil was its detection in the field, which was pricey with conventional methods. Nanotechnology, by exploiting the sole properties of nanomaterials, has developed nanosensors able of detecting pathogens at levels as low as parts per billion. Apart from detection, nanotechnology also has solutions for degrading determined chemicals into harmless and sometimes helpful components. Agricultural technology should take advantage of the powerful tools of nanotechnology for the benefit of mankind. The tools of nanotechnology can be employed to address the urgent issues of environmental protection and pollution. Nanotechnology can endeavor to provide and fundamentally streamline the technologies currently used in environmental detection, sensing, and remediation.

Finally, we could say that nanoencapsulation is currently the most promising technology for protection of host plants against insect pests. Thus, nanotechnology will develop agricultural production including pest management in the next few years. Over the next 2 decades, the Green Revolution would be accelerated by nanotechnology means.

References

Abduz Zahir, A., Bagavan, A., Kamaraj, C., Elango, G., Abdul Rahuman, A., 2012. Efficacy of plant-mediated synthesized silver nanoparticles against *Sitophilus oryzae*. J. Biopest. 5, 95–102.

Abracado, L.G., Esquivel, D.M.S., Alves, O.C., Wajnbergo, E., 2005. Magnetic material in head, thorax, and abdomen of *Solenopsis substituta* ants: a ferromagnetic resonance study. J. Magn. Reson. 175, 309–316.

Acosta-Avalos, D., Wajnberg, E., Oliveira, P., Leal, I., Farina, M., Esquivel, D.S., 1999. Isolation of magnetic nanoparticles from *Pachycondyla marginata*. J. Exp. Biol. 202, 2687–2692.

Allard, T., Menguy, N., Salomon, J., Calligaro, T., Weber, T., Calas, G., et al., 2004. Revealing forms of iron in river-borne material from major tropical rivers of the Amazon basin (Brazil). Geochim. Cosmochim. Acta 68, 3079–3094.

Almansa, A., Wogerer, C., Rempp, H., Gebauer, M., 2006. IPMMAN Roadmap for micro- and nano-manufacturing, Version 2. 10 August.

Anonymous, 2009. Nanotechnology and nano science applications: revolution in India and beyond. Strategic Applications Integrating Nano Science. Available from: www.sainsce.com

Ayutsede, J., Gandhi, M., Sukigara, S., Ko, F., 2008. Carbon Nanotube Reinforced *Bombyx mori* Nanofibers by the Electrospinning Process. Materials Research Society, Warrendale, PA, pp. 15086–7573.

Bariana, H.S., Shannon, A.L., Chu, P.W.G., Waterhouse, P.M., 1994. Detection of five seed borne legume viruses in one sensitive multiplex polymerase chain reaction test. Phytopathology 84, 1201–1205.

Barik, T.K., Sahu, B., Swain, V., 2008. Nanosilica—from medicine to pest control. Parasitol. Res. 103, 253–258.

Bhatkhande, D., Pangarkar, V., Beenackers, C., 2001. Photocatalytic degradation for environmental applications—a review. J. Chem. Technol. Biotechnol. 77, 102–116.

Bhattacharyya, A., 2009. Nanoparticles-from drug delivery to insect pest control. Akshar 1, 1–7.

Bhattacharyya, A., Debnath, N., 2008. Nano particles-a futuristic approach in insect population. In: Proceeding on UGC Sponsored National Seminar on Recent Advances in Genetics and Molecular Biology, Biotechnology and Bioinformatics, November 21st and 22nd, 2008. Jointly organized by department of Zoology and Botany, Vidyasagar College, Kolkata, West Bengal, Indian.

Bhattacharyya, A., Barik, B., Kundu, P., Mandal, D.N., Das, A., Sen, P., Rao, C.V., Mandal, S., 2007. Bioactivity of nanoparticles and allelochemicals on stored grain pest-*Sitophilus oryzae* (L) (Coleoptera: Curculionidae). Published in 27th Annual Session of The Academy of Environmental Biology and National Symposium of Biomarkers of Environmental Problems, October 26–28, 2007, Charan Singh University, Meerut, U.P., Indian.

Bhattacharyya, A., Gosh, M., Chinnaswamy, K.P., Sen, P., Barik, B., Kundu, P., Mandal, S., 2008. Nano-particle (allelochemicals) and silkworm physiology. In: Chinnaswamy, K.P., Vijaya Bhaskar Rao, A., (Eds.), In Recent Trends in Seribio-Technology. Bangalore Indian. pp. 58--63.

Bhattacharyya, A., Bhaumik, A., Rani, P.U., Mandal, S., Epidi, T.T., 2010. Nano-particles—a recent approach to insect pest control. Afric. J. Biotechnol. 9, 3489–3493.

Billen, J., 2006. Signal variety and communication in social insects. Proc. Neth. Entomol. Soc. Meet. 17, 9–17.

Binhi, V.N., 2004. Stochastic dynamics of magnetic nanoparticles and a mechanism of biological orientation in the geomagnetic field. arXiv: physics/0412158v1 [physics biol-ph], Moscow, Russia, December 27.

Boehm, A.L., Martinon, I., Zerrouk, R., Rump, E., Fessi, H., 2003. Nanoprecipitation technique for the encapsulation of agrochemical active ingredients. J. Microencapsul. 20, 433–441.

Chambarelli, L.L., Pinho, M.A., Abracado, L.G., Esquivel, D.M.S., Wajnberg, E., 2008. Temporal and preparation effects in the magnetic nanoparticles of *Apis mellifera* body parts. J. Magn. Magn. Mater. 320, 207–210.

Chaudhry, Q., Schroder, P., Werck-Reichhart, D., Grajek, W., Marecik, R., 2002. Prospects and limitations of pytoremediation for the removal of persistent pesticides in the environment. Environ. Sci. Pollut. Res. 4-9, 4–17.

Chinnamuthu, C.R., Boopathi, P.M., 2009. Nanotechnology and agroecosystem. Madras Agric. J. 96, 17–31.

Cho, E.K., Goodman, R.M., 1979. Strains of soybean mosaic virus: classification based on virulence in resistant soybean cultivars. Phytopathology 69, 467–470.

Colvin, V., 2003. The potential environmental impact of engineered nanomaterials. Nat. Biotechnol. 21, 1166–1170.

Corradini, E., Moura, M.R., Mattoso, L.H.C., 2010. A preliminary study of the incorporation of NPK fertilizer into chitosan nanoparticles eXPRESS. Polym. Lett. 4, 509–515.

Dawson, K., 2008. Bionano interactions—a rational approach to the interaction between nanoscale materials and living matter? Nanobioeurope 8, 1–2.

de Oliveira, J.F., Alves, O.C., Esquivel, D.M.S., Wajnberg, E., 2008. Ingested and biomineralized magnetic material in the prey *Neocapritermes opacus* termite: FMR characterization. J. Magn. Reson. 191, 112–119.

Debnath, N., Mitra, S., Das, S., Goswami, A., 2012. Synthesis of surface functionalized silica nanoparticles and their use as entomotoxic nanocides. Powder Technol. 221, 252–256.

DeRosa, M.C., Monreal, C., Schnitzer, M., Walsh, R., Sultan, Y., 2010. Nanotechnology in fertilizers. Nat. Nanotechnol. 5, 91.

Desoil, M., Gillis, P., Gossuin, Y., Pankhurst, Q.A., Hautot, D., 2005. Definitive identification of magnetite nanoparticles in the abdomen of the honeybee *Apis mellifera*. J. Phys. Conf. Ser. 17, 45–49.

Ding, W.K., Shah, N.P., 2009. Effect of various encapsulating materials on the stability of probiotic bacteria. J. Food Sci. 74, M100–M107.

Doorn, R.A., Szemes, M., Bonants, P., Kowalchuk, G.A., Salles, J.F., Ortenberg, E., et al., 2007. Quantitative multiplex detection of plant pathogens using a novel ligation probe based system coupled with universal, high-throughput real-time PCR on Open Arrays™. BMC Genomics 8, 276.

Duebendorf, St. G.T., 2008. How do nanoparticles behave in the environment? NanoEco-Empa organized international meeting on nanoparticles in the environment. Environ. Sci. Technol. Available from: http://pubs.acs.org/cgibin/ asap.cgi/esthag/asap/html/es7029637.html

Ehrlich, H., Janussen, D., Simon, P., Bazhenov, V.V., Shapkin, N.P., Erler, C., Mertig, M., Born, R.E., Heinemann, S., Hanke, T., Worch, H., Vournakis, J.N., 2008. Nanostructural organization of naturally occurring composites-Part II: silica-chitin-based biocomposites. J. Nanomater. 2008, 1–8.

Eijkel, K., Hruby, J., Kubiak, G., Scott, M., Brokaw, J., Saile, V., Walsh, S., White, C., Walsh, D., 2006. Commercial importance of a unit cell: nanolithographic patenting trends for microsystems, microfabrication, and nanotechnology. J. Microlithogr. Microfabr Microsyst. 5 (1), 011014.

Elek, N., Hoffman, R., Raviv, U., Resh, R., Ishaaya, I., Magdassi, S., 2010. Novaluron nanoparticles: Formation and potential use in controlling agricultural insect pests. Coll. Surf. A 372, 66–72.

El-Jaick, L.J., Acosta-Avalos, D., Esquivel, D.M., de, S., Wajnberg, E., Linhares, M.P., 2001. Electron paramagnetic resonance study of honeybee *Apis mellifera* abdomens. Eur. Biophys. J. 29, 579–586.

Esquivel, D.M.S., 2007. Magnetic nanoparticles in social insects: are they the geomagnetic sensors? Entomological Society of America Annual Meeting. December 10, 2007, NO-0574.

Esquivel, D.M.S., Wajnberg, E., Cernicchiaro, G.R., Acosta-Avalos, D., Garcia, B.E., 2002. Magnetic material arrangement in *Apis mellifera* abdomen. Mat. Res. Soc. Symp. Proc. 724, 1–4.

Esquivel, D.M.S., Wajnberg, E., Nascimento, F.S., de Pinho, M.B., Lins de Barros, G.P., Eizemberg, R., 2007. Do geomagnetic storms change the behaviour of the stingless bee guirucu (*Schwarziana qadripunctata*). Naturwissenschaften 94, 139–142.

Farmer, V.C., Adams, M.J., Fraser, A.R., Palmieri, F., 1983. Synthetic imogolite: properties, synthesis and possible applications. Clay Miner. 18, 459–472.

Farre, M.J., Franch, M.I., Ayllon, J.A., Peral, J., Domenech, X., 2007. Biodegradability of treated aqueous solutions of biorecalcitrant pesticides by means of photocatalytic by means of photocatalytic ozonation. Desalnation 211, 22–23.

Feynman, R.P., 1960. There's plenty of room at the bottom. Annual Meeting of the American Physical Society at Caltech and later published in Engineering and Science, 22–36.

Fiorito, S., 2008. Carbon nanotubes: Angels or demons? University La Sapienza Institute of Neurobiology and Molecular Medicine. CNR Rome, Italy.

Fletcher, J., Bender, C., Budowle, B., Cobb, W.T., Gold, S.E., Ishimaru, C.A., et al., 2006. Plant pathogen forensics: capabilities, needs, and recommendations. Microbiol. Mol. Biol. Rev. 70, 450–471.

Frederiksen, H.K., Kristensen, H.G., Pedersen, M., 2003. Solid lipid microparticle formulations of the pyrethroid gamma-cyhalothrin-incompatibility of the lipid and the pyrethroid and biological properties of the formulations. J. Control Release 86, 243–252.

Froggett, S., 2009. Nanotechnology and agricultural trade. In: OECD Conference on the Potential Environmental Benefits of Nanotechnology: Fostering Safe Innovation-Led Growth.

Fu, Z., Liu, H., Yang, Z., Ju, H., 2007. Recent developments in multianalyte immunoassay. Curr. Trends Biotechnol. Pharm. 1, 1–17.

Gabaldon, J.A., Maquieira, A., Puchades, R., 1999. Current trends in immunoassay based kits for pesticide analysis. Crit. Rev. Food Sci. Nutr. 39, 519–538.

Gajbhiye, M., Kesharwani, J., Ingle, A., Gade, A., Rai, M., 2009. Fungus mediated synthesis of silver nanoparticles and its activity against pathogenic fungi in combination of fluconazole. Nanomedicine 5, 282–286.

Gan, N., Yang, X., Xie, D., Wu, Y., Wen, W.A., 2010. Disposable organophosphorus pesticides enzyme biosensor based on magnetic composite nanoparticles modified screen printed carbon electrode. Sensors 10, 625–638.

Gao, X., Jackson, T.A., Lambert, K.M., Li, S., Hartman, G.L., Niblack, T.L., 2004. Detection and quantification of *Fusarium solani* f. sp. *glycines* with real-time quantitative polymerase chain reaction. Plant Dis. 88, 1372–1380.

Garboczi, E.J., 2009. Concrete nanoscience and nanotechnology: Definitions and applications. In : Bittnar, Z., Bartos, P.J.M., Nemecek, J., Smilauer, V., Zeman, J. (Eds.), Nanotechnology in construction: proceedings of the NICOM3 (3rd International Symposium Nanotechnology in Construction). Prague, Czech Republic p. 81–88.

Gha-Young, K., Joonmok, S., Min-Su, K., Seung-Hyeon, M., 2008. Preparation of a highly sensitive enzyme electrode using gold nanoparticles for measurement of pesticides at the ppt level. J. Environ. Monit. 10, 632–637.

Ghormade, V., Deshpande, M.V., Paknikar, K.M., 2011. Perspectives for nano-biotechnology enabled protection and nutrition of plants. Biotechnol. Advan. 29, 792–803.

Ghormade, V., Gholap, H., Kale, S., Kulkarni, V., Bhat, S., Paknikar, K.M., 2015. Fluorescent cadmium telluride quantum dots embedded chitosan nanoparticles: a stable, biocompatible preparation for bio-imaging. J. Biomater. Sci. Polym. Ed. 26, 42–56.

Giasuddin, A.B.M., Kanel, S.R., Choi, H., 2007. Adsorption of humic acid onto nanoscale zerovalent iron and its effect on arsenic removal. Environ. Sci. Technol. 41, 2022–2027.

Goldwasser, Y., Eizenberg, H., Golan, S., Kleifeld, Y., 2003. Control of *Orobanche crenata* and *Orobanche aegyptiaca* in parsley. Crop Prot. 22, 295–305.

Gorb, E.V., Gorb, S.N., 2009. Contact mechanics at the insect-plant interface: how do insects stick and how do plants prevent this? In: Borodich, F.M. (Ed.),

IUTAM Sympos. Scaling in Solid Mechanics, IUTAM Bookseries. Springer Science and Business Media B.V, p. 243.

Goswami, A., Roy, I., Sengupta, S., Debnath, N., 2010. Novel applications of solid and liquid formulations of nanoparticles pests and pathogens. Thin Solid Films 519, 1252–1257.

ETC Group, 2004. Down on the farm :impact of nano-scale technologies on food and agriculture.2004. Available from: http://www.etcgroup.org/upload/publication/80/02/etcdotfarm2004.pdf

Guan, H., Chi, D., Yu, J., Li, X., 2008. A novel photodegradable insecticide: preparation, characterization and properties evaluation of nano-imidacloprid pesticide. Biochem. Physiol. 92, 83–91.

Guo, Y.R., Liu, S.H., Gui, W.J., Zhu, G.N., 2009. Gold immune-chromatographic assay for simultaneous detection of carbofuran and triazophos in water samples. Anal. Biochem. 389, 32–39.

Hager, H., 2011. Nanotechnology in agriculture. Available from: http://www.topcropmanager.com/

Hee Joo, S.h, Cheng, I.F., 2006. Nanotechnology for environmental remediation. Springer, USA.

Hoffmann, M.R., Martin, S.T., Choi, W., Bahnemann, D.W., 1995. Environmental applications of semiconductor photocatalysis. Chem. Rev. 95, 69–96.

Hoyt, V.W., Mason, E., 2008. Nanotechnology emerging health issues. J. Chem. Health Saf. 15, 10–15.

Hsu, C.Y., Ko, F.Y., Li, C.W., Fann, K., Lue, J.T., 2007. Magnetoreception system in honeybees (*Apis mellifera*). PLoS One 2, 1–11.

Huck, W.T.S., 2008. Responsive polymers for nanoscale actuation. Mater. Today 11, 24–32.

Hui-Peng, Y., Xiao-Feng, W., Gokulamma, K., 2006. Antiviral activity in the mulberry silkworm *Bombyx mori* (L.). J. Zhejiang Univ. Sci. A. 2, 350–356.

Ishay, J.S., Barkay, Z., Eliaz, N., Plotkin, M., Volynchik, S., Bergman, D.J., 2008. Gravity orientation in social wasp comb cells (Vespinae) and the possible role of embedded minerals. Naturwissenschaften 95, 333–342.

Jain, R.K., McKern, N.M., Tolin, S.A., Hill, J.H., Barnett, O.W., Tosic, M., et al., 1992. Confirmation that fourteen potyvirus isolates from soybean are strains of one virus by comparing coat protein peptide profiles. Phytopathology 82, 294–299.

Jin, H.J., Chen, J., Karageorgiou, V., Altman, G.H., Kaplan, D.L., 2004. Human bone marrow stromal cell responses on electrospun silk fibroin mats. Biomaterials 25, 1039–1047.

Joel, D.M., 2000. The long-term approach to parasitic weeds control: manipulation of specific developmental mechanisms of the parasite. Crop Prot. 19, 753–758.

Joel, D.M., Hershenhorn, J., Eizenberg, H., Aly, R., Ejeta, G., Rich, P.J., et al., 2007. Biology and management of weedy root parasites. Hort. Rev. 33, 267–349.

Jones, P., 2006. A nanotech revolution in agriculture and the food industry. Information Systems for Biotechnology. Available from: http://www.isb.vt.edu/articles/jun0605.htm

Joseph, T., Morrison M., 2006. Nanotechnology in agriculture and food. A nanoforum report, Institute of Nanotechnology, May 2006. Available from: www.nanoforum.org.

Joshi, K.A., Tang, J., Haddon, R., Wang, J., Chen, W., Mulchandani, A., 2005. A disposable biosensor for organophosphorus nerve agents based on carbon nanotubes modified thick film strip electrode. Electroanalysis 17, 54–58.

Jurado-Expósito, M., Castejón-Muñoz, M., García-Torres, L., 1996. Broomrape (*Orobanche crenata*) control with imazethapyr applied to pea (*Pisum sativum*) seed. Weed Technol. 10, 774–780.

Jurado-Expósito, M., García-Torres, L., Castejón-Muñoz, M., 1997. Broadbean and lentil seed treatments with imidazolines for the control of broomrape (*Orobanche crenata*). J. Agr. Sci. 129, 307–314.
Kaushik, A., Solanki, P.R., Ansarib, A.A., Malhotra, B.D., Ahmad, S., 2009. Iron oxide-chitosan hybrid nanobiocomposite based nucleic acid sensor for pyrethroid detection. Biochem. Eng. J. 46, 132–140.
Kim, J., Grate, J.W., Wang, P., 2006. Nanostructures for enzyme stabilization. Chem. Engineer. Sci. 61, 1017–1026.
Kostoff, R.N., Schaller, R.R., 2001. Science and technology roadmaps. IEEE Trans. Eng. Manage. 48, 132–143.
Kostoff, R.N., Shlesinger, M.F., 2005. CAB: citation-assisted background. Scientometrics 62, 199–212.
Kostoff, R.N., Boylan, R., Simons, G.R., 2004. Disruptive technology roadmaps. Technol. Forecast. Soc. Change 71, 141–159.
Kostoff, R.N., Murday, J., Lau, C., Tolles, W., 2006. The seminal literature of global nanotechnology research. J. Nanopart. Res. 8, 193–213.
Kostoff, R.N., Koytcheff, R.G., Lau, C.G.Y., 2007. Global nanotechnology research literature overview. Technol. Forecast. Soc. Change 74, 1733–1747.
Kricka, L.J., 1992. Multianalyte testing. Clin. Chem. 38, 327–328.
Kumar, R., 2009. Nanotechnology in Agriculture. G.B. Pant University of Agriculture and Technology, Pantnagar, Uttrakhand.
Kuzma, J.R., VerHage P., 2006. Nanotechnology in agriculture and food production: anticipated applications. Project on emerging nanotechnologies, One Woodrow Wilson Plaza 1300 Pennsylvania Avenue, N.W. Washington, DC 20004-3027.
Lai, F., Wissing, S.A., Müller, R.H., Fadda, A.M., 2006. *Artemisia arborescens* L. essential oil-loaded solid lipid nanoparticles for potential agricultural application: preparation and characterization. AAPS Pharm. Sci. Tech. 7, 1–9.
Lam, C.W., James, J.T., McCluskey, R., Hunter, R.L., 2004. Pulmonary toxicity of single-wall carbon nanotubes in mice 7 and 90 days after intratracheal instillation. Toxicol. Sci. 77, 126–134.
Lawry, J.V., 2001. Insects separate diffusing particles in parallel. Nanotech. Model. Simul. Microsyst. 1, 254–257.
Li, Z.Z., Chen, J.F., Liu, F., Liu, A.Q., Wang, Q., Sun, H.Y., et al., 2007. Study of UV-shielding properties of novel porous hollow silica nanoparticle carriers for avermectin. Pest Manag. Sci. 63, 241–246.
Linton, J.D., 2004. Determining demand, supply, and pricing for emerging markets based on disruptive process technologies. Technol. Forecast. Soc. Change 71, 105–120.
Lisa, M., Chouhan, R.S., Vinayaka, A.C., Manonmani, H.K., Thakur, M.S., 2009. Gold nanoparticles based dipstick immuno-assay for the rapid detection of dichlorodiphenyltrichloroethane: an organochlorine pesticide. Biosens. Bioelectron. 25, 224–227.
Lister, R.M., 1978. Application of the enzyme-linked immunosorbent assay for detecting viruses in soybean seed and plants. Phytopathology 68, 1393–1400.
Liu, X.Y., Du, N., 2004. Zero-sized effect of nano-particles and inverse homogeneous nucleation. J. Biol. Chem. 279, 6124–6131.
Liu, Y., Yan, I., Heiden, P., Laks, P., 2001. Use of nanoparticles for controlled release of biocides in solid wood. J. Appl. Polym. Sci. 79, 458–465.
Liu, F., Wen, L.X., Li, Z.Z., Yu, W., Sun, H.Y., Chen, J.F., 2006. Porous hollow silica nanoparticles as controlled delivery system for water soluble pesticide. Mat. Res. Bull. 41, 2268–2275.
Liu, J., Wang, F.H., Wang, L.L., Xiao, S.Y., Tong, C.Y., Tang, D.Y., et al., 2008. Preparation of fluorescence starch-nanoparticle and its application as plant transgenic vehicle. J. Cent. South Univ. Technol. 15, 768–773.

López-Ráez, J.A., Matusova, R., Cardoso, C., Jamil, M., Charnikhova, T., Kohlen, W., et al., 2009. Strigolactones: ecological significance and use as a target for parasitic plant control. Pest Manag. Sci. 65, 471–477.

Lucano, M.J., Cernicchiaro, G., Wajnberg, E., Esquivel, D.M.S., 2006. Stingless bee antennae: a magnetic sensory organ? Biol. Metals. 19, 225–343.

Majumder, D., Banerjee, R., Ulrichs, C., Mewis, I., Samanta, A., Das, A., Mukhopadhayay, S., Adhikary, S., Goswami, A., 2006. Nanofabricated materials in cancer treatment and agri-biotech applications: buckyballs in quantum holy grails. IETE J. Res. 52, 339–356, (Special Issue: Nano-electronic devices and technology).

Moraru, C.I., Panchapakesan, C.P., Qingrong, H., Takhistov, P., Sean, L., Kokini, J.L., 2003. Nanotechnology: a new frontier in food science. Food Technol. 57, 24–29.

Mousavi, S.E., Rezaei, M., 2011. Nanotechnology in agriculture and food production. J. Appl. Environ. Biol. Sci. 1, 414–419.

Neethirajan, S., Gordon, R., Wang, L., 2009. Potential of silica bodies (phytoliths) for nanotechnology. Trends Biotechnol. 27, 461–467.

Nel, A., Xia, T., Madler, L., Li, N., 2006. Toxic potential of materials at the nanolevel. Science 311, 622–627.

Nowack, B., 2009. Is anything out there? What life cycle perspectives of nano-products can tell us about nanoparticles in the environment? Nano Today 4, 11–12.

Oberdorster, G., Sharp, Z., Atudorei, V., Elder, A., Gelein, R., Kreyling, W., Cox, C., 2004. Translocation of inhaled ultrafine particles to the brain. Inhal. Toxicol. 16, 437–445.

Oberdorster, G., Oberdorster, E., Oberdorster, J., 2005. Nanotoxicology: an emerging discipline evolving from studies of ultrafine particles. Environ. Health Perspect. 113, 823–839.

Owolade, O.F., Ogunleti, D.O., Adenekan, M.O., 2008. Titanium Dioxide affects disease development and yield of edible cowpea. EJEAF Chem. 7, 2942–2947.

Paknikar, K.M., Nagpal, V., Pethkar, A.V., Rajwade, J.M., 2005. Degradation of lindane from aqueous solutions using iron sulfide nanoparticles stabilized by biopolymers. Sci. Tech. Adv. Mat. 6, 370–374.

Palmer, A.G., Chena, M.C., Kinger, N.P., Lynn, D.G., 2009. Parasitic angiosperms, semagenesis and general strategies for plant–plant signalling in the rhizosphere. Pest Manag. Sci. 65, 512–519.

Panteghini, M., Ceriotti, F., Schumann, G., Siekmann, L., 2001. Establishing a reference system in clinical enzymology. Clin. Chem. Lab. Med. 39, 795–800.

Patil, S.A., 2009. Economics of agri poverty: nano-bio solutions. Indian Agric. Res. Institute, New Delhi, Indian.

Pérez-de-Luque, A., Rubiales, D., 2009. Nanotechnology for parasitic plant control. Pest Manag. Sci. 65, 540–545.

Phaal, R., Farrukh, C.J.P., Probert, D.R., 2004. Technology roadmapping—a planning framework for evolution and revolution. Technol. Forecast. Soc. Change 71, 5–26.

Popat, A., Liu, J., Hu, Q.H., et al., 2012. Adsorption and release of biocides with mesoporous silica nanoparticles. Nanoscale 4, 970–975.

Predicala, B., 2009. Nanotechnology: potential for agriculture. Prairie Swine Centre Inc., University of Saskatchewan, Saskatoon, SK, 123–134.

Ragaei, M., Sabry, A.H., 2014. Nanotechnology for insect pest control. Internat. J. Sci. Environ. Technol. 3, 528–545.

Rai, M., Ingle, A., 2012. Role of nanotechnology in agriculture with special reference to management of insect pests. Appl. Microbiol. Biotechnol. 94, 287–293.

Ramanathan, M., Luckarift, H.R., Sarsenova, A., Wild, J.R., Ramanculov, E.R., Olsen, E.V., et al., 2009. Lysozyme-mediated formation of protein–silica nanocomposites for biosensing applications. Colloid. Surf B 73, 58–64.
Rao, G.V., Tinkle, S., Weissman, D.N., Antonini, J.M., Kashon, M.L., Salmen, R., Battelli, L.A., Willard, P.A., Hoover, M.D., Hubbs, A.F., 2003. Efficacy of a technique for exposing the mouse lung to particles aspirated from the pharynx. J. Toxicol. Environ. Health A. 66, 1441–1452.
Royal Society and the Royal Academy of Engineering, 2004. Nanoscience and nanotechnologies: Opportunities and uncertainties. Royal Society and Royal Academy of Engineering, London, UK, 116 pp.
Sahayaraj, K., 2014. Nanotechnology and plant biopesticides: an overview. In advances in plant *Biopesticides* (pp. 279–293). Springer India.
Sanchez, F., Sobolev, K., 2010. Nanotechnology in concrete—a review. Constr. Build. Mater. 24, 2060–2071.
Sanguansri, P., Augustin, M.A., 2006. Nanoscale materials development—a food industry perspective. Trends Food Sci. Technol. 17, 547–556.
Sasson, Y., Levy-Ruso, G., Toledano, O., Ishaaya, I., 2007. Nanosuspensions: emerging novel agrochemical formulations. In: Ishaaya, I., Nauen, R., Horowitz, A.R. (Eds.), Insecticides Design Using Advanced Technologies. Springer-Verlag, Netherlands, pp. 1–32.
Schaad, N.W., Opgennorth, D., Gaush, P., 2002. Real-time polymerase chain reaction for one-hour on-site diagnosis of Pierce's disease of grape in early season asymptomatic vines. Phytopathology 92, 721–728.
Scott, N.R., 2007. Nanotechnology opportunities in agriculture and food systems. Biological and Environmental Engineering, Cornell University NSF Nanoscale Science and Engineering Grantees Conference December 5, 2007, Arlington, VA.
Scott, N., Chen, H., 2003. Nanoscale science and engineering for agriculture and food systems. A report submitted to cooperative state research, education and extension service, USDA, National Planning Workshop, Washington.
Scrinis, G., 2006a. Nanotechnology and the Environment: the nano-atomic reconstruction of nature. Chain React. 97, 23–26.
Scrinis, G., 2006b. When small isn't beautiful. Arena Magazine 83, 38–40.
Scrinis, G., Lyons, K., 2007. The emerging nano-corporate paradigm: nanotechnology and the transformation of nature, food and agri-food systems. Internat. J. Sociol. Food Agric. 15, 22–44.
Scrivener, K.L., Kirkpatrick, R.J., 2008. Innovation in use and research on cementitious material. Cem. Concr. Res. 38, 128–136.
Sharma, S., Goswami, A., Singh, N.J., Kabilan, L., Deodhar, S.S., 1996. Immunogenicity of the nonrepetitive regions of the circumsporozoite protein of *Plasmodium knowlesi*. Am. J. Trop. Med. Hyg. 55, 635–641.
Sharon, M., Choudhary, A.K., Kumar, R., 2010. Nanotechnology in agricultural diseases and food safety. J. Phytol. 2, 83–92.
Slowik, T.J., Green, B.L., Thorvilson, H.G., 1998. Detection of magnetism in the red imported fire ant (*Solenopsis invicta*) using magneticresonance imaging. Bioelectromagnetics 18, 396–399.
Stadler, T., Buteler, M., Weaver, D.K., 2010. Novel use of nanostructured alumina as an insecticide. Pest Manag. Sci. 66, 577–579.
Stephenson, G.R., 2003. Pesticide use and world food production: risks and benefits. In: Coats, J.R., Yamamoto, H. (Eds.), Environmental fate and effects of pesticides. ACS Symposium Series, Washington, 853, pp. 261–270.
Sukul, N.C., Singh, R.K., Sukul, (Chunari) S., Sen, P., Bhattacharyya, A., Sukul, A., Chakrabarty, R., 2009. Potentized drugs enhance growth of *Pigeon pea*. Environ. Ecol. 26, 1115–1118.

Susha, V.S., Chinnamuthu, C. R., Pandian, K., 2009. Remediation of herbicide atrazine through metal nano particle. Proceedings of International Conference on Magnetic Materials and their Applications in the 21st Century, October 21–23, 2008. Organized by the Magnetic Society of India, National Physical Laboratory, New Delhi.

Tai Kai, N.G., 2008. Structural analysis of crystalline and nanocrystalline materials. In Proc. of Dept of Physics, The Hong Kong University of Science and Technology, Clear Water Bay, Kowloon, Hong Kong.

Thomas, K., Sayre, P., 2005. Research strategies for safety evaluation of nanomaterials, part I: evaluating the human health implications of exposure to nanoscale materials. Toxicol. Sci. 87, 316–321.

Tilman, D., Cassman, K.G., Matson, P.A., Naylor, R., Polasky, S., 2002. Agricultural sustainability and intensive production practices. Nature 418, 671–677.

Torney, F. 2009. Nanoparticle mediated plant transformation. Emerging technologies in plant science research Interdepartmental Plant Physiology Major Fall Seminar Series. Physics, p. 696.

Torney, F., Trewyn, B.G., Lin, V.S., Wang, K., 2007. Mesoporous silica nanoparticles deliver DNA and chemicals into plants. Nat. Nanotechnol. 2, 295–300.

Tsuji, K., 2001. Microencapsulation of pesticides and their improved handling safety. J. Microencapsul. 18, 137–147.

Uddin, W., Viji, G., Schumann, G.L., Boyd, S.H., 2003. Detection of *Pyricularia grisea* causing gray leaf spot of perennial ryegrass turf by a rapid immuno-recognition assay. Plant Dis. 87, 772–778.

Ulrichs, C., Mewis, I., Goswami, A., 2005. Crop diversification aiming nutritional security in West Bengal—biotechnology of stinging capsules in nature's water-blooms. Annual Technical Issue of State Agriculture Technologists Service Association. pp. 1–18.

Ulrichs, C., Mewis, I., Goswami, A., Chatterjee, S.D., Banerjee, S.P., Adhikary, S., Bhattacharyya, A., 2006a. Biodiversity-Macro and micro: to be nano or not to be! Everyman's Science 11, 433–443.

Ulrichs, C., Entenmann, S., Goswami, A., Mewis, I., 2006b. Abrasive und hydrophil/lipophile Effekte unterschiedlicher inerter Stäube IM Einsatz gegen Schadinsekten am Beispiel des Kornkäfers *Sitophilus granarius* L. Gesunde Pflanze 58, 173–181.

Ulrichs, C., Krause, F., Rocksch, T., Goswami, A., Mewis, I., 2006c. Electrostatic application of inert silica dust based insecticides onto plant surfaces. Commun. Agric. Appl. Biol. Sci. 71, 171–178.

Ulrichs, C., Goswami, A., Mewis, I., 2007. Nano-structured silica-physical active pesticides for urban settings. In: Proceedings of the second international symposium on plant protection and plant health in Europe, DPG-BCPC, Berlin, May 10–12, 2007.

Vandergheynst, J., Scher, H., Guo, H.Y., Schultz, D., 2007. Water-in-oil emulsions that improve the storage and delivery of the biolarvacide *Lagenidium giganteum*. BioControl 52, 207–229.

Vidhyalakshmi, R., Bhakyaraj, R., Subhasree, R.S., 2009. Encapsulation "The Future of Probiotics"—a review. Adv. Biol. Res. 3, 96–103.

Vijayakumar, P.S., Abhilash, O.U., Khan, B.M., Prasad, B.L.V., 2010. Nanogold-loaded sharp-edged carbon bullets as plant-gene carriers. Adv. Funct. Mater. 20, 2416–2423.

Vinayaka, A.C., Basheer, S., Thakur, M.S., 2009. Bioconjugation of CdTe quantum dot for the detection of 2,4-dichlorophenoxyacetic acid by competitive fluoroimmunoassay based biosensor. Biosens. Bioelectron. 24, 1615–1620.

Vurro, M., Boari, A., Evidente, A., Andolfi, A., Zermane, N., 2009. Natural metabolites for parasitic weed management. Pest Manag. Sci. 65, 466–471.

Wajnberg, E., Cernicchiaro, G., Souza, D.M., de Esquivel, D.M.S., 2004. Antennae: the strongest magnetic part of the migratory ant. Bio. Metals 17, 467–470.
Walsh, S.T., 2004. Road mapping a disruptive technology: a case study-the emerging microsystems and top-down nanosystems industry. Technol. Forecast. Soc. Change 71, 161–185.
Wang, X., Wang, Y., Xiong, X., Li, T., Liang, J., Chen, J., 2004. Aqueous nano insecticide suspension and its preparation process. Chem. Abs. 142, 213751.
Wang, L., Li, Z., Zhang, G., Dong, J., Eastoe, J., 2007. Oil-in-water nanoemulsions for pesticide formulations. J. Colloid Interface Sci. 314, 230–235.
Wang, H., Wang, J., Choi, D., Tang, Z., Wu, H., Lin, Y., 2009. EQCM immunoassay for phosphorylated acetylcholinesterase as a biomarker for organophosphate exposures based on selective zirconia adsorption and enzyme-catalytic precipitation. Biosens. Bioelectron. 24, 2377–2383.
Warheit, D.B., Laurence, B.R., Reed, K.L., Roach, D.H., Reynolds, G.A., Webb, T.R., 2004. Comparative pulmonary toxicity assessment of single-wall carbon nanotubes in rats. Toxicol. Sci. 77, 117–125.
Watson, G.S., Watson, J.A., 2004. Natural nano-structures in insectspossible functions of ordered arrays characterized by atomic force microscopy. Appl. Surface Sci. 235, 139–144.
Waychunas, G.A., Kim, C.S., Banfield, J.F., 2005. Nanoparticulate iron oxide minerals in soils and sediments: unique properties and contaminant scavenging mechanisms. J. Nanopart. Res. 7, 409–433.
Weiss, J., Takhistov, P., McClements, J., 2006. Functional materials in food nanotechnology. J. Food Sci. 71, 107–116.
Wilkinson, J., 2002. Genetically modified organisms, organics and the contested construction of demand in the agrofood system. Internat. J. Sociol. Agric. Food 10, 3–11.
Wilson, M.A., Tran, N.H., Milev, A.S., Kannangara, G.S.K., Volk, H., Lu, G.H.M., 2008. Nanomaterials in soils. Geoderma 146, 291–302.
Yang, L., Watts, D.J., 2005. Particle surface characteristics may play an important role in phytotoxicity of alumina nanoparticles. Toxicol. Lett. 158, 122–132.
Yang, F.L., Li, S.G., Zhu, F., Lei, C.L., 2009. Structural characterization of nanoparticles loaded with garlic essential oil and their insecticidal activity against *Tribolium castaneum* (Herbst) (Coleoptera: Tenebrionidae). J. Agric. Food Chem. 57, 10156–10162.
Ying, J.Y., 2009. Nanobiomaterials. Nano Today 4, 1–2.
Yuen, G.Y., Xia, J.Q., Sutula, C.L., 1998. A sensitive ELISA for *Pythium ultimum* using polyclonal and species-specific monoclonal antibodies. Plant Dis. 82, 1029–1032.
Zhang, W.X., 2003. Nanoscale iron particles for environmental remediation: an overview. J. Nanopart. Res. 5, 323–332.
Zhang, J., Liu, Z., 2006. Cicada wings: a stamp from nature for nanoimprint. Lithography 2, 1440–1443.
Zhang, Y.Q., Shen, W.D., Xiang, R.L., Lan-Jian Zhuge, L.J., Gao, W.J., Wang, W.B., 2007. Formation of silk fibroin nanoparticles in water-miscible organic solvent and their characterization. J. Nanopart. Res. 9, 885–900.
Zhang, X., Zhang, J., Zhu, K.Y., 2010. Chitosan/double-stranded RNA nanoparticle-mediated RNA interference to silence chitin synthase genes through larval feeding in the African malaria mosquito (*Anopheles gambiae*). Insect Mol. Biol. 19, 683–693.
Zhao, X., Hilliard, L.R., Mechery, S.J., Wang, Y., Bagwe, R.P., Jin, S.A., 2004. Rapid bioassay for single bacterial cell quantitation using bioconjugated nanoparticles. Proc. Natl. Acad. Sci. 101, 15027–15032.

8

BOTANICAL PESTICIDES WITH VIRUCIDAL, BACTERICIDAL, AND FUNGICIDAL ACTIVITY

Luminita Marutescu, Marcela Popa*, Crina Saviuc*, Veronica Lazar**, Mariana Carmen Chifiriuc****

**Research Institute of the University of Bucharest-ICUB, Bucharest, Romania; **Faculty of Biology and Research Institute of the University of Bucharest - ICUB, University of Bucharest, Bucharest, Romania*

1 Introduction

Botanical pesticides belong to the category of biopesticides, and are defined as naturally occurring or derived materials from living organisms used for the pest control. Biopesticides include microbial products active against microbial and viral pests, biochemical, nontoxic compounds derived from different organisms (insects, plants, pheromones, etc.), and genetically modified plants incorporating protectants.

The advantages of biopesticides are that they are less toxic, prone to rapid biodegradation, are more targeted to a specific pest, exhibiting a specific mode of action and rather manage than eradicate, thus maintaining the ecological balance. However, they also have disadvantages as compared to conventional pesticides because they have a short shelf-life and therefore a limited field persistence, have a much narrower spectrum and a slower killing rate (Steinwand, 2008; O'Brien et al., 2009). Therefore, currently, there is much interest in the development of new pesticides both efficient, and also fulfilling the safety requirements for food security and human health (Diallo et al., 2011; Hynes et al., 2008).

Isolation of ethnobotanical biologically active substances has been a continuous concern of chemistry since its beginning, the first biologically active substances being the alkaloids. Depending on the chemical properties of the active compounds, several methods have been developed for obtaining them: (1) aqueous extracts (cold maceration at ambient temperature for 2–12 h, with

New Pesticides and Soil Sensors. http://dx.doi.org/10.1016/B978-0-12-804299-1.00009-6

periodic stirring, followed by filtration and immediate use; decoction is used for plant materials with hard consistency, such as roots, rhizomes, bark, some fruits, and seeds and consists in heating the minced plant material covered with a sufficient amount of water for 15–30 min on slow fire filtration while hot; infusion allows extraction from flower or other fragile plant parts, such as leaves, buds, aerial parts, and consists in adding boiled hot water over the minced vegetal material in a cover pot for 10–30 min, wherein the active substances of plant material pass into infusion, the obtained filtrate being used within 24 h); (2) hydroalcoholic extracts or tinctures are obtained without heating the active ingredients as compared to the corresponding aqueous extracts (Ionescu, 2014). However, despite their long history going back to ancient times, the use of plant extracts in agriculture stopped around the 1950s, due to the emergence and widespread use of synthetic insecticides manufactured at relatively low cost and industrial scale (Luko and Mora, 2006; Khan et al., 2013b).

Essential oils (EOs) or their major compounds, alone or in different combinations, as well as alcoholic or water plant extracts are widely used as biopesticides, some of them being classified as class II, III, or IV repellents, used as fumingants, antiquorum sensing agents, and so on. The existent scientific studies suggest that the plant organisms and derived compounds could represent valuable resources for the development of novel biopesticides formulations (Cervantes-Ceballos et al., 2015).

The plant extract and oils are included in the category of biochemical biopesticides, besides insect pheromones, plant growth regulators, and insect growth regulators. The second category of biopesticides is represented by the microbial pesticides, including the bacterial, fungal, viral, and other microbial biopesticides.

Compared to insect pheromones, the plant extracts and oils are highly diverse mixtures or compounds derived from plants, with a larger spectrum of target pests and mechanisms of action. Plant extracts and oils are most often used as insecticides, and also as herbicides. Products made from plant extracts and oils can be regulated as biopesticides or conventional pesticides depending on their mode of action and level of toxicity.

The active ingredient can be represented by a single molecule or a mixture of naturally occuring molecules or a synthetic analog to the naturally occurring substance. However, it must be taken into account that some phtyocompounds are not included in the category of biopesticides, but in that of conventional pesticides, due to their high toxicity (e.g., D-limonene), even though the containing EOs (citrus), are regulated as biopesticides (O'Brien et al., 2009).

In this chapter we will refer to the plant-derived biopesticides with activity against viral, bacterial, and fungal pests.

2 Plant Origin Pesticides: Antimicrobial Secondary Metabolites

Defense responses orchestrated by the plants' innate immunity before or after the contact with pathogen elicitors, include the phytoalexin and phytoanticipin production, secondary metabolites arresting the spread of pathogens (González-Lamothe et al., 2009). Some secondary metabolites of plant origin have been identified as potential chemotherapeutants in plant protection, that is, phenolics, terpenoids, and EOs, alkaloids, lectins, and polypeptides. However, the utilization of plant extracts as botanical pesticides is still limited by several factors, such as extraction methods standardization, stability and/or formulation of the active ingredient, complexity of the extracted mixture, and the difficulties in the purification steps, resistance development under selective pressure (Dwijendra, 2014; Bardin et al., 2015). On the other hand, nanotechnology applications in formulating, and the improvement of the techniques for identification and dosing of active compounds favored the expanding concerns for the use of botanical pesticides (Dwijendra, 2014). Nowadays, plant parts, such as fruit, leaf, bark, seed, and stem extracts have been used for synthesis of nanoparticles, as effective formulations for the phytopathogens control (Paulkumar et al., 2014).

2.1 Phenolics

As expected for natural compounds, plant phenolics are a wide group of substances (there are more than 8000 currently known phenolics) characterized by the presence of the hydroxyl radical. Their presentation is as conjugates, linked with mono- or oligosacharides, and according to the nature of the aglycone and the linker atom are classified as: simple phenolics or benzoquinones (C6), hydroxybenzoic acids (C6–C1), phenylacetic acids (C6–C2), phenylpropanoids (C6–C3), naphtoquinones (C6–C4), xanthones(C6–C1–C6), antraquinones (C6–C2–C6), flavonoids (C6–C3–C6), lignans (C6–C3), biflavonoids $(C6–C3–C6)_2$, tannins $(C6–C3–C6)_n$. This phenolics list from simple to complex reinforces the idea of structural diversity correlated with differrent oxidation state, degree of hydroxylation, and chirality centers, explaining their multiple biological properties (Balasundram et al., 2006). The activity of particular phenolic compounds depends on their structural diversity, acting as phytoalexins, or phytoanticipins altering the microbial cell coatings by interaction with membrane proteins, causing structural and functional impairment (Pusztahelyi et al., 2015; Mandal et al., 2010).

Different extraction procedures could be applied on fresh, frozen, or dried plants to obtain phenolics ubiquitous distributed in all their organs. Current pretreatment steps include milling, grinding, and homogenization of the samples, with direct impact on the quality and quantity of extracted compounds (Dai and Mumper, 2010; Abascal et al., 2005; Asami et al., 2003). However, there are no general procedures for extracting all types of phenolics. They could be optimized in terms of temperature, solvent and extraction method, taking into account the solubility and physicochemical properties of the extracted compounds. Solvent selection varies in a limited range, namely methanol, ethanol, acetone, ethyl acetate, and water, single or mixture of solvents being used, especially organic:water combinations with different polarities. Acidic pH of the solvent mixture could yield to a better solubility, stabilizing compounds, such as anthocyanin (Asami et al., 2003).

Some phenolic compounds associated with the antimicrobial activities from plants could be cited, that is, *simple phenolics*—coumarin and cathecol; *stilbenoids*—resveratrol; *phenolic acids*—gallic, *p*-coumaric, pherulic, sinapic, caffeic acid; *flavonoids*—catechin, naringerin, quercetin, rutin (Maddox et al., 2010). Due to their chemical diversity it is a difficult task to select and present general methods for obtaining and characterizing phenolics, but looking to the conjugated double and aromatic bonds, one could state that all phenolics exhibit a degree of UV absorbtion. However, hyphenated techniques, modern high-performance chromatographic techniques combined with instrumental analysis are the "state of the art" for the profiling and quantification of phenolic compounds (Dai and Mumper, 2010).

2.2 Alkaloids

Alkaloids are widely distributed in species belonging to several families within angiosperms. They are versatile heterocyclic nitrogen compounds with reported antimicrobial activity against fungal or bacterial phytopathogens. Furoquinoline alkaloids, quinolizidine alkaloid extracts, isoquinoline alkaloids (corynoline and acetylcorynoline), pyrrolizidine alkaloids have been mentioned as active compounds (Joosten and van Veen, 2011; Pérez-Laínez et al., 2008). The multitarget mechanisms of action are represented by the outer membrane or cytoplasmic membrane disruption, respiratory inhibition, the Z-ring perturbation, and nucleic acid synthesis/cell division inhibition (Bardin et al., 2015; Cushnie et al., 2014).

2.3 Essential Oils

Plant disease management with EOs has been applied as one of the ecofriendly controls. Plant EOs exhibit different levels of antimicrobial efficacies to various ranges of plant fungal or bacterial pathogens and they efficiently reduced the major diseases in crops (Hong et al., 2015). In fact, all the EOs have antimicrobial activity, in a concentration-dependent manner (Hammer and Carson, 2011). There are some specific constraints regarding the efficacy of the EOs as biopesticides. They require greater application rates (active ingredient or combination of actives in small quantity in the complex mixture) and may require frequent reapplication when used as out-of-door materials (Opender et al., 2008). The final product formulation as ready to use, as well as extraction yields could be limiting factors (Hüsnü can Başer and Buchbauer, 2009). Few processes have been described for the EOs formulation as biopesticides: chemical processes—molecular inclusion or interfacial polymerization; physicochemical techniques—coacervation and liposome encapsulation; physical processes—spray drying, spray chilling, or cooling, cocrystallization, extrusion, or fluidized-bed coating (Nollet and Singh Rathore, 2015).

EOs are obtained exclusively by physical methods (pressing, distillation, extraction simple, or continuous), using the whole plant or specific organs. Identification of constituents of EOs are recommended to be performed by chromatographic techniques, and their constituents belong to several classes of substances: (1) monoterpene hydrocarbons; (2) phenol and methyl ethers; (3) monoterpene alcohols; (4) sesquiterpene lactones; (5) monoterpene aldehydes and ketones; (6) ethers; (7) monoterpene oxides; (8) phthalides. Concerning the mechanism of antimicrobial action, a cascade of events, debuting with cellular coatings disruption and based on the mixture/compound lipophilicity, could be accepted.

2.4 Lectins and Polypeptides

Cationic peptides belonging to several classes of compounds, defensins, cathelicidins, and thrombocidins, have been described as antimicrobial molecules, and used as templates for drug discovery (Wimley and Hristova, 2011). Key features have been accepted for the antimicrobial peptides from plants belonging to different families, that is, the high content of cysteine and/or glycine, the presence of disulfide bridges, enhancing structural stability under stress conditions, and the positive charging of the amino acids, like arginine and/or lysine, and also the aspartic and glutamic acids. The interaction of the peptides with the microbial cells involves formation of membrane pores and future events, such as ion and metabolite leakage, depolarization, interruption of the respiratory processes, and cell death (Nawrot et al., 2014). It should be mentioned that antimicrobial peptides and proteins all have unique features, reflecting in specific protocols for extraction and purification of these molecules, also having common biochemical characteristics, such as low molecular mass (10 kDa), which may facilitate purification by size exclusion techniques, the positive charging, thus being separable from anionic species that comprise the majority of all proteins (Schaffer, 1997).

Lectins are clusters of glycoproteins that recognize specifically and bond reversibly to carbohydrates, mainly by the sugar moiety of glycoconjugates (Peumans and Van Damme, 1995; Ingale and Hivrale, 2013). The best-characterized family of plant lectins are Fabaceae, Poaceae, and Solanaceae; especially some of leguminous seeds have a remarkable amount of lectin. The lectin–carbohydrate recognition could result in cell agglutination and precipitation of glycoconjugates in vitro. Their specific interaction with carbohydrates is also involved in their antimicrobial role—preventing the bacterial adhesion/penetration into the host cell cytoplasm, blocking the movement of the motile bacteria, or inhibiting virulence features in bacteria. However, natural resistance to lectins was mentioned in virulent *Pseudomonas solanacearum* strains, that escaped for the specific lectin mediated recognition, and infected potato plants (Ingale and Hivrale, 2013).

3 Biopesticides With Activity Against Viral, Bacterial, and Fungal Pests

Viruses are always potentially pathogenic to the host, altering the cellular physiological activity. The viral pathogenicity is quantitatively expressed by viral virulence, which is a multifactorial property defining the ability of a virus to multiply, disseminate in the organism, successfully compete with the effect or immune response and produce pathological effects. Viral virulence is dependent on the number of sensitive cells and on the intensity and complexity of the host defense reactions, which cause elimination and inactivation of the virus and/or infected cells. Viruses with cytolytic (cytocidal) effects are extremely virulent, while the transformant ones have a moderate virulence (temperate viruses). In the infected cells, the accumulated viral components cause structural, biochemical, and functional changes. Sometimes, a hyperacute cytotoxic effect due to cell death before viral replication without progeny virus production can occur. In this case, cell death is the result of a toxic effect of viral proteins (Mihaescu et al., 2007).

Viral infections in plants (e.g., barley yellow dwarf, brome mosaic, soilborne wheat mosaic, wheat streak mosaic, tobacco mosaic, tomato bushy stunt, cucumber mosaic) are difficult to treat due to the fact that the host does not exhibit specific symptoms, the lesions being often mistaken with other physiological disorders or genetic diseases. Moreover, the transmission ways are very diverse, including soil, biological, and mechanical vectors. Total aqueous and ethanolic extracts, as well as isolated compounds, alone (flavonoids, terpenoids, pehnols) or in combinations have been demonstrated to exhibit inhibitory activity against plant viruses (Table 8.1).

Table 8.1 Botanical Biopesticides With Antiviral Activity

Plant Extract/Compound	Plant Species	Pest Species	References
Flavonoid quercetagetin 3′-methylether	*Centaurea rupestris* L.	Tomato bushy stunt virus	Rusak et al. (1997)
Callus	*Phytolacca americana*	Tobacco mosaic virus	Misawa et al. (1975)
Limonene, 1,8-cineole, and α-zingiberene/EOs, extracted from Chinese indigenous aromatic plants	Ginger, lemon, tea tree, tangerine peel, *Artemisia*, lemongrass	Tobacco mosaic virus	Lu et al. (2013)
Oxygenated sesquiterpene alpha-bisabolol	*Micromeria graeca*, Komiza	Satellite-associated cucumber mosaic virus	Vuko et al. (2012)
Beta-caryophyllene and caryophyllene oxide/EO	*Teucrium arduini* L.	Tobacco mosaic virus, cucumber mosaic virus	Dunkić et al. (2011)
Sesquiterpene hydrocarbons β-caryophyllen, germacrene D, β-pinene, α-pinene/EOs	*Teucrium polium*, *T. flavum*, *T. montanum*, *T. chamaedrys*	Cucumber mosaic virus	Bezić et al. (2011)
Tababiphenyls	*Nicotiana tabacum*	Tobacco mosaic virus	Shang et al. (2014)
Organic extracts Aqueous and ethanolic extracts Aqueous and ethanolic extracts	*Lessonia trabeculata* *Gracillaria chilensis* *Durvillaea antarctica*	Tobacco mosaic virus	Jiménez et al. (2011)

Bacterial plant pathogens (bacterial stripe, basal glume rot, bacterial spike blight) are spread by air, water, mechanical, or biological vectors. Transmission and infection are favored by moist environments and by the existence of previous tissue lesions. Stomatal openings can also be used for infection and penetration. After infection, such pathogens invade the vascular system or the intercellular spaces in host tissue; express their virulence potential by producing toxins or other enzymes leading to the tissue necrosis. Necrosis results from toxins produced or enzymatic activity of the bacteria (Table 8.2).

Table 8.2 Botanical Biopesticides With Antibacterial Activity

Plant Extract/Compound	Plant Species	Pest Species	References
Caffeine		*Ralstonia solanacearum, Clavibacter michiganesis* subsp. *Sepedonicus, Dickeya solani, Pectobacterium* (atrosepticum), *Pectobacterium carotovorum* subsp. (carotovorum), *Pseudomonas syringae* pv. tomato, *Xanthomonas campestris* subsp. campestri	Sledz et al. (2015)
Carvacrol, eugenol, terpineol, alpha-pinene		*Candidatus Phytoplasma mali*	Aldaghi et al. (2008)
Eugenol emulsion/EOs		*X. campestris* pv. phaseoli var. *Fuscans*	Lo Cantore et al. (2009)
Wastewaters from alpeorujo oil extraction	*Alpeorujo*	*Erwinia* spp., *Pseudomonas* spp., and *Clavibacter* spp.	Medina et al. (2011)
Antimicrobial peptide	*Apuleia leiocarpa*	*X. campestris*	Carvalho Ade et al. (2015)
Glucosinolates and glucosinolate hydrolysis products and leaf methanolic extracts of different GSL-enriched	*Brassica*	*X. campestris* pv. *campestris* and *P. syringae* pv. *maculicola* scletoriorum	Sotelo et al. (2015)

Table 8.2 Botanical Biopesticides With Antibacterial Activity (*cont.*)

Plant Extract/Compound	Plant Species	Pest Species	References
Glucosinolates (gsls), secondary metabolites found in *Brassica* vegetables	*Brassica*	*X. campestris* pv. *campestris*, *P. syringae* pv. *maculicola*	Sotelo et al. (2015)
Sap	*Calendula suffruticosa*	*P. syringae*, *P. fluorescens*, *X. campestris*, *Agrobacterium tumefaciens*	Radioza and Iurchak (2007)
Cytisine	*Calia secundiflora* (Ortega) Yakovlev (Fabaceae)	*Pseudomonas* sp., *X. campestris*, *Erwinia carotovora*	Pérez-Laínez et al. (2008)
EO components, coumarins, flavonoids, phenolic acids, and fatty acids	Chamomile	*P. syringae* pv. *maculicola*	Móricz et al. (2013)
EOs	*Cuminum cyminum* L. and *Carum carvi* L.	*Clavibacter*, *Curtobacterium*, *Rhodococcus*, *Erwinia*, *Xanthomonas*, *Ralstonia*, *Agrobacterium*	Iacobellis et al. (2005)
Invertase inhibitory protein	*Cyphomandra betacea*	*X. campestris* pvar. *vesicatoria*, *Pseudomonas solanacearum*, *Pseudomonas corrugata*, *P. syringae* pv. *Syringae*, *Erwinia carotovora* var. *carotovora*	Ordóñez et al. (2006)
Invertase inhibitory proteins	*C. betacea* Sendt. *Solanum tuberosum*	*X. campestris* pvar. *vesicatoria*, *Pseudomonas solanacearum*, *P. corrugata*, *P. syringae*, and *Erwinia carotovora* var *carotovora*	Isla et al. (2002)
Plant hairpin-like defense polypeptide	*Echinochloa crusgalli* L.	Phytopathogenic bacteria	Ryazantsev et al. (2013)
Fragarin	*Fragaria*	*Clavibacter michiganensis*	Filippone et al. (2013)
Antimicrobial proteins	*Hordeum vulgare* *Zea mays*	*C. michiganensis* subsp. *sepedonicus* *Pseudomonas solanacearum*	Molina et al. (1993)

(*Continued*)

Table 8.2 Botanical Biopesticides With Antibacterial Activity (*cont.*)

Plant Extract/Compound	Plant Species	Pest Species	References
Apigenin, 3,8′-biapigenin, quercetin, kaempferol, and linolenic acid	*Hypericum perforatum*	*P. syringae* pv. *maculicola*, *X. campestris* pv. *vesicatoria*	Jesionek et al. (2015a)
Honokiol and magnolol	*Magnolia dealbata*	*Clavibacter michiganensis* subsp. *michiganensis*	Jacobo-Salcedo Mdel et al. (2011)
Deoxymikanolide, scandenolide, dihydroscandenolide, mikanolide, dihydromikanolide, and *m*-methoxy benzoic acid	*Mikania micrantha*	*R. solanacearum*, *Xanthomonas oryzae* pv. *oryzae*, *X. campestris* pv. *Vesicatoria*, *X. campestris* pv. *citri*	Li et al. (2013)
Methanol, acetone, ethyl acetate, and petroleum spirit extracts	*Nymphaea nouchali*	*X. campestris*	Dash et al. (2013)
Limonin and imperatorin	*Poncirus trifoliata* Rafin	*Xanthomonas* spp.	Rahman et al. (2014)
Aqueous extracts	*Pyrus* spp.	*Erwinia amylovora*	Jin and Sato (2003)
Cationic peptide	*Robinia pseudoacacia*	*Corynebacterium michiganense*, *Erwinia carotovora* subsp. *Carotovora*, *P. syringae* pv *syringae*, *X. campestris* pv. *campestris*	Talas-Og˘ras¸ et al. (2005)
EOs (α-pinene, α-phellandrene, and D-limonene)	*Schinus terebinthifolius* *Schinus molle*	*Colletotrichum acutatum* and *Botrytis cinerea* *Bacillus megaterium*, *Bacillus mojavensis*, *Clavibacter michiganensis* *Escherichia coli*, *X. campestris*, *Pseudomonas savastanoi*, *and P. syringae* pv. *Phaseolicola*	Elshafie et al. (2010, 2016)
7,8-Dihdroxy-6-[3′-beta-D-glucopyranosyloxy-2′(xi)-hydroxy-3′-methylbutyl]-coumarin, 6-(2,3-dihydroxy-3-methylbutyl)-7-methoxycoumarin, skimmin, osthol, esculetin, and scopuletin	*Skimmia anquetelia* (Rutaceae)	*Agrobacterium tumefaciens*, *P. syringae*, *Pactobacterium carotovorum*	Sharma et al. (2008)

Table 8.2 Botanical Biopesticides With Antibacterial Activity (*cont.*)

Plant Extract/Compound	Plant Species	Pest Species	References
A 5-kDa polypeptide, pseudothionin	*Solanum tuberosum* L.	*Pseudomonas solanacearum*	Moreno et al. (1994)
Antimicrobial peptide Snakin-1	*S. tuberosum* L.	*Clavibacter michiganense* subsp. sepedonicus	Segura et al. (1999)
Potide-G	*S. tuberosum* L.	*C. michiganense* subsp. Michiganinse *Rhizoctonia solani*	Kim et al. (2005)
Trypsin-chymotrypsin protease inhibitor	*S. tuberosum* L.	*C. michiganense* subsp. Michiganinse *Rhizoctonia solani*	Segura et al. (1998)
Antimicrobial peptide	*Spinacia oleracea* cv. matador	*C. michiganensis*, *R. solanacearum*	Purnavab et al. (2015)
EO [α-pinene (25.769%) and myrcene (12.507)] and methanolic extract [sinapic acid (15.553 mg/g) and eugenol (6.805 mg/g)]	*T. polium*	*R. solanacearum*, *Pantoea agglomerans*, *Brennaria nigrifluens*	Ordóñez et al. (2011)
2′,4′-Dihydroxychalcone	*Tucumán propolis*	*Erwinia carotovora* spp. *carotovora*, *P. syringae* pvar. tomato, *P. corrugata*, *X. campestris* pvar vesicatoria	Körpe et al. (2013)
Methanol and aqueous extracts	*Urtica dioica* L. *Urtica pilulifera* L.	*C. michiganensis* *Xanthomonas vesicatoria*	Duvick et al. (1992)
Antimicrobial proteins	*Z. mays*	*C. michiganense* ssp. Nebraskense	Jesionek et al. (2015b)
Apigenin and α-linolenic acid	*Matricaria recutita* L. and *Achillea millefolium* L.	*P. syringae* pv. Maculicola, *X. campestis* pv. vesicatoria	Soberón et al. (2014)
Flavonol mono- and diglycosides, and gallic acid	*Ligaria cuneifolia* *Jodina rhombifolia*	*P. syringae*	Soberón et al. (2014)
Petroleum ether and ethyl acetate extracts	*Viola yedoensis*, *V. Prionantha*, *Corydalis bungeana*, and *Gueldenstaedtia verna*	*P. syringae*	Xie et al. (2004)

(*Continued*)

Table 8.2 Botanical Biopesticides With Antibacterial Activity (*cont.*)

Plant Extract/Compound	Plant Species	Pest Species	References
Plant extracts	*Feronia limonia, Xanthium strumarium, Glossocardia bosvellia*	*X. campestris*	Mehta et al. (1983)
Culture filtrates of six different edible mushroom species	*Hericium erinaceus, Lentinula edodes Grifola frondosa,* and *Hypsizygus marmoreus*	*Pectobacterium carotovorum* subsp. *Carotovorum, Agrobacterium tumefaciens, R. solanacearum, Xanthomonas oryzae* pv. *oryzae, X. campestris* pv. *campestris, X. Axonopodis* pv. *vesicatoria, X. Axonopodis* pv. *citiri,* and *X. axonopodis* pv. glycine	
Ethyl acetate, methanol, cold water, and boiling water extracts	*Coccinia adoensis, Cineraria grandiflora, Pavonia urens, Marattia fraxinea, Clutia abyssinica* var. *Usambarica,* and *Vangueria infausta*	*Candida albicans, Aspergillus fumigatus, Fusarium culmorum, Staphylococcus aureus, P. syringae, Erwinia amylovora*	de Boer et al. (2005)

Fungal diseases in plant are very diverse and affecting all parts of the plant, that is, crown (e.g., common root rot, crown rot, sclerotium wilt), stem or sheath (e.g., eyespot, stem rust), leaves (e.g., leaf blight, rust, powdery mildew), spikes (e.g., ergot), and seeds (e.g., black point, carnal bunt) (Table 8.3).

4 Conclusions

The chemical diversity and lack of or reduced secondary effects justify the enhancement of the research efforts for developing alternative biological control means, more efficient and safer than chemical pesticides, in conformity with the current EU regulations (Lynch, 1995; Manole et al., 2005). Efforts should be directed for the identification and purification of the efficient compounds, which can be further used alone or in various mixtures to obtain commercially available formulations for agricultural

Table 8.3 Botanical Biopesticides With Antifungal Activity

	Plant Species	Pest Species	References
Dehydroeffusol (18–21 μg/mL)	*Juncus effusus* L. Medulla	*Venturia ineaqualis, Phytophthora infestans, Plasmopara viticola*	Thuerig et al. (2015)
Oxygenated monoterpene	*Citrus aurantium* L.		Metoui et al. (2015)
Grape marc extract		*Phytophthora parasitica* var. Nicotianae	Benouaret and Goupil (2015)
5-Methylmellein	*Biscogniauxia mediterranea*	*Phomopsis obscurans*	Silva-Hughes et al. (2015)
Fatty acids methyl esters, lupeol, and naphthoquinones, such as lapachol, α-lapachone, naphtho[2,3-*b*]furan-4,9-dione, 2-isopropyl- and avicenol-C (1 and 1.5 mg/mL)	*Avicennia schaueriana*	*Cladosporium sphaerospermum, Cladosporium cladosporioides, Colletotrichum lagenarium*	Fardin and Young (2015)
O-Methylcapaurine	*Zanthoxylum rhoifolium*	*B. cinerea, Sclerotinia sclerotiorum, A. alternata, Colletotrichum gloeosporioides, Clonostachys rosea*	Carotenuto et al. (2015)
5-*n*-Alkylresorcinol	*Triticum* spp.	*Fusarium graminearum, Fusarium culmorum, Fusarium avenaceum, Fusarium poae*	Ciccoritti et al. (2015)
Prosapogenins	*Medicago sativa*	*Pyricularia oryzae*	Abbruscato et al. (2014)
Ellagitannin	*Euphorbia antisyphilitica* (*E. antisyphilitica*)	*A. alternata, Fusarium oxyzporum, Colletotrichum gloeosporoides, Rhizoctnia solani*	Ascacio-Valdés et al. (2013)
Cadinan-3-ene-2,7-dione, 7-hydroxycadinan-3-ene-2-one, 5,6-dihydroxycadinan-3-ene-2,7-dione, cadinan-3,6-diene-2,7-dione and 2-acetyl-cadinan-3,6-diene-7-one	*Eupatorium adenophorum*	*Rhizoctonia solani Sclerotium rolfsii*	Kundu et al. (2013)

(*Continued*)

Table 8.3 Botanical Biopesticides With Antifungal Activity (*cont.*)

	Plant Species	Pest Species	References
Petroleum ether extracts and chloroformic extract	*Inula viscosa*, *Asteriscus graveolens*, *Bubonium odorum*, *Thymus leptobotrys*, and *Anvillea radiata*	*Penicillium italicum*	Askarne et al. (2013)
Curcumin, demethoxycurcumin, and bisdemethoxy-curcumin(30 μm)	*Curcuma longa*	*Phomopsis obscurans*, *Phomopsis viticola*	
Erythro-(7R,8R)-Δ(8′)-4,7-dihydroxy-3,3′,5′-trimethoxy-8-O-4′-neolignan, erythro-(7R,8R)-Δ8′-7-acetoxy-3,4,3′,5′-tetra-methoxy-8-O-4′-neolignan, and 5-hydroxy-eugenol(>30 μm)	*Myristica*	*P. obscurans*, *P. viticola*	
Pullulan coatings containing meadowsweet flowers	*Filipendula ulmaria*	*Rhizopus arrhizus*	Synowiec et al. (2014)
Wightianines A–E/methanolic extract of *Parnassia wightiana* (0.78 μg/mL)	*Parnassia wightiana*	*Cytospora* sp.	Wang et al. (2014)
Mixtures of isorhamnetin/dunnione/kaempferol/ferulic/gallic acid in various combinations MFC: 10–50 μg/mL Quercetin MIC: 15 μg/mL	*Calceolaria integrifolia*	*Aspergillus niger*, *Fusarium moniliforme*, *Fusarium sporotrichum*, *Rhizoctonia solani*, and *Trichophyton mentagrophytes*	Céspedes et al. (2014)
Volatile sulfur compounds derived from garlic (*Allium sativum*) extracts	*A. sativum*	*B. cinerea*	Gándara-Ledezma et al. (2015)
7-hydroxycalamenene (MIC: 19.53–2500 μg/mL)	*Croton cajucara*	*Absidia cylindrospora*, *Cunninghamella elegans*, *Mucor circinelloides*, *Mucor circinelloides* f. Circinelloides, *Mucor mucedo*, *Mucor plumbeus*, *Mucor ramosissimus*, *Rhizopus microsporus*, *Rhizopus oryzae*, and *Syncephalastrum racemosum*	Azevedo et al. (2014)

Table 8.3 Botanical Biopesticides With Antifungal Activity (*cont.*)

	Plant Species	Pest Species	References
Aliphatic and aromatic isothiocyanates/hydrated dry Brassicaceae shoot tissues	Brassicaceae	*Aphanomyces euteiches*	Hossain et al. (2014)
Pseudolaric acid A, ethyl pseudolaric acid B, pseudolaric acid B, pseudolaric acid B-O-β-D-glucoside, piperonylic acid, propionic acid, 3-hydroxy-4-methoxybenzoic acid, and 4-(3-formyl-5-methoxyphenyl) butanoic acid/ethanol extracts of *Cortex pseudolaricis* (5 μg/mL)	*Cortex pseudolaricis*	*Colletotrichum gloeosporioides*	Zhang et al. (2014)
Medicinal plant extracts *Adhatoda vasica, Eucalyptus globulus, Lantana camara, Nerium oleander,* and *Ocimum basilicum*		*Fusarium oxysporum* f. Sp. Lycopersici race 3	Isaac and Abu-Tahon (2014)
Plant latex extracts containing alkaloids, flavonoids, glycosides, phenols, saponins, steroids, tannins, and terpenoids	*Thevetia peruviana, Artocarpus heterophyllus, Manilkara zapota*	*Aspergillus fumigatus, A. niger, A. terreus, F. solani, P.digitatum, R. arrhizus*	Sibi et al. (2013)
Methanolic extracts	*Asparagus stipularis, Cyperus capitatus, Stipagrostis lanata*	*Alternaria solani, Aspergillus niger, Rhizopus stolonifer*	Maswada and Abdallah (2013)
Citronella oil		*A. alternata*	Chen et al. (2014)
B-Sitosterol and β-sitosteryl linoleate misc of 250 and 500 μg/mL	*Anadenanthera colubrina*	*A. alternata*	Campos et al. (2014)
EO of *Melaleuca alternifolia*, EO of *Syzygium aromaticum* and extract from *Mimosa tenuiflora*	*Melaleuca alternifolia, Syzygium aromaticum, Mimosa tenuiflora*	*A. alternata, B. cinerea,* and *F. oxysporum* f. Sp. Lycopersici (races 1 and 2)	La Torre et al. (2014)
Alliospiroside A (ALA) and alliospiroside B/*n*-butanol extract of *Allium cepa*	*N*-butanol extract of *A. cepa*	*C. gloeosporioides*	Teshima et al. (2013)

(*Continued*)

Table 8.3 Botanical Biopesticides With Antifungal Activity (*cont.*)

	Plant Species	Pest Species	References
Methanolic extract	*Desmodium elegans*	*F. solani*	Khan et al. (2013a)
Ampelopsin A, hopeaphenol, trans-resveratrol, ampelopsin H, ε-viniferin, and E-vitisin B/methanolic and ethanolic crude extracts of canes	*Vitis vinifera*	*Plasmopara viticola, Erysiphe necator, B. cinerea*	Schnee et al. (2013)
Methanol extracts (0.156–1.25 mg/mL)	*Cistus villosus, Ceratonia siliqua, Halimium umbellatum*	*Geotrichum candidum*	Talibi et al. (2012)
EOs (0.05–0.11 μg/mL)	*A. cepa* L., *A. sativum*	*Aspergillus versicolor*	Kocić-Tanackov et al. (2012)
4-Hydroxy-5,6-dimethoxynaphthalene-2-carbaldehyde, 12,13-didehydro-20,29-dihydrobetulin, 7-methyljuglone, diospyrin, isodiospyrin, shinanolone, lupeol, betulin, betulinic acid, betulinaldehyde, and ursolic acid	*Diospyros virginiana*	*Colletotrichum fragariae, C. gloeosporioides, C. acutatum, B. cinerea, F. oxysporum, Phomopsis obscurans, P. viticola*	Wang et al. (2011a)
7(2E)-4(4,5-dihydro-3-methylene-2-oxo-5-furanyl)-3-methylbut-2-enyloxy) coumarin	*Clausena excavata*	*Rhizoctonia solani* and *S. sclerotiorum*	Kumar et al. (2011)
Squamocin, squamocin-G, and squamostatin-A	*Annona squamosa*	*Phytophthora infestans, Puccinia recondita*	Dang et al. (2011)
Ethanol extracts	*Armoracia rusticana* and *A. sativum* L.	*Sclerotium rolfsii* Sacc., *F. oxysporum Schlecht.*, and *F. culmorum* (Wm.G. Sm) Sacc. *B. cinerea* Pers., *S. rolfsii*	Tedeschi et al. (2011)
Organic extracts Aqueous and ethanolic extracts Aqueous and ethanolic extracts	*Lessonia trabeculata* *Gracillaria chilensis* *Durvillaea antarctica*	*B. cinerea* *Phytophthora cinnamomi* Tobacco mosaic virus (TMV) in tobacco leaves	Jiménez et al. (2011)
Garden cress seed, pomegranate peel, and olive leaf extracts		*Aspergillus flavus* and *A. ochraceus*	Tayel et al. (2011)

Table 8.3 Botanical Biopesticides With Antifungal Activity (*cont.*)

	Plant Species	Pest Species	References
Isothiocyanates	Brassicaceae (*Brassica juncea*, *B. carinata*, *B. nigra*, and *Sinapis* spp.)	*S. sclerotiorum*	Kurt et al. (2011)
Antifungal protein CkTLP	*Cynanchum komarovii*	*Verticillium dahliae*, *F. oxysporum*, *Rhizoctonia solani*, *B. cinerea*, *Valsa mali*	Wang et al. (2011b)
Hexane, ethyl acetate, and methanol extracts	*Parmelia reticulata*	*Sclerotium rolfsii*, *Rhizoctonia solani*, *R. bataticola*, *Fusarium udum*, *Pythium aphanidermatum*, *P. debaryanum*	Goel et al. (2011)
Ethanol extract	*Solanum nigrum*	*Alternaria brassicicola*	Lin et al. (2011)
Ursane-type triterpene saponins (30 μm)	*Zygophyllum coccineum* L.	*Phomopsis viticola*	Amin et al. (2011)
Volatile oil	*Atractylodes lancea*	*Rhodotorula glutinis* and *Saprolegnia*, *Rhizopus*, *Absidia*, *Trichoderma viride*, *Aspergillus niger*	Wang et al. (2009)
EOs	*Zataria multiflora*, *Thymus migricus*, *Satureja hortensis*, *Foeniculum vulgare*, *Carum capticum*	*Aspergillus* sp.	Alizadeh et al. (2010)
Ethanolic plant extract	*Glycyrrhiza glabra*	*Phytophthora infestans* *Pseudoperonospora cubensis* *Podosphaera xanthii* *Uromyces appendiculatus*	
EOs (α-pinene, α-phellandrene, and D-limonene)	*Schinus terebinthifolius* *Schinus molle*	*Colletotrichum acutatum and B. cinerea* *Bacillus megaterium*, *Bacillus mojavensis* and *Clavibacter michiganensis* *Escherichia coli*, *Xanthomonas campestris*, *Pseudomonas savastanoi*, *Pseudomonas syringae* pv. *Phaseolicola*	Elshafie et al. (2016)

(*Continued*)

Table 8.3 Botanical Biopesticides With Antifungal Activity (*cont.*)

	Plant Species	Pest Species	References
Dimeric sesquiterpene (mics = 1–32 μg/mL)	*Chloranthus henryi* Hemsl.	*Alternaria kikuchiana*, *B. cinerea*, *Colletotrichum lagenarium*, *Magnaporthe grisea*, *Pythium ultimum*, *Phytophthora infestans*	Lee et al. (2009)
Dichloromethane extract	*Euphorbia helioscopia* L. (Euphorbiaceae)	*F. solani*	Uzair et al. (2009)

use (Luko and Mora, 2006; Oerke et al., 1994; Răbonțu, 2010). To achieve this goal, several steps must be followed, that is, the identification of the most appropriate plant organ(s) and methods that will be used for the extraction, isolation, identification, and characterization of the active compounds with good yields, followed by the demonstration of the biological effects of the obtained bioproducts and finally their certification for use in agriculture (Lenteren, 2003). Also, elucidating the biosynthesis metabolic pathways will be of great interest for the development of new biotechnologies. Moreover, the knowledge of their specific mechanisms of action and targets will greatly help to establish synergistic or antagonistic associations.

References

Abascal, K., Ganora, L., Yarnell, E., 2005. The effect of freeze-drying and its implications for botanical medicine: a review. Phytother. Res. 19, 655–660.

Abbruscato, P., Tosi, S., Crispino, L., Biazzi, E., Menin, B., Picco, A.M., Pecetti, L., Avato, P., Tava, A., 2014. Triterpenoid glycosides from *Medicago sativa* as antifungal agents against *Pyricularia oryzae*. J Agric Food Chem. 62 (46), 11030–11036.

Aldaghi, M., Massart, S., Druart, P., Bertaccini, A., Jijakli, M.H., Lepoivre, P., 2008. Preliminary evaluation of antimicrobial activity of some chemicals on in vitro apple shoots infected by "*Candidatus phytoplasma* mali". Commun. Agric. Appl. Biol. Sci. 73 (2), 335–341.

Alizadeh, A., Zamani, E., Sharaifi, R., Javan-Nikkhah, M., Nazari, S., 2010. Antifungal activity of some essential oils against toxigenic *Aspergillus* species. Commun. Agric. Appl. Biol. Sci. 75 (4), 761–767.

Amin, E., El-Hawary, S.S., Fathy, M.M., Mohammed, R., Ali, Z., Tabanca, N., Wedge, D.E., Becnel, J.J., Khan, I.A., 2011. Triterpenoidal saponins: bioactive secondary metabolites from *Zygophyllum coccineum*. Planta Med. 77 (5), 488–491.

Asami, D.K., Hong, Y.J., Barrett, D.M., Mitchell, A.E., 2003. Comparison of the total phenolic and ascorbic acid content of freeze-dried and air-dried marionberry, strawberry, and corn grown using conventional, organic, and sustainable agricultural practices. J. Agric. Food Chem. 51, 1237–1241.

Ascacio-Valdés, J., Burboa, E., Aguilera-Carbo, A.F., Aparicio, M., Pérez-Schmidt, R., Rodríguez, R., Aguilar, C.N., 2013. Antifungal ellagitannin isolated from *Euphorbia antisyphilitica* Zucc. Asian Pac. J. Trop. Biomed. 3 (1), 41–46.

Askarne, L., Talibi, I., Boubaker, H., Boudyach, E.H., Msanda, F., Saadi, B., Ait Ben Aoumar, A., 2013. Use of Moroccan medicinal plant extracts as botanical fungicide against citrus blue mould. Lett. Appl. Microbiol. 56 (1), 37–43.

Azevedo, M.M., Almeida, C.A., Chaves, F.C., Campos-Takaki, G.M., Rozental, S., Bizzo, H.R., Alviano, C.S., Alviano, D.S., 2014. Effects of 7-hydroxycalamenene isolated from Croton cajucara essential oil on growth, lipid content and ultrastructural aspects of *Rhizopus oryzae*. Planta Med. 80 (7), 550–556.

Balasundram, N., Sundram, K., Samman, S., 2006. Phenolic compounds in plants and agri-industrial by-products: antioxidant activity, occurrence, and potential uses. Food Chem. 99, 191–203.

Bardin, M., Ajouz, S., Comby, M., 2015. Is the efficacy of biological control against plant diseases likely to be more durable than that of chemical pesticides? Front. Plant Sci. 6, 566.

Benouaret, R., Goupil, P., 2015. Grape Marc extract-induced defense reactions and protection against *Phytophthora parasitica* are impaired in NahG tobacco plants. J. Agric. Food Chem. 63 (30), 6653–6659.

Bezić, N., Vuko, E., Dunkić, V., Ruščić, M., Blažević, I., Burčul, F., 2011. Antiphytoviral activity of sesquiterpene-rich essential oils from four croatian teucrium species. Molecules 16 (9), 8119–8129.

Campos, V.A., Perina, F.J., Alves, E., Sartorelli, J., Moura, A.M., Oliveira, D.F., 2014. *Anadenanthera colubrina* (Vell.) Brenan produces steroidal substances that are active against *Alternaria alternata* (Fr.) Keissler and that may bind to oxysterol-binding proteins. Pest Manag. Sci. 70 (12), 1815–1822.

Carotenuto, G., Carrieri, R., Tarantino, P., Alfieri, M., Leone, A., De Tommasi, N., Lahoz, E., 2015. Fungistatic activity of *Zanthoxylum rhoifolium* Lam. bark extracts against fungal plant pathogens and investigation on mechanism of action in *Botrytis cinerea*. Nat Prod Res. 29 (23), 2251–2255.

Carvalho Ade, S., da Silva, M.V., Gomes, F.S., Paiva, P.M., Malafaia, C.B., da Silva, T.D., Vaz, A.F., da Silva, A.G., Arruda, I.R., Napoleão, T.H., Carneiro-da-Cunha, M.d., Correia, M.T., 2015. Purification, characterization and antibacterial potential of a lectin isolated from *Apuleia leiocarpa* seeds. Int. J. Biol. Macromol. 75, 402–408.

Cervantes-Ceballos, L., Caballero-Gallardo, K., Olivero-Verbel, J., 2015. Repellent and anti-quorum sensing activity of six aromatic plants occurring in Colombia. Nat. Prod. Commun. 10 (10), 1753–1757.

Céspedes, C.L., Salazar, J.R., Ariza-Castolo, A., Yamaguchi, L., Avila, J.G., Aqueveque, P., Kubo, I., Alarcón, J., 2014. Biopesticides from plants: *Calceolaria integrifolia* s.l. Environ. Res. 132, 391–406.

Chen, Q., Xu, S., Wu, T., Guo, J., Sha, S., Zheng, X., Yu, T., 2014. Effect of citronella essential oil on the inhibition of postharvest *Alternaria alternata* in cherry tomato. J. Sci. Food Agric. 94 (12), 2441–2447.

Ciccoritti, R., Pasquini, M., Sgrulletta, D., Nocente, F., 2015. Effect of 5-n-alkylresorcinol extracts from durum wheat whole grain on the growth of fusarium head blight (FHB) causal agents. J. Agric. Food Chem. 63 (1), 43–50.

Cushnie, T.P.T., Cushnie, B., Lamb, A.J., 2014. Alkaloids: an overview of their antibacterial, antibiotic-enhancing and antivirulence activities. Int. J. Antimicrob. Agents. 44 (5), 377–386.

Dai, J., Mumper, R., 2010. Plant phenolics: extraction, analysis and their antioxidant and anticancer properties. Molecules 15, 7313–7352.

Dang, Q.L., Kim, W.K., Nguyen, C.M., Choi, Y.H., Choi, G.J., Jang, K.S., Park, M.S., Lim, C.H., Luu, N.H., Kim, J.C., 2011. Nematicidal and antifungal activities of annonaceous acetogenins from *Annona squamosa* against various plant pathogens. J. Agric. Food Chem. 59 (20), 11160–11167.

Dash, B.K., Sen, M.K., Alam, K., Hossain, K., Islam, R., Banu, N.A., Rahman, S., Jamal, A.H., 2013. Antibacterial activity of *Nymphaea nouchali* (Burm. f) flower. Ann. Clin. Microbiol. Antimicrob. 12, 27.

de Boer, H.J., Kool, A., Broberg, A., Mziray, W.R., Hedberg, I., Levenfors, J.J., 2005. Anti-fungal and anti-bacterial activity of some herbal remedies from Tanzania. J Ethnopharmacol. 96 (3), 461–469.

Diallo, S., Crépin, A., Barbey, C., Orange, N., Burini, J.F., Latour, X., 2011. Mechanisms and recent advances in biological control mediated through the potato rhizosphere. FEMS Microbiol. Ecol. 75 (3), 351–364.

Dunkić, V., Bezić, N., Vuko, E., 2011. Antiphytoviral activity of essential oil from endemic species *Teucrium arduini*. Nat. Prod. Commun. 6 (9), 1385–1388.

Duvick, J.P., Rood, T., Rao, A.G., Marshak, D.R., 1992. Purification and characterization of a novel antimicrobial peptide from maize (*Zea mays* L.) kernels. J. Biol. Chem. 267 (26), 18814–18820.

Dwijendra, S., 2014. Advances in Plant Biopesticides. Springer, New Delhi.

Elshafie, H.S., Ghanney, N., Mang, S.M., Ferchichi, A., Camele, I., 2010. *Glycyrrhiza glabra* extract protects plants against important phytopathogenic fungi. Commun. Agric. Appl. Biol. Sci. 75 (4), 531–540.

Elshafie, H.S., Ghanney, N., Mang, S.M., Ferchichi, A., Camele, I., 2016. An in vitro attempt for controlling severe phytopathogens and human pathogens using essential oils from Mediterranean plants of *Genus schinus*. J. Med. Food. 19 (3), 266–273.

Fardin, K.M., Young, M.C., 2015. Antifungal potential of *Avicennia schaueriana* Stapf & Leech. (*Acanthaceae*) against *Cladosporium* and *Colletotrichum* species. Lett. Appl. Microbiol. 61 (1), 50–57.

Filippone, M.P., Diaz-Ricci, J.C., Castagnaro, A.P., Farías, R.N., 2013. A novel hairpin-like antimicrobial peptide from barnyard grass (*Echinochloa crusgalli* L.) seeds: structure-functional and molecular-genetics characterization. Biochimie 99, 63–70.

Gándara-Ledezma, A., Corrales-Maldonado, C., Rivera-Domínguez, M., Martínez-Téllez, M.Á., Vargas-Arispuro, I., 2015. Post-harvest control of gray mold in table grapes using volatile sulfur compounds from *Allium sativum*. J. Sci. Food Agric. 95 (3), 497–503.

Goel, M., Dureja, P., Rani, A., Uniyal, P.L., Laatsch, H., 2011. Isolation, characterization and antifungal activity of major constituents of the Himalayan lichen *Parmelia reticulata* Tayl. J. Agric. Food Chem. 59 (6), 2299–2307.

González-Lamothe, R., Mitchell, G., Gattuso, M., Diarra, M.S., Malouin, F., Bouarab, K., 2009. Plant antimicrobial agents and their effects on plant and human pathogens. Int. J. Mol. Sci. 10 (8), 3400–3419.

Hammer, K.A., Carson, C.F., 2011. Lipids and essential oils as antimicrobial agents. Ed. John Wiley & Sons Ltd, Chichester, p. 256–293.

Hong, J.K., Yang, H.J., Jung, H., Yoon, D.J., Sang, M.K., Jeun, Y.-C., 2015. Application of volatile antifungal plant essential oils for controlling pepper fruit anthracnose by *Colletotrichum gloeosporioides*. Plant Pathol. J. 31 (3), 269–277.

Hossain, S., Bergkvist, G., Berglund, K., Glinwood, R., Kabouw, P., Mårtensson, A., Persson, P., 2014. Concentration- and time-dependent effects of isothiocyanates produced from Brassicaceae shoot tissues on the pea root rot pathogen *Aphanomyces euteiches*. J. Agric. Food Chem. 62 (20), 4584–4591.

Hüsnü can Başer, K., Buchbauer, G., 2009. Handbook of essential oils. science, technology and applications. Ed. CRC Press Taylor & Francis Group, Boca Raton.

Hynes, R.K., Leung, G.C., Hirkala, D.L., Nelson, L.M., 2008. Isolation, selection, and characterization of beneficial rhizobacteria from pea, lentil, and chickpea grown in western Canada. Can. J. Microbiol. 54 (4), 248–258.

Iacobellis, N.S., Lo Cantore, P., Capasso, F., Senatore, F., 2005. Antibacterial activity of *Cuminum cyminum* L. and *Carum carvi* L. essential oils. J. Agric. Food Chem. 53 (1), 57–61.

Ingale, A.G., Hivrale, A.U., 2013. Plant as a plenteous reserve of lectin. Plant Signal. Behav. 8 (12), e26595.

Ionescu, I., 2014. Ecological protection means in the integrated control of medicinal and aromatic plants pests. PhD thesis. Bucharest University of Agronomical Sciences and Veterinary Medicine.

Isaac, G.S., Abu-Tahon, M.A., 2014. In vitro antifugal activity of medicinal plant extract against *Fusarium oxysporum* f. sp. lycopersici race 3 the causal agent of tomato wilt. Acta. Biol. Hung. 65 (1), 107–118.

Isla, M.I., Ordóñez, R.M., Moreno, M.I., Sampietro, A.R., Vattuone, M.A., 2002. From the antibiogram to prescription, second ed. bioMérieux, p. 80–10.

Jacobo-Salcedo Mdel, R., Gonzalez-Espindola, L.A., Alonso-Castro, A.J., Gonzalez-Martinez Mdel, R., Domínguez, F., Garcia-Carranca, A., 2011. Antimicrobial activity and cytotoxic effects of *Magnolia dealbata* and its active compounds. Nat. Prod. Commun. 6 (8), 1121–1124.

Jesionek, W., Móricz, Á.M., Alberti, Á., Ott, P.G., Kocsis, B., Horváth, G., Choma, I.M., 2015a. TLC-Direct bioautography as a bioassay guided method for investigation of antibacterial compounds in *Hypericum perforatum* L. J. AOAC Int. 98 (4), 1013–1020.

Jesionek, W., Móricz, Á.M., Ott, P.G., Kocsis, B., Horváth, G., Choma, I.M., 2015b. TLC-direct bioautography and lc/ms as complementary methods in identification of antibacterial agents in plant tinctures from the Asteraceae family. J. AOAC Int. 98 (4), 857–861.

Jiménez, E., Dorta, F., Medina, C., Ramírez, A., Ramírez, I., Peña-Cortés, H., 2011. Anti-phytopathogenic activities of macro-algae extracts. Mar. Drugs. 9 (5), 739–756.

Jin, S., Sato, N., 2003. Benzoquinone, the substance essential for antibacterial activity in aqueous extracts from succulent young shoots of the pear *Pyrus* spp. Phytochemistry 62 (1), 101–107.

Joosten, L., van Veen, J.A., 2011. Defensive properties of pyrrolizidine alkaloids against microorganisms. Phytochem. Rev. 10 (1), 127–136.

Khan, A., Usman, R., Rauf, A., Wang, M.L., Muhammad, N., Aman, A., Tahir, T.H., 2013a. In vitro biological screening of the stem of *Desmodium elegans*. Asian Pac. J. Trop. Biomed. 3 (9), 711–715.

Khan, H.M., Ahmad, N., Rashdi, S.M.M., Rauf, I., Ismail, M., Tofique, M., 2013b. Management of sucking complex in bt cotton through the application of different plant products. PJLS 01 (01), 42–48.

Kim, J.Y., Park, S.C., Kim, M.H., Lim, H.T., Park, Y., Hahm, K.S., 2005. Antimicrobial activity studies on a trypsin-chymotrypsin protease inhibitor obtained from potato. Biochem. Biophys. Res. Commun. 330 (3), 921–927.

Kocić-Tanackov, S., Dimić, G., Lević, J., Tanackov, I., Tepić, A., Vujičić, B., Gvozdanović-Varga, J., 2012. Effects of onion (*Allium cepa* L.) and garlic (*Allium sativum* L.) essential oils on the *Aspergillus versicolor* growth and sterigmatocystin production. J. Food. Sci. 77 (5), M278–M284.

Körpe, D.A., İşerı, Ö.D., Sahin, F.I., Cabi, E., Haberal, M., 2013. High-antibacterial activity of *Urtica* spp. seed extracts on food and plant pathogenic bacteria. Int. J. Food Sci. Nutr. 64 (3), 355–362.

Kumar, R., Saha, A., Saha, D., 2011. A new antifungal coumarin from *Clausena excavata*. Fitoterapia 83 (1), 230–233.

Kundu, A., Saha, S., Walia, S., Shakil, N.A., Kumar, J., Annapurna, K., 2013. Cadinene sesquiterpenes from *Eupatorium adenophorum* and their antifungal activity. J. Environ. Sci. Health B 48 (6), 516–522.

Kurt, S., Güneş, U., Soylu, E.M., 2011. In vitro and in vivo antifungal activity of synthetic pure isothiocyanates against *Sclerotinia sclerotiorum*. Pest Manag. Sci. 67 (7), 869–875.

La Torre, A., Caradonia, F., Gianferro, M., Molinu, M.G., Battaglia, V., 2014. Activity of natural products against some phytopathogenic fungi. Commun. Agric. Appl. Biol. Sci. 79 (3), 439–449.

Lee, Y.M., Moon, J.S., Yun, B.S., Park, K.D., Choi, G.J., Kim, J.C., Lee, S.H., Kim, S.U., 2009. Antifungal activity of CHE-23C, a dimeric sesquiterpene from *Chloranthus henryi*. J. Agric. Food Chem. 57 (13), 5750–5755.

Lenteren, J.C., 2003. Quality Control and Production of Biological Control Agents—Theory and Testing Procedures Cabi Publishing, Wageningen University, The Netherlands, pp. 1–19, 167–191.

Li, Y., Li, J., Li, Y., Wang, X.X., Cao, A.C., 2013. Antimicrobial constituents of the leaves of *Mikania micrantha* H.B.K. PLoS One 8 (10), e76725.

Lin, T.C., Fan, M.C., Wang, S.Y., Huang, J.W., 2011. Identification of the *Solanum nigrum* extract component involved in controlling cabbage black leaf spot disease. J. Agric. Food Chem. 59 (5), 1667–1672.

Lo Cantore, P., Shanmugaiah, V., Iacobellis, N.S., 2009. Antibacterial activity of essential oil components and their potential use in seed disinfection. J. Agric. Food Chem. 57 (20), 9454–9461.

Lu, M., Han, Z., Xu, Y., Yao, L., 2013. In vitro and in vivo anti-tobacco mosaic virus activities of essential oils and individual compounds. J. Microbiol. Biotechnol. 23 (6), 771–778.

Luko, H.G., Mora, A., 2006. Advances in phytomedicine. Naturally occurring bioactive compounds. 3, 379-403.

Lynch, M.R., 1995. Strategies and criteria for the mutual recognition of authorizations in the context of the European regulatory system for plant protection products. XIII-th Int. Plant Prot. Congr. Hague, Netherlands, July 2–7, 1995, ref. 874.

Maddox, C.E., Laur, L.M., Tian, L., 2010. Antibacterial activity of phenolic compounds against the phytopathogen *Xylella fastidiosa*. Curr. Microbiol. 60 (1), 53–58.

Mandal, S.M., Chakraborty, D., Dey, S., 2010. Phenol ic acids act as signaling molecules in plant-microbe symbioses. Plant Signal. Behav. 5 (4), 359–368.

Manole, T., Iamandei, M., Rădulescu, G., 2005. Evaluarea potențialului insecticid al produsului "NICOTOX 5" asupra unor specii de insecte dăunătoare aplicat în condiții controlate (I). An. ICDPP, XXXIII, pp. 202–211.

Maswada, H.F., Abdallah, S.A., 2013. In vitro antifungal activity of three geophytic plant extracts against three post-harvest pathogenic fungi. Pak. J. Biol. Sci. 16 (23), 1698–1705.

Medina, E., Romero, C., de Los Santos, B., de Castro, A., Garcia, A., Romero, F., Brenes, M., 2011. Antimicrobial activity of olive solutions from stored Alpeorujo against plant pathogenic microorganisms. J. Agric. Food Chem. 59 (13), 6927–6932.

Mehta, P., Chopra, S., Mehta, A., 1983. Antimicrobial properties of some plant extracts against bacteria. Folia Microbiol. (Praha) 28 (6), 467–469.

Metoui, N., Gargouri, S., Amri, I., Fezzani, T., Jamoussi, B., Hamrouni, L., 2015. Activity antifungal of the essential oils; aqueous and ethanol extracts from *Citrus aurantium* L. Nat. Prod. Res. 29 (23), 2238–2241.

Mihaescu, G., Chifiriuc, C., Ditu, L.M., 2007. General Microbiology. University of Bucharest House, Bucharest, 552 p.

Misawa, M., Hayashi, M., Tanaka, H., 1975. Production of plant virus inhibitor by *Phytolacca americana* suspension culture. Biotechnol. Bioeng. 17 (9), 1335–1347.

Molina, A., Segura, A., García-Olmedo, F., 1993. Lipid transfer proteins (nsLTPs) from barley and maize leaves are potent inhibitors of bacterial and fungal plant pathogens. FEBS Lett. 316 (2), 119–122.

Moreno, M., Segura, A., García-Olmedo, F., 1994. Pseudothionin-St1, a potato peptide active against potato pathogens. Eur. J. Biochem. 223 (1), 135–139.

Móricz, A.M., Ott, P.G., Alberti, A., Böszörményi, A., Lemberkovics, E., Szoke, E., Kéry, A., Mincsovics, E., 2013. Applicability of preparative overpressured layer chromatography and direct bioautography in search ofantibacterial chamomile compounds. J. AOAC Int. 96 (6), 1214–1221.

Nawrot, R., Barylski, J., Nowicki, G., Broniarczyk, J., Buchwald, W., Goździcka-Józefiak, A., 2014. Plant antimicrobial peptides. Folia Microbiol. (Praha) 59 (3), 181–196.

Nollet, L., Singh Rathore, H., 2015. Biopesticides handbook. Ed. CRC Press Taylor & Francis Group, Boca Raton.

O'Brien, K.P., Franjevic, S., Jones, J., 2009. Green Chemistry and Sustainable Agriculture: The Role of Biopesticides. Springer, New Delhi, Heidelberg, New York, Dordrecht, London.

Oerke, E.C., Dehne, H.W., Schönbeck, F., Webber, A., 1994. Crop production and crop protection—estimated losses in major food and cash crops. Elsevier Science, pp. 543–654.

Opender, K., Suresh, W., Dhaliwal, G.S., 2008. Essential oils as green pesticides: potential and constraints. Biopestic. Int. 4 (1), 63–84.

Ordóñez, R.M., Ordóñez, A.A., Sayago, J.E., Nieva Moreno, M.I., Isla, M.I., 2006. Antimicrobial activity of glycosidase inhibitory protein isolated from *Cyphomandra betacea* Sendt. Fruit Peptides 27 (6), 1187–1191.

Ordóñez, R.M., Zampini, I.C., Moreno, M.I., Isla, M.I., 2011. Potential application of Northern Argentine propolis to control some phytopathogenic bacteria. Microbiol. Res. 166 (7), 578–584.

Paulkumar, K., Gnanajobitha, G., Vanaja, M., Rajeshkumar, S., Malarkodi, C., Pandian, K., Annadurai, G., 2014. *Piper nigrum* leaf and stem assisted green synthesis of silver nanoparticles and evaluation of its antibacterial activity against agricultural plant pathogens. Scientific World J. 2014, 829894.

Pérez-Laínez, D., García-Mateos, R., San Miguel-Chávez, R., Soto-Hernández, M., Rodríguez-Pérez, E., Kite, G., 2008. Bactericidal and fungicidal activities of *Calia secundiflora* (Ort.) Yakovlev. Z. Naturforsch C. 63 (9–10), 653–657.

Peumans, W.J., Van Damme, E.J., 1995. Lectins as plant defense proteins. Plant Physiol. 109 (2), 347–352.

Purnavab, S., Ketabchi, S., Rowshan, V., 2015. Chemical composition and antibacterial activity of methanolic extract and essential oil of Iranian *Teucrium polium* against some of phytobacteria. Nat. Prod. Res. 29 (14), 1376–1379.

Pusztahelyi, T., Holb, I.J., Pócsi, I., 2015. Secondary metabolites in fungus-plant interactions. Front. Plant Sci. 6, 573.

Răbonțu, C., 2010. Food safety and its role in the evolution of food trade. An. Univ. "Constantin Brâncuşi" 2, 161–172.

Radioza, S.A., Iurchak, L.D., 2007. Antimicrobial activity of Calendula L. Plants. Mikrobiol. Z. 69 (5), 21–25.

Rahman, A., Islam, R., Al-Reza, S.M., Kang, S.C., 2014. In vitro control of plant pathogenic *Xanthomonas* spp. using *Poncirus trifoliata* Rafin. EXCLI J. 13, 1104–1110.

Rusak, G., Krajacić, M., Plese, N., 1997. Inhibition of tomato bushy stunt virus infection using a quercetagetin flavonoid isolated from *Centaurea rupestris* L. Antiviral Res. 36 (2), 125–129.

Ryazantsev, D.Y., Rogozhin, E.A., Dimitrieva, T.V., Drobyazina, P.E., Khadeeva, N.V., Egorov, T.A., Grishin, E.V., Zavriev, S.K., 2013. A novel hairpin-like antimicrobial peptide from barnyard grass (*Echinochloa crusgalli* L.) seeds: structure-functional and molecular-genetics characterization. Biochimie 99, 63–70.

Schaffer, W., 1997. Antibacterial Peptide Protocols. Humana Press, Totowa, New Jersey.

Schnee, S., Queiroz, E.F., Voinesco, F., Marcourt, L., Dubuis, P.H., Wolfender, J.L., Gindro, K., 2013. Vitis vinifera canes, a new source of antifungal compounds against *Plasmopara viticola, Erysiphe necator*, and *Botrytis cinerea*. J. Agric. Food Chem. 61 (23), 5459–5467.

Segura, A., Moreno, M., Molina, A., García-Olmedo, F., 1998. Novel defense in subfamily from spinach (*Spinacia oleracea*). FEBS Lett. 435 (2-3), 159–162.

Segura, A., Moreno, M., Madueño, F., Molina, A., García-Olmedo, F., 1999. Snakin-1, a peptide from potato that is active against plant pathogens. Mol. Plant Microb. Interact. 12 (1), 16–23.

Shang, S.Z., Xu, W.X., Lei, P., Zhao, W., Tang, J.G., Miao, M.M., Sun, H.D., Pu, J.X., Chen, Y.K., Yang, G.Y., 2014. Biphenyls from *Nicotiana tabacum* and their anti-tobacco mosaic virus. Fitoterapia 99, 35–39.

Sharma, R.K., Negi, D.S., Gibbons, S., Otsuka, H., 2008. Chemical and antibacterial constituents of *Skimmia anquetelia*. Planta Med. 74 (2), 175–177.

Sibi, G., Wadhavan, R., Singh, S., Shukla, A., Dhananjaya, K., Ravikumar, K.R., Mallesha, H., 2013. Plant latex: a promising antifungal agent for post harvest disease control. Pak. J. Biol. Sci. 16 (23), 1737–1743.

Silva-Hughes, A.F., Wedge, D.E., Cantrell, C.L., Carvalho, C.R., Pan, Z., Moraes, R.M., Madoxx, V.L., Rosa, L.H., 2015. Diversity and antifungal activity of the endophytic fungi associated with the native medicinal cactus *Opuntia humifusa* (Cactaceae) from the United States. Microbiol Res. 175, 67–77.

Sledz, W., Los, E., Paczek, A., Rischka, J., Motyka, A., Zoledowska, S., Piosik, J., Lojkowska, E., 2015. Antibacterial activity of caffeine against plant pathogenic bacteria. Acta Biochim. Pol. 62 (3), 605–612.

Soberón, J.R., Sgariglia, M.A., Dip Maderuelo, M.R., Andina, M.L., Sampietro, D.A., Vattuone, M.A., 2014. J Antibacterial activities of *Ligaria cuneifolia* and *Jodina rhombifolia* leaf extracts against phytopathogenic and clinical bacteria. Biosci. Bioeng. 118 (5), 599–605.

Sotelo, T., Lema, M., Soengas, P., Cartea, M.E., Velasco, P., 2015. In vitro activity of glucosinolates and their degradation products against brassica-pathogenic bacteria and fungi. Appl. Environ. Microbiol. 81 (1), 432–440.

Steinwand, B., 2008. Biopesticide Ombudsman. US Environmental Protection Agency, Washington DC. Personal Communication.

Synowiec, A., Gniewosz, M., Kraśniewska, K., Chlebowska-Śmigiel, A., Przybył, J.L., Bączek, K., Węglarz, Z., 2014. Effect of meadowsweet flower extract-pullulan coatings on rhizopus rot development and postharvest quality of cold-stored red peppers. Molecules 19 (9), 12925–12939.

Talas-Oğraş, T., Ipekçi, Z., Bajroviç, K., Gözükirmizi, N., 2005. Antibacterial activity of seed proteins of *Robinia pseudoacacia*. Fitoterapia 76 (1), 67–72.

Talibi, I., Askarne, L., Boubaker, H., Boudyach, E.H., Msanda, F., Saadi, B., Ben Aoumar, A.A., 2012. Antifungal activity of Moroccan medicinal plants against citrus sour rot agent *Geotrichum candidum*. Lett. Appl. Microbiol. 55 (2), 155–161.

Tayel, A.A., Salem, M.F., El-Tras, W.F., Brimer, L., 2011. Exploration of Islamic medicine plant extracts as powerful antifungals for the prevention of mycotoxigenic *Aspergilli* growth in organic silage. J. Sci. Food Agric. 91 (12), 2160–2165.

Tedeschi, P., Leis, M., Pezzi, M., Civolani, S., Maietti, A., Brandolini, V., 2011. Insecticidal activity and fungitoxicity of plant extracts and components of horseradish (*Armoracia rusticana*) and garlic (*Allium sativum*). J. Environ. Sci. Health B. 46 (6), 486–490.

Teshima, Y., Ikeda, T., Imada, K., Sasaki, K., El-Sayed, M.A., Shigyo, M., Tanaka, S., Ito, S., 2013. Identification and biological activity of antifungal saponins from shallot (*Allium cepa* L. Aggregatum group). J. Agric. Food Chem. 61 (31), 7440–7445.

Thuerig, B., Ramseyer, J., Hamburger, M., Oberhänsli, T., Potterat, O., Schärer, H.J., Tamm, L., 2015. Efficacy of a Juncus effusus extract on grapevine and apple plants against Plasmopara viticola and Venturia inaequalis, and identification of the major active constituent. Pest Manag Sci.

Uzair, M., Loothar, B.A., Choudhary, B.A., 2009. Biological screening of *Euphorbia helioscopia* L. Pak. J. Pharm. Sci. 22 (2), 184–186.

Vuko, E., Dunkić, V., Bezić, N., Ruscić, M., Kremer, D., 2012. Chemical composition and antiphytoviral activity of essential oil of *Micromeria graeca*. Nat. Prod. Commun. 7 (9), 1227–1230.

Wang, Y., Dai, C.C., Chen, Y., 2009. Antimicrobial activity of volatile oil from *Atractylodes lancea* against three species of endophytic fungi and seven species of exogenous fungi. Ying Yong Sheng Tai Xue Bao. 20 (11), 2778–2784.

Wang, Q., Li, F., Zhang, X., Zhang, Y., Hou, Y., Zhang, S., Wu, Z., 2011a. Purification and characterization of a CkTLP protein from *Cynanchum komarovii* seeds that confers antifungal activity. PLoS One 6 (2), e16930.

Wang, X., Habib, E., León, F., Radwan, M.M., Tabanca, N., Gao, J., Wedge, D.E., Cutler, S.J., 2011b. Antifungal metabolites from the roots of *Diospyros virginiana* by overpressure layer chromatography. Chem. Biodivers. 8 (12), 2331–2340.

Wang, D.M., Zhang, C.C., Zhang, Q., Shafiq, N., Pescitelli, G., Li, D.W., Gao, J.M., 2014. Wightianines A-E, dihydro-β-agarofuran sesquiterpenes from *Parnassia wightiana*, and their antifungal and insecticidal activities. J. Agric. Food Chem. 62 (28), 6669–6676.

Wimley, W.C., Hristova, K., 2011. Antimicrobial peptides: successes, challenges and unanswered questions. J. Membr. Biol. 239 (1–2), 27–34.

Xie, C., Kokubun, T., Houghton, P.J., Simmonds, M.S., 2004. Antibacterial activity of the Chinese traditional medicine. Zi Hua Di Ding. Phytother Res. 18 (6), 497–500.

Zhang, J., Yan, L.T., Yuan, E.L., Ding, H.X., Ye, H.C., Zhang, Z.K., Yan, C., Liu, Y.Q., Feng, G., 2014. Antifungal activity of compounds extracted from Cortex pseudolaricis against Colletotrichum gloeosporioides. J. Agric. Food Chem. 62 (21), 4905–4910.

9

PRESENT AND PERSPECTIVES IN PESTICIDES BIOSENSORS DEVELOPMENT AND CONTRIBUTION OF NANOTECHNOLOGY

Irina Gheorghe, Ilda Czobor, Veronica Lazar, Mariana Carmen Chifiriuc

Faculty of Biology and Research Institute of the University of Bucharest - ICUB, University of Bucharest, Bucharest, Romania

1 Introduction

Anthropic activities generate the release of contaminants, such as pesticides and other pollutants, in the aquatic environment, which present a real threat to ecosystems and human health. Thus, monitoring tools become essential for water managers to detect these chemicals before the occurrence of adverse effects (Durrieu et al., 2016).

Pesticides, due to their pest removal properties, are largely used in agricultural fields for crop production enhancement. Due to their lucrative outcomes, pesticides of various classes have been designed to persist in the environment over a longer duration after their application to achieve maximum effectiveness. Apart from their recalcitrant structure and agricultural benefits, pesticides also exhibit acute toxicological effects onto the other various life forms. Their accumulation in the living systems can be detrimental if accumulated in higher concentrations. Pesticides also became a main concern for food safety. Thus, their prompt and accurate analysis is a crucial matter of concern. Conventional techniques like chromatographic techniques (high-performance liquid chromatography, capillary electrophoresis, and mass spectrometry) are effective for the analysis of pesticides in the environment but have certain limitations, such as complexity, time-consuming sample preparation,

New Pesticides and Soil Sensors. http://dx.doi.org/10.1016/B978-0-12-804299-1.00010-2

and the requirement of expensive apparatus and trained persons to operate used for pesticides (Pundir and Chauhan, 2012). So there is an acute need for the development of new rapid, cost-effective, sensitive, specific, and easy to use methods which can detect these compounds in the field (Verma and Bhardwaj, 2015; Liu et al., 2013a). The rapid detection of toxic pesticides would allow taking immediate decision on efficient decontamination procedures and could prevent further damage and potential casualties. These goals can be achieved by using biosensors that detect pesticide residues (Jokar et al., 2016). The purpose of this chapter is to present the current state and perspectives in the development of pesticides biosensors and the contribution of nanotechnology.

Biosensors are used in a wide range of applications for the quick and easy detection of pesticides and water contaminants, such as heavy metal ions, organophosphates (OPs), biological warfare agents, and pathogens, drug residues in food, determining levels of toxic substances before and after bioremediation, to drug discovery and evaluation of biological activity of new compounds, and so on. The advantages of biosensors over other screening methods, such as radioimmunoassay, enzyme-linked immunosorbent assay, fluorescence immunoassay, and luminescence immunoassay, with respect to food analysis, include automation, improved reproducibility, speed of analysis, and real-time analysis. Biosensors currently have an important role in food safety, which will be well reinforced by further advances in the technology, reagents, and sample handling (McGrath et al., 2012).

A biosensor is an analytical device, used for the detection of an analyte, combining a biological component (bioreceptor represented by biomolecules or synthetic molecules obtained using biological scaffolds) with a physico-chemical detector, as well as an associated electronic system, which amplifies, process and display the detected signal. A successful biosensor must use a highly specific biocatalyst, stable in various stirring, pH, and temperature conditions (most often enzymes) (Schöning and Poghossian, 2002); give a dose-dependent and, desirably, real-time response; be cost-effective, portable, easy to use (Grieshaber et al., 2008).

The advent of nanotechnology offers promising ways for the optimization and miniaturization of biosensing devices. The higher surface:volume ratio of nanosized objects increases their electrical properties and thus their sensitivity to external conditions variations. Moreover, the nanometer size is close to that of target biomolecules, increasing thus their sensitivity. Nanostructured materials (nanoparticles, nanowires, nantubes, nanorods) show therefore a promising potential in the design of biosensors, being used as labels for affinity biosensors, biomolecule immobilization platforms, and biocatalysts in various applications (Merkoci, 2007; Grieshaber et al., 2008).

2 Electrochemical Biosensing Techniques Used for Pesticides Detection

In electrochemical biosensing the generated signal will be detected by measuring the current (amperometric methods, such as voltammetry, chronoamperometry), the potential or charge accumulation (potentiometric), the conductive properties (conductometric methods, such as those using field-effect transistors) (Schöning and Poghossian, 2002), impedance (impedimetric methods, including electrochemical impedance spectroscopy) (Grieshaber et al., 2008; Katz and Willner, 2003; Gosser and Cyclic Voltammetry, 1994; Eggins, 2002). The electrochemical methods can be combined with optical ones, in order to obtain highly sensitive, real-time, in situ, nondestructive and label-free analysis of different solutions or bulk materials (e.g., optical waveguide light-mode spectroscopy, surface plasmon resonance (SPR), ellipsometry, gravimetric techniques like quartz crystal microbalance, and imaging techniques, such as AFM), confocal laser scanning microscopy (Grieshaber et al., 2008). Different variants of magnetic resonance imaging (MRI) can also be used in combination with electrochemistry for biosensing. A novel biosensing approach using the detection of magnetoresistive effect is the bead array counter (BARC) that could be used as multianalyte biosensor for the detection and identification of biological warfare agents (Baselt et al., 1998; Rifea et al., 2003; Edelstein et al., 2000).

2.1 Acetylcholinesterase -Based Biosensors and Enzymatic Immobilization Methods

OPs, amongst the most toxic substances known, are used widely in agriculture around the world. Their extensive use, however, has resulted in their occurrence in the water and food supply threatening humans and animals. Therefore, there is a need for determination of these neurotoxic compounds sensitively, selectively, and rapidly in the field (Mulchandani, 2011).

Acetylcholinesterase (AChE) is the biological regulator of the ACh neurotransmitter. It degrades the acetylcholine and generates choline and acetate acid. The activity of AChE is inhibited by OP and carbamate pesticides, compromising the degradation of the neurotransmitter. Therefore, a growing interest has been shown for the development of more and more faster and sensitive detection systems for pesticides that include this enzyme (Dhull et al., 2013; Schena and Johnsson, 2014). The inhibition of AChE parameter can be used as a "toxicological index", defined as the amount of compound, which causes a certain percentage of cholinesterase inhibition equivalent to a known amount of a reference compound causing the same percentage inhibition (Bernabei et al., 1993).

An electrochemical biosensor based on AChE immobilized on a ZnO nanorod interface has been proposed to detect the presence of the fungicide captan residues in fruits (apples), that could cause acute toxicity (eye and skin irritation, dermatitis, conjunctivitis, and vomiting) in humans. The obtained bioelectrode showed a high sensitivity with a very low limit of detection (LOD) of 10^7 nM (Nesakumar et al., 2015).

An enzyme inhibition-based homogeneous electrochemical biosensing strategy was designed for the detection of the organophosphorus pesticides, such as diazinon. OPs are among the most and largely used pesticides. They are organic compounds that contain a phosphoryl or a thiophosphoryl bond. Their detection is normally performed by GC– and LC–MS, which are very sensitive, but not appropriate for on site and real time detection. Another assay exploited the resistance of a mercury ion-mediated helper probe (HP) to nuclease–catalyzed digestion. The mercury ion-mediated T–$Hg^{(2+)}$–T base pairs facilitate the HP labeled with methylene blue (MB) to fold into a hairpin structure, preventing its digestion by exonuclease I, and thus resulting in a decreased electrochemical response. The competitive removal of mercury from the base pairs by the thiol groups (–SH), provided by AChE, cause a nuclease–catalyzed digestion, and the increase of the electrochemical response increase. The detection limit of this biosensor for diazinon using real samples is very low (0.25 μg/L) (Wang et al., 2016).

An AChE biosensor based on unsubstituted pillar[5]arene (P[5]A) as electron mediator was successfully used for a highly sensitive detection of OP and carbamate pesticides. The AChE was immobilized by carbodiimide binding on carbon black (CB) placed on glassy carbon electrode (GCE) and the signal was detected in the chronoamperometric mode, providing very low detection limits of 4×10^{-12} M formalaoxon, 5×10^{-9} M for methyl-paraoxon, 2×10^{-11} for carbofuran and 6×10^{-10} foraldicarb with 10 min incubation. This biosensor was tested for the analysis of pesticide residuals in spiked samples of peanut and beetroot (Shamagsumova et al., 2015).

A cobalt phthalocyanine-modified carbon epoxy composite electrode coupled with acetylcholinesterase or butyrylcholinesterase immobilized by covalent bounding was designed for pesticides detection with the limits of 1.5 and 8.4 μg/mL for paraoxon and heptenophos, in less than 3 min (Skladal and Mascini, 1992).

One-step modification using single-walled carbon nanotubes and cophtalocyanine has been proposed to decrease the working potential and to increase the signal of thiocholine oxidation. The biosensor proved to be useful for pesticides detection in samples of sparkling and tap waters (Ivanov et al., 2011).

A sensitive electrochemical AChE biosensor was successfully developed on polyaniline (PANI) and multiwalled carbon nanotubes (MWCNTs) core–shell modified GCE, and used to detect carbamate pesticides in fruit and vegetables (apple, broccoli, and cabbage) using chronoamperometry (Cesarino et al., 2012).

A conductometric biosensor based on AChE was developed for detecting different classes of toxic compounds (organophosphorus pesticides, heavy metal ions, surfactants, aflatoxin, glycoalkaloids) in complex multicomponent aqueous samples (Stepurska et al., 2015).

2.2 AChE Immobilization Approaches

The solvent tolerance of immobilized enzymes is important for many biosensing applications. AChE was immobilized onto a GCE with the aid of Cu–Mg–Al calcined layered double hydroxide (CLDH), which provided a bigger effective surface area for AChE loading, which could improve the precision and stability of AChE biosensor. In order to effectively compensate the poor electroconductibility of CLDHs, graphene–gold nanocomposites (GN–AuNPs) were used for improving the electron transfer rate (Zhai et al., 2014). A novel AChE biosensor based on Ag NPs, carboxylic graphene (CGR) and nafion (NF) hybrid modified glass GCE has been also successfully used for AchE immobilization. Ag NPs–CGR–NF possessed predominant conductivity, catalysis, and biocompatibility and provided a hydrophilic surface for AChE adhesion. chitosan (CS) was used to immobilize AChE on the surface of Ag NPs–CGR–NF/GCE to keep the AChE activities (Liu et al., 2014a). In another study, AchE was electroimmobilized into a thick conducting layer of polypyrrole. Porcine skin gelatin and gluteraldehyde mixture was used for stabilizing the system. Polypyrrole catalyzed the electrochemical oxidation of thiocholine and promoted the electron transfer, thus lowering the oxidation potential and increasing the detection sensitivity. The sensor was applied to detect the sample organophosphate pesticide ethylparaoxon and organocarbamate pesticide carbofuran (Dutta and Puzari, 2014).

AChE was immobilized on silica sol–gel (SiSG) on a carbon paste electrode (CPE) and used as working electrode, shoeing a good linearity range for malathion and acephate (Raghu et al., 2014).

Another sensitive amperometric AChE biosensor based on NiO nanoparticles (NiO NPs), CGR, and NF modified GCE has been developed. NiO NPs–CGR–NF nanocomposites with excellent conductivity, catalysis, and biocompatibility offered an extremely hydrophilic surface for AChE adhesion (Yang et al., 2013a).

A sensitive amperometric AChE biosensor based on platinum nanoparticles (Pt NPs), CGR, and NF-modified GCE has been described (Yang et al., 2013b). The Pt NPs–CGR–NF nanocomposites with excellent conductivity, catalysis, and biocompatibility offered an extremely hydrophilic surface for AChE adhesion. CS was used as cross-linker to immobilize the AChE on Pt–CGR–NF-modified GCE. NF was used as a protective membrane of the AChE biosensors (Yang et al., 2013b).

An amperometric AChE biosensor, based on SnO_2 nanoparticles (SnO_2 NPs), CGR and NF modified GCE for the detection of methyl parathion and carbofuran has been developed (Zhou et al., 2013). The nanocomposites of SnO_2 NPs and CGR was synthesized and characterized by scanning electron microscopy (SEM), X-ray diffraction (XRD), and Fourier transform infrared spectroscopy (FTIR). CS was used to immobilize AChE on SnO_2 NPs–CGR–NF/GCE and to improve electronic transmission between AChE and SnO_2 NPs–CGR–NF/GCE. NF was used as the protective membrane for the AChE biosensor. The SnO_2 NPs–CGR–NF nanocomposites with excellent conductivity, catalysis, and biocompatibility offered an extremely hydrophilic surface for AChE adhesion. The AChE biosensor showed favorable affinity to acetylthiocholine chloride (ATCl). The biosensor exhibited low applied potential, high sensitivity, and acceptable stability, thus providing a promising tool for analysis of pesticides. Another amperometric AChE biosensor was developed based on the nanocomposite of MWCNTs, tin oxide (SnO_2) nanoparticles, and chitosan (CS). AChE and NF were immobilized onto the nanocomposite film to prepare AChE biosensor for pesticide residues detection (Chen et al., 2015). The morphologies and electrochemistry properties of the surface modification were investigated using cyclic voltammetry, differential pulse voltammetry, and SEM, respectively. Compared with individual MWCNTs–CS, SnO_2–CHIT and bare gold electrode, this nanocomposite showed the most obvious electrochemical signal in the presence of $[Fe(CN)_6]^{(3-/4-)}$ as a redox couple. Based on the inhibition of pesticides on the AChE activity, using chlorpyrifos as model pesticide, the proposed biosensor exhibited a wide range, low detection limit, good reproducibility, and high stability. Using cabbages, lettuces, leeks, and bok choy as model samples, acceptable recovery of 98.7–105.2% was obtained. The proposed method was proven to be a feasible quantitative method for chlorpyrifos analysis, which may open a new door ultrasensitive detection of chlorpyrifos residues in vegetables and fruits.

An amperometric biosensor for the detection of OP compounds has been constructed, based on rat brain AChE immobilized onto nanocomposite of ZnS-nanoparticles (ZnSNPs) and poly(indole-5-carboxylic acid) electrodeposited on Au electrode. In the presence of ATCl as a substrate, ZnSNPs promoted electron transfer reactions at a lower potential and catalyzed electrochemicaloxidation of enzymatically formed thiocholine, thus increasing detection sensitivity. The biosensor determined malathion and chlorpyrifos in spiked tap water samples with a 95–100% accuracy (Chauhan et al., 2011a).

An AChE purified from rat brain was immobilized onto gold nanoparticles (AuNPs) assembled on the surface of porous calcium carbonate ($CaCO_3$) microsphere. The resulting AChE–AuNPs–$CaCO_3$ bioconjugate was mounted on the surface of Au electrode with the help of SiSG matrix to prepare the working electrode (Chauhan et al., 2011b). This electrode was connected to Ag/AgCl (3M/saturated KCl) as standard and Pt wire as an auxiliary electrode through a potentiostat to construct an organophosphorus (OP) biosensor. The biosensor was based on inhibition of AChE by OP compounds/insecticides. The biosensor exhibited good reusability (50 times without considerable loss) and storage stability (50% within 60 days, when stored at 4°C).

New AChE sensor based on Ag nanoparticles decorated with macrocyclic ligand has been developed and successfully used for highly sensitive detection of organophosphate and carbamate pesticides (Evtugyn et al., 2014). AChE was immobilized by carbodiimide binding on CB layer deposited on a GCE. The AChE sensor was tested for the detection of residual amounts of pesticides in spiked samples of peanut and grape juice. The protecting effect of new macrocyclic compounds bearing quaternary ammonia fragments was shown on the example of malaoxon inhibition.

A highly sensitive biosensor was obtained by using GCE modified with CS on which hollow gold nanospheres (HGNs) were absorbed based on the strong electrostatic adsorption affinity. After that, L-cysteine was assembled on HGNs through Au—S bond and, AChE was immobilized with covalent binding via –COOH groups of L-cysteine onto the modified GCE. The AChE biosensor proved to be suitable for trace detection of pesticide residues in vegetables and fruits (Sun et al., 2013).

An AChE biosensor with superior accuracy and sensitivity was successfully developed based on interdigitated array microelectrodes (IAMs) constituted of a series of parallel microband electrodes connected with alternating microbands. CS was used for AchE immobilization material and carbaryl as model compound (Gong et al., 2014).

SiO_2 nanosheets (SNS)–NF nanocomposites proved to be an extremely hydrophilic surface for biomolecule adhesion. CS was used as a cross-linker to immobilize AChE, and NF was used as a protective membrane to improve the stability of the AChE biosensor (Yang et al., 2013c).

Exfoliated graphene oxide (GO) was functionalized by a diazonium reaction to introduce abundant carboxyl groups. Then, *Nα,Nα*-bis(carboxymethyl)-L-lysine hydrate (NTA–NH_2) and $Ni^{(2+)}$ were anchored onto the GO based materials step by step. AChE was immobilized on the functionalized graphene oxide (FGO) through the specific binding between Ni–NTA and His–tag (Zhang et al., 2014).

Another nanohybrid of gold nanoparticles, polypyrrole, and reduced GO sheets (Au–PPy–rGO) was used for the design of an AChE biosensor. AChE was encapsulated in a silica matrix and immobilized on the Au–PPy–rGO nanocomposite by codeposition with $(NH4)_2SiF_6$. The Au–PPy–rGO nanocomposite showed excellent conductivity and exhibited a high electrocatalytic activity and specific affinity for thiocholine, and thus an improved detection sensitivity. Since AChE molecules were protected by the circumambient silica matrix, which provided a biocompatible environment and facilitated mass transport, the fabricated AChE biosensor displayed high stability and excellent activity together with a fast response to OPs pesticides (Yang et al., 2014).

On the basis of the AChE inhibition principle, a novel on-chip enzymatic microreactor based on AChE adsorbed on GO magnetic nanocomposites was designed through an in situ chemical deposition strategy for analyzing dimethoate, an OP pesticide (Liang et al., 2013).

A highly sensitive and rapid amperometric biosensor for OPs was based on immobilization of AChE on a novel TiO_2-decorated graphene (TiO_2–G) nanohybrid (Wang et al., 2011).

An ultrasensitive amperometric AChE biosensor for the detection of monocrotophos, a typical highly toxic organophorous pesticide was fabricated by controlled immobilization of AChE on gold nanoparticles/poly(dimethyldiallylammonium chloride) protected prussian blue nanocomposite modified electrode surface for the detection of OPs (Wu et al., 2011).

A biosensor based on AChE and carbon nanosphere (CNS) immobilized on a GCE was developed for the detection of carbofuran and fenitrothion, with high sensitivity and low detection limits (Cai et al., 2014).

It has been also reported a site-specific affinity immobilization of $(His)_6$-tagged AChE onto Ni/NiO nanoparticles for the development of an electrochemical screen-printed biosensor for the detection of OPs (Ganesana et al., 2011). AChE and choline oxidase (ChO) were coimmobilized onto the conducting polymer poly(4-(2,5-di(thiophen-2-yl)-1H-pyrrol-1-yl)benzenamine) films using covalent binding technique and the designed biosensor was tested for the determination of paraoxon-ethyl in spiked tap water samples (Kanik et al., 2013). The layered double hydroxides (LDHs) provided a biocompatible microenvironment for the immobilization of AChE, preserving its bioactivity and utility for the detection of methyl parathion used as model (Gong et al., 2013). The AChE immobilized on ionic liquid-functionalized graphene was used for modifying a GCE providing a new and promising tool for the analysis of enzyme inhibitors (Li and Han, 2012). An amperometric biosensor, fabricated by immobilizing AChE on MWCNTs-chitosan nanocomposites modified GCE, provided a high sensitivity owing to the excellent conductivity and favorable biocompatibility of MWCNTs-CS nanocomposites. The sensitivity of the biosensor was further enhanced using the electrochemical reduction signal of DTNB for determination. Moreover, the proposed protocol was successfully employed for the determination of methyl parathion in water and soil samples (Dong et al., 2013). AchE specific antibodies were immobilized on multiwalled carbon nanotubes-gold (MWCNTs-Au) nanocomposites modified screen-printed carbon electrode (SPCE) (Chen et al., 2012a). An acetylcholinesterase-immobilized sensor unit can be successfully obtained by encapsulating the enzyme within hybrid mesoporous silica membranes successfully detected with high sensitivity for detecting dichlorvos, aldicarb and parathion (Itoh et al., 2014).

An AChE biosensor based on CS that exhibited high solvent resistance and enabled sensitive detection of pesticides in the presence of a high content of organic solvents (25% methanol, 15% acetonitrile, and 100% cyclohexane) has been developed. The detection limits of the biosensor for paraoxon ranged from 2.5 μM in 100% cyclohexane to 100 nM in 15% acetonitrile (Warner and Andreescu, 2016). Another highly sensitive biosensor for the detection of organophosphorus pesticides employing the cobalt(II) 4,4,4,4-tetrasulfo-phthalocyanine (CoTSPc) macrocycle complex, carbon nanotubes (CNT), and 1-methyl-3-octylimidazolium tetrafluoroborate (OMIM[BF4]) involved the immobilization of AChE on the composite electrode surface by cross-linking with glutaraldehyde and CS. The detection rates of different organophosphorus pesticides (fenitrothion, malathion, dichlorvos ranged from

1 to 16 pmol/L (Pereira et al., 2015). The AChE was immobilized onto amino functionalized carbon nanotubes (CNT–NH_2), to obtain highly sensitive and practical organophosphorus pesticide biosensors. The AChE was adsorbed in high amounts on the surface of CNT–NH_2 and the biosensor achieved a low detection limit of 0.08 nM for paraoxon, with satisfactory reproducibility and stability for the determination of low concentrations of pesticides in real vegetable samples (Yu et al., 2015).

2.3 Electrochemical Bienzymatic Biosensor

A bienzymatic biosensor composed of laccase (LACC), tyrosinase (TYR) and AuNPs entrapped in a CS polymeric matrix (LACC–TYR–AuNPs–CS/GPE) was developed in a single step by electrodeposition of a hybrid film onto a graphene doped CPE and used for carbamates detection (Oliveira et al., 2014).

2.4 Potentiometric Butyrylcholine (BuCh) Sensor

A highly sensitive potentiometric butyrylcholine (BuCh) sensor based on plasticized poly(vinyl chloride) membrane was fabricated using tetrakis(3,5-bis[2-methoxy-hexafluoro-methyl] phenyl) borate (HFPB) as a cation exchanger and used for the organophosphate pesticides, 2,2-dichlorovinyldimethylphosphate ando-(4-bromo-2-chlorophenyl)o-ethyl S-propylphosphothiolate) detection in micromole and subnanomole range (Ishibashi, 1995).

2.5 Potentiometric Biosensor Based on SiO_2 Nanoparticles

A potentiometric biosensor for the detection the organophosphate pesticide methamidophos has been developed. The biosensor is based on a self-assembled platform formed by poly(allylamine) hydrochloride (PAH) and silicon dioxide nanoparticles (SiO_2–Np) that contains the immobilized enzyme AChE. After quantifying ACh, the inhibition of AChE in the presence of methamidophos was determined. This biosensor is simple to obtain and operate, appropriate for production at an industrial scale, at a low processing cost (Arruda et al., 2014).

2.6 Biosensors Based on Carbon Nanostructures

Carbon allotropes such as graphene and carbon nanotubes, have been incorporated in electrochemical biosensors for highly sensitive and selective detection of various analytes, due to their many advantages for such applications, like high carrier mobility, ambipolar electric field effect, high surface area, flexibility and compatibility with microfabrication techniques. These biosensors are suitable for the design of portable and point-of-use/field -deployable assay kits (Ramnani et al., 2016).

Benomyl is an agricultural pesticide with toxicity on human health and for the environment. A simple and sensitive electroanalytical method for cyclic voltammetry and differential pulse voltammetry determination using a magnetic nickel ferrite ($NiFe_2O_4$)/MWCNTs nanohybrid-modified GCE has been developed. The detection limit in phosphate-buffered saline at pH 6.0 was 2.51×10^{-8} mol/L but the method was also used to detect benomyl in real samples with satisfactory results (Wang et al., 2015a).

The Prussian blue nanocubes/reduced graphene oxide (PBNCs/rGO) nanocomposite was used to design a novel AChE biosensor for detection of OPs. The PBNCs/rGO hybrids nanocomposite exhibited high electrocatalytic activity towards the oxidation of thiocholine, which lead to the sensitive detection of OP pesticides (Zhang et al., 2012a).

2.7 Piezoelectric Biosensors

Immunosensors based on acoustic waves are of emerging interest because of their good sensitivity, real-time monitoring capability, and experimental simplicity (Jia et al., 2012). Piezoelectric systems have emerged as ones of the most attractive biosensing assays for the biopesticides detection due to their simplicity, low instrumentation costs, possibility for real-time and label-free detection and generally high sensitivity. Piezoelectric crystals such as quartz vibrate with characteristic resonant frequency depending on their thickness and cut under the influence of an electric field. The resonant frequency will modify when different molecules adsorb or desorb from the surface of the crystal, and the induced changes are detected by an electronic circuit. Biosensors based on the quartz crystal microbalance have been reported in the literature for organophosphate and carbamate pesticide analysis (Marrazza, 2014). A piezoelectric crystal immunobiosensor has been developed for the assay of atrazine herbicides in drinking water with a detection limit of 0.03–100 μg/L (Guilbault et al., 1992). An AChE-coated thin film bulk acoustic resonator has been developed for the detection of organophosphorus pesticides (Chen et al., 2012b; Chen et al., 2013).

3 Optical and Imaging Biosensing Methods

3.1 Quantum Dots Based Sensors

A sensitive photoelectrochemical (PEC) biosensor for detection of OPs using the nanocomposite of CdSe@ZnS quantum dots (QDs) and graphene deposited on the ITO coated glass electrode as a photoactive electrode has been described (Li et al., 2015). Under visible light irradiation, the AChE–CdSe@ZnS/graphene nanocomposite can generate a stable photocurrent and the photocurrent is found to be inversely dependent on the concentration of OPs.

A label free silicon quantum dots (SiQDs)-based sensor was designed for ultrasensitive detection of pesticides carbaryl, parathion, diazinon, and phorate in food samples (Yi et al., 2013).

An optical biosensing method using CdTe QDs and bienzyme-immobilized eggshell membranes for the determination of OPs has been developed. Increasing amounts of OPs led to a decrease of the enzymatic activity and thus a decrease in the production of hydrogen peroxide, which can quench the fluorescence of the CdTe QDs. The detection limits for OPs were very low, that is, 4.3×10^{-12} mol/L for paraoxon and 2.47×10^{-12} mol/L for parathion and the method proved to be adequate for Ops detection in real fruit samples and showed good repeatability. Moreover, the bienzyme-immobilized eggshell membrane demonstrated a long shelf-life of at least 2 months and the results (Xue et al., 2016). A biofunctional AChE-graphene nanosheets (GNs)–CdTe quantum dots QDs hybrid was used ad cathodic ECL emitters for OPs sensing (Liang et al., 2014). A novel visible light photoelectrochemical platform coupled with enzyme-inhibition for rapid and sensitive determination of OPs was constructed based on a dual functional Cd0.5Zn0.5S-RGO nanocomposite (Liu et al., 2014b).

In this selective method for detection of OPs the generated H_2O_2 can quench the fluorescence of Mn:ZnSe d-dots. When paraoxon are introduced in solution, it can interact with the active centers of AChE and decrease the enzyme activity. This leads to the decrease of the H_2O_2 production and then the fluorescence quenching rate of Mn:ZnSe d dots. The proposed biosensor has been employed for quick determination of paraoxon in tap water and milk samples with satisfactory reproducibility and accuracy. This nanobiosensor was proved to be sensitive, rapid, simple and tolerance of most interfering substances (Gao et al., 2012).

A simple and sensitive fluorescent sensor for methyl parathion based on L-tyrosine methyl ester functionalized carbon dots (Tyr–CDs) exhibiting strong and stable photoluminescence and tyrosinase system was developed. Tyrosinase can catalyze the oxidation of tyrosine methyl ester on the surface of carbon dots to corresponding quinone products, which can quench the fluorescence of carbon dots. When organophosphorus pesticides, such as methyl parathion are introduced in system, they can decrease the enzyme activity, thus decrease the fluorescence quenching rate. The enzyme inhibition rate was proportional to the logarithm of the methyl parathion concentration and the detection limit was 4.8×10^{-11} M. This sensing system has been successfully used for the analysis of cabbage, milk and fruit juice samples (Hou et al., 2015).

3.2 Meso-Tetra (4-Sulfonatophenyl) Porphine (TPPS4) and 2-Hydroxyquinoxaline Based Biosensor

Since all of the OPs inhibit the cholinesterases with a common mechanism, many detection methods use the inhibition-based biosensors. The interaction of quinalphos with plant-esterase involves besides the decrease in the enzymatic activity, the cleavage of quinalphos with the release of 2-hydroxyquinoxaline that could became an ideal biomarker. The 2-hydroxyquinoxaline and meso-tetra (4-sulfonatophenyl) porphine ($TPPS_4$) as an optical probe have been used for the detection of quinalphos, by registering the spectral responses of TPPS4 with a detection limit of 0.01 mg/kg (Yang et al., 2015).

3.3 Fluorescent Biosensors

Fluorescent molecularly imprinted polymers, which were designed for the selective recognition and fluorescence detection of λ-cyhalothrin (LC), were synthesized via fluorescein 5(6)-isothiocyanate (FITC) and 3-aminopropyltriethoxysilane (APTS)/ SiO_2 particles. The SiO_2@FITC–APTS polymer was deposited as an imprinted polymer film of about 100 nm thickness which successfully detected LC in Chinese spirits with a detection limit of 9.17 nM/L (Wang et al., 2015b). Core–shell magnetic Fe3O4/SiO_2–MPS [(methacryloxyl) propyl trimethoxysilane molecularly imprinted polymers] were also used for for optical sensitive detection of LC (Gao et al., 2014). A core–shell structured nanocomposite (YVO4:$Eu^{(3+)}$@MIPs), composed of lanthanide doped YVO4:$Eu^{(3+)}$ as fluorescent signal and surface molecular imprinted polymers as molecular selective recognition sites were designed for the detection of LC with a detection limit of 1.76 μM (Liu et al., 2014c).

A novel label-free, rapid, cost-effective, and highly sensitive fluorometric sensor has been constructed for the detection of AChE activity and its inhibitor based on the fluorescence quenching of DNA-templated copper/silver nanoclusters (DNA–Cu/AgNCs). This method was also used to detect spiked OPs in agricultural products successfully (Li et al., 2013).

AChE and CdTe were immobilized onto the surface of quartz in a self-assembled multilayer film for the fluorimetric detection of pesticides (Sun et al., 2011a).

A screen printed carbon electrode was integrated into a flow cell while AchE was immobilised on cobalt(II) phthalocyanine modified electrodes by entrapment in aphotocrosslinkable polymer The automated flow-based biosensor wassuccessfully used to quantify three OPs in milksamples in less than 15 min (Mishra et al., 2012).

Peptide nanotubes (PNTs) encapsulating horseradish peroxidase and surface coated with AChE were attached to gold screen printed electrodes to construct a novel gas phase OP biosensor (Baker et al., 2014).

A disposable evanescent wave fiber optic sensor was obtained by coating a molecularly imprinted polymer containing a fluorescent signaling group (naphthalimide-based fluorescent monomer which shows fluorescence enhancement upon binding with carboxyl-containing molecules) on a polystyrene optical waveguide. The sensing element was interrogated with a fiber-coupled spectrofluorimeter. The fiber optic sensor specifically detected the targets represented by the herbicide 2,4-dichlorophenoxyacetic acid and the mycotoxin citrinin in the low nM range (Ton et al., 2015).

The inherent peroxidase-like nanozyme activity of gold nanoparticles was combined with the high affinity and specificity of an acetamiprid-specific S-18 aptamer to design a rapid, specific and sensitive biosensor used to detect this neurotoxic pesticide with a detection limit of 0.1 ppm within 10 min. Similar to an enzymatic competitive inhibition process, in the presence of a cognate target, these aptamer molecules leave the gold nanoparticles surface in a target concentration-dependent manner, reactivating their nanozyme activity. This reversible inhibition of the gold nanoparticles nanozyme activity can either be directly visualized in the form of color change of the peroxidase reaction product or can be quantified using UV-visible absorbance spectroscopy (Weerathunge et al., 2014).

A biosensor based on the oligonucleotide ss-DNA aptamer in the receptor role, silver nanoparticles as optical sensors and salt as the aggregative inducer of AgNPs was used to detect the presence of Acetamiprid. The selective detection of Acetamiprid was performed with a detection limit of 89.8 nM (Jokar et al., 2016).

3.4 Nanosensors Based on Upconversion Nanoparticles (UCNPs) and Gold Nanoparticles (AuNPs)

A novel nanosensor for the detection of organophosphorus pesticides in real food samples with good sensitivity, stability based on the fluorescence resonance energy transfer (FRET) between NaYF4:Yb,Er upconversion nanoparticles (UCNPs) and gold nanoparticles (AuNPs) has been developed. The detection mechanism is based on the fact that AuNPs quench the fluorescence of UCNPs and the organophosphorus pesticide inhibits the activity of AChE. Under optimized conditions the detection limits of parathion-methyl, monocrotophos and dimethoatewere 0.67, 23, and 67 ng/L, respectively (Long et al., 2015a).

A biosensor based on nanomagnet-silica core–shell conjugated to organophosphorous hydrolase (OPH) enzyme was designed for detection of paraoxon, using coumarin1, a competitive inhibitor of the OPH enzyme, as a fluorescence-generating molecule. Upon excitation of cumarin1 located at the active site of the OPH enzyme, the emitted radiations were intensified due to the mirroring effect of the nanomagnet–silica core–shell conjugated to the enzyme. In presence of paraoxon and consequent competition with the fluorophore in occupying enzyme's active site, a significant dose-dependentsignal reduction was observed. This assay allowed the detection of paraoxon in the 10–250 nM concentration range with a detection limit of 5×10^{-6} μM (Khaksarinejad et al., 2015).

p-Phenyleneethynylene oligomers with bear pendant charged groups making them ideal for sensing. A biosensor based on one anionic and one cationic oligomer combined with substrates that are susceptible to enzymatic degradation by phospholipases or acetylcholinesterases was designed. The fluorescence quantum yields of thesensors enhanced from 30 to 66 times compared to the oligomers without substrate (Hill et al., 2015).

High throughput screening of protein-small molecule binding interactions using label-free optical biosensors is challenging, as the detected signals are often similar in magnitude to experimental noise. A self-referencing external cavity laser ECL biosensor approach with high resolution and sensitivity was used to demonstrate detection of binding between small molecules and a variety of immobilized protein targets with binding affinities or inhibition constants in the subnanomolar to low micromolar range. This biosensor has the ability to perform specific detection in the presence of interfering compounds (Meng Zhang et al., 2014).

3.5 Colorimetric Assays

Using a Cu (I)-catalyzed click chemistry as the colorimetric signal amplification process improved colorimetric sensitivity for OPs detection by the AChE inhibition system (Fu et al., 2013).

Gold nanoparticles have been used as signal-enhancing detection probes in the field of pesticides detection biosensors (diazinon, iprobenfos, and edifenpho) in part-per-billion (ppb) concentrations in water samples (Kim et al., 2015a). Self-assembly modulation of gold nanorods (AuNRs) was achieved by enzymatic reaction, and further employed for colorimetric assays of AChE and organophosphate pesticides in human blood. The resulting thiols then react with the tips of the AuNRs by S–Au conjunction and prevent subsequent cysteine-induced AuNR end-to-end (EE) self-assembly. Correspondingly, the AuNR SPR is regulated, which results in a distinctly ratiometric signal output. As ChE is incubated with OPs, the enzymatic activity is inhibited. So, the cysteine-induced assembly is observed again. On the basis of this principle, OPs can be well determined ranging from 0.12 to 40 pM with a 0.039 pM detection limit, which is at least 500 and respectively 7000 times lower than those of previous colorimetric methods (Lu and Xia, 2015).

A colorimetric sensor array comprising five inexpensive and commercially available thiocholine and H_2O_2 sensitive indicators for the simultaneous detection and identification of OPs and carbamates was developed. In the presence of OPs and carbamates the activity of AChE in inhibited, preventing production of thiocholine and H_2O_2 from S-acetylthiocholine and acetylcholine and thus resulting in decreased or no color reactions to thiocholine and H_2O_2 sensitive indicators. Thisassay could discriminate between OPs and carbamates and fromother kinds of pesticides (Qian and Lin, 2015).

The sensitive detection of iprobenfos (IBF) and edifenphos (EDI) was successfully conducted by using a new aptamer-based colorimetric multiaptasensor, with a detection limit of 10 and 5 nM, respectively. The detection of the respective pesticides in spiked paddy and polished rice samples using this multiaptasensor was around 80 and 90%, respectively (Kwon et al., 2015).

A colorimetric method for the detection of dichlorvos is based on polydiacethylene and AChE inhibition. The blue-to-red color transition of poly(10,12-pentacosadynoic acid) vesicles can be induced by myristoylcholine which is enzymatically hydrolyzed by acetylcholinesterase to myristic acid and choline to prevent the color transition. In the presence of dichlorvos, the hydrolytic activity of the enzyme is inhibited that the blue-to-red color transition is restored with a linear correlation to the dichlorvos concentration (Pimsen et al., 2014).

3.6 Nanobiosensors Based on Atomic Force Microscopy

Nanosensors based on atomic force microscopy (AFM) tips are useful for detecting agrochemicals because they provide higher sensitivity with operation at the nanometer scale. The specific interactions between AFM tips functionalized with the enzyme acetolactate synthase (ALS) have been exploited to detect the ALS-inhibitor herbicides metsulfuron-methyl and imazaquin. Using atomic force spectroscopy (AFS) the adhesion force between tip and substrate could be measured and proved to be considerably higher with approximately 250% and 160% for metsulfuron-methyl and imazaquin, respectively, when the ALS-functionalized tip (nanobiosensor) was used, in comparison to unfunctionalized probes. The specific biorecognition force plays a crucial role in the higher sensitivity of the nanobiosensor, thus opening the way for the design of similarly engineered tips for detecting herbicides and other analytes (da Silva et al., 2014).

3.7 Surface-Enhanced Raman Spectroscopy (SERS) -Based Biosensors for Rapid Detection of Pesticides

Biological silver nanoparticles could be an advantageous alternative to build newer and safer tools against biological vectors (Suresh et al., 2015). The detection of the organochlorine pesticides aldrin, dieldrin, lindane, and α-endosulfan has been performed by using surface-enhanced Raman spectroscopy (SERS) and optimization of the SERS-sensing substrate. In order to overcome the low affinity of pesticides, the silver nanoparticles metal surface was functionalized with alkyl dithiols in order to induce the nanoparticle linkage and create interparticle junctions where sensitive hot spots needed for SERS enhancement are present and to create a specific environment in the nanogaps between silver and gold nanoparticles, making them suitable for the assembly and SERS detection of the analyzed pesticides. The obtained results confirmed the high sensitivity of SERS for the detection of the organochlorine pesticides with a LOD reaching 10^{-8} M, thus providing a promising way for the design of suitable nanosensors for the identification and quantitative analysis of these compounds (Kubackova et al., 2015).

The size- and shape-dependent SERS activities of plasmonic core–shell nanoparticles towards detection of the pesticide thiram were investigated. Monodisperse Au@Agnanocubes (NCs) and Au@Ag nanocuboids (NBs) with Ag shell thickness adjusted from ~1 to ~16 nm were synthesized and used as SERS substrates for thiram detection. The Raman intensities with three different lasers (514, 633 and 782 nm) were recorded and compared. The results show that the excitation wavelength discriminated particle shapes regardless of particle sizes and for the optimized laser wavelength, the maximum Raman enhancement was achieved at a certain threshold of particle size (or silver coating thickness). By exciting particles at their optimized sizes with the corresponding optimized laser wavelengths, the detection limit of for thiram were 100 and 80 pM for NCs and NBs, respectively (Guo et al., 2015).

The Agnanoparticle (AgNP) decorated ZnO–mesoporous-nanosheets (NSs) grafted on a flexible carbon fiber cloth (CFC) have proven to be sensitive, flexible and reproducible SERS substrates. The composite SERS-substrates were achieved by a combination of atomic layer deposition of ZnO-seeds on each fiber of the CFC (denoted as ZnO-seeds@CFC), chemical bath deposition and subsequent pyrolysis for the creation of ZnO–mesoporous-NSs grafted on ZnO-seeds@CFC, and ion-sputtering of AgNPs on the ZnO–mesoporous-NSs. As abundant SERS "hot spots" are generated from the electromagnetic coupling of the densely distributed AgNPs, and the semiconducting ZnO–mesoporous-NSs also have chemical supporting enhancement and distinct molecule adsorbing abilities, the composite SERS-substrates demonstrate high SERS-sensitivity with good signal reproducibility. The composite SERS-substrates were successfully used to detect pesticides and highly toxic polychlorinated biphenyls (PCBs), at low concentrations of 10^{-7} M for methyl parathion and 5×10^{-6} M for PCB-77, showing promising potential for the SERS-based rapid detection of toxic organic pollutants in the environment (Wang et al., 2014).

4 Immunosensors

The development of immunosensors for the detection of small molecules is of great interest because of their simplicity, high sensitivity and extended analytical range.

4.1 Immunoelectrodes

Due to their small size, pesticides cannot be simultaneously recognized by two antibodies impeding their detection by noncompetitive two-site immunoassays, which are superior to competitive ones in terms of sensitivity, kinetics, and working range. Testing for traces of different pesticides (triazinic, OPs and chlorurates), present in hydrophobic matrices such as sunflower oil was checked using new immunosensors working in organic solvent mixtures (OPIEs). The competitive process took place in an *n*-hexane-chloroform 75% (V/V) mixture, while the subsequent final enzymatic measurement was performed in decane using tert-butylhydroperoxide as substrate of the enzymatic reaction. A Clark electrode was used as transducer and peroxidase enzyme as marker. A linear response of between about 10 nM and 4 μM was usually obtained in the presence of sunflower oil. Immunosensors show satisfactory selectivity and precision and recovery tests carried out on commercial sunflower oil samples gave excellent results (Martini et al., 2015a).

Using immunosensors (with Clark electrode as transducer and peroxidase enzyme as marker) active in organic solvent mixtures made possible the detection of different pesticides (triazinic, OPs and chlorurates) found in traces in hydrophobic matrices such as olive oil (Martini et al., 2015b).

A novel optical biosensor device using recombinant methyl parathion hydrolase (MPH) enzyme immobilized on agarose by metal-chelate affinity to detect OP compounds with a nitrophenyl group. The biosensor principle is based on the optical measurement of the product of OP catalysis by MPH (*p*-nitrophenol) (Lan et al., 2012).

A magneto–electrochemical immunosensor for the herbicide molinate proved to be more rapid and exhibited a mwider linear range when compared to the conventional ELISA (Arévalo et al., 2012).

An immunosensor for the detection of the pesticide atrazine in environmental samples was obtained by using the self-assembling process of the disulfide derivative of the pesticide atrazine on a gold substrate (Hromadová et al., 2013).

An electrochemical immunosensor based on IAMs with immobilized chlorpyrifos monoclonal antibodies was developed for sensitive, specific and rapid detection of chlorpyrifos. Electrochemical impedance spectroscopy was used in conjunction with the fabricated sensor to detect chlorpyrifos, proving to be a valuable tool for screening pesticide presence in environmental, agricultural and pharmaceutical samples due to its rapidity, sensitivity and low cost (Cao et al., 2015).

A novel multianalyte electrochemical immunosensor based on the assembly of patterned SWNTs on glassy carbon (GC) substrates was developed for simultaneous detection of endosulfan and paraoxon, proving high repeatability, reproducibility, stability and selectivity (Liu et al., 2014d).

A disposable electrochemical immunosensor for the determination of phenyl urea herbicide-diuron has been developed using low cost laser ablated gold electrodes fabricated on polystyrene substrate, deposited with prussian blue–gold nanoparticle (PB–GNP) film (Sharma et al., 2011).

An electrochemical impedance immunosensor was designed for the detection of phenoxy acid herbicide 2,4-Dichlorophenoxybutyric acid (2,4-DB)(Zhang et al., 2012b).

A disposable amperometric immunosensor for detection of chlorpyrifos-methyl (CM) has been developed by combining dual signal amplification of screen-printed carbon electrodes (SPCE) with an enzymatic catalytic reaction. The immobilization of albumin conjugated chlorpyrifos-methyl antigen (BSA–Ag) and platinum colloid on the electrodes was achieved into SiSG (Wei et al., 2012).

An amperometric immunosensor based on multiwall carbon nanotubes (MWCNTs) and graphene sheets-ethyleneimine polymer-Au (GS–PEI–Au) nanocomposites self-assembled onto the surface of a glass carbon electrode (GCE) for the detection of carbofuran was developed. The nanocomposites can increase the surface area of the GCE to capture a large amount of antibody, as well as produce a synergistic effect in the electrochemical performance (Zhu et al., 2013). An amperometric immunosensor based on MWCNTs–thionine–chitosan nanocomposite film as electrode-modified material was developed for the detection of chlorpyrifos residues (Sun et al., 2012). A label-free immunosensor based on SWNTs modified GC electrodes has been developed for the direct detection of paraoxon (Liu et al., 2013b).

An amperometric immunosensor modified with protein A/ deposited gold nanocrystals (DpAu) exhibiting high specificity, reproducibility, stability, and regeneration performance was developed for the detection of carbofuran residues (Sun et al., 2011b). In another study, the anticarbofuran monoclonal antibody was directly immobilized on the surface of a GCE using SiSG technology (Sun et al., 2011c).

An immunosensor for the detection of parathion was achieved by the photonic immobilization technique consisting in activating an antibody solution by breaking the disulfide bridge in the triad Trp/Cys–Cys through absorption of ultrashort UV laser pulses. The free thiol groups so produced interact with gold lamina making the antibody oriented upside, that is, with its variable parts exposed to the environment, thereby greatly increasing the detection efficiency (Funari et al., 2013).

4.2 Optofluidics-Based Biosensing Platform

The adsorption of pesticides in soil is a key process that affects transport, degradation, mobility, and bioaccumulation of these substances. To obtain extensive knowledge regarding the adsorption processes of pesticides in the environment, the new green assay technologies for the rapid, sensitive, field-deployable, and accurate quantification of pesticides are required. An evanescent wave-based optofluidics biosensing (EWOB) platform was developed by combining advanced photonics and microfluidics technology for the rapid sensitive immunodetection and adsorption kinetics assay of pesticides. The robustness, reusability, and accuracy of the EWOB allow an enhanced prediction of pesticide adsorption kinetics in soil. Therefore, proposed EWOB system provides a simple, green, and powerful tool to investigate the transport mechanism and fate of pesticide residues (Long et al., 2015b).

4.3 Immunosensors Based on Surface Plasmon Resonance

The SPR method combined with immune reactions has been used to detect coumaphos with high sensitivity and specificity. The required equipments are simple, environmental friendly, and easy to control (Li et al., 2014).

A very sensitive SPR competitive immunoassay using a PH–BSA immobilized sensor chip was developed to measure phosmet in food samples (Song et al., 2013).

A SPR immunoassay for on-line detection of the strobilurin fungicide pyraclostrobin in apple, grape, and cranberry samples untreated fruit juices was described (Mauriz et al., 2012).

A highly sensitive and specific SPR-based competitive immunoassay where TBZ-protein conjugate is immobilized onto gold surfaces for the detection of thiabendazole (TBZ) has been developed (Estevez et al., 2012).

A new surface-initiated polymerization based on pasting the initiator on a sensor chip surface was applied to prepare a malachite green (MG) imprinted ultrathin film on a SPR sensor. The MIP modified SPR sensor showed high sensitivity and selectivity, as well as good stability in detecting MG (Dong et al., 2012).

A new approach that combines SPR sensor technology with Fe_3O_4 magnetic nanoparticles (MNPs) conjugated with antibodies specific to antigen assays was developed for directly detecting of deltamethrin in soybean. The excellent selectivity of the present biosensor was also confirmed by two kinds of pesticides (fenvalerate and atrazine) as controls. This magnetic separation and amplification strategy has great potential for detection of other small analytes in trace level concentration, with high selectivity and sensitivity by altering the target-analyte-capture agent labeled to the carboxyl-coated Fe_3O_4 MNPs (Liu et al., 2014e).

It has also been reported a SPR biosensor decorated with an oligopeptide, TPFDLRPSSDTR for online detection of glyphosate (Ding and Yang, 2013).

A direct competitive enzyme-linked immunosorbent assay (dc-ELISA) and an immunosensor based on SPR-sensor were developed for the fungicide boscalidassay in horticultural crops. Recovery of the spiked boscalidat the maximum residue limit of 1–40 mg/kg was 85–109% by the SPR-sensor and 100–124% by the dc-ELISA. On real tomato samples, the results obtained by both of these immunoassays correlated well with the results obtained by high-performance liquid chromatography (Hirakawa et al., 2015a).

An immunosensor based on SPR-sensor was developed to analyze chlorothalonil (CTN) residues in vegetables. Conjugates of *N*-(pentachlorophenoxyacetyl)glycine and bovine serum albumin were covalently coated on the sensor chip. The SPR-sensor quantitatively determined CTN at concentrations ranging from 8.0 to 44 ng/mL, using TPN9A, a monoclonal antibody to CTN. CTN spiked in vegetables was recovered at 90–118% within 1 day and at 90–115% across 3 days, correlating with HPLC results (Hirakawa et al., 2015b).

A new SPR immunodevice for triazine pesticide determination was compared with two other amperometric (conventional and screen-printed) "competitive" assays and provided comparable results, but the measurement time was much shorter and the assay much easier to perform (Tomassetti et al., 2015).

4.4 Immunochromatographic Assay

A novel bare-eye based one-step signal amplified semiquantitative immunochromatographic competitive assay (SAS–ICA) was developed for detection of the pesticide imidacloprid. Signal amplification was achieved by dual labeling of the test lines (TLs) on the strip using high affinity nanogold-biotinylated anti-imidaclopridmAb (BAb) and nanogold-streptavidin (Sa) probes. The relative color intensities of three TLs on a nitrocellulose (NC) membrane were used for directvisual analysis. The sensitivity and semiquantitative analytical capacity of the SAS–ICA strip were 10-fold and 160-fold higher than those of traditional ICA, respectively. The developed SAS–ICA strip was applied to the analysis of spiked and authentic contaminated Chinese cabbage samples in the laboratory and under field conditions, and the results were validated by HPLC (Fang et al., 2015).

4.5 Microflow-Injection Analysis (μFIA) Immunoassay

As a part of developing new systems for continuously monitoring the presence of pesticides in groundwater, a microfluidic amperometric immunosensor was developed for detecting the herbicide residue 2,6-dichlorobenzamide (BAM) in water. A competitive immunosorbent assay served as the sensing mechanism and amperometry was applied for detection. Both the immunoreaction chip (IRC) and detection (D) unit are integrated on a modular microfluidic platform with in-built microflow-injection analysis (μFIA) function. The immunosorbent, immobilized in the channel of the IRC, was found to have high long-term stability and withstand many regeneration cycles, both of which are key requirements for systems utilized in continuous monitoring. Detection of BAM standard solutions was performed in the concentration range 0.0008–62.5 μg/L, which demonstrate the potential of the constructed μFIA immunosensor as an atline monitoring system for controlling the quality of groundwater supply (Uthuppu et al., 2015).

4.6 Multicomponent Lateral-Flow Assay Based on Antibody–Antigen Reaction

A multicomponent lateral-flow assay based on an antibody–antigen reaction was designed for the rapid and simultaneous detection of trace contaminants in water, including a heavy metal (Pb(II), the algal toxinmicrocystin–leucine–arginine (MC–LR), the antibiotic chloramphenicol (CAP), the hormone testosterone (T), and the pesticide CTN. Samples or standards containing the five analytes were preincubated with the freeze-dried colloidal-gold-labeled monoclonal antibody conjugates to improve the sensitivity of the assay. The results were obtained within 20 min with a paper-based sensor. The cut-off values for the strip test were 4 ng/mL for Pb(II), 1 ng/mL for MC–LR, 0.1 ng/mL for CAP, 5 ng/mL for T, and 5 ng/mL for CTN. The assay was evaluated using spiked water samples, and the accuracy and reproducibility of the results were good, proving that this lateral-flow device provides an effective and rapid method for the onsite detection of multiple contaminants in water samples, with no treatment or devices required (Xing et al., 2015).

4.7 Magnetoelectrochemical Immunosensors Combined With Noncompetitive Immunoassays

Although graphenes and related materials are among the most promising for research in electrochemical sensors, their applications are limited by the insufficient sensitivity of these nanohybrids for trace molecules. However, this disadvantage could be surpassed by signal amplification strategies, such as those based on magnetoelectrochemical immunoassay which assures a good sensitivity by the electrochemical bursting of MNPs into a large number of metal ions (Sharma et al., 2012). The advantages of magneto-electrochemical immunosensors have been combined with the improved sensitivity and direct proportional signal of noncompetitive immunoassays to develop a new phage antiimmunocomplex electrochemical immunosensor (PhAIEI) for the detection of the herbicide atrazine. The noncompetitive assay is based on the use of recombinant M13 phage particles bearing a peptide that specifically recognizes the immunocomplex of atrazine with an antiatrazine monoclonal antibody. The PhAIEI performed with a LOD of 0.2 pg/mL, which is 200-fold better than the LOD obtained using the same antibody in an optimized conventional competitive ELISA, with a large increase in working range. The developed PhAIEI was successfully used to assay undiluted river water samples with no pretreatment and excellent recoveries. Apart from the first demonstration of the benefits of integrating phage antiimmunocomplex particles into electrochemical immunosensors, the extremely low and environmentally relevant detection limits of atrazine attained with the PhAIEIS may have direct applicability to fast and sensitive detection of this herbicide in the environment (González-Techera et al., 2015).

5 Whole-Cell Based Biosensors

5.1 Bacterial Cells

An amperometric biosensor, incorporating the cyanobacterium *Synechococcus* as the biocatalyst has been developed for on-line herbicide detection at concentrations down to 20 μg/L (Rawson et al., 1989). In whole-cell based biosensors, spectrophotometry is one of the most commonly used methods for detecting OPs due to its simplicity and reliability. The sensor performance is directly affected by the cell immobilization method because it determines the amount of cells, the mass transfer rate, and the stability. An immobilization method, based on the attachment of the microbe on single-walled carbon nanotube film, has been applied to whole-cell-based organophosphate sensors to increase specificity, rapidity, and stability. Cryoimmobilized, recombinant *Escherichia coli* cells capable of hydrolyzing a wide spectrum of OP pesticides and chemical warfare agents by organophosphate hydrolase were used for the detection of OP neurotoxins (Rainina et al., 1996). *E. coli* expressing organophosphorus hydrolase (OPH) in the periplasmic space and single-walled carbon nanotubes were attached to the device which was further used to hydrolyze paraoxon, and detected by measuring the concentration of the enzymatic reaction product, *p*-nitrophenol. The specific activity of this device was over 2.5 times that reported previously for other whole-cell organophosphate sensors (Kim et al., 2015b). The immobilization of OPH on environmentally friendly supports is of great importance for developing stabilized enzymes for degradation of organophosphorus compounds.

Bacillus subtilis spores were used as immobilizing matrix for OPH, which was covalently bound to the spores by using EDC–NHS as coupling reagents. The immobilized enzyme hydrolyzed the pesticide paraoxon with a yield was six times higher than the immobilized enzyme. Therefore, *B. subtilis* spores can represent an environmentally and cost-effective alternative for the design of biosensors for the monitoring and biodegradation of organophosphate contaminants in the environment and detoxification processes in bioreactors with high reusability without decrease in the activity (Falahati-Pour et al., 2015). A new approach for the identification of organophosphorous compounds was based on the high-affinity binding of these compounds with the esterase two from *Alicyclobacillus acidocaldarius*. The quenching of the tryptophan residues after esterase two binding with the organophosphate pesticides, such as paraoxon, parathion, chlorpyriphos, and other organophosphate thio-derivatives, was detected by fluorescence spectroscopy. The changes in the fluorescence signals permitted an immediate and quantitative identification of these compounds from nano- to picomolar concentrations. Therefore, the exploitation of fluorescence technology in combination with a sensitive and very stable bioreceptor could represent a successful approach for the development of sensitive and specific biosensors (Carullo et al., 2015).

5.2 Fungal Cells

A potentiometric biosensor for the detection of permethrin in treated wood based on immobilized cells of the fungus *Lentinus sajor* (caju) proved to have a performance similar to that of HPLC (Arip et al., 2013).

5.3 Algal Cells

Algal cell biosensors, based on the photosystem II activity measurement, have been designed for the detection of chemicals in urban rainwaters. An immobilization technique of algal cells was performed in order to improve the performance of such biosensors. Immobilization was achieved by encapsulation in a hybrid alginate/silica translucid hydrogel (Durrieu et al., 2016). In another study the AChE was immobilized on a functional support constituted of a graphite paste modified with tetracyanoquinodimethane mediator, along with the use of *Cladaphropsis membranous* macroalgae, assurring an enhanced stability and sensitivity of the biosensor for the detection of methyl parathion OP insecticide in water samples, the results being similar to those obtained with GC–MS techniques (Nunes et al., 2014). The *Dictyosphaerium chlorelloides* microalgae cells were immobilized into porous silicone films and the inhibition of their photosynthetic activity by herbicides was monitored with an integrated robust luminescent O_2 sensor. This biosensing device detected in situ herbicide concentrations of 12 μg/L (Haigh-Flórez et al., 2014). The marine green alga *Ostreococcus tauri* was used as a free-living eukaryotic cell luminescent biosensor for assessing the presence of two degradation products of diuron in marine (Sanchez-Ferandin et al., 2013).

5.4 Mammalian Cells

Water is a renewable resource but yet finite. Its sustainable usage and the maintenance of a good quality are essential for an intact environment, human life, and a stable economy. Emerging technologies aim for a continuous monitoring of water quality, overcoming periodic analytical sampling, and providing information on the current state of inshore waters in real time. The rat liver cells (RLC-18) were used for the design of a cell-based sensor system capable to detect small variations in the water quality and to indicate a possible physiological damage caused. The integrated signals are represented by cellular metabolism, oxygen consumption, and morphological integrity. The water contamination with the organophosphate pesticide chlorpyrifos and with tetrabromobisphenol A, a flame retardant was followed by the occurrence of a very specific response, but the toxicity is mitigated if both chemicals are present at once (Guijarro et al., 2015).

5.5 Animal Models

Transgenic fish models, such as zebrafish (*Danio rerio*) lineage, expressing a destabilized fluorescent protein driven by the myosin light chain promoter were used for detecting the growth-related effects of pollutants even at the lower, environmentally acceptable concentration (Almeida et al., 2014).

6 Conclusions

The permanent and release of high amounts of contaminants, such as pesticides and other pollutants, in soil and the aquatic environment, presents a real threat both to ecosystems and human health. Thus, the development of rapid, cost-effective, accurate, and real time monitoring tools is crucial and would allow taking immediate decision on efficient decontamination procedures and could prevent further damage and potential casualties. Biosensors can overcome the limits of conventional techniques used for pesticides detection which are highly expensive and time consuming, while the advent of nanotechnology offers promising ways for the optimization and miniaturization of biosensing devices.

References

Alméida, D.V., Vaz, B., Azevedo Figueiredo, M., Junior, A.S., Marins, L.F., 2014. Fluorescent transgenic zebrafish as a biosensor for growth-related effects of methyl parathion. Aquat. Toxicol. 152, 147–151.

Arévalo, F.J., González-Techera, A., Zon, M.A., González-Sapienza, G., Fernández, H., 2012. Ultra-sensitive electrochemical immunosensor using analyte peptidomimetics selected from phage display peptide libraries. Biosens. Bioelectron. 32 (1), 231–237.

Arip, M.N., Heng, L.Y., Ahmad, M., Ujang, S., 2013. A cell-based potentiometric biosensor using the fungus *Lentinus sajor*-caju for permethrin determination in treated wood. Talanta 116, 776–781.

Arruda, I.G., Guimarães, F.E., Ramos, R.J., Vieira, N.C., 2014. Self-assembly of SiO_2 nanoparticles for the potentiometric detection of neurotransmitter acetylcholine and its inhibitor. J. Nanosci. Nanotechnol. 14 (9), 6658–6661.

Baker, P.A., Goltz, M.N., Schrand, A.M., Yoon do, Y., Kim, D.S., 2014. Organophosphate vapor detection on gold electrodes using peptide nanotubes. Biosens. Bioelectron. 61, 119–123.

Baselt, D.R., Lee, G.U., Natesan, M., Metzger, S.W., Sheehan, P.E., Colton, R., 1998. A biosensor based on magnetoresistance technology. J. Biosens. Bioelectron. 13 (7–8), 731–739.

Bernabei, M., Chiavarini, S., Cremisini, C., Palleschi, G., 1993. Anticholinesterase activity measurement by a choline biosensor: application in water analysis. Biosens. Bioelectron. 8 (5), 265–271.

Cai, JR(1), Zhou, L.N., Han, E., 2014. A sensitive amperometric acetylcholine biosensor based on carbon nanosphere and acetylcholinesterase modified electrode for detection of pesticide residues. Anal. Sci. 30 (6), 669–673.

Cao, Y., Sun, X., Guo, Y., Zhao, W., Wang, X., 2015. An electrochemical immunosensor based on interdigitated array microelectrode for the detection of chlorpyrifos. Bioproc. Biosyst. Eng. 38 (2), 307–313.

Carullo, P., Cetrangolo, G.P., Mandrich, L., Manco, G., Febbraio, F., 2015. Fluorescence spectroscopy approaches for the development of a real-time organophosphate detection system using an enzymatic sensor. Sensors 15 (2), 3932–3951.

Cesarino, I., Moraes, F.C., Lanza, M.R., Machado, S.A., 2012. Electrochemical detection of carbamate pesticides in fruit and vegetables with a biosensor based on acetylcholinesterase immobilised on a composite of polyaniline-carbon nanotubes. Food Chem. 135 (3), 873–879.

Chauhan, N., Narang, J., Pundir, C.S., 2011a. Immobilization of rat brain acetylcholinesterase on ZnS and poly(indole-5-carboxylic acid) modified Au electrode for detection of organophosphorus insecticides. Biosens. Bioelectron. 29 (1), 82–88.

Chauhan, N., Narang, J., Pundir, C.S., 2011b. Immobilization of rat brain acetylcholinesterase on porous gold-nanoparticle-$CaCO_3$ hybrid material modified Au electrode for detection of organophosphorous insecticides. Int. J. Biol. Macromol. 49 (5), 923–929.

Chen, A., Du, D., Lin, Y., 2012a. Highly sensitive and selective immuno-capture/electrochemical assay of acetylcholinesterase activity in red blood cells: a biomarker of exposure to organophosphorus pesticides and nerve agents. Environ. Sci. Technol. 46 (3), 1828–1833.

Chen, D., Wang, J., Xu, Y., Zhang, L., 2012b. A thin film electro-acoustic enzyme biosensor allowing the detection of trace organophosphorus pesticides. Anal. Biochem. 429 (1), 42–44.

Chen, D., Wang, J., Xu, Y., Li, D., Zhang, L., Li, Z., 2013. Highly sensitive detection of organophosphorus pesticides by acetylcholinesterase-coated thin film bulk acoustic resonator mass-loading sensor. Biosens. Bioelectron. 41, 163–167.

Chen, D., Sun, X., Guo, Y., Qiao, L., Wang, X., 2015. Acetylcholinesterase biosensor based on multi-walled carbon nanotubes-SnO_2-chitosan nanocomposite. Bioproc. Biosyst. Eng. 38 (2), 315–321.

da Silva, A.C., Deda, D.K., Bueno, C.C., Moraes, A.S., Da Roz, A.L., Yamaji, F.M., Prado, R.A., Viviani, V., Oliveira, Jr., O.N., Leite, F.L., 2014. Nanobiosensors exploiting specific interactions between an enzyme and herbicides in atomic force spectroscopy. J. Nanosci. Nanotechnol. 14 (9), 6678–6684.

Dhull, V., Gahlaut, A., Dilbaghi, N., Hooda, V., 2013. Acetylcholinesterase biosensors for electrochemical detection of organophosphorus compounds: a review. Biochem. Res. Int. 2013, 731501.

Ding, X., Yang, K.L., 2013. Development of an oligopeptide functionalized surface plasmon resonance biosensor for online detection of glyphosate. Anal. Chem. 85 (12), 5727–5733.

Dong, J., Peng, Y., Gao, N., Bai, J., Ning, B., Liu, M., Gao, Z., 2012. A novel polymerization of ultrathin sensitive imprinted film on surface plasmon resonance sensor. Analyst 137 (19), 4571–4576.

Dong, J., Fan, X., Qiao, F., Ai, S., Xin, H., 2013. A novel protocol for ultra-trace detection of pesticides: combined electrochemical reduction of Ellman's reagent with acetylcholinesterase inhibition. Anal Chim Acta. 761, 78–83.

Durrieu, C., Ferro, Y., Perullini, M., Gosset, A., Jobbágy, M., Bilmes, S.A., 2016. Feasibility of using a translucid inorganic hydrogel to build a biosensor using immobilized algal cells. Environ. Sci. Pollut. Res. Int. 23 (1), 9–13.

Dutta, R.R., Puzari, P., 2014. Amperometric biosensing of organophosphate and organocarbamate pesticides utilizing polypyrrole entrapped acetylcholinesterase electrode. Biosens. Bioelectron. 52, 166–172.

Edelstein, R.L., Tamanaha, C.R., Sheehan, P.E., Miller, M.M., Baselt, D.R., Whitman, L.J., Colton, R.J., 2000. The barc biosensor applied to the detection of biological warfare agents. Biosens. Bioelectron. 14 (10–11), 805–813.

Eggins, B., 2002. Chemical Sensors and Biosensors (Analytical Techniques in the Sciences). John Wiley & Sons, West Sussex.

Estevez, M.C., Belenguer, J., Gomez-Montes, S., Miralles, J., Escuela, A.M., Montoya, A., Lechuga, L.M., 2012. Indirect competitive immunoassay for the detection of fungicide Thiabendazole in whole orange samples by Surface Plasmon Resonance. Analyst 137 (23), 5659–5665.

Evtugyn, G.A., Shamagsumova, R.V., Padnya, P.V., Stoikov, I.I., Antipin, I.S., 2014. Cholinesterase sensor based on glassy carbon electrode modified with Ag nanoparticles decorated with macrocyclic ligands. Talanta 127, 9–17.

Falahati-Pour, S.K., Lotfi, A.S., Ahmadian, G., Baghizadeh, A., 2015. Covalent immobilization of recombinant organophosphorus hydrolase on spores of *Bacillus subtilis*. J. Appl. Microbiol. 118 (4), 976–988.

Fang, Q., Wang, L., Cheng, Q., Cai, J., Wang, Y., Yang, M., Hua, X., Liu, F., 2015. A bare-eye based one-step signal amplified semiquantitative immunochromatographic assay for the detection of imidacloprid in Chinese cabbage samples. Anal. Chim. Acta. 881, 82–89.

Fu, G., Chen, W., Yue, X., Jiang, X., 2013. Highly sensitive colorimetric detection of organophosphate pesticides using copper catalyzed click chemistry. Talanta 103, 110–115.

Funari, R., Della Ventura, B., Schiavo, L., Esposito, R., Altucci, C., Velotta, R., 2013. Detection of parathion pesticide by quartz crystal microbalance functionalized with UV-activated antibodies. Anal. Chem. 85 (13), 6392–6397.

Ganesana, M., Istarnboulie, G., Marty, J.L., Noguer, T., Andreescu, S., 2011. Site-specific immobilization of a $(His)_6$-tagged acetylcholinesterase on nickel nanoparticles for highly sensitive toxicity biosensors. Biosens. Bioelectron. 30 (1), 43–48.

Gao, X., Tang, G., Su, X., 2012. Optical detection of organophosphorus compounds based on Mn-doped ZnSe D-dot enzymatic catalytic sensor. Biosens. Bioelectron. 36 (1), 75–80.

Gao, L., Wang, J., Li, X., Yan, Y., Li, C., Pan, J., 2014. A core-shell surface magnetic molecularly imprinted polymers with fluorescence for λ-cyhalothrin selective recognition. Anal. Bioanal. Chem. 406 (28), 7213–7220.

Gong, J., Guan, Z., Song, D., 2013. Biosensor based on acetylcholinesterase immobilized onto layered double hydroxides for flow injection/amperometric detection of organophosphate pesticides. Biosens. Bioelectron. 39 (1), 320–323.

Gong, Z., Guo, Y., Sun, X., Cao, Y., Wang, X., 2014. Acetylcholinesterase biosensor for carbaryl detection based on interdigitated array microelectrodes. Bioproc. Biosyst. Eng. 37 (10), 1929–1934.

González-Techera, A., Zon, M.A., Molina, P.G., Fernández, H., González-Sapienza, G., Arévalo, F.J., 2015. Development of a highly sensitive noncompetitive electrochemical immunosensor for the detection of atrazine by phage anti-immunocomplex assay. Biosens. Bioelectron. 64, 650–656.

Gosser, D.K., Cyclic Voltammetry, 1994. Simulation and Analysis of Reaction Mechanisms. VHC Publishers, Inc..

Grieshaber, D., MacKenzie, R., Vörös, J., Reimhult, E., 2008. Electrochemical biosensors—sensor principles and architectures. Sensors 8 (3), 1400–1458.

Guijarro, C., Fuchs, K., Bohrn, U., Stütz, E., Wölfl, S., 2015. Simultaneous detection of multiple bioactive pollutants using a multiparametric biochip for water quality monitoring. Biosens. Bioelectron. 72, 71–79.

Guilbault, G.G., Hock, B., Schmid, R., 1992. A piezoelectric immunobiosensor for atrazine in drinking water. Biosens. Bioelectron. 7 (6), 411–419.

Guo, P., Sikdar, D., Huang, X., Si, K.J., Xiong, W., Gong, S., Yap, L.W., Premaratne, M., Cheng, W., 2015. Plasmonic core-shell nanoparticles for SERS detection of the pesticide thiram: size- and shape-dependent Raman enhancement. Nanoscale 7 (7), 2862–2868.

Haigh-Flórez, D., de la Hera, C., Costas, E., Orellana, G., 2014. Microalgae dual-head biosensors for selective detection of herbicides with fiber-optic luminescent O_2 transduction. Biosens. Bioelectron. 54, 484–491.

Hill, E.H., Zhang, Y., Evans, D.G., Whitten, D.G., 2015. Enzyme-specific sensors via aggregation of charged *p*-phenylene ethynylenes. ACS Appl. Mater. Interfaces 11, 5550–5560.

Hirakawa, Y., Yamasaki, T., Harada, A., Ohtake, T., Adachi, K., Iwasa, S., Narita, H., Miyake, S., 2015a. Analysis of the fungicide boscalid in horticultural crops using an enzyme-linked immunosorbent assay and an immunosensor based on surface plasmon resonance. J. Agric. Food Chem. 63 (36), 8075–8082.

Hirakawa, Y., Yamasaki, T., Watanabe, E., Okazaki, F., Murakami-Yamaguchi, Y., Oda, M., Iwasa, S., Narita, H., Miyake, S., 2015b. Development of an immunosensor for determination of the fungicide chlorothalonil in vegetables, using surface plasmon resonance. J. Agric. Food Chem. 63 (28), 6325–6330.

Hou, J., Dong, J., Zhu, H., Teng, X., Ai, S., Mang, M., 2015. A simple and sensitive fluorescent sensor for methyl parathion based on L-tyrosine methyl ester functionalized carbon dots. Biosens. Bioelectron. 68, 20–26.

Hromadová, M., Pospíšil, L., Sokolová, R., Bulíčková, J., Hof, M., Fischer-Durand, N., Salmain, M., 2013. Atrazine-based self-assembled monolayers and their interaction with anti-atrazine antibody: building of an immunosensor. Langmuir 29 (52), 16084–16092.

Ishibashi, N., 1995. Potentiometric butyrylcholine sensor for organophosphate pesticides. Imato T(1). Biosens. Bioelectron. 10 (5), 435–441.

Itoh, T., Shimomura, T., Hayashi, A., Yamaguchi, A., Teramae, N., Ono, M., Tsunoda, T., Mizukami, F., Stucky, G.D., Hanaoka TA, 2014. Electrochemical enzymatic biosensor with long-term stability using hybrid mesoporous membrane. Analyst 139 (18), 4654–4660.

Ivanov, A.N., Younusov, R.R., Evtugyn, G.A., Arduini, F., Moscone, D., Palleschi, G., 2011. Acetylcholinesterase biosensor based on single-walled carbon nanotubes—Co phtalocyanine for organophosphorus pesticides detection. Talanta 85 (1), 216–221.

Jia, K., Toury, T., Ionescu, R.E., 2012. Fabrication of an atrazine acoustic immunosensor based on a drop-deposition procedure. IEEE Trans Ultrason. Ferroelectr. Freq. Control 9 (9), 2015–2021.

Jokar, M., Safaralizadeh, M.H., Hadizadeh, F., Rahmani, F., Kalani, M.R., 2016. Design and evaluation of an apta-nano-sensor to detect Acetamiprid in vitro and in silico. J. Biomol. Struct. Dyn. 17, 1–13.

Kanik, F.E., Kolb, M., Timur, S., Bahadir, M., Toppare, L., 2013. An amperometric acetylcholine biosensor based on a conducting polymer. Int. J. Biol. Macromol. 59, 111–118.

Katz, E., Willner, I., 2003. Probing biomolecular interactions at conductive and semiconductive surfaces by impedance spectroscopy: routes to impedimetric immunosensors, dna-sensors, and enzyme biosensors. Electroanalysis 15 (11), 913–947.

Khaksarinejad, R., Mohsenifar, A., Rahmani-Cherati, T., Karami, R., Tabatabaei, M., 2015. An organophosphorus hydrolase-based biosensor for direct detection of paraoxon using silica-coated magnetic nanoparticles. Appl. Biochem. Biotechnol. 176 (2), 359–371.

Kim, M.S., Kim, G.W., Park, T.J., 2015a. A facile and sensitive detection of organophosphorus chemicals by rapid aggregation of gold nanoparticles using organic compounds. Biosens. Bioelectron. 67, 408–412.

Kim, I., Kim, G.H., Kim, C.S., Cha, H.J., Lim, G., 2015b. Optical detection of paraoxon using single-walled carbon nanotube films with attached organophosphorus hydrolase-expressed *Escherichia coli*. Sensors 15 (6), 12513–12525.

Kubackova, J., Fabriciova, G., Miskovsky, P., Jancura, D., Sanchez-Cortes, S., 2015. Sensitive surface-enhanced Raman spectroscopy (SERS) detection of organochlorine pesticides by alkyl dithiol-functionalized metal nanoparticles-induced plasmonic hot spots. Anal. Chem. 87 (1), 663–669.

Kwon, Y.S., Nguyen, V.T., Park, J.G., Gu, M.B., 2015. Detection of iprobenfos and edifenphos using a new multi-aptasensor. Anal. Chim. Acta. 868, 60–66.

Lan, W., Chen, G., Cui, F., Tan, F., Liu, R., Yushupujiang, M., 2012. Development of a novel optical biosensor for detection of organophosphorus pesticides based on methyl parathion hydrolase immobilized by metal-chelate affinity. Sensors (Basel) 12 (7), 8477–8490.

Li, Y., Han, G., 2012. Ionic liquid-functionalized graphene for fabricating an amperometric acetylcholinesterase biosensor. Analyst. 137 (13), 3160–3165.

Li, W., Li, W., Hu, Y., Xia, Y., Shen, Q., Nie, Z., Huang, Y., Yao, S., 2013. A fluorometric assay for acetylcholinesterase activity and inhibitor detection based on DNA-templated copper/silver nanoclusters. Biosens. Bioelectron. 47, 345–349.

Li, Y., Ma, X., Zhao, M., Qi, P., Zhong, J., 2014. Quick and label-free detection for Coumaphos by using surface plasmon resonance biochip. PLoS One 9 (8), e104689.

Li, X., Zheng, Z., Liu, X., Zhao, S., Liu, S., 2015. Nanostructured photoelectrochemical biosensor for highly sensitive detection of organophosphorous pesticides. Biosens. Bioelectron. 64, 1–5.

Liang, R.P., Wang, X.N., Liu, C.M., Meng, X.Y., Qiu, J.D., 2013. Construction of graphene oxide magnetic nanocomposites-based on-chip enzymatic microreactor for ultrasensitive pesticide detection. J. Chromatogr. A 1315, 28–35.

Liang, H., Song, D., Gong, J., 2014. Signal-on electrochemiluminescence of biofunctional CdTe quantum dots for biosensing of organophosphate pesticides. Biosens. Bioelectron. 53, 363–369.

Liu, S., Zheng, Z., Li, X., 2013a. Advances in pesticide biosensors: current status, challenges, and future perspectives. Anal. Bioanal. Chem. 405 (1), 63–90.

Liu, G., Song, D., Chen, F., 2013b. Towards the fabrication of a label-free amperometric immunosensor using SWNTs for direct detection of paraoxon. Talanta 104, 103–108.

Liu, Y., Wang, G., Li, C., Zhou, Q., Wang, M., Yang, L., 2014a. A novel acetylcholinesterase biosensor based on carboxylic graphene coated with silver nanoparticles for pesticide detection. Mater. Sci. Eng. C Mater. Biol. Appl. 35, 253–258.

Liu, Q., Cai, J., Huan, J., Dong, X., Wang, C., Qiu, B., Wang, K., 2014b. A visible light photoelectrochemical biosensor coupling enzyme-inhibition for organophosphates monitoring based on a dual-functional Cd(0.5)Zn(0.5) S-reduced graphene oxide nanocomposite. Analyst 139 (5), 1121–1126.

Liu, C., Song, Z., Pan, J., Yan, Y., Cao, Z., Wei, X., Gao, L., Wang, J., Dai, J., Meng, M., Yu, P., 2014c. A simple and sensitive surface molecularly imprinted polymers based fluorescence sensor for detection of λ-Cyhalothrin. Talanta 125, 14–23.

Liu, G., Guo, W., Song, D., 2014d. A multianalyte electrochemical immunosensor based on patterned carbon nanotubes modified substrates for detection of pesticides. Biosens. Bioelectron. 52, 360–366.

Liu, X., Li, L., Liu, Y.Q., Shi, X.B., Li, W.J., Yang, Y., Mao, L.G., 2014e. Ultrasensitive detection of deltamethrin by immune magnetic nanoparticles separation coupled with surface plasmon resonance sensor. Biosens. Bioelectron. 59, 328–334.

Long, Q., Li, H., Zhang, Y., Yao, S., 2015a. Upconversion nanoparticle-based fluorescence resonance energy transfer assay for organophosphorus pesticides. Biosens. Bioelectron. 68, 168–174.

Long, F., Zhu, A., Shi, H., Sheng, J., Zhao, Z., 2015b. Adsorption kinetics of pesticide in soil assessed by optofluidics-based biosensing platform. Chemosphere 120, 615–620.

Lu, L., Xia, Y., 2015. Enzymatic reaction modulated gold nanorod end-to-end self-assembly for ultrahigh sensitively colorimetric sensing of cholinesterase and organophosphate pesticides in human blood. Anal. Chem. 87 (16), 8584–8591.

Marrazza, G., 2014. Piezoelectric biosensors for organophosphate and carbamate pesticides: a review. Biosensors (Basel) 4 (3), 301–317.

Martini, E., Tomassetti, M., Campanella, L., 2015a. Determination of traces of several pesticides in sunflower oil using organic phase immuno electrodes (OPIEs). Talanta 132, 503–512.

Martini, E., Merola, G., Tomassetti, M., Campanella, L., 2015b. Agent orange herbicides, organophosphate and triazinic pesticides analysis in olive oil and industrial oil mill waste effluents using new organic phase immunosensors. Food Chem. 169, 358–365.

Mauriz, E., García-Fernández, C., Mercader, J.V., Abad-Fuentes, A., Escuela, A.M., Lechuga, L.M., 2012. Direct surface plasmon resonance immunosensing of pyraclostrobin residues in untreated fruit juices. Anal. Bioanal. Chem. 404 (10), 2877–2886.

McGrath, T.F., Elliott, C.T., Fodey, T.L., 2012. Biosensors for the analysis of microbiological and chemical contaminants in food. Anal. Bioanal. Chem. 403 (1), 75–92.

Meng Zhang, Peh, J., Hergenrother, P.J., Cunningham, B.T., 2014. Detection of protein-small molecule binding using a self-referencing external cavity laser biosensor. Conf. Proc. IEEE Eng. Med. Biol. Soc.

Merkoci, A., 2007. Electrochemical biosensing with nanoparticles. Febs. Journal. 274 (2), 310–316.

Mishra, R.K., Dominguez, R.B., Bhand, S., Muñoz, R., Marty, J.L., 2012. A novel automated flow-based biosensor for the determination of organophosphate pesticides in milk. Biosens. Bioelectron. 32 (1), 56–61.

Mulchandani, R.A., 2011. Microbial biosensors for organophosphate pesticides. Appl. Biochem. Biotechnol. 165 (2), 687–699.

Nesakumar, N., Sethuraman, S., Krishnan, U.M., Rayappan, J.B., 2015. Cyclic voltammetric acetylcholinesterase biosensor for the detection of captan in apple samples with the aid of chemometrics. Anal. Bioanal. Chem. 407 (16), 4863–4868.

Nunes, G.S., Lins, J.A., Silva, F.G., Araujo, L.C., Silva, F.E., Mendonça, C.D., Badea, M., Hayat, A., Marty, J.L., 2014. Design of a macroalgae amperometric biosensor; application to the rapid monitoring of organophosphate insecticides in an agroecosystem. Chemosphere 111, 623–630.

Oliveira, T.M., Barroso, M.F., Morais, S., Araújo, M., Freire, C., de Lima-Neto, P., Correia, A.N., Oliveira, M.B., Delerue-Matos, C., 2014. Sensitive bi-enzymatic biosensor based on polyphenoloxidases-gold nanoparticles-chitosan hybrid film-graphene doped carbon paste electrode for carbamates detection. Bioelectrochemistry 98, 20–29.

Pereira, Nd, de Oliveira, F.M., Pereira, N.R., Verly, R.M., Souto, D.E., Kubota, L.T., Tanaka, A., Damos, F.S., Luz Rde, C., 2015. Ultrasensitive biosensor for detection of organophosphorus pesticides based on a macrocycle complex/carbon nanotubes composite and 1-methyl-3-octylimidazolium tetrafluoroborate as binder compound. Anal. Sci. 31 (1), 29–35.

Pimsen, R., Khumsri, A., Wacharasindhu, S., Tumcharern, G., Sukwattanasinitt, M., 2014. Colorimetric detection of dichlorvos using polydiacetylene vesicles with acetylcholinesterase and cationic surfactants. Biosens. Bioelectron. 62, 8–12.

Pundir, C.S., Chauhan, N., 2012. Acetylcholinesterase inhibition-based biosensors for pesticide determination: a review. Anal. Biochem. 429 (1), 19–31.

Qian, S., Lin, H., 2015. Colorimetric sensor array for detection and identification of organophosphorus and carbamate pesticides. Anal. Chem. 87 (10), 5395–5400.

Raghu, P., Madhusudana Reddy, T., Reddaiah, K., Kumara Swamy, B.E., Sreedhar, M., 2014. Acetylcholinesterase based biosensor for monitoring of Malathion and Acephate in food samples: a voltammetric study. Food Chem. 142, 188–196.

Rainina, E.I., Efremenco, E.N., Varfolomeyev, S.D., Simonian, A.L., Wild, J.R., 1996. The development of a new biosensor based on recombinant *E. coli* for the direct detection of organophosphorus neurotoxins. Biosens. Bioelectron. 11 (10), 991–1000.

Ramnani, P., Saucedo, N.M., Mulchandani, A., 2016. Carbon nanomaterial-based electrochemical biosensors for label-free sensing of environmental pollutants. Chemosphere 143, 85–98.

Rawson, D.M., Willmer, A.J., Turner, A.P., 1989. Whole-cell biosensors for environmental monitoring. Biosensors 4 (5), 299–311.

Rifea, J.C., Miller, M.M., Sheehan, P.E., Tamanaha, C.R., Tondra, M., Whitman, L., 2003. Design and performance of GMR sensors for the detection of magnetic microbeads in biosensors. J. Sensors Actuat. Phys. 107 (3), 209–218.

Sanchez-Ferandin, S., Leroy, F., Bouget, F.Y., Joux, F., 2013. A new, sensitive marine microalgal recombinant biosensor using luminescence monitoring for toxicity testing of antifouling biocides. Appl. Environ. Microbiol. 79 (2), 631–638.

Schena, A., Johnsson, K., 2014. Sensing acetylcholine and anticholinesterase compounds. Angew. Chem. Int. Ed. Engl. 53 (5), 1302–1305.

Schöning, M.J., Poghossian, A., 2002. Recent advances in biologically sensitive field-effect transistors (BioFETs). Analyst 127 (9), 1137–1151.

Shamagsumova, R.V., Shurpik, D.N., Padnya, P.L., Stoikov, I.I., Evtugyn, G.A., 2015. Acetylcholinesterase biosensor for inhibitor measurements based on glassy carbon electrode modified with carbon black and pillar[5]arene. Talanta 144, 559–568.

Sharma, P., Sablok, K., Bhalla, V., Suri, C.R., 2011. A novel disposable electrochemical immunosensor for phenyl urea herbicide diuron. Biosens. Bioelectron. 26 (10), 4209–4212.

Sharma, P., Bhalla, V., Dravid, V., Shekhawat, G., Jinsong-Wu, Prasad, E.S., Suri, C.R., 2012. Enhancing electrochemical detection on graphene oxide-CNT nanostructured electrodes using magneto-nanobioprobes. Sci. Rep. 2, 877.

Skladal, P., Mascini, M., 1992. Sensitive detection of pesticides using amperometric sensors based on cobalt phthalocyanine-modified composite electrodes and immobilized cholinesterases. Biosens Bioelectron 7 (5), 335–343.

Song, Y., Liu, M., Wang, S., 2013. Surface plasmon resonance sensor for phosmet of agricultural products at the ppt detection level. J. Agric. Food Chem. 61 (11), 2625–2630.

Stepurska, K.V., Soldatkin, C.O., Kucherenko, I.S., Arkhypova, V.M., Dzyadevych, S.V., Soldatkin, A.P., 2015. Feasibility of application of conductometric biosensor based on acetylcholinesterase for the inhibitory analysis of toxic compounds of different nature. Anal. Chim. Acta. 854, 161–168.

Sun, X., Liu, B., Xia, K., 2011a. A sensitive and regenerable biosensor for organophosphate pesticide based on self-assembled multilayer film with CdTe as fluorescence probe. Luminescence 26 (6), 616–621.

Sun, X., Zhu, Y., Wang, X., 2011b. Amperometric immunosensor based on a protein A/deposited gold nanocrystals modified electrode for carbofuran detection. Sensors (Basel) 11 (12), 11679–11691.

Sun, X., Du, S., Wang, X., Zhao, W., Li, Q., 2011c. A label-free electrochemical immunosensor for carbofuran detection based on a sol-gel entrapped antibody. Sensors (Basel) 11 (10), 9520–9531.

Sun, X., Cao, Y., Gong, Z., Wang, X., Zhang, Y., Gao, J., 2012. An amperometric immunosensor based on multi-walled carbon nanotubes-thionine-chitosan nanocomposite film for chlorpyrifos detection. Sensors (Basel) 12 (12), 17247–17261.

Sun, X., Zhai, C., Wang, X., 2013. A novel and highly sensitive acetyl-cholinesterase biosensor modified with hollow gold nanospheres. Bioproc. Biosyst. Eng. 36 (3), 273–283.

Suresh, U., Murugan, K., Benelli, G., Nicoletti, M., Barnard, D.R., Panneerselvam, C., Kumar, P.M., Subramaniam, J., Dinesh, D., Chandramohan, B., 2015. Tackling the growing threat of dengue: *Phyllanthus niruri*-mediated synthesis of silver nanoparticles and their mosquitocidal properties against the dengue vector *Aedes aegypti* (Diptera: Culicidae). Parasitol. Res. 114 (4), 1551–1562.

Tomassetti, M., Martini, E., Campanella, L., Favero, G., Sanzó, G., Mazzei, F., 2015. A new surface plasmon resonance immunosensor for triazine pesticide determination in bovine milk: a comparison with conventional amperometric and screen-printed immunodevices. Sensors (Basel) 15 (5), 10255–10270.

Ton, X.A., Acha, V., Bonomi, P., Tse Sum Bui, B., Haupt, K., 2015. A disposable evanescent wave fiber optic sensor coated with a molecularly imprinted polymer as a selective fluorescence probe. Biosens. Bioelectron. 64, 359–366.

Uthuppu, B., Heiskanen, A., Kofoed, D., Aamand, J., Jørgensen, C., Dufva, M., Jakobsen, M.H., 2015. Micro-flow-injection analysis (μFIA) immunoassay of herbicide residue 2,6-dichlorobenzamide—towards automated at-line monitoring using modular microfluidics. Analyst 140 (5), 1616–1623.

Verma, N., Bhardwaj, A., 2015. Biosensor technology for pesticides—a review. Appl. Biochem. Biotechnol. 175 (6), 3093–3119.

Wang, K., Li, H.N., Wu, J., Ju, C., Yan, J.J., Liu, Q., Qiu, B., 2011. TiO_2-decorated graphene nanohybrids for fabricating an amperometric acetylcholinesterase biosensor. Analyst. 136 (16), 3349–3354.

Wang, Z., Meng, G., Huang, Z., Li, Z., Zhou, Q., 2014. Ag-nanoparticle-decorated porous ZnO-nanosheets grafted on a carbon fiber cloth as effective SERS substrates. Nanoscale 6 (24), 15280–15285.

Wang, Q., Yang, J., Dong, Y., Zhang, L., 2015a. One-step fabrication of a multifunctional magnetic nickel ferrite/multi-walled carbon nanotubes nanohybrid-modified electrode for the determination of benomyl in food. J. Agric. Food Chem. 163 (19), 4746–4753.

Wang, J., Gao, L., Han, D., Pan, J., Qiu, H., Li, H., Wei, X., Dai, J., Yang, J., Yao, H., Yan, Y., 2015b. Optical detection of λ-cyhalothrin by core-shell fluorescent molecularly imprinted polymers in Chinese spirits. J. Agric. Food Chem. 63 (9), 2392–2399.

Wang, X., Dong, S., Hou, T., Liu, L., Liu, X., Li, F., 2016. Exonuclease I-aided homogeneous electrochemical strategy for organophosphorus pesticide detection based on enzyme inhibition integrated with a DNA conformational switch. Analyst 141 (5), 1830–1836.

Warner, J., Andreescu, S., 2016. An acetylcholinesterase (AChE) biosensor with enhanced solvent resistance based on chitosan for the detection of pesticides. Talanta 146, 279–284.

Weerathunge, P., Ramanathan, R., Shukla, R., Sharma, T.K., Bansal, V., 2014. Aptamer-controlled reversible inhibition of gold nanozyme activity for pesticide sensing. Anal. Chem. 86 (24), 11937–11941.

Wei, W., Zong, X., Wang, X., Yin, L., Pu, Y., Liu, S., 2012. A disposable amperometric immunosensor for chlorpyrifos-methyl based on immunogen/platinum doped silica sol–gel film modified screen-printed carbon electrode. Food Chem. 135 (3), 888–892.

Wu, S., Lan, X., Zhao, W., Li, Y., Zhang, L., Wang, H., Han, M., Tao, S., 2011. Controlled immobilization of acetylcholinesterase on improved hydrophobic gold nanoparticle/Prussian blue modified surface for ultra-trace organophosphate pesticide detection. Biosens. Bioelectron. 27 (1), 82–87.

Xing, C., Liu, L., Song, S., Feng, M., Kuang, H., Xu, C., 2015. Ultrasensitive immunochromatographic assay for the simultaneous detection of five chemicals in drinking water. Biosens. Bioelectron. 66, 445–453.

Xue, G., Yue, Z., Bing, Z., Yiwei, T., Xiuying, L., Jianrong, L., 2016. Highly-sensitive organophosphorus pesticide biosensors based on CdTe quantum dots and bi-enzyme immobilized eggshell membranes. Analyst 141 (3), 1105–1111.

Yang, L., Wang, G., Liu, Y., Wang, M., 2013a. Development of a biosensor based on immobilization of acetylcholinesterase on NiO nanoparticles-carboxylic graphene-nafion modified electrode for detection of pesticides. Talanta 113, 135–141.

Yang, L., Wang, G., Liu, Y., 2013b. An acetylcholinesterase biosensor based on platinum nanoparticles-carboxylic graphene-nafion-modified electrode for detection of pesticides. Anal. Biochem. 437 (2), 144–149.

Yang, L., Wang, G.C., Liu, Y.J., An, J.J., Wang, M., 2013c. Development of a stable biosensor based on a SiO_2 nanosheet-Nafion-modified glassy carbon electrode for sensitive detection of pesticides. Anal. Bioanal. Chem. 405 (8), 2545–2552.

Yang, Y., Asiri, A.M., Du, D., Lin, Y., 2014. Acetylcholinesterase biosensor based on a gold nanoparticle-polypyrrole-reduced graphene oxide nanocomposite modified electrode for the amperometric detection of organophosphorus pesticides. Analyst 139 (12), 3055–3060.

Yang, L., Han, J., Liu, W., Li, J., Jiang, L., 2015. Conversion of inhibition biosensing to substrate-like biosensing for quinalphos selective detection. Anal. Chem. 87 (10), 5270–5277.

Yi, Y., Zhu, G., Liu, C., Huang, Y., Zhang, Y., Li, H., Zhao, J., Yao, S., 2013. A label-free silicon quantum dots-based photoluminescence sensor for ultrasensitive detection of pesticides. Anal. Chem. 85 (23), 11464–11470.

Yu, G., Wu, W., Zhao, Q., Wei, X., Lu, Q., 2015. Efficient immobilization of acetylcholinesterase onto amino functionalized carbon nanotubes for the fabrication of high sensitive organophosphorus pesticides biosensors. Biosens. Bioelectron. 68, 288–294.

Zhai, C., Guo, Y., Sun, X., Zheng, Y., Wang, X., 2014. An acetylcholinesterase biosensor based on graphene-gold nanocomposite and calcined layered double hydroxide. Enzyme Microb. Technol. 58–59, 8–13.

Zhang, L., Zhang, A., Du, D., Lin, Y., 2012a. Biosensor based on Prussian blue nanocubes/reduced graphene oxide nanocomposite for detection of organophosphorus pesticides. Nanoscale 4 (15), 4674–4679.

Zhang, L., Wang, M., Wang, C., Hu, X., Wang, G., 2012b. Label-free impedimetric immunosensor for sensitive detection of 2,4-dichlorophenoxybutyric acid (2,4-DB) in soybean. Talanta 101, 226–232.

Zhang, H., Li, Z.F., Snyder, A., Xie, J., Stanciu, L.A., 2014. Functionalized graphene oxide for the fabrication of paraoxon biosensors. Anal. Chim. Acta. 827, 86–94.

Zhou, Q., Yang, L., Wang, G., Yang, Y., 2013. Acetylcholinesterase biosensor based on SnO_2 nanoparticles-carboxylic graphene-nafion modified electrode for detection of pesticides. Biosens. Bioelectron. 49, 25–31.

Zhu, Y., Cao, Y., Sun, X., Wang, X., 2013. Amperometric immunosensor for carbofuran detection based on MWCNTs/GS-PEI-Au and AuNPs-antibody conjugate. Sensors (Basel) 13 (4), 5286–5301.

10

PESTICIDES AND ANTIMICROBIAL RESISTANCE: FROM ENVIRONMENTAL COMPARTMENTS TO ANIMAL AND HUMAN INFECTIONS

Carmen Curutiu, Veronica Lazar, Mariana Carmen Chifiriuc
Faculty of Biology and Research Institute of the University of Bucharest - ICUB, University of Bucharest, Bucharest, Romania

1 Introduction

The ability of microorganisms to develop resistance to the majority of current antibiotics is a very common, increasing, and threatening phenomenon, especially for the clinical field. In fact, most of the antibiotics which were used at the beginning of the so-called "antibiotic era" are no longer used clinically because many bacterial species are now tolerant to them. Instead, other antibiotics were developed, but bacteria do not let their guard down and continue to defend, finding new ways to become resistant to these new classes of substances.

Moreover, some multidrug-resistant (MDR) forms evolved. So called "superbugs" are showing high levels of resistance to different antibiotic classes due to multiple mutations, being responsible for high rates of morbidity and mortality; the treatment of these bacteria is difficult, requiring longer hospital stays and high healthcare costs. For example, in case of tuberculosis (TB), an archetypical human pathogen, the administration of a combination of anti-TB drugs has become essential for this disease treatment yet multidrug resistance still continues to be a problem in TB treatment. Some *Mycobacterium tuberculosis* strains resistant to four or more of the front-line treatments (i.e., extremely drug-resistant [XDR] strains) (Shah et al., 2007; Sotgiu et al., 2009),

New Pesticides and Soil Sensors. http://dx.doi.org/10.1016/B978-0-12-804299-1.00011-4

and even worse, totally drug resistant [TDR] strains have occurred (Velayati et al., 2009). In *M. tuberculosis* case, no horizontal gene transfer (HGT) is implicated but spontaneous mutation is responsible for antibiotic resistance (Smith and Coast, 2002).

Another threat is that of methicillin-resistant *Staphylococcus aureus* (MRSA) strains, which are resistant not only to methicillin (introduced for penicillinase-producing *S. aureus*) but could also be resistant to aminoglycosides, tetracyclines, macrolides, chloramphenicol, or lincosamides, and moreover also to disinfectants, being more and more implicated in hospital-acquired infections. For such resistant strains, vancomycin represents the last option, but resistance to vancomycin in *Enterococcus* species is common and alarming because of the risk of its transmission to MRSA strains by HGT. Such MRSA strains resistant to vancomycin are already found, but are still rare (de Lencastre et al., 2007).

Acinetobacter baumannii and pseudomonads are naturally resistant to many antibiotics having a suite of "r" genes and pathogenicity determinants. Recent studies showed that some derivatives have at least 28 genomic islands encoding antibiotic resistance determinants (Davies and Davies, 2010).

Recent data resulting after bacterial genome sequencing showed the existence of more than 20,000 potential resistance genes (r genes) of nearly 400 different types, but fortunately, the number of functional resistance determinants in pathogens is much smaller (Smith and Coast, 2002).

Today, the medical world is aware of the magnitude of the antibiotic problem, and huge efforts are being made to change the way that antibiotics are used and prescribed, and to slow bacterial evolution regarding antibiotic resistance, but solutions found thus far are not very efficient. This is the reason why microbiologists continue to learn and study bacterial evolution, in order to anticipate the bacterial response to medical treatment and to stop the progression of resistance (Haddix et al., 2000).

Due to many different modes of action of antibiotics, bacterial resistance to them can evolve in different ways. Briefly, three principal mechanisms could be involved: (1) changes in the permeability of the cellular membrane that either impede the entrance of the antibiotic into the cell or determine the efflux of antibiotic out of the cell, (2) degradation and/or inactivation of the antibiotic, and (3) acquisition of a mutation that induces changes to the target which is no longer sensitive. The resistance genes could appear spontaneously in a population as a result of mutations or as a result of the horizontal gene transfer, meaning exchanging genes between related or unrelated microbial species (Haddix et al., 2000).

The capacity of the resistance genes to move into other bacteria is a major contribution in the dissemination of antibiotic resistance. There are many possible mechanisms of this dissemination, each one amplifying the resistance, that is: (1) plasmidial transfer, (2) chromosomal/or plasmid-associated resistance gene transfer mediated by bacteriophages, (3) incorporation into new strains of naked DNA, released from dead bacteria, as in the case of pneumococci or *Haemophilus* spp. (Nikaido, 2009).

The misuse of antimicrobial substances is the factor that mostly contributes to the appearance and development of AMR. The selective pressure appears not as a natural process, but as the result of human applications of antibiotics (underuse, overuse, and misuse). Unfortunately, the high use of these substances had a significant environmental downside. From their introduction, millions of tons of antibiotics have been produced; these huge quantities become toxic for the environment and contribute to the selection of resistant microbial strains (Smith and Coast, 2002).

About 100,000 tons of antibiotics are manufactured every year in the entire world and used for human therapy, for animal growth, and even in aquaculture. Large quantities of antibiotics (mostly penicillins and tetracyclines) are used as growth promoters for food animals, and also as pesticides in agriculture (tetracyclines and streptomycin). Although, the therapeutic use of antibiotics is predominant, antimicrobial agents are used also as: (1) growth factors/prophylactic use in animals; (2) therapeutic/prophylactic use for humans; (3) therapeutic/prophylactic use in fish culture; (4) therapeutic/prophylactic use for pets; (5) pest control/cloning of plants and agriculture; (6) biocides in toiletries, and in handcare and household cleaning products; (7) biocide for instrumental and medical surfaces in hospitals, and (8) culture sterility, cloning, and selection in research and industry. All these anthropogenic activities have been determined to be major environmental sources of resistance and, most probably, of virulence genes (Smith and Coast, 2002).

Compared to the medical field, the emergence of resistant bacteria in agriculture represents a small part of the total microbial resistance pool, but constitutes a good example of how the long exposure of microorganisms to antibiotics determines a selective pressure permitting adaptation of some bacteria to environmental growth inhibitor agents. Since the microorganisms that contain transposons or other protection mechanisms succeed and continue to survive, there will be selected multiresistant microorganisms in the environment. Moreover, these microorganisms possess only a few mechanisms by which they can totally destroy the antibiotic, like the presence of β-lactamases, acetylases for chloramphenicol, esterases for macrolides, and aminoglyoside-inactivating enzymes. By any other mechanism, the antibiotic is released from the cell, but it is not destroyed. It is only released into the environment, where it continues to exert its selective pressure by accumulating at low concentration, perfect for selecting resistant individuals.

Many other antibiotic-like substances known as "antibacterials" are used in different products, from solvents or disinfectants for medical or pharmaceutical fields to soap, floor cleaners, or dish-washing detergents. The principal components of these compounds are represented by triclosan or quaternary ammonium compounds (QACs), such as benzalkonium chloride.

There are concerns that the widespread use of these substances will select multiresistant bacterial strains, and although mechanisms for resistance to antibiotics are known, mechanisms for resistance to biocides are not fully understood. High concentrations of biocides are regularly microbicidal, but the use of these substances in different products at low concentrations may influence the prevalence of antibiotic-resistant bacteria. Some studies investigated the resistance patterns of the QAC-resistant strains to some antibiotics and the results indicated a correlation between antibiotic resistance and environments where QACs are regularly used. There are studies revealing similarities regarding resistance mechanisms between biocides and antibiotics that shared the same target site, involving genes for multidrug pumps, plasmide-encoded in Gram-positive bacteria or chromosome-encoded in Gram-negative bacteria (Webber and Piddock, 2003).

It is well-known that biocides could determine an adaptive multiple-antibiotic resistance phenotype, either due to an increase in the expression of efflux pumps, or to a reduced synthesis of outer membrane porins.

A related phenomenon is coresistance, which appears when the genetic mutation that made the pest resistant to one pesticide also makes it resistant to others, often those with a similar mechanism of action (Daly et al., 1998). This process could also occur not only between different classes of pesticides, but also between pesticides and heavy metals or antibiotics, and when it occurrs this mechanism could be mediated physiologically (cross-resistance) or genetically (coresistance). Coresistance appears when two or more related resistance genes are located next to each other on one mobile genetic element. Cross-resistance represents the mechanism by which bacteria become tolerant to more antimicrobial substances like antibiotics and heavy metals (Chapman, 2003). In this category we could include some multidrug efflux pumps that mediate rapid elimination of the toxic agent (antibiotic/metallic ion) out of the cell (Martinez et al., 2009).

Efflux pumps are represented by proteins localized in cellular membranes, used by bacteria to pump out unwanted toxic substances. For example, the AcrAB efflux system from *Escherichia coli*, a pump that is under the control of the regulon mar (the multiple antibiotic resistances) is used by bacteria to pump out bile acids and fatty acids to decrease their toxicity. But among their physiological role, efflux mechanisms have a big impact on antimicrobial resistance. Both antibiotic-susceptible and antibiotic-resistant bacteria have and express efflux genes, encoded by chromosomal genes that contribute to intrinsic (natural) resistance, or plasmids being responsible for acquired resistance, respectively. Efflux pump genes can be maintained in unfavorable environments, allowing selection of mutants that overexpress these genes. Their presence on mobile genetic elements permit their distribution to other species, thus spreading antibiotic resistance.

The principal bacterial efflux pumps based on the structure and the energy sources are divided into six superfamilies: major facilitator superfamily (MFS), multidrug and toxic compound extrusion family (MATE), ATP-binding cassette superfamily (ABC), small multidrug resistance family (SMR), resistance-nodulation-cell division superfamily (RND), and drug metabolite transporter (DMT) superfamily (Webber and Piddock, 2003; Piddock, 2006).

Pseudomonas aeruginosa is well recognized for its intrinsic resistance to a large panel of substances due to the presence of multidrug efflux pumps. For example, MexAB-OprM pump is responsible for increased resistance to some antibiotics, such as aztreonam, gentamicin, tetracycline, and tobramycin in biofilm structures of *P. aeruginosa* biofilms. The level of expression of OprR, correlates also with resistance of *P. aeruginosa* to QACs (Tabata et al., 2003). The same AcrAB pump from *E. coli* and other *Enterobacteriacaeae* members, responsible for some antibiotic resistance, pump out different biocides (e.g., triclosan, QACs, chlorhexidine) (Levy, 2002a). Overexpression of the AcrAB pump in some strains of *E. coli* isolated from clinical fields or overexpression of efflux pump in *Pseudomonas* strains contributed to resistance to antibiotics, and also cross-resistance to triclosan (McMurry et al., 1998a; Chuanchuen et al., 2001). SmeDEF multidrug efflux pump from *Stenotrophomonas maltophilia* confer resistance of this specie to triclosan (Sanchez et al., 2005), and genes responsible for resistance to QACs were observed in MRSA strains (Fraise, 2002). Another researcher's group showed a link between resistance to antibiotics and resistance to triclosan and QACs in the case of *Pseudomonas stutzeri* strains (Levy, 2002b).

Resistance to triclosan or isoniazid could occur through multidrug efflux pumps, but is also conferred by a mutation in the enzyme. Triclosan inhibited enoyl (acyl carrier protein) reductase (FabI) in *E. coli*, targeting fatty acid synthesis, and the mutation in this gene conferred resistance to triclosan. Some studies made on *E. coli* mutants resistant to triclosan proved the genetic target of triclosan, namely the product of the *fabI* gene, enoyl reductase, the same protein that also represents the target for isoniazid, an antibiotic used against *M. tuberculosis* (McMurry et al., 1998b). The same FabI gene is also involved in resistance to triclosan in *S. aureus*. In *Mycobacterium* species, the target is the same—enoyl reductase, but encoded by InhA gene, the mycobacterial homolog of *E. coli* FabI. Mutations in this gene were found to be responsible for decreased isoniazid sensitivity of *Mycobacterium smegmati*, but not of *M. tuberculosis* (Parikh et al., 1999).

Correlation between antibiotic and biocide resistance was observed in *E. coli* mutants resistant to pine oil that overexpressed the marA gene (multiple antibiotic resistance), which also presented low-level resistance to some antibiotics (tetracycline, ampicillin, nalidixic acid, and chloramphenicol) (Moken et al., 1997). In *E. coli* a low-level cross-resistance between didecyldimethylammonium chloride, eugenol, and thymol and antibiotics (chloramphenicol) was also observed. Mutants of *S. aureus* that presented resistance to pine oil cleaner also demonstrated reduced susceptibility to vancomycin and oxacillin (Price et al., 2002). MRSA strains resistant to benzalkonium chloride also presented an increased resistance to some β-lactam antibiotics (Akimitsu et al., 1999), but this higher resistance was not observed in cases of other classes of antibiotics, suggesting that resistance to oxacillin and benzalkonium were connected.

In healthcare settings, biocides are largely used for proper disinfection in order to keep a hospital-acquired infection from spreading. For eliminating the possibility and to determine any change in antibiotic susceptibility, biocides should be used at concentrations and conditions that enable a rapid and effective kill of bacteria. MIC values increase or decrease as a result of exposure to sublethal doses of biocides and this has consequences both for the medical field and also for environmental pollution. Adaptive low-level resistance as a result of increases in MIC values has medical implications, causing failure therapy. Moreover, the probability of spontaneous mutations becomes higher, which finally leads to high-level changes in the susceptibility of microbial populations exposed to both biocides and antibiotics. Biocides that decrease the MIC value of an antibiotic make that antibiotic a significant selection factor at low concentrations. Exposure to low concentrations of biocides may select bacteria with efflux genes and the occurrence of antimicrobial resistance, aspects that should be kept in mind in case of development of new antibacterial agents, in order to minimize the risk of resistance occurrence.

Biocides that evaporate (alcohols) or reactive biocides (e.g., peroxide and hypochlorite bleach) should be used because they are eliminated rapidly and the risk of developing tolerance is minimal (Webber and Piddock, 2003).

Reducing antibiotics use is not sufficient for stopping antibiotic resistance and its spread in the clinical field or environment (Salyers and Amábile-Cuevas, 1997). Contamination of the environment with heavy metals by human activities, such as aquaculture or agricultural practices (Burridge et al., 2010; Han et al., 2002; Nicholson et al., 2003), is another huge problem, contributing to pollution due to the presence of metals in feed additives, fertilizers, pesticides, and antifouling products. For example, in aquaculture, antibiotics and metal-containing products are frequently used to prevent fouling, and also for feeding or treating fish in order to limit some infections (Burridge et al., 2010). Therefore, bacterial species of aquacultures are exposed to heavy metals and antibiotics, exposure that increases the possibility of the occurrence of resistance selection and coselection phenomena. Not all heavy metals are equally toxic to bacteria. Toxicity depends on heavy metals chemical affinity to the thiol groups, and to their solubility under physiological conditions. For example, the elements Fe, Mn, and molybdenum (Mo) have limited toxicity; Zn, Ni, Cu, Co, Cr, vanadium (V), and tungsten (W) are toxic elements with metabolic relevance; and Ag, Cd, Hg, Pb, antimony (Sb), and uranium (U) are exhibiting a strong toxicity (Nies, 1999). But bacteria do succeed in developing some mechanisms to protect against metal ions that could cause cellular damage. There are three general mechanisms described in bacteria for heavy metal resistance: (1) the first mechanism is represented by sequestration of toxic metals, minimizing in this way the concentration of the free toxic ions in the cytoplasm. Cell membrane, cell wall, and extracellular polymeric substance (EPS) of biofilms could absorb toxic metals, explaining the enhanced metal tolerance of the bacteria embedded into biofilms (Harrison et al., 2007); (2) another mechanism of resistance to heavy metals is represented by the detoxification through reduction of intracellular ions. For example, some species present an enzyme, mercury reductase, encoded by the *merA* gene. With this enzyme, Hg^{2+} is reduced to the less toxic compound, Hg^0 that diffuses out of the cell, due to its low evaporation point (Nies, 1999); (3) the third mechanism is represented by the presence of efflux systems by which bacteria eliminate antibiotics and other substances from the biocides category, and also toxic ions (Nies and Silver, 1995). *Alcaligenes eutrophus* has such an efflux system, called the cation/proton antiporter Czc, that confers tolerance to Cd^{2+}, Zn^{2+}, and Co^{2+} by extrusion of metals from the cytoplasm into the environment. The bacterial population's metal tolerance is increased by persister cells that mediate time-dependent tolerance to toxic metal ions due to upregulation of resistance and stress response genes (Harrison et al., 2007).

In recent years, researchers concluded that resistance to heavy metals could be selected indirectly by coselection with antibiotic resistance. Such an example was observed in an aquatic bacterium carrying a plasmid with genes conferring resistance to both antibiotics and metals (Cr and Co) (Osman et al., 2010). Due to their close disposition, it is clear that in the case of HGT, these genes will be both transmitted. Another example was observed in the case of an *Enterococcus faecium* strain isolated from farm animals—a genetic linkage of Cu resistance conferred by *tcrB* gene, observed resistance encoded by [*erm*(B)], and glycopeptide resistance due to *vanA* gene were present (Hasman and Aarestrup, 2002). Macrolides are widely administrated in veterinary medicine (Grave et al., 2010) and glycopeptide antibiotics were also used for animals in the past, but as growth promoters. Thus, this genetic linkage could be an example of how heavy metals induce the spread of resistance to antibiotics, with great impact in veterinary and human medicine. At present, glycopeptide antibiotics, such as vancomycin, represent one of the last-resort antibiotics for human medicine. Another example of coresistance can be observed in the case of *Aeromonas salmonicida* subsp. *salmonicida* isolated from Atlantic salmon (*Salmo salar*) from aquaculture facilities. This species was identified as carrying Hg (*mer* operon) and multiple antibiotic resistance genes (*aadA7, sulI, sulII, floR, tetA, tetR, strA, strB*, and bla_{CMY-2}) on plasmid IncA/C, this being the first finding of plasmid associated with resistance to florfenicol (*floR*), an antibiotic that treats furunculosis in aquacultures.

Integrons are genetic elements capable of acquiring and exchanging DNA. Class 1 integrons are involved in coselection because they are frequently found in contaminated environments and contain gene cassettes that mediate resistance to antibiotics. It seems that the presence of integrons confer a selective advantage to bacteria to stressful environmental conditions, a good example being the toxic metals. Some studies confirmed that class 1 integrons in aquatic environments contaminated with heavy metals were discovered (Rosewarne et al., 2010). Class 1 integrons which are closely located to genes codifying for the multidrug efflux pump czcA, a pump known to extrude the metal ions Zn^{2+}, Cd^{2+}, and Co^{2+}, were found in bacteria isolated from fresh water (Stokes et al., 2006).

AcrAB efflux system in *E.coli* is regulated by the soxS protein. When *soxS* is upregulated, for example, under oxidative stress, caused by several metal ions like $Cr_2O_7^-$ and Cu^{2+}, an increased production of the AcrAB efflux system additionally mediates enhanced tolerance toward antibiotics, such as chloramphenicol, tetracyclin, novobiocin, nafcillin, and oxacillin. On the contrary, other studies indicate that increased heavy metal concentrations conducted to a decreased antibiotic resistance. The minimum inhibitory concentration (MIC) for some tested antibiotics was decreased when the testing procedure was conducted with the addition of mercury chloride. The same observations were also made by other researchers; a decreased resistance to aminoglycosides in an environment with a high level of Hg was registered (Seiler and Berendonk, 2012).

Antibiotics are not the only substances against which bacteria must protect itself. Insecticides and herbicides introduced in the 1940s and 1950s soon exerted selective pressure that increased the number of resistant varieties of plants and insects.

Pesticide resistance could be described as a lower susceptibility of a pest population to a pesticide that was efficient against it before. Resistance to pesticide is based on a genetic mechanism. When a pest population is exposed to a pesticide, most of the pests are killed, but some pests from that population survive. Natural selection occurs: only the most resistant pests survive and transmit their genetic features to descendants. Even higher concentrations or more frequent applications are not efficient to kill the entire population. The descendants of those pests who have managed to survive will have the ability, like their parents, to resist to the action of that pesticide. And this process takes place with every generation, and taking into account that most of the pests have a new generation in a few weeks, it is clear that with increasing frequency of application, the number of resistant pests will be higher, until the entire population will become resistant.

The Insecticide Resistance Action Committee (IRAC) defines pesticide resistance as a heritable change in the sensitivity of a pest population, meaning the repeated failure of a pesticide to achieve the expected level of control when it is administrated according to the recommendation for that pest species. So, at present, pests represent a real threat for human health, due to their involvement in medical or agricultural fields. For example, some pests which are very resistant to pesticides are vectors for some human pathogens that are also resistant to conventional drugs used for treating the respective diseases. Recent studies indicate that more than 500 species of insects and mites, 270 weed species,

150 plant pathogens, and many rat species are now resistant to pesticides that once were efficient against them. Similar to antibiotics, multiple resistance (resistance to more pesticides from different chemical classes) appeared (IRAC, 2007). This multiple resistance occurs when pesticides are used sequentially, a new class of pesticides replacing another one to which pests already manifest resistance (Table 10.1).

Herbicides are used throughout the entire world and could be present in food supply, humans, atmosphere, pets, and homes. At the origin, their use is directed against plants, but their applications for gardens or agricultural crops increases the risk of exposure of the potential pathogens for humans or domestic animals. Usually, before being released in the market, herbicides are tested for their toxicity, but not for their sublethal effects on microorganisms, which might conduct to greater tolerances to antibiotics. Kurenbach et al. (2015) investigated the exposure of *E. coli* and *Salmonella enterica* serovar *typhimurium* to commercial formulations of three herbicides—dicamba (3,6-dichloro-2-methoxybenzoic acid; Kamba), 2,4-dichlorophenoxyacetic acid (2,4-D), and glyphosate [*N*-(phosphonomethyl) glycine; Roundup], and also to salicylic acid, a substance that presents some structural similarities with the first two herbicides. The results revealed the modification of the behavior of these strains to antibiotics from different classes: ampicillin (Amp), ciprofloxacin (Cip), kanamycin (Kan), tetracycline (Tet), and chloramphenicol (Cam). The results varied by species, herbicides, and antibiotics. *S. typhimurium* exposure to sublethal concentrations of Kamba and 2,4-D determined an increased tolerance to Amp, Cam, Cip, and Tet but a greater susceptibility to Kan. Roundup significantly increased the tolerance to Kan and Cip. Exposure of *E. coli* to Kamba and 2,4-D, showed similar effects, but no increase in the tolerance to Amp. After exposure to Roundup, tolerance to Kan and Cip was increased. Surprisingly, a greater effect was obtained in cases of simultaneous exposure of the strains to antibiotics and herbicides, a possible explanation being the modification of target exposure to the antibiotic, by an increase or decrease in efflux, or permeability. For example, activation of the same AcrAB-TolC efflux pump in *E. coli* and *S. typhimurium* determines a lower susceptibility to fluoroquinolones, lactams, tetracycline, and chloramphenicol. After exposure to salicylic acid (a known inducer of AcrAB-TolC) an increased susceptibility to aminoglycosides was noticed. Likewise, after exposure to Kamba or 2,4-D, an increased susceptibility to kanamycin was observed but exposure to Roundup determines reduced susceptibility to aminoglycosides. MIC values of the antibiotics could increase up to 3 times in the presence of herbicides,

Table 10.1 Principal Classes of Pesticides Based on Their Active Ingredient

Class of Pesticide	Chemical Structure	Pesticide
Pyrethroids	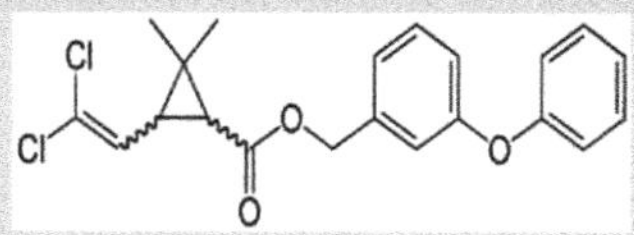 Permethrin	Bifenthrin, Cypermethrin, Deltamethrin, Permethrin, Resmethrin, Sumithrin
Organophosphates	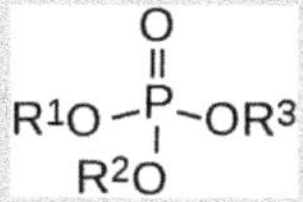	Chlorfenvinphos, Chlorpyriphos, Chlorpyriphos-Methyl, Dimethoate, Omethoate, Phosalone, Pirimiphos-Methyl, Triazophos
Organochlorines	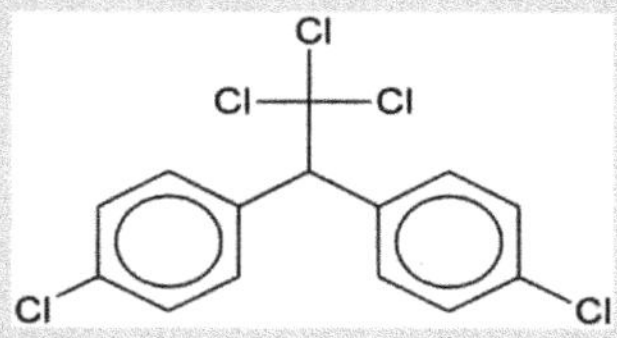 DDT	Chlorothalonil, a-Endosulfan, ß-Endosulfan, Endosulfan-Sulfate, Lindane, Tetradifon, p.p.-DDT, p.p. -DDE
Carbamates	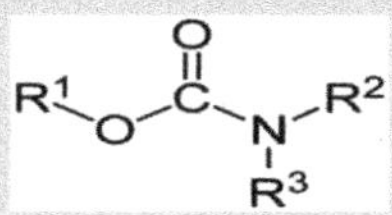	Carbaryl, Fenoxycarb
Dicarboximides	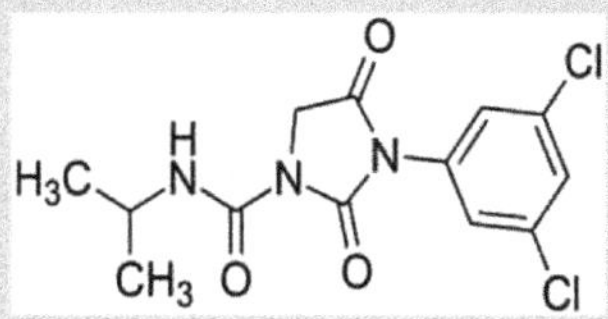 Iprodione	Captan, Iprodione
Organonitrogen	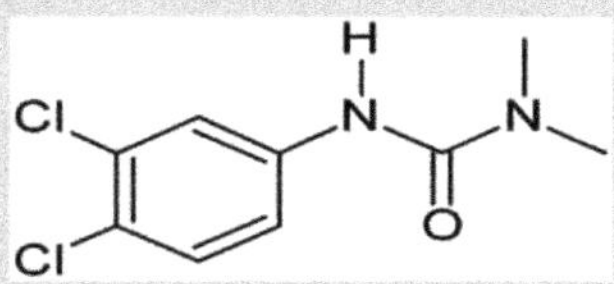 Diuron	Aldicarb, Benomyl, Carbendazim, Carbofuran, Chlorprophan, Diuron (herbicide), Formetanate, Methiocarb, Methomyl, Oxamyl, Propham, Propoxur, Thiobencarb A
Others		Bromopropylate (Benzilate, Acaricide); Buprimate (Pyrimidine, Fungicide); Metalaxyl (Acylalanine, Fungicide); Thiophanate-Methyl (Fungicide)

Adapted from http://www.sigmaaldrich.com/analytical-chromatography/air-monitoring/applications/agricultural-contaminants.html.

which significantly influences the treatment of bacterial infections (Kurenbach et al., 2015).

In environments that are already polluted with low, sublethal concentrations of antibiotics, adding a herbicide makes those concentrations reach a level high enough to select resistant strains.

Studies proved that the quantity of herbicides needed to determine the maximum response to an antibiotic is higher than the maximum residue limits (MRLs) permitted by international trading laws. That means the human or animal food containing lower MRLs should not be capable of inducing changes in gut microbiota. But the quantity of herbicides needed to determine a detectable antibiotic response was much lower than the specified herbicide application rate, and because herbicide-induced antibiotic response is cumulative when substances that determine similar phenotypic changes are combined (e.g., Kamba and salicylic acid), the real range of exposure proves to be much higher. It is thus evident that testing each component of a biocide against some microorganisms only for their severe effects (as is done currently for evaluating herbicides) is not sufficient and does not take into account their role in the appearance of a resistant phenotype (Kurenbach et al., 2015).

Environmental exposure to herbicides occurs in urban and agricultural settings, in waterways, small animals, and insects. The latest ones being treated with antibiotics (e.g., honeybee) create perfect conditions to induce tolerance. Bee products, including honey, are subjected to different sources of contamination from the environment, such as pesticides, heavy metals, bacteria, and radioactive materials. Pesticides in bee products mean a lower quality. According to the European Union regulations, honey should be free of chemicals. Pesticide residues are responsible for genetic mutations and cellular degradation.

Antibiotics used in honey and other bee products are represented by those used in veterinary settings, such as streptomycin, sulfonamide, and chloramphenicol. Antibiotics are used for treating infections at relatively high doses or as "growth promoters" at low doses. Due to the fact that no MRLs have been established for pesticides in honey, it is difficult to evaluate the level of contamination with pesticides and to determine its possible effects on human health. However, systemic contact of pesticides with nectar and pollen could directly affect honey bee health and ultimately contaminate honey-containing food with pesticides. The extensive use of antibiotics determined an accumulation of antibiotic residues in honey, conducting to decreased quality and difficulty in marketing. The problem arises from the fact that antibiotic residues have a relatively long half-life and could have direct toxic effects on humans. Antibiotic residues in honey result mostly from the environment and inadequate use in beekeeping. Some international reports declare residues of oxytetracycline and chloramphenicol, above the regulatory standards, found in honey. Some analyzed honey samples from Turkey showed erythromycin residues. Another study revealed lincomycin residue in honey collected after a period of 41-weeks after bee colonies were treated with antibiotics (Granja et al., 2009; Adams et al., 2009).

In some countries from the European Community, the use of antibiotics in beekeeping is illegal. In Switzerland, the United Kingdom, and Belgium, action limits for antibiotics in honey were established, ranging between 0.01 and 0.05 mg/kg for each antibiotic group.

A proof of cross-resistance was found in Switzerland in bees that collected nectar from meadows treated with the asulam, a herbicide. Honey produced by those bees was not only contaminated by asulam but also by sulfanilamide, its degradation product. So, it is clear that the use of herbicides could determine the appearance of residues of sulfonamide drugs in food (Al-Waili et al., 2012).

Many studies are conducted on antifungal herbicides. Azoles, besides dithiocarbamates, strobilurins, and benzimidazoles are widely applied in the field for their antimycotic activity against many species of fungi for plant protection. Large quantities of azoles are used annually, and about 100 g/ha should be administrated once in the field, multiple applications per year being sometimes required. One important characteristic of azoles is their long-lasting stability. They could remain active for many months in certain ecological niches, such as soil and water. For example, the half-time of triadimenol, a primary metabolite of triadimefon, ranges from 110 to 375 days in soil (Tomlin, 1997). This explains why azole residues were found in various foods, such as strawberry samples, grapes, peppermint, or carrots up to 0.5–0.8 mg/kg. Although the level of the pesticide residues found in food were not so high as to reach toxic levels for consumers, the amount of such remnant pesticides could, however, be important.

The mechanism of action of all azoles—irrespective of their chemical structure and variable biological properties—consists of affecting the activity of fungal enzyme encoded by *Cyp51A* gene, lanosterol 14 alpha-demethylase. This enzyme determines the transformation of lanosterol in ergosterol, an essential component of the cytoplasmatic membrane. The inhibition of the enzyme means the inhibition of ergosterol formation, resulting in cell membrane disorganization and impairment of fungal growth. Because of this, azoles are fungistatic rather than fungicidal substances, so concerns for their capacity to exert selective pressure are justified (Bowyer and Denning, 2014).

Many species of fungi are primarily susceptible to azoles, but not all. Some of them are naturally resistant because ergosterol (the target of azoles) is not required for their cell wall and membrane formation (such as *Pneumocystis* spp). Besides this, at least three resistance mechanisms were identified in case of azoles: (1) exclusion or active efflux from the cell, (2) structural alterations in the target fungal enzyme, and (3) overproduction of the target fungal enzyme. Efflux pumps found in fungi belong to the CDR family (members of the ATP-binding cassette transporters) and MDR1 (a major facilitator) (Prasad and Rawal,2014).

Many CDR1 genes were identified in a fungal cell and some of them are involved in azole resistance. Some susceptible strains could become resistant if genetic alterations occur, and in the end permanent resistant phenotype could result. On the other hand, the modifications could be transient. It was observed that the production of CDR1 mRNA varied in different growth phases and physiological conditions (Lyons and White, 2000).

It is well known that the existence of a persistent antimicrobial pressure on a population will select resistant individuals, especially if the antimicrobial substance has a microbiostatic, and not microbicid effect. The problem is that the excessive use of azoles in agriculture will also affect the saprophytic species and even human pathogenic fungi, not just the plant pathogenic species. Those strains that succeeded in surviving will benefit from the selective pressure, acquiring azole resistance. For the medical field, the risk that patients will encounter such resistant strains will be increased.

Azole resistance also represents a serious problem for patients treated for yeast infections; from this category, *Candida glabrata* became a major concern. Patients may present azole-resistant fungi in three ways: (1) the infecting or colonizing strain is susceptible but suffers mutation and becomes azole resistant; (2) the patient was infected with a heterogeneous population and selected resistant variant during treatment and exposure to antimycotics; or (3) the patient acquires an inherently resistant strain from the external environment (White et al., 1998).

So, the resistance of the fungal strain to treatment can appear in patients after long administration of azoles. But resistant fungi can also develop in the external environment, and those species can infect the human host in the future. For example, azole-resistant *Candida* from patients that were not exposed to antifungal agents before were isolated. Also, some data revealed that some AIDS patients or other immunocompromised patients were infected with some resistant cryptococci prior to drug treatment (Hof, 2001). *Candida krusei* and some molds are also naturally resistant to some azoles because of a low uptake of it into the cell. Some of the efflux pumps that confer resistance to azole could confer resistance to a broad spectrum of other antifungals as well, such as cycloheximide, benztriazoles, and other agents. Moreover, other cellular functions could be affected, so an increased resistance to azole could determine an increased virulence for the respective strain. Some azole-resistant variants of *Candida albicans* produced more extracellular aspartic proteinases, an important virulence factor. Also, some yeast capable of forming hyphae in the presence of azoles were isolated (Fekete-Forgacs et al., 2000).

Another question that arises is about the influence of azole administration on the normal fungal microbiota of humans. The level of azole residue intake is not so high as to be toxic for consumers (in this case the use of azole would be forbidden), but it is enough to exert a selective pressure on the autochthonous *Candida* species.

Other studies that evaluate the risk of cross-resistance emergence in clinical *Aspergillus fumigatus* due to the massive use of azole pesticide in agriculture were realized. A study by Faria-Ramos et al. (2014) aimed to investigate whether Prochloraz (PCZ), an azole extensively used in agriculture, could be associated with the development of cross-resistance to clinical azoles among *A. fumigatus*, a saprophytic mold known to be cause of some allergic syndromes, noninvasive infections, and invasive aspergillosis, a condition associated with significant morbidity and mortality in humans; natural habitat of this strain is represented by the environment, including soil and plants. The study revealed that besides the emergence of cross-resistance, exposure to PCZ determines a series of phenotypic changes: the decrease and depigmentation of colonies from green to white and a progressive absence of conidiation, modifications that could lead to a misidentification of the species in the clinical field. In the case of PCZ, the high MIC values were maintained at the same levels even after the selective pressure was removed. For voriconazole (VRC) and posaconazole (POS), other antifungals tested, after 30 days without selective pressure, the MIC value decreased. In case of itraconazole, in the absence of selective pressure of PCZ, the MIC value reverted to the initial level, and conidiation and also typical mature green colonies reappeared.

In a more recent report, Le Pape et al. (2016) also link the use of fungicides in agriculture to the presence of triazole-resistant *A. fumigatus* among azole-naive persons. These strains presented the TR34/L98H and TR46/Y121F/T289A mutations in the *CYP51A* gene and its promoter region, this mechanism of resistance being reported both in samples isolated from the environment and clinical samples from Europe, Asia, and Africa. On the other hand, some clinical strains from United States and Latin America show no fungicide-driven resistance in *A. fumigatus,* although the use of pesticides is a frequent practice in the Americas. In a study from 2015, 60 soil samples from flower fields and greenhouses in Columbia were analyzed. *Aspergillus* strains were tested for azole-resistance on media supplemented with itraconazole (4 mg/L) or voriconazole (4 mg/L). Twenty *A. fumigatus* strains were resistant and tested for *CYP51A* gene alterations. Results showed that the strains had great diversity in molecular resistance, TR46/Y121F/T289A ($n = 17$), TR34/L98H ($n = 1$), and TR53 ($n = 1$) mutations being observed (Le Pape et al., 2016).

The incidence of multiazole resistance in *A. fumigatus* due to the TR34/L98H mutations is high in Europe and Asia, being responsible for treatment failures. The clinical strains could be regarded as two distinct groups. One group of strains is represented by those isolated from noninvasive diseases including patients with allergic bronchopulmonary aspergillosis (ABPA), aspergilloma, and chronic pulmonary aspergillosis (CPA). These patients received long-term azole therapy (especially itraconazole) and developed resistance to that fungicide after 1–30 months of treatment. The mechanism of resistance consists of mutations in the cyp51A gene, which proves that *A. fumigatus* strains are capable of rapidly adapting to azole drugs in patients treated for a long time. The strains isolated from patients with chronic aspergillosis, that were initially susceptible and later become resistant, had the same genotype; changes appear only in the specific mutations conferring azole resistance, a fact that sustains the occurrence of resistance developed from azole therapy.

The second group is represented by strains isolated from patients with acute aspergillosis but that probably did not come in contact with azole drugs before. Unlike the first group in which resistance development occurs by de novo mutation of the strains in cavitary lesions, the second group acquired resistance to azole drugs from external environments. And unfortunately, this is the situation most frequently encountered, as about 50% of the patients with invasive aspergillosis with azole-resistant *A. fumigatus* strains are azole-naïve. For these cases, a high percentage of mortality was registered (88%). TR34/L98H mutations, seem to be responsible for the resistance. That confers resistance to itraconazole and intermediate susceptibility or resistance to voriconazole, posaconazole, or both.

So it is clear that the irrational use of azole could determine azole-resistance and cross-resistance and could compromise the utility of these substances for clinical strains in the future (Faria-Ramos et al., 2014).

Researchers are still looking for a better approach. More studies are necessary to elucidate all the aspects, but until then, more care should be taken regarding the use of azoles in agriculture, especially because their use in the clinical field is absolutely necessary, since there are not many alternatives that can be administrated to patients for treatment of fungal infections, which tend to become more and more frequent (Hof, 2001).

2 Conclusions

Increasing pesticide use in agriculture is clearly responsible for the selection and emergence of multiple-antibiotic resistant phenotypes in pathogenic strains. The modified phenotype occurs after the exposure of strains to antibiotics and to different chemical substances that could exert a selective pressure. The uncontrolled use of antimicrobials will increase the possibility of spontaneous mutations, leading ultimately to higher levels of resistance that in the end will undermine the efficiency of antibiotic therapy. Although it is clear that we cannot afford a life without antibiotics or pesticides, a balance must be maintained and a more and more judicious use of these substances will be absolutely necessary.

Acknowledgments

The financial support of the research project PN-II-RU-TE- 2014-4-2037 is gratefully acknowledged.

References

Adams, S.J., Fussell, R.J., Dickinson, M., Wilkins, S., Sharman, M., 2009. Study of the depletion of lincomycin residues in honey extracted from treated honeybee (*Apis mellifera* L.) colonies and the effect of the shook swarm procedure. Anal. Chim. Acta 637 (1–2), 315–320.

Akimitsu, N., Hamamoto, H., Inoue, R., et al., 1999. Increase in resistance of methicillin resistant *Staphylococcus aureus* to β-lactams caused by mutations conferring resistance to benzalkonium chloride, a disinfectant widely used in hospitals. Antimicrob. Agents Chemother. 43 (12), 3042–3043.

Al-Waili, N., Salom, K., Al-Ghamdi, A., Ansari, M.J., 2012. Antibiotic, pesticide, and microbial contaminants of honey: human health hazard. Sci. World J. 2012, 930849, p 9.

Bowyer, P., Denning, D.W., 2014. Environmental fungicides and triazole resistance in Aspergillus. Pest Manag. Sci. 70, 173–178.

Burridge, L., Weis, J.S., Cabello, F., Pizarro, J., Bostick, K., 2010. Chemical use in salmon aquaculture: a review of current practices and possible environmental effects. Aquaculture 306, 7–23.

Chapman, J.S., 2003. Disinfectant resistance mechanisms, cross-resistance, and co-resistance. Int. Biodeterior. Biodegrad. 51, 271–276.

Chuanchuen, R., Beinlich, K., Hoang, T.T., Becher, A., Karkhoff-Schweitzer, R., Schweitzer, H.P., 2001. Cross-resistance between triclosan and antibiotics in Pseudomonas aeruginosa is mediated by multidrug efflux pumps: exposure of a susceptible mutant strain to triclosan selects nfxB mutants overexpressing MexCD-OprJ. Antimicrob. Agents Chemotherapy 45, 428–432.

Daly, H., Doyen, J.T., Purcell, III, A.H., 1998. Introduction to Insect Biology and Diversity, second ed. Oxford University Press, New York, New York, 279–300 (Chapter 14).

Davies, J., Davies, D., 2010. Origins and evolution of antibiotic resistance. Microbiol. Mol. Biol. Rev. 74 (3), 417–433.

de Lencastre, H., Oliveira, D., Tomasz, A., 2007. Antibiotic resistant *Staphylococcus aureus*: a paradigm of adaptive power. Curr. Opin. Microbiol. 10, 428–435.

Faria-Ramos, I., Farinha, S., Neves-Maia, J., Tavares, P.R., Miranda, I.M., Estevinho, L.M., Pina-Vaz, C., Rodrigues, A.G., 2014. Development of cross-resistance by *Aspergillus fumigatus* to clinical azoles following exposure to prochloraz, an agricultural azole. BMC Microbiol. 14, 155.

Fekete-Forgacs, K., Gyüre, L., Lenkey, B., 2000. Changes of virulence factors accompanying the phenomenon of induced fluconazole resistance in *Candida albicans*. Mycoses 43, 273–279.

Fraise, A.P., 2002. Susceptibility of antibioticresistant cocci to biocides. J. Appl. Microbiol. 92 (Suppl.), 158S–162S.

Granja, R., Niño, A.M., Zucchetti, R., Niño, R.M., Patel, R., Salerno, A.G., 2009. Determination of erythromycin and lyiosin residues in honey by LC/MS/MS. J. AOAC Int. 92 (3), 975–980.

Grave, K., Torren-Edo, J., Mackay, D., 2010. Comparison of the sales of veterinary antibacterial agents between 10 European countries. J. Antimicrob. Chemother. 65, 2037–2040.

Haddix, P.L., Paulsen, E.T., Werner, T.F., 2000. Natural selection and evolution of antibiotic resistance in bacteria. Bioscene 26, 1–21.

Han, F.X., Banin, A., Su, Y., Monts, D.L., Plodinec, J.M., Kingery, W.L., et al., 2002. Industrial age anthropogenic inputs of heavy metals into the pedosphere. Naturwissenschaften 89, 497–504.

Harrison, J.J., Ceri, H., Turner, R.J., 2007. Multimetal resistance and tolerance in microbial biofilms. Nat. Rev. Microbiol. 5, 928–938.

Hasman, H., Aarestrup, F.M., 2002. tcrB, a gene conferring transferable copper resistance in Enterococcus faecium: occurrence, transferability, and linkage to macrolide and glycopeptide resistance. Antimicrob. Agents Chemother. 46, 1410–1416.

Hof, H., 2001. Critical annotations to the use of azole antifungals for plant protection. Antimicrob. Agents Chemother. 45 (11), 2987–2990.

IRAC, 2007. Resistance Management for Sustainable Agriculture and Improved Public Health, Insecticide Resistance Action Committee.

Kurenbach, B., Marjoshi, D., Amábile-Cuevas, C.F., Ferguson, G.C., Godsoe, W., Gibson, P., Heinemann, J.A, 2015. Sublethal exposure to commercial formulations of the herbicides dicamba, 2,4-dichlorophenoxyacetic acid, and glyphosate cause changes in antibiotic susceptibility in Escherichia coli and Salmonella enterica serovar Typhimurium. mBio 6 (2), e00009–e00015.

Le Pape, P., Lavergne, R.-A., Morio, F., Alvarez-Moreno, C., 2016. Fungicide-driven alterations in azole-resistant *Aspergillus fumigatus*, Colombia, 2015. Emerg. Infect. Dis. 22 (1), 156–157.

Levy, S.B., 2002a. Active efflux, a common mechanism for biocide and antibiotic resistance. J. Appl. Microbiol. 92 (Suppl.), 65S–71S.
Levy, S.B., 2002b. Factors impacting on the problem of antibiotic resistance. J. Antimicrob. Chemother. 49 (1), 25–30.
Lyons, C.N., White, T.C., 2000. Transcriptional analyses of antifungal drug resistance in *Candida albicans*. Antimicrob. Agents Chemother. 44, 2296–2303.
Martinez, J.L., Sánchez, M.B., Martínez-Solano, L., Hernandez, A., Garmendia, L., Fajardo, A., et al., 2009. Functional role of bacterial multidrug efflux pumps in microbial natural ecosystems. FEMS Microbiol. Rev. 33, 430–449.
McMurry, L.M., Oethinger, M., Levy, S.B., 1998a. Overexpression of marA, soxS or acrAB produces resistance to triclosan in *Escherichia coli*. FEMS Microbiol. Lett. 166, 305–309.
McMurry, L.M., Oethinger, M., Levy, S.B., 1998b. Triclosan targets lipid synthesis. Nature 394, 531–532.
Moken, M.C., McMurray, L.M., Levy, S.B., 1997. Selection of multiple antibiotic-resistant (mar) mutants of *Escherichia coli* by using the disinfectant pine oil: roles of the mar and acrAB loci. Antimicrob. Agents Chemother. 41 (12), 2770–2772.
Nicholson, F.A., Smith, S.R., Alloway, B.J., Carlton-Smith, C., Chambers, B.J., 2003. An inventory of heavy metals inputs to agricultural soils in England and Wales. Sci. Total Environ. 311, 205–219.
Nies, D.H., 1999. Microbial heavy-metal resistance. Appl. Microbiol. Biotechnol. 51, 730–750.
Nies, D.H., Silver, S., 1995. Ion efflux systems involved in bacterial metal resistances. J. Ind. Microbiol. 14, 186–199.
Nikaido, H., 2009. Multidrug resistance in bacteria. Annu. Rev. Biochem. 78, 119–146.
Osman, O., Tanguichi, H., Ikeda, K., Park, P., Tanabe-Hosoi, S., Nagata, S., 2010. Copper-resistant halophilic bacterium isolated from the polluted Maruit Lake, Egypt. J. Appl. Microbiol. 108, 1459–1470.
Parikh, S., Moynihan, D.P., Xiao, G., Tonge, P.J., 1999. Roles of tyrosine 158 and lysine 165 in the catalytic mechanism of InhA, the enoylACP reductase from *Mycobacterium tuberculosis*. Biochemistry 38 (41), 13623–13634.
Piddock, L.J., 2006. Clinically relevant chromosomally encoded multidrug resistance efflux pumps in bacteria. Clin. Microbiol. Rev. 19, 382–402.
Prasad, R., Rawal, M.K., 2014. Efflux pump proteins in antifungal resistance. Front Pharmacol. 5, 202.
Price, C.T.D., Singh, V.K., Jayaswal, R.K., Wilkinson, B.J., Gustafason, J.E., 2002. Pine oil cleaner-resistant *Staphylococcus aureus*: reduced susceptibility to vancomycin and oxacillin and involvement of SigB. Appl. Environ. Microbiol. 68 (11), 5417–5421.
Rosewarne, C.P., Pettigrove, V., Stokes, H.W., Parsons, Y.M., 2010. Class 1 integrons in benthic bacterial communities: abundance, association with Tn402-like transposition modules and evidence for coselection with heavy-metal resistance. FEMS Microbiol. Ecol. 72, 35–46.
Salyers, A.A., Amábile-Cuevas, C.F., 1997. Why are antibiotic resistance genes so resistant to elimination? Antimicrob. Agents Chemother. 41, 2321–2325.
Sanchez, P., Moreno, E., Martinez, J.L., 2005. The biocide triclosan selects Stenotrophomonas maltophiliamutants that overproduce the Sme DEF multidrug efflux pump. Antimicrob. Agents Chemother. 49 (2), 781–782.
Seiler, C., Berendonk, T.U., 2012. Heavy metal driven co-selection of antibiotic resistance in soil and water bodies impacted by agriculture and aquaculture. Front. Microbiol. 3, 399.

Shah, N.S., Wright, A., Bai, G.H., Barrera, L., Boulahbal, F., Martin-Casabona, N., Drobniewski, F., Gilpin, C., Havelkova, M., Lepe, R., Lumb, R., Metchock, B., Portaels, F., Rodrigues, M.F., Rusch-Gerdes, S., Deun, A.V., Vincent, V., Laserson, K., Wells, C., Cegielski, J.P., 2007. Worldwide emergence of extensively drug-resistant tuberculosis. Emerg. Infect. Dis. 13, 380–387.

Smith, R.D., Coast, J., 2002. Antimicrobial resistance: a global response. Bull. World Health Organ. 80, 126–133.

Sotgiu, G., Ferrara, G., Matteelli, A., Richardson, M.D., Centis, R., Ruesch-Gerdes, S., Toungoussova, O., Zellweger, J.-P., Spanevello, A., Cirillo, D., Lange, C., Migliori, G.B., 2009. Epidemiology and clinical management of XDR-TB: a systematic review by TBNET. Eur. Respir. J. 33, 871–881.

Stokes, H.W., Nesbo, C.L., Holley, M., Bahl, M.I., Gillings, M.R., Boucher, Y., 2006. Class 1 integrons potentially predating the association with Tn402-like transposition genes are present in a sediment microbial community. J. Bacteriol. 188, 5722–5730.

Tabata, A., Nagamune, H., Maeda, T., Murakami, K., Miyake, Y., Kourai, H., 2003. Correlation between resistance of *Pseudomonas aeruginosato* quaternary ammonium compounds and expression of outer membrane protein OprR. Antimicrob. Agents Chemother. 47 (7), 2093–2099.

Tomlin, C.D.S. (Ed.), 1997. The Pesticide Manual. eleventh ed. British Crop Protection Council, Surrey, United Kingdom.

Velayati, A.A., Masjedi, M.R., Farnia, P., Tabarsi, P., Ghanavi, J., ZiaZarifi, A.H., Hoffner, S.E., 2009. Emergence of new forms of totally drug-resistant tuberculosis bacilli: super extensively drug-resistant tuberculosis or totally drug-resistant strains in Iran. Chest 136, 420–425.

Webber, M.A., Piddock, L.J.V., 2003. The importance of efflux pumps in bacterial antibiotic resistance. J. Antimicrob. Chemother. 51, 9–11.

White, T.C., Marr, K.A., Bowden, R.A., 1998. Clinical, cellular, and molecular factors that contribute to antifungal drug resistance. Clin. Microbiol. Rev. 11, 382–402.

11

MOLECULAR MECHANISMS OF PESTICIDES TOXICITY

Luminita Marutescu, Mariana Carmen Chifiriuc
Faculty of Biology and Research Institute of the University of Bucharest - ICUB, University of Bucharest, Bucharest, Romania

1 Introduction

Environmental pollutants, including pesticides could have a major impact on the public health. However, little information is known about the mechanisms of their toxicity at cellular and molecular level (Braconi et al., 2011). A pesticide is represented by any substance or mixture of substances used for preventing, destroying, or controlling any pest (vectors of human or animal diseases, undesired species of plants, animals, insects, arachnids, or other pests). Despite their beneficial effects chemical pesticides could also be toxic or even lethal for other organisms and pollutants for the environments. Pesticides are exhibiting different degrees of toxicity to human beings, being classified by the World Health Organization (WHO) and the International Agency for Research on Cancer (IARC), in class Ia, extremely hazardous; class Ib, highly hazardous; class II, moderately hazardous; class III, slightly hazardous; class IV, products unlikely to present acute hazard in normal use. Pesticides can induce acute toxicity after immediate exposure to a single dose, or subchronic, chronic, or delayed toxicity, after repeated or continuous exposure. The exposure routes can be represented by dermal or digestive, respiratory and conjunctive mucosa. Pesticides almost always occur in mixtures with other ones. The combined toxicological effects of two or more components of a pesticide mixture can take one of three forms: independent, dose addition, or interaction. Not all mixtures of pesticides with similar chemical structures produce additive effects; thus, if they act on multiple sites their mixtures may produce different toxic effects. The additive approach also fails when evaluating mixtures that involve a secondary chemical that changes the

New Pesticides and Soil Sensors. http://dx.doi.org/10.1016/B978-0-12-804299-1.00012-6

toxicokinetics of the pesticide as a result of its increased activation or decreased detoxification, which is followed by an enhanced or reduced toxicity, respectively (Hernández et al., 2013).

There have been identified more than 95 biochemical targets of pesticides, which could also be impaired in humans and animals, such as enzymes [e.g., acetylcholinesterase (AChE), cytochrome *c* reductase], ion channels, receptors [acetylcholine, esterase, gamma-aminobutyric acid, aryl hydrocarbon receptor (AhR), and estrogen receptor α], cytoskeleton (tubulin biosynthesis). Therefore, knowing, defining, and testing pestcides toxicity can become critical for both food production and human health (Casida, 2009). Currently debated and investigated issues in the pesticides toxicology include: possible long-term effects of chronic low-level exposures; genetic susceptibility to pesticides toxicity; developmental toxicity and neurotoxicity; molecular targets and mechanisms of action and of toxicity (Costa, 2006).

The establishment of guidelines for pesticides toxicity should address cost-effective, large-scale assessment routine tests. This requires a multilevel approach using cell culture, invertebrates, or nonmammalian models, followed by the more specific investigation of certain processes in mammalian models (Slotkin, 2004).

The 1-methyl-4-phenyl-1,2,3,6-tetrahydropyridine, chlorpyrifos (CPF), rotenone, and paraquat induced behavioral alterations, in both adult and larval zebrafish, suggesting the usefulness of this experimental model to establish the toxic doses and for dissecting the molecular mechanisms underlying the pesticides neurotoxicity (Bretaud et al., 2004; Sledge et al., 2011; Levin et al., 2004).

Caenorhabiditis elegans is also an attractive experimental platform model for studying the neurotoxicity and antioxidant stress responses induced by pesticides (Avila et al., 2012), and to assess the toxicitty levels and interaction of binary mixtures of pesticides, while *Biomphalaria alexandrina* snails hemocytes can be used as models for studying the toxicity of herbicides (Mohamed, 2011; Svendsen et al., 2010). *C. elegans* was used to investigate the effects of phosphine, a fumigant on mitochondria, which induced a rapid perturbation of mitochondrial morphology, drastic decrease of oxidative respiration and of themitochondrial membrane potential (DeltaPsim) (Zuryn et al., 2008). *Daphnia magna* microarray is of great further value for the elucidation of molecular mechanisms of toxicity and for the future development of specific biomarkers for hazard characterization (Soetaert et al., 2007). Freshwater algae models can be used to assess the risk of aquatic toxicity of chemical mixtures, acting either synergically or indenpedently (Faust et al., 2003). Cotolerance between environmental and chemical stressors might be expected for similarly acting stressors due to common defense mechanisms. Acclimatization of green alga *Chlamydomonas reinhardtii* to UV radiation and subsequently exposure toward chemicals that share a common physiological target showed that acclimated algae were not co-tolerant to the herbicides paraquat and diuron, suggesting that the fast physiological and biochemical defense mechanisms that conferred tolerance of algae toward higher UVR levels were related to singlet oxygen defense. Thus, knowledge of the molecular toxicity mechanisms of chemicals, rather than their general physiological target, is needed in order to predict cotolerance between environmental and chemical stressors (Korkaric et al., 2015; Zhao et al., 2016). The brain proteins array in male fathead minnows (*Pimephales promelas*) exposed to permethrin, terbufos or their combination has shown the utility of this methodological approach to understand the molecular and cellular mechanisms of pesticides toxicity and to appreciate their cumulative effects (Biales et al., 2011). The invertebrate models, such as *Tigriopus*, a harpacticoid copepod have an important role in the evaluation of pesticides toxicity (assessing endocrine-disruption, assessing whole-animal bioassay and gene expression studies (Raisuddin et al., 2007). A custom-designed chamber for safely containing phosphine gas has been designed to be utilized in a screening program with *C. elegans* for identifying phosphine synergists but also for toxicity studies (Valmas and Ebert, 2006). The yeast *Saccharomyces cerevisiae* represents a well-consolidated and widely used eukaryotic model, with a number of features that make it an ideal organism to carry out functional toxicological studies. Regarding the analysis of the effects of pesticides on yeast much still remains to be done. Furthermore, a deeper knowledge of the effects of environmental pollutants on biotechnological processes associated with the use of yeasts is to be hoped (Braconi et al., 2015).

A panel of different chemical stressors (pesticide, pesticide degradation compounds, polycyclic aromatic hydrocarbon, and heavy metal) mimicking environmental pollution conditions was used for studying plant functioning under chemical stress conditions. Seed-level or root-level subtoxic exposure of the C3 grass *Lolium perenne* produced physiological perturbations and complex metabolic shifts involving stressor-specific effects, indicating multilevel mechanisms of action, such as the effects of glyphosate and its degradation product aminomethylphosphonic acid on quinate levels. Furthermore, major modifications of nitrogen metabolism, especially affecting asparagine, and of photorespiration, especially affecting alanine and glycerate were evidenced (Serra et al., 2015).

A simple and rapid in vitro toxicological assay, utilizing submitochondrial particles (SMP) has been developed for the quantitative evaluation of the toxicity of compounds with different mechanisms of action: uncouplers, inhibitors of the enzyme complexes involved in reverse electron transfer and in oxidative phosphorylation and chemicals that alter the membrane structure (Argese et al., 2005).

As the induction of oxidative stress is one of the most often inquired mechanism of toxicity, redox proteomics which identify posttranslationally oxidized proteins can be an important tool for the evaluation of pesticides toxicity (Braconi et al., 2011).

Bioinformatic approaches, such as 3D-QSAR, Docking, Local Binding Energy, and GRID methods can be integrated in a tool for predicting pesticides toxicity and studying their mechanisms of action, including endocrine disruptor activity (Fratev et al., 2007). Chemical and structural parameters could be useful in modeling chemical reactivity and predicting level of toxicity within homologous series of pesticides compounds, as already demonstrated for 43 organophosphorous (OP) compounds (Yan et al., 2006).

Analysis of 976 chemicals (including failed pharmaceuticals, alternative plasticizers, food additives, and pesticides) was performed in Phases I and II of the US EPA's ToxCast project across 331 cell-free enzymatic and ligand-binding high-throughput screening (HTS) assays. A large inventory of chemical–biological interactions can inform read-across methods, as well as link potential targets to molecular initiating events in adverse outcome pathways for diverse toxicities (Sipes et al., 2011).

The development of sensitive, specific, simple to assay in noninvasive samples biochemical biomarkers of the exposure of organisms to environmental chemicals and of their toxic effects is also needed. These could be represented by the assay of: enzymes (e.g., inhibition of serum "B" esterases to monitor exposure of birds to OP insecticides), DNA damage (induced by aromatic hydrocarbons), transthyretin-retinol binding protein complex (affected by a metabolite of 3,4,3′,4′,tetrachlorobiphenyl), precursors of clotting proteins (Walker, 1995), genes experession (chronic exposure to pesticides might affect the expression of genes implicated in AhR—estrogen receptor α crosstalk that could represent an important biomarker to assess long-term effects of pesticides on human health) (L'Héritier et al., 2014).

2 Organophosphorus Pesticides

OP or organophosphates compounds are toxic chemicals commonly used as pesticides and herbicides in agriculture, industry, and the home. Some OPs are highly toxic to humans and have been used in warfare and terrorist attacks.

The primary mechanism mediating the acute neurotoxicity of these pesticides is the inhibition of target AChE activity in neuromuscular junctions and the central nervous system.

AChE inhibitors are widely used as pesticides and drugs. Their primary effect is the overstimulation of cholinergic receptors, which results in an improper muscular function. During vertebrate embryonic development nerve activity and intracellular downstream events are critical for the regulation of muscle fiber formation. The transcriptomic response of a known AChE inhibitor, the organophosphate azinphos-methyl (APM), in zebrafish embryos was compared to response with two non-AChE inhibiting unspecific control compounds, 1,4-dimethoxybenzene (DMB) and 2,4-dinitrophenol (DNP). A highly specific cluster of APM induced gene transcripts was identified and a subset of strongly regulated genes was analyzed in more detail. The small heat shock protein hspb11 was found to be the most sensitive induced gene in response to AChE inhibitors. Comparison of expression in wild-type, ache and sop (fixe) mutant embryos revealed that hspb11 expression was dependent on the nicotinic acetylcholine receptor (nAChR) activity. Furthermore, modulators of intracellular calcium levels within the whole embryo led to a transcriptional upregulation of hspb11, which suggests that elevated intracellular calcium levels may regulate the expression of this gene. During early zebrafish development, hspb11 was specifically expressed in muscle pioneer cells and Hspb11 morpholino-knockdown resulted in effects on slow muscle myosin organization (Klüver et al., 2011).

However, not all OPs are potent inhibitors of the AChE. The widespread use of OPs has heightened concern regarding their toxicity in man, with numerous reports linking OPs to various forms of delayed neuropathy encompassing a range of neurodegenerative, psychological, and neurobehavioral effects. There is mounting evidence to suggest that subacute levels of OPs have the ability to interact directly with a range of target proteins in addition to AChE (i.e., noncholinergic targets), causing major disruption of membrane and protein turnover, protein phosphorylation, mitochondrial dysfunction, oxidative stress, and cytoskeletal reorganization. Major advances have been made in the study of one OP binding protein neuropathy target esterase (NTE) in terms of its true physiological role.

Additionally, there is increasing evidence for the ability of OPs to cause disruption in a number of metabolic and cell-signaling pathways that affect neuronal cell proliferation, differentiation, and survival and to interact direct with nonesterase proteins, such as tubulin (Hargreaves, 2012).

Doses of CPF and diazinon OP insecticides, which do not produce significant AChE inhibition affect instead cholinergic and serotonergic neurotransmitter systems supporting memory function in rats (Timofeeva et al., 2008).

Another noncholinergic pathway involved in the organophosphate pesticides neurotoxiciy is the enzyme acylpeptide hydrolase, which can be considered as a new biomarker for the neurotoxicity of these pesticides (Pancetti et al., 2007).

OP pesticides could cause airway hyperreactivity due to noncholinergic mechanisms of their neurotoxicity (Proskocil et al., 2010).

There is significant experimental evidence that acute OP intoxication elicits a robust inflammatory response, and emerging evidence suggests that chronic repeated low-level OP exposure also upregulates inflammatory mediators. A critical question that is just beginning to be addressed experimentally is the pathophysiologic relevance of inflammation in either acute or chronic OP intoxication (Banks and Lein, 2012).

Gene expression analysis revealed that neuroblastoma cells treated with the high doses of *CPF, dichlorvos* and *methamidophos* markedly activated cell apoptosis and inhibited cell growth and proliferation genes, which would most likely lead to the process of cell death. Interestingly, the analysis also revealed significant decrease in expressions of many genes in a specific spliceosome pathway in cells treated with the low doses of all three different OPs. The change of spliceosome pathway may represent an important mechanism of injury in neuronal cells exposed to low doses of various OPs. In addition to unraveling a potentially different form of OP pathogenesis, this finding could provide a new diagnostic marker in assessing OP-associated injury in cells or tissues. In addition, these results could also contribute to the development of new prevention and/or therapeutic regimens against OP toxicity (Li et al., 2012).

Monocrotophos, a commonly used OP pesticide induced increased levels of caspase-3 and -9, Bax, p53, p21, Puma, and cytochrome *c* in PC12 cells and decreased those of Bcl(2), Bcl(w), and Mcl1, demonstrating the proapoptotic effect which, after long-term exposure is replaced by a necrotic one (Kashyap et al., 2010).

The effect of OPs (frequent substances spilled in aquatic ecosystems) on the immune system of fishes and in immunotoxicology was recently reviewed (Díaz-Resendiz et al., 2015). Some cellular and molecular mechanisms that might be involved in immunoregulation mechanisms of OP pesticides are also discussed (Díaz-Resendiz et al., 2015).

Environmental pollutants, such as OP and organochloride pesticides have been also associated with changes in sperm parameters (Lu, 2015).

There is increasing evidence reporting that OPs impair glucose homeostasis and cause insulin resistance and type 2 diabetes. Insulin resistance is a complex metabolic disorder that defies explanation by a single etiological pathway. Formation of advanced glycation end products, accumulation of lipid metabolites, activation of inflammatory pathways, and oxidative stress have all been implicated in the pathogenesis of insulin resistance. Ultimately, these molecular processes activate a series of stress pathways involving a family of serine kinases, which in turn have a negative effect on insulin signaling. Experimental and clinical data suggest an association between these molecular mechanisms and OPs compounds. It was first reported that OPs induce hyperglycemia. Then a concomitant increase of blood glucose and insulin was pointed out. For some years only, we have begun to understand that OPs promote insulin resistance and increase the risk of type 2 diabetes (Lasram et al., 2014).

Biological mechanisms underlying subchronic *CPF* neurotoxicity were investigated on rats. Potential mediators, CRHBP and NPY, were found elevated in the CA1 region of the hippocampus at a level that inhibits hippocampal cholinesterase to less than 20% of control while subchronic exposure to CPF at a level that produces more moderate inhibition (approximately 50% of control) does not produce a discernable change in gene expression. Gene ontology–enrichment analysis suggested association of these genes with receptor-mediated cell survival signaling pathways. miR132/212 was also elevated in the CA1 hippocampal region, which may play a role in the disruption of neurotrophin-mediated cognitive processes after CPF administration (Lee et al., 2016). CPF exposure of zebrafish embryos decreased expression of six proteins mainly involved in cytoskeleton structure, protein translation, signal transduction and lipoprotein metabolism (Liu et al., 2015b).

Oxidative stress may be induced by pesticides and it could be the cause of health alteration mediated by pollutants exposure. A large number of registered products containing CPF is used to control pest worldwide. CPF exposure leads to various neurological disorders adverting disturbance in molecular pathways and normal brain functions. Major complications arise when these potent nerve agents access neuronal mechanisms causing adverse effect on AChE and brain lipids with generation of reactive oxygen species. CPF elicits chronic intoxication leading to redox disturbance with irreversible brain damage and oxidative stress. Neuroprotective and antiapoptotic effects of eugenol (EO), a phenolic antioxidant, against CPF-induced neurotoxicity were explored on rat brain. Experimental results indicated that alterations caused by neurotoxic effects of CPF were attenuated by EO administration with decreased protein expressions of caspase-3. Thus, through its antioxidant and antiapoptotic activities, EO showed protective effect against CPF-induced neuronal damage.

CPF (50 μM) induces redox imbalance altering the antioxidant defense system in breast cancer cells. The main mechanism involved in the inhibition of cell proliferation induced by CPF is an increment of p-ERK1/2 levels mediated by H_2O_2 in breast cancer cells (Ventura et al., 2015). Evaluation of CPF neurotoxicity on human neural precursor cells derived from human embryonic stem cells in showed that the pesticide induced cell death in part through NF-κB activation via ROS generation, enabling the interaction of p53 with Bcl-2 and Bax and subsequent release of cytochrome *c*. These data suggest that CPF may affect neurodevelopment in a manner similar to that of several known and suspected neurotoxicants (Lee et al., 2011).

Neurobehavioral disorders, such as anxiety, autism, and attention deficit hyperactivity disorders are typically influenced by genetic and environmental factors. Although several genetic risk factors have been identified in recent years, little is known about the environmental factors that either cause neurobehavioral disorders or contribute to their progression in genetically predisposed individuals. One environmental factor that has raised concerns is CPF, found ubiquitously in the environment. Subchronic exposure to 0.01 or 0.1 μM CPF during development induces specific behavioral defects in 7-day-old zebrafish larvae. The larvae displayed decreases in swim speed and thigmotaxis, yet no changes in avoidance behavior were seen. Exposure to 0.001 μM CPF did not affect swimming, thigmotaxis, or avoidance behavior and exposure to 1 μM CPF induced behavioral defects, but also induced defects in larval morphology. Since thigmotaxis, a preference for the edge, is an anxiety-related behavior in zebrafish larvae, we propose that subchronic CPF exposure interferes with the development of anxiety-related behaviors (Richendrfer et al., 2012).

Toxicity of *dichlorvos* (DDVP), one of the most widely used OPs, was investigated on goldfish (*Carassius auratus*). The results have revealed severe organ impairment. Also, DDVP influenced different metabolites, dose-dependently, involved with imbalance of neurotransmitters, oxidative stress, and disorders of energy and amino acid metabolism (Liu et al., 2015a).

Pesticides, such as *parathion* and carbaryl cause hyperstimulation of cholinergic receptors and an increase in excitatory neurotransmission. Glutamatergic hyperstimulation can occur after exposure to excitatory amino acid toxins, such as the marine toxin domoic acid. Cytochrome P450 2B has an important role in methyl-parathion activation in the rat brain in vitro, suggesting that metabolic activation is important for the organ specific toxicity to the central nervous system of this pesticide (Albores et al., 2001). Parathion has been shown to possess the highest antiandrogen activity, as compared to permethrin and cypermethrin.

Malathion and diazinon OP insecticides affected the viability of mouse oocytes during the early oogenesis, by modulating the expression of genes encoding proteins involved in transcription (BP75), translation (ribosomal protein S5), and mitochondrial function (cytochrome oxidase subunits I and III) (Bonilla et al., 2008). Malathion increases reactive oxygen species generation in fish, by the modulation of the antioxidant enzymes, catalase, gluthatione peroxidase, glutathione reductase, and glutathione-S-transferase, which can be used as biomarkers of toxic exposure to malathion (Huculeci et al., 2009). Gene expression assay in pig fertilized morular embryos exposed for 96 h to high concentrations of malathion pesticide revealed changes in the expression of genes involved in the mitochondrial metabolism, such as cytochrome *c*, major histocompatibility complex I and a hypothetical protein related with a splicing (Salazar et al., 2007).

Other pesticides, such as lindane and strychnine do not affect excitatory neurotransmission directly, but rather, they block the inhibitory regulation of neurotransmission by antagonism of inhibitory GABA and glycine synapses (Jett, 2012).

Using microarray it was demonstrated that *lindane* modified the expression of genes involved in several key signaling pathways, including detoxification (CYP3A4, Gsta2, CYP4A1), apoptosis (Eif2b3, Eif2b4, PKC), PKC activity and redox status in primary cultured rat hepatocytes, that could explain the acute and chronic toxic effects of lindane (Zucchini-Pascal et al., 2011).

Pesticide exposure has repeatedly been associated with cancers. However, molecular mechanisms are largely undetermined. *Diazinon*, a common organophosphate, has been associated with cancers. Genome-wide DNA methylation analyses on DNA samples obtained from human hematopoietic K562 cell exposed to diazinon and ethanol provided direct experimental evidence that diazinon may modify gene promoter DNA methylation levels, which may play a pathological role in cancer development (Zhang et al., 2012a). Diazinon induced modulation of the major pro- and antiinflammatory cytokines, revealed by the decrease of IL-2, IL-4, IL-10, IL-12, and IFN-gamma levels in the mouse splenocytes cultures. However, in in vivo studies, the level of IL-2 increased in CD4 T, IL-10 in CD4 and CD8 T cells and B cells was, whereas INF-gamma was significantly decreased in B cells (Alluwaimi and Hussein, 2007).

Methamidophos is one of the most toxic OP compounds. It acts via phosphorylation of a serine residue in the active site of AChE and butyrylcholinesterase, leading to enzyme inactivation.

Exposure to a nonneuropathic OP compound induced an increased activity of the MAPK pathway whereas exposure to neuropathic OP compounds prevented upregulation of the pathway. Since this pathway is integral to neurite outgrowth and cell survival, this study has revealed molecular mechanisms implicated in neuronal response after exposure to neuropathic OP compound compounds (Pomeroy-Black and Ehrich, 2012).

Methyl parathion (MP) is an extensively used OP pesticide, which has been associated with a wide spectrum of toxic effects on environmental organisms. Proteomic approaches were used for studying the alterations of membrane protein profiles in zebrafish liver (ZFL) cell line exposed to MP for 24 h two-dimensional gel electrophoresis revealed a total of 13 protein spots, whose expression levels were significantly altered by MP. These differential proteins were identified to be membrane proteins, among which seven were upregulated, while two were downregulated. In addition, the mRNA levels corresponding to these differential membrane proteins were further analyzed by quantitative real-time PCR. And the differential expression of arginase-2 was specially validated via Western blotting. Regarding the physiological functions, these proteins are involved in molecular chaperon, cytoskeleton system, cell metabolism, signal transduction, transport, and hormone receptor respectively, suggesting the complexity of MP-mediated toxicity to ZFL cell. These data could provide useful insights for better understanding the hepatotoxic mechanisms of MP and develop novel protein biomarkers for effectively monitoring MP contamination level in aquatic environment.

The acute phase response induced by the OP compounds *soman* and *paraoxon* consists in macrophage activation, stimulation of glucocorticoid, acute phase proteins and the immunomodulatory alpha(1)-acid glycoprotein secretion. These effects suggest the induction of a negative feedback mechanism that prevents overstimulation of the immune system (Ivanović-Matić et al., 2008).

The subchronic administration of the OP insecticide *methidathion* induced irregularities and breaks of the elastic fibers from the aortic wall media, demonstrating the vascular toxicity of this pesticide (Yavuz et al., 2005).

3 Organochlorine Pesticides

Organochlorine, similar to organophosphate pesticides are compounds that can be detected in human populations as a result of occupational or residential exposure. Despite their occurrence in considerably low levels in humans, their biological effects are hazardous since they interact with a plethora of enzymes, proteins, receptors, and transcription factors. The mechanism of pesticide-mediated toxicity is a combination of various enzyme-inhibitory, metabolic, and transcriptional events acting at the cellular and molecular level (Androutsopoulos et al., 2013).

Hexachlorobenzene (HCB) is a widespread environmental pollutant, and a liver tumor promoter in rodents. Experimental studies have showed that HCB-induced HepG2 proliferation and cell cycle progression depend on ERK1/2 phosphorylation, which is mediated by the AhR, a ligand-activated transcription factor that is involved in drug and xenobiotic metabolism (de Tomaso Portaz et al., 2015).

Accumulation of environmental toxins, such as pesticides and metals, are suggested risk factors for the development of typical late onset PD, although genetic factors seem to be substantial in early onset cases. Pesticides are environmental risk factors in genesis of idiopathic Parkinson's disease (PD) and other neurological syndromes. The etiology of most neurodegenerative disorders is multifactorial and consists of an interaction between environmental factors and genetic predisposition. The role of pesticide exposure in neurodegenerative disease has long been suspected, but the specific causative agents and the mechanisms underlying are not fully understood. For the main neurodegenerative diseases, such as PD, Alzheimer's disease and amyotrophic lateral sclerosis there are evidences linking their etiology with long-term/low-dose exposure to pesticides, such as paraquat, maneb, dieldrin, pyrethroids and organophosphates. Most of these pesticides share common features, namely the ability to induce oxidative stress, mitochondrial dysfunction, α-synuclein fibrillization and neuronal cell loss. Small genetic alterations can sensitize cells to metal-induced cell death, a finding that may revive the interest in exogenous factors in the etiology of PD. Mutations of DJ-1 are known to cause a form of recessive early onset Parkinson disease, highlighting an important functional role for DJ-1 in early disease prevention (Björkblom et al., 2013).

The incidence of PD correlates with environmental exposure to pesticides, such as the organochlorine insecticide, *dieldrin*. Previous studies found an increased concentration of the pesticide in the striatal region of the PD patient's brain and also that dieldrin adversely affects cellular processes associated with PD. These processes include mitochondrial function and reactive oxygen species production. However, the mechanism and specific cellular targets responsible for dieldrin-mediated cellular dysfunction and the structural components of dieldrin contributing to its toxicity (toxicophore) have not been fully defined. For this purpose comparisons of the toxicity profiles for different dieldrin analog (including aldrin, endrin, and *cis*-aldrin diol) were investigated. Results indicated a structure-specific effect important for elucidating the mechanisms of dieldrin neurotoxicity (Allen et al., 2013a,b).

Exposure to organochlorinated pesticides, such as *dieldrin* has been linked to Parkinson's and Alzheimer's diseases, endocrine disruption, and cancer. Functional genomics approach in the model eukaryote *Saccharomyces cerevisiae* showed that dieldrin alters leucine availability. Additionally, appropriate negative regulation of the Ras/protein kinase A pathway, along with an intact pyruvate dehydrogenase complex, is required for dieldrin tolerance. Many yeast genes described in this study have human orthologs that may modulate dieldrin toxicity in humans (Gaytán et al., 2013).

Heptachlor alters the dopamine transport, this being one of the molecular basis for the increased incidence of PD after pesticides exposure (Miller et al., 1999).

Dieldrin and *trans-nonachlor* treatments of human monocytes in vitro resulted in increasing intracellular superoxide levels via a NADPH oxidase-dependent mechanism that relies on elevated intracellular arachidonic acid levels. Chronic activation of monocytes induced by organochlorine insecticides exposure might contribute to pathogenic oxidative stress and inflammation (Mangum et al., 2015).

The detailed mechanisms of free radicals in triggering *pentachlorophenol (PCP)/tetrachlorohydroquinone (TCHQ)*-mediated tumor promotion and toxicity are still not completely determined. However PCP and TCHQ (formed during PCP metabolism) proved to be mild tumor promoters in two-stage tumorigenesis models, in which the possible mechanism could be through ROS generation and changes in Bcl-2 gene expression. Also, the findings revealed that TCHQ can induce DNA lesions and glutathione depletion in mammalian cells. Mitogen-activated protein kinase (MAPK) activation is involved in PCP/TCHQ-triggered cytotoxicity, as evidenced by the finding that higher doses of TCHQ could lead to necrosis of freshly isolated splenocytes through the production of a large amount of ROS and sustained ERK activation. These results could explain partly the underlying molecular mechanisms contributing to the tumorigenesis induced by PCP (Chen et al., 2015a).

PCP causes a Warburg-like effect on zebrafish embryos during gastrulation, and the affected embryos had the phenotype of developmental delay. PCP acts as an inhibitor of oxidative phosphorylation (Xu et al., 2008). PCP has been shown to induce systemic toxicity, carcinogenesis, and endocrine-disrupting activities in fish, as evidenced by the up regulation of the 125-kDa vitellogenin protein the hepatocytes of male channel catfish (Dorsey and Tchounwou, 2004). PCP has been shown to induce systemic toxicity and carcinogenesis in several experimental studies. Using human liver carcinoma cells it has been shown that PCP modulated the expression of cellular proteins, including CYP1A1 in a dose-response relationship (Dorsey and Tchounwou, 2003).

Functional approach in the model eukaryote *Saccharomyces cerevisiae* exposed to *toxaphene* demonstrated that the insecticide affects yeast mutants defective in processes associated with transcription elongation and nutrient utilization. Synergistic growth defects were observed upon exposure to both toxaphene and the known transcription elongation inhibitor mycophenolic acid. Several of the yeast genes identified in this study have human homologs, warranting further investigations into the potentially conserved mechanisms of toxaphene toxicity (Gaytán et al., 2013).

Chloropicrin is an aliphatic volatile nitrate compound that is mainly used as a pesticide. It has several toxic effects in animals and can cause irritating and other health problems in exposed humans. The cytotoxicity of chloropicrin in the retinal pigment epithelium is postulated to be associated with oxidative stress and perturbation of the endoplasmic reticulum functions, which are possibly among the mechanisms involved in oculotoxicity of chloropicrin (Pesonen et al., 2012).

The organochlorine *methoxychlor* induced a significant increase in the levels of cytosolic cytochrome *c* and procaspase-9 after 6 h of exposure to a single dose, as well as of Fas, FasL, pro- and cleaved caspase-3 were observed, demonstrating the induction of testicular apoptosis in adult rats (Vaithinathan et al., 2010). Methoxychlor also increased the levels of heat shock proteins, clusterin, and oxidative stress-related parameters in the testis of adult male rats (Vaithinathan et al., 2009).

Endosulfan is an organochlorine pesticide commonly used in agriculture yet classified by the Stockholm Convention in 2011 as a persistent organic pollutant (POP). Its potential toxicity makes its continued use a major public health concern. The phenotypical effects of endosulfan on HepG2 liver cells were investigated. It was revealed that endosulfan profoundly alters the phenotype of liver cells by inducing cell detachment and partial the induction of the epithelial to mesenchymal process, as well as disrupting the anoikis process. These events account, at least in part, for the carcinogenic potential of endosulfan in liver (Peyre et al., 2012). The impact of *endosulfan* in clams, *Ruditapes philippinarum* was also investigated. The results offers information for the characterization of potential molecular biomarkers that may be used in future environmental monitoring and to investigate the mechanisms of stress to endosulfan in clams/marine invertebrates (Tao et al., 2013).

1,1,1-Trichloro-2,2-bis (2-chlorophenyl-4-chlorophenyl) ethane (o,p′-DDT) is an organochlorine pesticide and endocrine disruptor known to activate the estrogen receptor. Systematic comparative gene expression assessments were used for the identification of comparable temporal phenotypic responses in animal studies, which are valuable for elucidating conserved and divergent estrogen signaling mechanisms in rodent uterotrophy (Kwekel et al., 2013).

Dichlorodiphenyltrichloroethane (DDT) is a widely used organochlorine pesticide ubiquitous in the environment and a xenoestrogen that promotes rodent hepatomegaly and tumors. It has been shown significant correlation between DDT serum concentration and liver cancer incidence in humans, but the underlying mechanisms remain elusive. An experimental rat model study has indicated that DDT treatment may result in cell cycle progression and apoptosis inhibition through CAR- and ERα-mediated gene activation in mouse liver. Thus proliferative and antiapoptotic conditions induced by CAR and ERα activation may be important contributors to the early stages of hepatocarcinogenesis as produced by DDT in rodent livers (Kazantseva et al., 2013).

DDT has been shown to activate the complement system through the alternative pathway in the absence of any pathogen, enhancing the susceptibility to infections, to increase the level of tumor necrosis factor-alpha (TNF-alpha) and nitric oxide in macrophages bursting inflammatory reactions, to induce cytokine imbalance and immune-dysregulation, as well as macrophages apoptosis (Dutta et al., 2008).

The exposure to DDT and its related pesticides has long been linked to endocrine disruption. Probing the molecular recognition of DDT analogs by targeted receptors at the atomic level is critical for deciphering this mechanism. Molecular dynamics simulation was applied to probe the molecular recognition process of DDT and its five analogs, including dichlordiphenyldichloroethylene (DDE), dichlorodiphenyldichloroethane (DDD), methoxychlor (MXC), p,p'-hydroxy-DDT (HPTE), and dicofol by human estrogen receptor (ER) α, and human ER-related receptor (ERR) γ. Van der Waals interactions mainly drive the interactions of DDT analogs with ERα ligand-binding domain (LBD) and ERRγ LBD. Minor structural changes of DDT analogs in the number and position of chlorine and phenolic hydroxyl moiety cause differences in binding modes through aromatic stacking and hydrogen bonding and thus affect differently conformational changes of ERα LBD and ERRγ LBD. The binding of DDT analogs affects the helix 12 orientation of ERα LBD but causes no rearrangement of helix 12 of ERRγ LBD (Zhuang et al., 2012).

The p,p′-Dichlorodiphenyldichloroethylene (DDE), the most stable metabolite of DDT induced apoptosis in peripheral blood mononuclear cells by activating both extrinsic and intrinsic apoptotic pathways involving caspase-8, Bid, caspase-9 and caspase-3, degradation of PARP and ubiquitination (Alegría-Torres et al., 2009).

The fungicide *N-(3,5-dichlorophenyl)succinimide* and its metabolites have been shown to induce nephrotoxicity manifested as acute polyuric renal failure and proximal tubular necrosis. The in vitro studies revealed that there the toxicity depends on the accumulation of sulfate conjugates and on genders (Rankin et al., 2001).

POPs are degradation-resistant anthropogenic chemicals that accumulate in the food chain and in adipose tissue. Transcriptomic analysis of rat liver tissues after exposure to six different POPs (toxaphene, hexachlorobenzene, chlordane, mirex, dieldrin, and heptachlor) was performed. The data from large-scale gene expression analysis of a different POP exposure in rat model suggest that characteristic expression profiles exist in liver hepatic cells and multiclassification of POP-specific molecular signatures can discriminate each toxicant at an early exposure time. The use of these molecular markers may be more widely implemented in combination with more traditional techniques for assessment and prediction of toxicity exposure to POPs from an environmental (Jung et al., 2012). Positive correlations have been reported between blood or peritumoral adipose tissue levels of persistent organic compounds acting as endocrine disruptors and inuctors of breast cancer risk (Fénichel and Brucker-Davis, 2008; Clapp et al., 2008).

4 Pyrethroids

Pyrethroids, insecticides, which affect sodium channels in neurons, are widely used to control insect pests for domestic and agricultural purposes and are found to be toxic to many organ systems including the male reproductive system. Brain-derived neurotrophic factor (BDNF) plays a fundamental role in neuronal synaptic plasticity. A decrease of plasticity in the brain may be related to the pathogenesis of neurodegenerative or psychiatric disorders. Type I and II pyrethroid insecticides affect similar metabolic pathways, which induced hepatotoxicity and nephrotoxicity (Liang et al., 2013).

D-allethrin exhibited a dose-dependent cytotoxicity on Leydig cell carcinoma cells, the cytotoxicity being associated with generation of reactive oxygen species, increased lipid peroxidation, alterations in antioxidant enzyme status and presence of apoptotic bodies. Allethrin induced apoptosis was associated with voltage-gated calcium channel mediated intracellular calcium release (Madhubabu and Yenugu, 2014). *Bifenthrin,* a pyrethroid insecticide with escalating usage, downregulates a number of estrogen-related transcripts, particularly at the lowest exposure level. Exposure of *Menidia beryllina* (inland silverside) to increasing concentrations of bifenthrin (ng/L) decreased reproductive output, which was consistent with changes in endocrine-related gene expression and choriogenin production (0.5 ng/L) (Brander et al., 2016).

Proteomic approach and mass spectrometry were used in order to analyze changes in protein expression profiles after 48 h of exposure of cladoceran *Daphnia magna* to *deltamethrin,* a class II alpha-cyano pyrethroid insecticide commonly used in agriculture. Deltamethrin inhibition site is located between the mitochondrial complexes II and III, causing perturbations in lipid–lipid and lipid–protein interactions, in transport mechanisms, and alters the membrane permeability and mitochondrial enzyme activities (Braguini et al., 2004).

The deregulated proteins belonged to 12 biological processes (i.e., metabolic processes, apoptosis and stimulus response) and 5 molecular functions (i.e., catalytic activity, binding, structural molecular activity, antioxidant, and receptor activities).

Transcription factor NF-E2-related factor 2 (Nrf2) is important for cell protection against chemical-induced oxidative stress. In PC12 cells, Nrf2 can be triggered by *deltamethrin,* a commonly used pyrethroid insecticide. Studies regarding molecular mechanisms behind Nrf2 activation by deltamethrin showed that cell glutathione depletion is not necessary for the activation of Nrf2/ARE by deltamethrin in PC12 cells, and that GCLC and HO-1 expression can increase through other signaling pathways (Li et al., 2013). It was found that deltamethrin (DM), a type II pyrethroid, increased brain-derived neurotrophic factorBDNF mRNA expression in cultured rat cortical neurons (Matsuya et al., 2012). The subcutaneous treatment with deltamethrin produces a dose- and exposure time–dependent arrest of spermatogenesis, an imbalance of sex hormones and increased malondialdehyde levels in rats demonstrating its gonads toxicity (Issam et al., 2009).

Lambda-cyhalothrin (LTC) is a synthetic pyrethroid with a broad spectrum of insecticidal and acaricidal activities used to control a wide range of insect pests in a variety of applications. Metabolomics approach revealed implication of glutamate–glutamine–gamma-aminobutyric axis in lambda-cyhalothrin–induced toxicity in goldfish *C. auratus*. Lambda-cyhalothrin exposure influenced levels of many metabolites (e.g., leucine, isoleucine, and valine in brain and kidney; lactate in brain, heart, and kidney; alanine in brain and kidney; choline in brain, heart, and kidney; taurine in brain, heart, and kidney; *N*-acetylaspartate in brain; myo-inositol in brain; phosphocreatine in brain and heart; 2-oxoglutarate in brain; *cis*-aconitate in brain, etc.), and broke the balance of neurotransmitters and osmoregulators, evoked oxidative stress, disturbed metabolisms of energy and amino acids.

Rat exposure to LTC (1/10DL50 = 6.23 mg/kg) for a period of 7, 14, and 21 days induced a noticeable genotoxic effect in rat peripheral blood evidenced by a significant increase in the frequency of micronuclei, a significant increase in ROS contents, nitrite formation, protein carbonyl levels, and lipid peroxidation in erythrocytes were observed at different times of treatments, suggesting the implication of oxidative stress in its toxicity (Fetoui et al., 2015).

Rotenone is an environmental neurotoxin that induces degeneration of dopaminergic neurons in substantia nigra pars compacta (SNpc), which ultimately results in Parkinsonism. Rotenone induces mitochondrial respiratory chain complex I dysfunctions, which can lead to the degeneration of retinal ganglion cells in Leber's optic neuropathy, attesting the role of environmental pesticides in neurodegenerative diseases (Zhang et al., 2006). Studies have showed that p38(MAPK)/p53-dependent induction of Bax contributes to rotenone's neurotoxicity in rat models of PD (Wu et al., 2013). Rotenone activation of the p38 and JNK pathways is responsible of the apoptosis of human dopaminergic SH-SY5Y cells (Newhouse et al., 2004). The cDNA microarray analysis of 1-methyl-4-phenyl-pyridinium toxicity in the same neural cells revealed the decresed expression levels of c-Myc and RNA-binding protein 3 (Conn et al., 2003). Prostaglandin A1 protected against rotenone-induced cell death by inducing HSPs and blocking nuclear translocation of NF-kappaB (Wang et al., 2002).

Oxidative stress is one of the mechanisms implicated to play a significant role in the pathophysiology of PD. It has been shown that an aqueous extract of *Selaginella delicatula* (SDAE) offered robust neuroprotection against rotenone in a *Drosophila* model (Chandran and Muralidhara, 2013). Some species of fish are more tolerant to rotenone, than others. The mechanism at which a fish handles oxidative stress plays an important role in the tolerance to rotenone (Amberg et al., 2012).

5 Dithiocarbamates

Intensive use of pesticides, particularly *dithiocarbamates,* in agriculture often leads to contamination of freshwater ecosystems. Tattoo exposure perturbs free radical processes, that is, induces mild oxidative stress and enhances the activity of certain antioxidant and associated enzymes in goldfish gills. It was concluded that goldfish respond to the presence of waterborne pesticide by adjusting antioxidant defenses through upregulation of activities of antioxidant and associated enzymes (Kubrak et al., 2012). *Propineb* affected the acetylcholine release and the molecular mechanisms involved in rat pheochromocytoma cells differentiated by NGF (PC12), probably by affecting the cytoskeletal actin (Viviani et al., 2008). *Carbofuran* neurotoxic effects could occur through noncholinergic mechanisms, due to changes in mitochondrial oxidative stress and functions associated with impaired cognitive and motor functions in rats (Kamboj et al., 2008). The endocrine disruptor activity of the fungicide *mancozeb,* an ethylenedithiocarbamate composed of a polymeric complex of manganese ethylenebisdithiocarbamate with zinc salt has been shown to impair mouse oocyte and further embryo development and meiosis, suggesting a role for in the infertility in exposed human populations (Cecconi et al., 2007). Mancozeb has been shown to induce immunosuppressant effects in agricultural workers as revealed by the decrease of lipopolysaccharide-induced tumor necrosis factor-alpha production in leukocytes and in vitro, in the promyelocytic cell line THP-1, by preventing IkappaB degradation and NF-kappaB nuclear translocation (Corsini et al., 2006).

The *CS2* and *methyl isothiocyanate* compounds resulted from the decomposition of *N-methyldithiocarbamate* proved the ability of interacting covalently with biological macromolecules and to effect covalent cross-linking, thus contributing to the carbamate pesticides toxicity (Valentine et al., 1995).

4-Vinylcyclohexene (VCH) is a dimer of 1,3-butadiene produced as a by-product of pesticides, plastic, rubber, flame retardants, and tire production. VCH mechanism of toxicity was studied using a *Drosophila melanogaster* model. The results indicated that VCH toxicity is associated with oxidative damage, as evidenced by the alteration in the oxidative stress–antioxidant balance, and possible neurotoxic consequences due to decreased AChE activity, and impairments in negative geotaxic behavior (Abolaji et al., 2014).

6 Herbicides

Atrazine (2-chloro-4-ethytlamino-6-isopropylamine-1,3,5-triazine) is the most commonly detected pesticide contaminant in ground and surface water, it is a member of the triazine class of herbicides. Atrazine is frequently found to contaminate potable water supplies above the maximum contaminant level of 3 μg/L as defined by the US Environmental Protection Agency. Previous studies have shown that atrazine is an endocrine disruptor owing to its adverse effects on the male reproductive system in several vertebrates. Studies suggest that the reproductive toxicity of atrazine may be the result of disruption of tight junctions and metabolic signaling pathways and/or induction of apoptosis in germ cells (Chen et al., 2015b).

Exposure to atrazine of zebrafish embryos has demonstrated the developmental origins of neurological alterations observed in adult female zebrafish (Wirbisky et al., 2015). Investigations regarding the molecular mechanisms underlying atrazine neurotoxicity indicated that this widely used broad-spectrum herbicide, may induce autophagy- and apoptosis-related changes in dopaminergic neurons. Moreover, this induction may be regulated by the Beclin-1 and Bcl-2 autophagy and apoptosis pathways (Song et al., 2015).

MALDI-TOF MS/MS analysis identified several differentially expressed phosphoproteins and total proteins in human breast epithelial MCF-10A cells after being exposed to environmentally relevant concentrations of atrazine. The expression of different proteins belonging to various cellular compartments (nucleus, cytosol, membrane) and varied in function, including those regulating the stress response, such as peroxiredoxin I, HSP70 and HSP27; structural proteins, such as tropomyosin and profilin 1; and oncogenesis proteins, such as ANP32A was observed. The results revealed that ANP32 expression after atrazine treatment increased dose and time dependently and was primarily located in the nucleus (Huang et al., 2014). Experimental or predictive results showed that atrazine and its metabolites in the three-hydrolysis paths (dealkylation, deamination, and Cl substitution, respectively) were carcinogenic.

Atrazine, a herbicide commonly applied to agricultural areas and a common contaminant of potable water supplies, is implicated as an endocrine-disrupting chemical (EDC) and potential carcinogen. Risk assessments suggest that intermediate and long-term exposure to triazine herbicides and its metabolites through water can cause severe damage to human health.

Studies show that EDCs can cause irreversible changes in tissue formation, decreased reproductive potential, obesity, and cancer. The US Environmental Protection Agency considers an atrazine concentration of ≤3 ppb in drinking water safe for consumption. Morphological alteration (significant increase in head length), altered genes associated with neuroendocrine and reproductive system development, function, and disease, cell cycle control and carcinogenesis and protein alterations were identified. These data will help to further define the biological pathways and mechanisms of toxicity (Weber et al., 2013).

Studies are indicating that DNA methylation might be involved in the toxicity caused by atrazine and CPF long exposure (>40 days) in the common carp (Wang et al., 2014).

Changes in gene expression of *Enchytraeus albidus* were significantly altered after 2 days exposure to three pesticides—atrazine, dimethoate (insecticide), and carbendazim (fungicide) in a dose-related manner. The mechanisms of response were comparable with the ones for mammals, suggesting conserved modes of action across species. Dimethoate, atrazine, and carbendazim significantly affected biological processes, like translation, regulation of the cell cycle or general response to stress. Intracellular signaling and microtubule-based movement were affected by dimethoate and carbendazim, whereas atrazine affected lipid and steroid metabolism (also by dimethoate) or carbohydrate metabolism (also by carbendazim). Response to DNA damage/DNA repair was exclusively affected by carbendazim (Novais et al., 2012).

Investigation of the possible effects of atrazine on Wistar rats submitted to subacute treatment showed an increase of catalase levels and maintenance of the expression of antioxidant enzymes (SOD and GST). In addition, lipid peroxidation, hepatic tissue degeneration, activation of HSP90, increased levels of connexin mRNA, and genotoxicity were observed. In conclusion, atrazine induced early hepatic oxidative stress that triggered defense mechanisms to maintain the morphophysiological integrity of the liver. Further studies are needed to better understand the effects of this herbicide on human health (Campos-Pereira et al., 2012).

Simazine is also an herbicide of the triazine class. Gene expression analysis was used to investigate the reproductive toxicity of *simazine* on male *Xenopus laevis* (0.1, 1.2, 11.0 and 100.9 μg/L for

100 days). The results indicated alteration and significantly down-regulation of genes involved in the cell cycle control, and amino acid metabolism pathways (Sai et al., 2015).

Exposure to *Sencor* (herbicidal component: *metribuzin*) on goldfish (*C. auratus* L.), induced various histopathological changes in goldfish kidney, such as hypertrophy of intertubular hematopoietic tissue, small and multiple hemorrhages, glomerular shrinkage, and also decreased activities of kindey enzymes: catalase, glutathione peroxidase, glutathione reductase, and AChE. However, glucose-6-phosphate dehydrogenase and lactate dehydrogenase activities increased after treatment. Thus induction of oxidative stress is one of the mechanisms responsible for Sencor toxicity to fish (Husak et al., 2014).

TGx microarray data revealed major signaling pathways and cell processes affected in *propiconazole* (PPZ) and phenobarbital (PB) mouse treated livers. Propiconazole produced an increase incidence of liver tumors in male CD-1 mice only at a dose that exceeded the maximum tolerated dose (2500 ppm). Additional studies show that the postulated key event of hepatocellular proliferation was observed in CD-1 mice for both PPZ and PB, and that PPZ is also a potent activator of the mouse CAR nuclear receptor. Thus, with regard to the events which are hallmarks of CAR-induced effects that are key events in the mode of action of mouse liver carcinogenesis with PB, PPZ-induced tumors can be viewed as being promoted by a similar PB-like CAR-dependent mode of action (Currie et al., 2014).

Conazole fungicides toxicity was investigated using the *Dunaliella Tertiolecta* alga model and have been shown to induce an increase of cellular volume and total lipid content, proving their interference with ergosterol biosynthesis (Baird and DeLorenzo, 2010).

The broad spectrum *demethylase inhibitors* fungicides have been shown to disrupt the endocrine-mediated processes in different organisms and to inhibit ecdysteroid biosynthesis in arthropods. Their chronic toxicity to *Daphnia magna* was evaluated and resulted in a decrease of the reproductive success by delaying molting and development and by causing severe developmental abnormalities among offspring (Hassold and Backhaus, 2009).

In *Daphnia,* the antiecdysteroidal fungicide *fenarimol* induced a set of proteolytic enzymes-including different serine proteases and carboxypeptidases and decreased different cuticula proteins. The embryo development related gene vitellogenin was differentially expressed with a significant increase in embryo abnormalities in the offspring (Soetaert et al., 2007).

The dicarboximide fungicide *iprodione* causes oxidative damage by the generation of free oxygen radicals and induces cytochrome P4501A3 (CYP1A3) that involves the activation of the AhR complex via phosphorylation-dephosphorylation reactions in cultured rainbow trout hepatocytes (Ferraris et al., 2005).

The sublethal effects of a commonly used insecticide, the *phenylpyrazole fipronil*, on larval fathead minnow (*Pimephales promelas*) was assessed utilizing a quantitative transcriptomic approach. Different mechanisms of toxicity were apparent over the course of the experiment, with short-term responses indicating neurotoxic effects. After 6 days of recovery, endocrine effects were observed with vitellogenin being upregulated 90-fold at 61 μg/L fipronil. Principal component analysis demonstrated a significant increase in gene transcription changes over time andduring the recovery period (Beggel et al., 2012).

Nitrofen, a diphenyl ether herbicide can produce fetal abnormalities in rodents. Prenatal exposure to nitrofen in mice induced sumptoms similar to those reported in the human genetic Fryns syndrome characterized by lung hypoplasia, diaphragmatic hernia, craniofacial malformations, skeletal malformations, cardiovascular malformations, and genitourinary malformations (Acosta et al., 2001). Using the undifferentiated P19 teratocarcinoma cells it has been shown that this pesticide induced a p38-independent, but caspase-3–dependent apoptosis, an increase of reactive oxygen species associated with a decrease of reduced/ oxidized glutathione, indicating that nitrofen alters the cellular redox (Kling et al., 2005).

Paraquat (*dipyridylium*, *N,N′*-dimethyl-4,4′-bipyridinium dichloride, PQ) is a highly toxic weed killer once promoted by the United States for use in Mexico to destroy marijuana plants. Research found that this herbicide was dangerous to workers who applied it to the plants. Investigations regarding the molecular mechanisms underlying delayed progressive pulmonary fibrosis showed the involvement of epithelial-mesenchymal transition, such as cellular response in both fibrogenesis and resistance to cell death during subacute paraquat poisoning of pulmonary epithelial cells (Yamada et al., 2015). Paraquat mainly accumulates in the lung where affects the polyamine transport system from the alveolar cells membrane, the redox cycling and the intracellular oxidative stress generation (Dinis-Oliveira et al., 2008). Investigation of the molecular mechanisms of paraquat-induced damage using cultured human fetal lung fibroblasts (MRC-5 cells) have indicated that exposure to paraquat led to a significant and time-dependent increase in tissue growth factor expression and induced changes in the morphology and biomechanical characteristics of the cells. These findings may represent useful targets of improved molecular-based therapies for paraquat poisoning. PQ significantly decreases cell viability, increases sub-G1 hypodiploids DNA contents and caspase 3/7 activity in lung alveolar epithelial cell-derived L2 cells, which also caused mitochondrial dysfunction, and decreased the mRNA expression of Bcl-2 and increased that of Bax, Bak, and p53. Moreover, the protein expressions of Bax and Bak were increased in PQ-treated cells. In addition, when PQ was exposed to L2 cells, the expressions of ER stress-related signaling genes (including Grp78, CHOP, and caspase-12 mRNA) and proteins (including phospho-eIF-2α, CHOP, Grp78, calpain I and -II, and caspase-12) were significantly increased. PQ also decreased the protein expressions of procaspase-9/7/3. In L2 cells, PQ induced Nrf-2 translocation from the cytosol to the nucleus. Cells transfected with Nrf-2 siRNA significantly reversed the PQ-induced toxicity, including depolarization of MMP, increased the Bax, Bak, p53 mRNAs expression, decreased the Bcl-2 mRNA expression, increased the caspase 3/7 activity, Grp78, CHOP, and caspase-12 mRNAs and protein expression, and decreased that of pro-caspase-3. Taken together, these results suggest that Nrf-2-regulated mitochondria and ER stress-related pathways are involved in the PQ-induced alveolar epithelial cell injury (Chen et al., 2012a).

Paraquat also induces cytoskeletal disruption (microtubules and microfilaments), generating very short actin polymers, which tend to aggregate one to another (Milzani et al., 1997).

Paraquat is also capable of generating oxidative stress and producing brain damage after chronic exposure. An in vivo experimental model of paraquat neurotoxicity suggested that the release of apoptogenic proteins from mitochondria to cytosol after paraquat treatment would be the consequence of an alteration in mitochondrial membrane permeability due to the presence of high superoxide anion levels. Also, under chronic exposure, striatal mitochondria became more sensitive to paraquat oxidative damage than cortical mitochondria (Czerniczyniec et al., 2013). Overexpression of a group of microRNAs (miRs) affects the antioxidant promoting factor, Nrf2 and related glutathione-redox homeostasis in SH-SY5Y dopaminergic neurons. Further studies showed a critical role for oxidant mediated miR153-Nrf2/ARE pathway interaction in paraquat neurotoxicity (Narasimhan et al., 2014).

Since their discovery, Parkinsonian toxins (6-hydroxydopamine, MPP+, paraquat, and rotenone) have been widely employed as in vivo and in vitro chemical models of PD. Alterations in mitochondrial homeostasis, protein quality control pathways, and more recently, autophagy/mitophagy have been implicated in neurotoxin models of PD (Dagda et al., 2009). The neurotoxin 1-methyl-4-phenylpyridinium (MPP+) and other mitochondrial inhibitors (e.g., rotenone or 3-nitropropionic acid) elicited apoptosis in cerebellar granule cell cultures via stimulation of autocrine excitotoxicity, cysteine proteases involved in the execution of cell death: caspases and calpains and subsequent neuronal apoptosis (Leist et al., 1998). A variety of neuroreceptors and ion channels have been identified as the major target sites of these neurotoxic insecticides causing various forms of hyperexcitation and paralysis in animals (Narahashi et al., 1998).

The *snca* and *mapt* genes and environmental factors are important risk factors of PD, the second-most common neurodegenerative disease. The agrichemicals maneb and paraquat selectively target dopaminergic neurons, leading to Parkinsonism, through ill-defined mechanisms. The ability of maneb and paraquat, separately and together, to induce synucleinopathy and tauopathy in wild type mice was investigated. Results showed that paraquat is much more toxic than maneb, via its inhibitory effects on proteasomes and autophagy, which lead to accumulation of α-synuclein and p-Tau (Wills et al., 2012).

Due to its capacity to induce dopaminergic neuron death PQ is used as a PD mimetic; however, its mechanism remains contradictory. The neuropathological effects of PQ in substantia nigra (SN), frontal cortex (FC), and hippocampus of the progressive mouse (adult Swiss albino) model of PD-like neurodegeneration were revealed using immunohistochemistry, western blots, and histological and biochemical analyses. PQ induces ROS production and differential α-synuclein expression that promotes neuroinflammation in microglia-dependent or -independent manners, and produces different patterns of dopaminergic neurotoxicity in three different regions of mouse brain (Mitra et al., 2011).

Minocycline is a second-generation tetracycline and is undergoing clinical trials for treating PD with an unresolved mechanism. The molecular mechanism of minocycline in preventing PQ-induced cytotoxicity have been studied and have shown that minocycline was effective in preventing PQ-induced apoptotic cell death, which involves the cleavages of poly (ADP-ribose) polymerase (PARP) and caspase-3 and increased fluorescence intensity of annexin V-FITC. In addition, PQ also quickly induced alterations of unfolded protein responses (UPRs) and subsequently dysfunction of the mitochondria (such as the decrease in membrane potential and increase in membrane permeability and superoxide formation). Finally, the mechanism of minocycline in preventing PQ-induced apoptosis might be mediated by attenuating endoplasmic reticulum stress and mitochondrial dysfunction, which respectively results in caspase-12 activation and the release of H_2O_2, HtrA2/Omi, and Smac/Diablo. Thus, minocycline could possibly be used to treat other neurodegenerative disorders with similar pathologic mechanisms (Huang et al., 2012).

Treatment with paraquat induced apoptosis in HK-2 cells, as evidenced by accumulation of sub-G1 cell population, chromatin condensation, DNA fragmentation, and translocation of phosphatidylserine. Mitochondria-mediated apoptosis pathway contributed importantly to PQ-induced apoptosis, as revealed by the activation of caspase-3/-9, cleavage of PARP, depletion of mitochondrial membrane potential regulated by Bcl-2 family members, and overproduction of reactive oxygen species. Moreover, treatments of PQ strongly inhibited the expression of Nrf2 and the downstream effectors, HO1 and NQO1 (Hong et al., 2013).

Oxidative stress is one of the major players in the pathogenesis of maneb and paraquat-induced disorders. *N*-Acetyl cysteine, a glutathione precursor and silymarin, a naturally occurring antioxidant protects maneb and/or paraquat-induced hepatotoxicity by reducing oxidative stress, inflammation and by modulating xenobitic metabolizing machinery and silymarin seems to be more effective (Ahmad et al., 2013). Paraquat toxicity involves the generation of superoxide anion by affecting the NADPH-cytochrome P450 oxidoreductase. Moreover, it has been shown that individuals carrying the functional variant POR alleles may have an altered susceptibility to paraquat exposure (Han et al., 2006).

The β-hydroxybutyrate has a renoprotective ability against paraquat-induced kidney injury.

Diquat (1,1′-ethylene-2,2′-bipyridilium), a nonselective bipyridyl herbicide, related structurally to paraquat, is a potent redox cycler being readily converted to a free radical which, in reaction with molecular oxygen, generating superoxide anions and subsequently other redox products. These products can induce lipid peroxidation in cell membranes, and potentially cause cell death (Jones and Vale, 2000).

Fluazinam, a fungicide from the pyridinamine group used to control the blight caused by *Phytophthora infestans* in potatoes was cytotoxic to SH-SY5Y neuronal cells, significantly increasing the reactive oxygen species (ROS) generation and induction of apoptosis revealed by the increase of cytochrome *c* into the cytosol, activation of caspase-3, decrease of Bcl-2 and increase of Bax.

Glyphosate, the active ingredient in Roundup formulations, is the most widely used herbicide worldwide, and as a result it contaminates surface waters and has been detected in food residues, drinking water and human urine, raising concerns for potential environmental and human health impacts.

This broad-spectrum herbicide glyphosate is reported to induce neural defects and craniofacial malformations, affecting the early morphogenesis. *Xenopus laevis* and chicken embryos treated with commercial glyphosate showed important alterations in cephalic and neural crest development. Using a reporter gene assay it has been shown that these impairments could be related to the increase of endogenous retinoic acid activity (Paganelli et al., 2010). The pesticide inhibited steroidogenesis by disrupting steroidogenic acute regulatory-StAR protein expression, demonstrating the susceptibility of StAR to environmental pollutants (Walsh et al., 2000).

Molecular mechanisms underlying the toxicity of glyphosate and Roundup in the liver of brown trout (*Salmo trutta*) was investigated using RNA-seq. The results indicated transcriptional changes that included the transcripts encoding components of the antioxidant system, a number of stress-response proteins and proapoptotic signaling molecules. Functional analysis also revealed overrepresentation of pathways involved in regulating of cell-proliferation and turnover, and upregulation of energy metabolism and other metabolic processes. Significant alterations in transcript expression were detected at the lowest concentrations tested (0.01 mg/L) thus raising concerns for the potential toxicity of this herbicide to fish populations inhabiting contaminated rivers (Uren Webster and Santos, 2015).

The investigation of subchronic exposure to glyphosate in juvenile oysters, *Crassostrea gigas*, a nontarget-organism disclosed significantly increased gene expression suggesting an activation of defense mechanisms at the molecular level. Individual biomarkers (glutathione-S-transferase, catalase activities, and malondialdehyde content) revealed only slight effects (Mottier et al., 2015).

The mechanism of glyphosate-induced occupational lung disease (asthma and rhinitis among farmers) is unknown. Exposure of murine models to to glyphosate-rich air samples, as well as glyphosate alone increased: eosinophil and neutrophil counts, mast cell degranulation, and production of IL-33, TSLP, IL-13, and IL-5 (Kumar et al., 2014).

It was demonstrated that the subchronic administration of low doses of Toc or α-Toc, glyphosate and zineb to rats (i.p. 1/250 LD50, 3 times a week for 5 weeks) provoked severe oxidative stress in testicles. These effects were also reflected in plasma (Astiz et al., 2013).

Linuron [3-(3,4-dichlorophenyl)-1-methoxy-1-methylurea] is used worldwide, and has been detected in surface waters, as well as in food and drinking water. Toxicological studies have reported that linuron acts as an antiandrogen in vitro and in vivo and disrupts mammalian male reproductive function. RNA-seq analysis of the hepatic transcriptional response of mature male brown trout exposed for 4 days to 1.7, 15.3, and 225.9 μg/L linuron revealed a decrease in the expression of transcripts encoding the majority of enzymes involved in the cholesterol biosynthesis pathway and an increased expression of a number of transcripts involved in cellular stress responses, including cyp1a (up to 560-fold), molecular chaperones, and antioxidant enzymes. Inhibition of cholesterol biosynthesis might result from the disruption of androgen signaling by linuron (Uren Webster and Santos, 2015).

Butachlor is an herbicide of the acetanilide class. Studies have showed that butachlor causes kidney and liver injuries in *C. auratus*. (1)H-NMR–based metabolomics approach disclosed metabolic changes that were related to the toxic effects of butachlor including oxidative stress, disorder of energy metabolism and amino acids metabolism, and disturbance of neurotransmitter balance in butachlor exposed goldfish (Xu et al., 2015). Butachlor has adverse effects on fecundity and disrupts sex hormone homeostasis in adult zebrafish. Butachlor does not cause significant alteration in the expression of genes involved estrogen receptors (ERα, ERβ1, and ERβ2), vitellogenins (VTG I), and cytochrome P450 aromatase after 30 days of exposure, whereas the transcription of VTG II gene was significantly upregulated in zebrafish exposed to 100 μg/L butachlor. It is suggested that butachlor may be a weak estrogen, and more endpoints need to be investigated to assess the effects of butachlor on the hypothalamus-pituitary-gonadal axis of zebrafish (Chang et al., 2012).

Acetochlor, a member of the chloroacetanilide family of herbicides, is widely used globally and is very frequently detected in watersheds of agricultural lands and fresh water streams. The principal mechanism underlying acetochlor-mediated cytotoxicity is likely to be through signal-regulated kinase-mediated intrinsic pathway of apoptosis (Zerin et al., 2015).

The pesticide *3,4-dichloropropionanilide* from the acetanilide class could affect immunity by inducing thymic atrophy and splenomegaly, decreasing T- and B-cell populations development in thymus and bone marrow and inhibiting the macrophages respiratory burst. The molecular mechanisms include alterations in nuclear factor (NF)-kappaB transcription factor activity and intracellular Ca(2+) signaling (Salazar et al., 2008).

2,4-Dichlorophenoxyacetic acid promotes oxidative and nitrosative stress, causing disturbances in the actin cytoskeleton, thereby affecting the dynamics of peroxisomes and some other organelles, such as the mitochondria, with xanthine dehydrogenase being involved in ROS production under these conditions. These structural changes in turn appear to be responsible for the leaf epinasty of *Arabidopsis plants* (Rodríguez-Serrano et al., 2014).

2,6-dichlorobenzonitrile herbicide produces severe lesions of mouse olfactory neuroepithelium and respiratory metaplasia. A role for IL-6 in suppressing olfactory receptor neuron regeneration in 2,6-dichlorobenzonitrile–treated mice was rejected by the failure of the antiinflammatory drug dexamethasone to prevent the subsequent respiratory metaplasia in the dorsal medial meatus, suggesting that other factors lead to horizontal basal cells neuroincompetence (Xie et al., 2013).

Exposure of the Pacific oyster *Crassostrea gigas* to *diuron* alone or within a mixture causes early effects on molecular, biochemical, and cellular parameters (Luna-Acosta et al., 2012).

The toxicity of the commonly used herbicide *alachlor* was evaluated using the eukaryotic model *Saccharomyces cerevisiae* and the genome-wide expression profiling which has shown that more than 100 genes involved in metabolism, transmembrane transport, cell defense, and detoxification were modulated. From these, candidate biomarkers sharing homology with proteins from ecologically relevant eukaryotic species can be established (Gil et al., 2011).

Ziram is a dimethyldithiocarbamate fungicide which can cause intraneuronal calcium [Ca(2+)] dysregulation and subsequently neuronal death. Study of signaling mechanisms underlying ziram-induced Ca(2+) dyshomeostasis and neurotoxicity revealed that NCX3 genetic deletion protects against ziram-induced neurotoxicity. Moreover, NCX3 and its downstream molecular pathways might be key factors involved in ziram toxicity (Jin et al., 2014).

The molecular mechanisms by which environmental pollutants including 2,3,7,8-*tetrachlorodibenzo-p-dioxin* (TCDD) or the widely used imidazole fungicide prochloraz display their toxic effects in vertebrates are still not well understood. Computer analysis studies identified nuclear AhR binding sites termed "dioxin response elements" (DREs) in the 5′-untranslated region (5′-UTR) of efflux transporter ABCG2 from the bovine mammary gland. These regulatory motifs mediate regulation of target genes by AhR agonists including TCDD and prochloraz. Identification of mammary ABCG2 as a novel target gene of pesticide prochloraz and dioxin could further help to improve the protection of breast-feeding infants and the consumer of dairy products (Halwachs et al., 2013).

The insecticide *buprofezin* exhibited genotoxicity in cultured Syrian hamster embryo cells as revealed by increased frequencies of morphologically transformed colonies and of micronuclei, in the absence of DNA damage proving its interaction with the mitotic apparatus (Herrera et al., 1993).

Octylphenol is the degradative product of alkylphenol ethoxylates that are widely used to produce rubber, pesticides, and paints. It is a chemically stable substance and demonstrates estrogenic effects, toxicity and carcinogenic effects in the environment. The toxin accumulates rapidly in the liver where it exerts most of its damage. The molecular-based approach identified several genes involved in apoptosis, signal transduction, cytoskeletal remodeling, innate immunity, material and energy metabolism, translation and transcription after exposure to octylphenol of the frog (*Rana chensinensis*).

Biopesticides based on *Bacillus thuringiensis israelensis* are the most used and most successful around the world. Decrease of *B. thuringiensis israelensis* insecticidal activity is linked with the deletion of cry4Aa and cry10Aa genes from the 128-kb pBtoxis plasmid and the early protease degradation of Cry toxins mainly due to some amino acids substitutions evidenced in Cry4Ba and Cry11Aa δ-endotoxins (Elleuch et al., 2015).

Chiral pesticides are ubiquitous in the aquatic environment, and their enantioselectivities in aquatic toxicity are known to be complicated.

The difference in enantioselective effects between enantiomers may sometimes differ by approximately 100-fold or more, which makes it important to incorporate enantioselective effects into the risk assessment of chiral pesticides. The different degrees of cytotoxicity was shown for the enantiomers of the chiral pesticide isocarbophos, an organophosphorus pesticide, using hepatocyte cells, affecting differently the apopotosis pathways and the reactive oxygen species production, the same behavior being observed for interaction with AChE of fenamiphos and of bifenthrin enantiomers induced oxidative stress and apoptosis mediated by the mitogen-activated protein kinase (MAPK) signaling (Liu et al., 2009, 2010; Wang et al., 2010; Lu et al., 2011).

Given the widespread use of chiral pesticides, a more comprehensive understanding of the significance of enantioselective aquatic toxicity will be very helpful in improving risk assessment and regulation of chiral pesticides (Zhang et al., 2012b).

Previous studies have showed that some *chiral pesticides* with estrogenic activity possess enantioselectivity in endocrine disruption. Despite the assessment of enantioselectivity in the estrogenic potential of chiral pesticides, which deserves particular attention, there has been limited research into their molecular mechanisms of human health risk. The role of enantioselectivity in the endocrine disruption and potential human maternal-fetal health risk of acetofenate (AF), an organochlorine insecticide, were investigated in both MCF-7 and JEG-3 cells. The results also demonstrated that S-(+)-AF possesses the strongest potential effects in disruption of hormone secretion, maternal immune tolerance, and steroidogenesis in the trophoblast (Chen et al., 2012b).

Recent studies have shown that *chiral pesticides* could enantioselectively induce cytotoxicity and genotoxicity. Investigation of the role of oxidative stress in enantiomer-specific, profenofos (PFF)-induced cytotoxicity and genotoxicity demonstrated that PFF enantioselectively reduced cell viability and induced DNA damage in PC12 cells. A concentration- and time-dependent significant induction of reactive oxygen species (ROS), malondialdehyde and gene expression encoding antioxidant enzyme (Cu-Zn-SOD, GST, and CAT) and stress protein (HSP 70 and HSP 90) was observed in (−)-PFF, whereas (+)-PFF and rac-PFF exhibited these effects to lesser degrees. PFF-dependent ROS accumulation, MDA release and oxidative stress gene expression preceded the loss of cell viability and induction of DNA damage, and already significantly changed at concentrations which are not yet cytotoxic or genotoxic. These results indicate that oxidative stress may contribute to PFF-induced toxicity and that it was not a consequence of it (Lu et Yu, 2014).

7 Endocrine Disruption—A Major Mechanism of Pesticides Toxicity

The effects of 13 pesticides (2-methyl-4-chlorophenoxyacetic acid, terbuthylazine, iodosulfuron-methyl-sodium, mesosulfuron-methyl, metsulfuron-methyl, chlormequat chloride, bitertanol, propiconazole, prothioconazole, mancozeb and its metabolite ethylene thiourea, cypermethrin, tau-fluvalinate, and malathion (currently banned in Denmark) used in Denmark on the function of thyroid hormone and AhR in cell culture were investigated. The data suggested that these pesticides can interfere with thyroid hormone signaling and AhR function in vitro and might have the potential to cause endocrine disruption (Ghisari et al., 2015).

Several endocrine Disrupting Chemicals (EDCs), such as pesticides, bisphenol A, phthalates, dioxins, and phytoestrogens, can interact with the female reproductive system and lead to endocrine disruption. Initially, it was assumed that EDCs exert their effects by binding to hormone receptors and transcription factors, but it is currently known that they may also alter the expression of enzymes involved in the synthesis or catabolism of steroids. The hexachlorocyclohexanes are widely used synthetic pesticides have been shown to act as GABAA channel blockers and to induce changes in calcium homeostasis by acting on different voltage-gated Ca^{2+} channel, alter genomic integrity and are endocrine disrupters, interfering with steroidogenesis, due to their estrogen like activity, also reported for pyrethroids (Olivero-Verbel et al., 2011; Taylor et al., 2010). Endocrine disruptive pesticides targeting estrogen receptor alpha and beta could induce potential adverse effects on human health (Swedenborg et al., 2010). Delta-Hexachlorocyclohexane interacts with cardiac ryanodine-sensitive Ca2+ channels and has ionophore activity, finally increasing the ionic permeability of phospholipid membranes (Buck and Pessah, 1999).

Biomonitoring studies have identified these compounds in adults, children, pregnant women, and fetuses. Among the diseases of the female reproductive tract associated with EDCs exposure are the following: precocious puberty, polycystic ovary syndrome, and premature ovarian failure. The different populations of the world are exposed to a great number of chemicals through different routes of infection; despite the various available studies, there is still much doubt regarding the additive effect of a mixture of EDCs with similar mechanisms of action (Costa, 2006).

Some chemicals used in consumer products or manufacturing (e.g. plastics, surfactants, pesticides, resins) have estrogenic activities, being called xenoestrogens (XEs). They chemically resemble physiological estrogens and are one of the major categories of synthesized compounds that disrupt endocrine actions. Potent rapid actions of XEs via nongenomic mechanisms contribute significantly to their disruptive effects on functional endpoints (e.g. cell proliferation/death, transport, peptide release). Membrane-initiated hormonal signaling in our pituitary cell model is predominantly driven by mERα with mERβ and GPR30 participation. We visualized ERα on plasma membranes using many techniques in the past (impeded ligands, antibodies to ERα) and now add observations of epitope proximity with other membrane signaling proteins. A range of rapid signals/protein activations by XEs has been demonstrated including a range of including: calcium channels, cAMP/PKA, MAPKs, G proteins, caspases, and transcription factors. XEs can cause disruptions of the oscillating temporal patterns of nongenomic signaling elicited by endogenous estrogens. Mixtures of XEs, commonly found in contaminated environments, disrupt the signaling actions of physiological estrogens even more severely than do single XEs. Understanding the features of XEs that drive these disruptive mechanisms will allow us to redesign useful chemicals that exclude estrogenic or antiestrogenic activities.

Aromatase enzyme plays a central role in steroidogenesis by converting androgens to estrogens and has been proposed as an important molecular target for many environmental endocrine disrupters chemicals (Laville et al., 2006).

Lipoic acid administration is a promising therapeutic strategy for coping with disorders suspected to be caused by OS generators—such as pesticides—in male reproductive system (Astiz et al., 2013).

The role of essential trace elements as the promising and efficient preventive prophylactic agents without any toxicity and side effects in attenuating the adverse effects caused by pesticides, have been reported by various scientists, the world over. In this perspective, zinc, a key constituent of more than 300 mammalian enzymes and many transcription factors has proved its protective potential in various models of animal toxicity. The hepatoprotective potential of zinc has been proved during various toxic states including pesticide toxicity. However, zinc warrants further examination with regard to documentation of specific molecular pathways to establish the exact mechanisms for zinc-mediated protection during pesticide toxicity. This novel finding facilitates the understanding of molecular mechanisms and to develop appropriate management alternatives to counteract PQ-induced neuronal pathogenesis.

8 Conclusions

Environmental pollutants, including pesticides could have a major impact on the public health, requiring a better knowledge and understanding of the mechanisms of their toxicity at cellular and molecular level is urgently needed. Many of the biochemical targets of pesticides could also be impaired in humans and animals, such as enzymes, ion channels, receptors, cytoskeleton. As pesticides often occur in mixture, they could induce enhanced toxicological effects. Therefore, knowing, defining, and testing pesticides toxicity can become critical for the human health. The establishment of guidelines for pesticides toxicity should address the development of simple and rapid toxicological assays that could be applied routinely, on large scale for the assessment of sensitive and specific biomarkers of the organisms' exposure to environmental chemicals.

References

Abolaji, A.O., Kamdem, J.P., Lugokenski, T.H., Nascimento, T.K., Waczuk, E.P., Farombi, E.O., Loreto, É.L., Rocha, J.B., 2014. Involvement of oxidative stress in 4-vinylcyclohexene-induced toxicity in Drosophila melanogaster. Free Radic Biol Med. 71, 99–108.

Acosta, J.M., Chai, Y., Meara, J.G., Bringas, Jr., P., Anderson, K.D., Warburton, D., 2001. Prenatal exposure to nitrofen induces Fryns phenotype in mice. Ann. Plast. Surg. 46 (6), 635–640.

Ahmad, I., Shukla, S., Kumar, A., Singh, B.K., Kumar, V., Chauhan, A.K., Singh, D., Pandey, H.P., Singh, C., 2013. Biochemical and molecular mechanisms of N-acetyl cysteine and silymarin-mediated protection against maneb- and paraquat-induced hepatotoxicity in rats. Chem. Biol. Interact. 201 (1–3), 9–18.

Albores, A., Ortega-Mantilla, G., Sierra-Santoyo, A., Cebrián, M.E., Muñoz-Sánchez, J.L., Calderón-Salinas, J.V., Manno, M., 2001. Cytochrome P450 2B (CYP2B)-mediated activation of methyl-parathion in rat brain extracts. Toxicol. Lett. 124 (1–3), 1–10.

Alegría-Torres, J.A., Díaz-Barriga, F., Gandolfi, A.J., Pérez-Maldonado, I.N., 2009. Mechanisms of p,p'-DDE-induced apoptosis in human peripheral blood mononuclear cells. Toxicol. In Vitro 23 (6), 1000–1006.

Allen, E.M., Florang, V.R., Davenport, L.L., Jinsmaa, Y., Doorn, J.A., 2013a. Cellular localization of dieldrin and structure-activity relationship of dieldrin analogues in dopaminergic cells. Chem. Res. Toxicol. 26 (7), 1043–1054.

Allen, E.M.G., Florang, V.R., Davenport, L.L., Jinsmaa, Y., Doorn, J.A., 2013b. Cellular localization of dieldrin and structure-activity relationship of dieldrin analogues in dopaminergic cells. Chem. Res. Toxicol. 26 (7), 1043–1054.

Alluwaimi, A.M., Hussein, Y., 2007. Diazinon immunotoxicity in mice: modulation of cytokines level and their gene expression. Toxicology 236 (1–2), 123–131.

Amberg, J.J., Schreier, T.M., Gaikowski, M.P., 2012. Molecular responses differ between sensitive silver carp and tolerant bighead carp and bigmouth buffalo exposed to rotenone. Fish Physiol. Biochem. 38 (5), 1379–1391.

Androutsopoulos, V.P., Hernandez, A.F., Liesivuori, J., Tsatsakis, A.M., 2013. A mechanistic overview of health associated effects of low levels of organochlorine and organophosphorous pesticides. Toxicology 307, 89–94.

Argese, E., Bettiol, C., Marchetto, D., De Vettori, S., Zambon, A., Miana, P., Ghetti, P.F., 2005. Study on the toxicity of phenolic and phenoxy herbicides using the submitochondrial particle assay. Toxicol. In Vitro 19 (8), 1035–1043.

Astiz, M., Hurtado de Catalfo, G.E., García, M.N., Galletti, S.M., Errecalde, A.L., de Alaniz, M.J., Marra, C.A., 2013. Pesticide-induced decrease in rat testicular steroidogenesis is differentially prevented by lipoate and tocopherol. Ecotoxicol. Environ. Saf. 91, 129–138.

Avila, D., Helmcke, K., Aschner, M., 2012. The *Caenorhabiditis elegans* model as a reliable tool in neurotoxicology. Hum. Exp. Toxicol. 31 (3), 236–243.

Baird, T.D., DeLorenzo, M.E., 2010. Descriptive and mechanistic toxicity of conazole fungicides using the model test alga *Dunaliella tertiolecta* (Chlorophyceae). Environ. Toxicol. 25 (3), 213–220.

Banks, C.N., Lein, P.J., 2012. A review of experimental evidence linking neurotoxic organophosphorus compounds and inflammation. Neurotoxicology 33 (3), 575–584.

Beggel, S., Werner, I., Connon, R.E., Geist, J.P., 2012. Impacts of the phenylpyrazole insecticide fipronil on larval fish: time-series gene transcription responses in fathead minnow (*Pimephales promelas*) following short-term exposure. Sci. Total Environ. 426, 160–165.

Biales, A.D., Bencic, D.C., Flick, R.L., Blocksom, K.A., Lazorchak, J.M., Lattier, D.L., 2011. Proteomic analysis of a model fish species exposed to individual pesticides and a binary mixture. Aquat. Toxicol. 101, 196–206.

Björkblom, B., Adilbayeva, A., Maple-Grødem, J., Piston, D., Ökvist, M., Xu, X.M., Brede, C., Larsen, J.P., Møller, S.G., 2013. Parkinson disease protein DJ-1 binds metals and protects against metal-induced cytotoxicity. J. Biol. Chem. 288 (31), 22809–22820.

Bonilla, E., Hernández, F., Cortés, L., Mendoza, M., Mejía, J., Carrillo, E., Casas, E., Betancourt, M., 2008. Effects of the insecticides malathion and diazinon on the early oogenesis in mice in vitro. Environ. Toxicol. 23 (2), 240–245.

Braconi, D., Bernardini, G., Santucci, A., 2011. Linking protein oxidation to environmental pollutants: redox proteomic approaches. J. Proteomics 74 (11), 2324–2337.

Braconi, D., Bernardini, G., Santucci, A., 2015. Saccharomyces cerevisiae as a model in ecotoxicological studies: a post-genomics perspective. J. Proteomics 137, 19–34.

Braguini, W.L., Cadena, S.M., Carnieri, E.G., Rocha, M.E., de Oliveira, M.B., 2004. Effects of deltamethrin on functions of rat liver mitochondria and on native and synthetic model membranes. Toxicol. Lett. 152 (3), 191–202.

Brander, S.M., Jeffries, K.M., Cole, B.J., DeCourten, B.M., White, J.W., Hasenbein, S., Fangue, N.A., Connon, R.E., 2016. Transcriptomic changes underlie altered egg protein production and reduced fecundity in an estuarine model fish exposed to bifenthrin. Aquat. Toxicol. 174, 247–260.

Bretaud, S., Lee, S., Guo, S., 2004. Sensitivity of zebrafish to environmental toxins implicated in Parkinson's disease. Neurotoxicol. Teratol. 26 (6), 857–864.

Buck, E.D., Pessah, I.N., 1999. Mechanisms of delta-hexachlorocyclohexane toxicity: II. Evidence for Ca2+-dependent K+-selective ionophore activity. J. Pharmacol. Exp. Ther. 289, 486–493.

Campos-Pereira, F.D., Oliveira, C.A., Pigoso, A.A., Silva-Zacarin, E.C., Barbieri, R., Spatti, E.F., Marin-Morales, M.A., Severi-Aguiar, G.D., 2012. Early cytotoxic and genotoxic effects of atrazine on Wistar rat liver: a morphological, immunohistochemical, biochemical, and molecular study. Ecotoxicol. Environ. Saf. 78, 170–177.

Casida, J.E., 2009. Pest toxicology: the primary mechanisms of pesticide action. Chem. Res. Toxicol. 22 (4), 609–619.

Cecconi, S., Paro, R., Rossi, G., Macchiarelli, G., 2007. The effects of the endocrine disruptors dithiocarbamates on the mammalian ovary with particular regard to mancozeb. Curr. Pharm. Des. 13 (29), 2989–3004.

Chandran, G., Muralidhara, 2013. Neuroprotective effect of aqueous extract of *Selaginella delicatula* as evidenced by abrogation of rotenone-induced motor deficits, oxidative dysfunctions, and neurotoxicity in mice. Cell. Mol. Neurobiol. 33 (7), 929–942.

Chang, J., Gui, W., Wang, M., Zhu, G., 2012. Effects of butachlor on estrogen receptor, vitellogenin and P450 aromatase gene expression in the early life stage of zebrafish. J. Environ. Sci. Health A Tox. Hazard Subst. Environ. Eng 47 (11), 1672–1677.

Chen, Y.W., Yang, Y.T., Hung, D.Z., Su, C.C., Chen, K.L., 2012a. Paraquat induces lung alveolar epithelial cell apoptosis via Nrf-2-regulated mitochondrial dysfunction and ER stress. Arch. Toxicol. 86 (10), 1547–1558.

Chen, F., Zhang, Q., Wang, C., Lu, Y., Zhao, M., 2012b. Enantioselectivity in estrogenicity of the organochlorine insecticide acetofenate in human trophoblast and MCF-7 cells. Reprod. Toxicol. 33 (1), 53–59.

Chen, X., Wang, J., Zhu, H., Ding, J., Peng, Y., 2015a. Proteomics analysis of *Xenopus laevis* gonad tissue following chronic exposure to atrazine. Environ. Toxicol. Chem. 34 (8), 1770–1777.

Chen, H.M., Lee, Y.H., Wang, Y.J., 2015b. ROS-triggered signaling pathways involved in the cytotoxicity and tumor promotion effects of pentachlorophenol and tetrachlorohydroquinone. Chem. Res. Toxicol. 28 (3), 339–350.

Clapp, R.W., Jacobs, M.M., Loechler, E.L., 2008. Environmental and occupational causes of cancer: new evidence 2005-2007. Rev. Environ. Health. 23, 1–37.

Conn, K.J., Ullman, M.D., Larned, M.J., Eisenhauer, P.B., Fine, R.E., Wells, J.M., 2003. cDNA microarray analysis of changes in gene expression associated with MPP+ toxicity in SH-SY5Y cells. Neurochem. Res. 28 (12), 1873–1881.
Corsini, E., Viviani, B., Birindelli, S., Gilardi, F., Torri, A., Codecà, I., Lucchi, L., Bartesaghi, S., Galli, C.L., Marinovich, M., Colosio, C., 2006. Molecular mechanisms underlying mancozeb-induced inhibition of TNF-alpha production. Toxicol. Appl. Pharmacol. 212 (2), 89–98.
Costa, L.G., 2006. Current issues in organophosphate toxicology. Clin. Chim. Acta 366 (1–2), 1–13.
Currie, R.A., Peffer, R.C., Goetz, A.K., Omiecinski, C.J., Goodman, J.I., 2014. Phenobarbital and propiconazole toxicogenomic profiles in mice show major similarities consistent with the key role that constitutive androstane receptor (CAR) activation plays in their mode of action. Toxicology 321, 80–88.
Czerniczyniec, A., Lores-Arnaiz, S., Bustamante, J., 2013. Mitochondrial susceptibility in a model of paraquat neurotoxicity. Free. Radic. Res. 47 (8), 614–623.
de Tomaso Portaz, A.C., Caimi, G.R., Sánchez, M., Chiappini, F., Randi, A.S., Kleiman de Pisarev, D.L., Alvarez, L., 2015. Hexachlorobenzene induces cell proliferation, and aryl hydrocarbon receptor expression (AhR) in rat liver preneoplastic foci, and in the human hepatoma cell line HepG2. AhR is a mediator of ERK1/2 signaling, and cell cycle regulation in HCB-treated HepG2 cells. Toxicology 336, 36–47.
Dagda, R.K., Zhu, J., Chu, C.T., 2009. Mitochondrial kinases in Parkinson's disease: converging insights from neurotoxin and genetic models. Mitochondrion 9 (5), 289–298.
Díaz-Resendiz, K.J., Toledo-Ibarra, G.A., Girón-Pérez, M.I., 2015. Modulation of immune response by organophosphorus pesticides: fishes as a potential model in immunotoxicology. J. Immunol. Res. 2015, 213836.
Dinis-Oliveira, R.J., Duarte, J.A., Sánchez-Navarro, A., Remião, F., Bastos, M.L., Carvalho, F., 2008. Paraquat poisonings: mechanisms of lung toxicity, clinical features, and treatment. Crit. Rev. Toxicol. 38, 13–71.
Dorsey, W.C., Tchounwou, P.B., 2003. CYP1a1, HSP70, P53, and c-fos expression in human liver carcinoma cells (HepG2) exposed to pentachlorophenol. Biomed. Sci. Instrum. 39, 389–396.
Dorsey, W.C., Tchounwou, P.B., 2004. Pentachlorophenol-induced cytotoxic, mitogenic, and endocrine-disrupting activities in channel catfish, *Ictalurus punctatus*. Int. J. Environ. Res. Public Health 1 (2), 90–99.
Dutta, R., Mondal, A.M., Arora, V., Nag, T.C., Das, N., 2008. Immunomodulatory effect of DDT (bis[4-chlorophenyl]-1,1,1-trichloroethane) on complement system and macrophages. Toxicology 252 (1–3), 78–85.
Elleuch, J., Zribi Zghal, R., Lacoix, M.N., Chandre, F., Tounsi, S., Jaoua, S., 2015. Evidence of two mechanisms involved in *Bacillus thuringiensis israelensis* decreased toxicity against mosquito larvae: genome dynamic and toxins stability. Microbiol. Res. 176, 48–54.
Faust, M., Altenburger, R., Backhaus, T., Blanck, H., Boedeker, W., Gramatica, P., Hamer, V., Scholze, M., Vighi, M., Grimme, L.H., 2003. Joint algal toxicity of 16 dissimilarly acting chemicals is predictable by the concept of independent action. Aquat. Toxicol. 63, 43–63.
Fénichel, P., Brucker-Davis, F., 2008. Environmental endocrine disruptors and breast cancer: new risk factors? Gynecol. Obstet. Fertil. 36 (10), 969–977.
Ferraris, M., Flora, A., Chiesara, E., Fornasari, D., Lucchetti, H., Marabini, L., Frigerio, S., Radice, S., 2005. Molecular mechanism of the aryl hydrocarbon receptor activation by the fungicide diprodione in rainbow trout (*Oncorhynchus mykiss*) hepatocytes. Aquat. Toxicol. 72 (3), 209–220.

Fetoui, H., Feki, A., Salah, G.B., Kamoun, H., Fakhfakh, F., Gdoura, R., 2015. Exposure to lambda-cyhalothrin, a synthetic pyrethroid, increases reactive oxygen species production and induces genotoxicity in rat peripheral blood. Toxicol. Ind. Health 31 (5), 433–441.

Fratev, F., Lo Piparo, E., Benfenati, E., Mihaylova, E., 2007. Toxicity study of allelochemical-like pesticides by a combination of 3D-QSAR, docking, Local Binding Energy (LBE) and GRID approaches. SAR QSAR Environ. Res. 18 (7–8), 675–692.

Gaytán, B.D., Loguinov, A.V., Lantz, S.R., Lerot, J.M., Denslow, N.D., Vulpe, C.D., 2013. Functional profiling discovers the dieldrin organochlorinated pesticide affects leucine availability in yeast. Toxicol. Sci. 132 (2), 347–358.

Ghisari, M., Long, M., Tabbo, A., Bonefeld-Jørgensen, E.C., 2015. Effects of currently used pesticides and their mixtures on the function of thyroid hormone and aryl hydrocarbon receptor in cell culture. Toxicol. Appl. Pharmacol. 284 (3), 292–303.

Gil, F.N., Gonçalves, A.C., Jacinto, M.J., Becker, J.D., Viegas, C.A., 2011. Transcriptional profiling in Saccharomyces cerevisiae relevant for predicting alachlor mechanisms of toxicity. Environ. Toxicol. Chem. 30 (11), 2506–2518.

Halwachs, S., Wassermann, L., Lindner, S., Zizzadoro, C., Honscha, W., 2013. Fungicide prochloraz and environmental pollutant dioxin induce the ABCG2 transporter in bovine mammary epithelial cells by the arylhydrocarbon receptor signaling pathway. Toxicol. Sci. 131 (2), 491–501.

Han, J.F., Wang, S.L., He, X.Y., Liu, C.Y., Hong, J.Y., 2006. Effect of genetic variation on human cytochrome p450 reductase-mediated paraquat cytotoxicity. Toxicol. Sci. 91, 42–48.

Hargreaves, A.J., 2012. Neurodegenerations induced by organophosphorous compounds. Adv. Exp. Med. Biol. 724, 189–204.

Hassold, E., Backhaus, T., 2009. Chronic toxicity of five structurally diverse demethylase-inhibiting fungicides to the crustacean *Daphnia magna*: a comparative assessment. Environ. Toxicol. Chem. 28 (6), 1218–1226.

Hernández, A.F., Parrón, T., Tsatsakis, A.M., Requena, M., Alarcón, R., López-Guarnido, O., 2013. Toxic effects of pesticide mixtures at a molecular level: their relevance to human health. Toxicology 307, 136–145.

Herrera, L.A., Ostrosky-Wegman, P., Schiffmann, D., Chen, Q.Y., Ziegler-Skylakakis, K., Andrae, U., 1993. The insecticide buprofezin induces morphological transformation and kinetochore-positive micronuclei in cultured Syrian hamster embryo cells in the absence of detectable DNA damage. Mutat. Res. 303 (3), 121–125.

Hong, G.L., Liu, J.M., Zhao, G.J., Wang, L., Liang, G., Wu, B., Li, M.F., Qiu, Q.M., Lu, Z.Q., 2013. The reversal of paraquat-induced mitochondria-mediated apoptosis by cycloartenyl ferulate, the important role of Nrf2 pathway. Exp. Cell. Res. 319 (18), 2845–2855.

Huang, C.L., Lee, Y.C., Yang, Y.C., Kuo, T.Y., Huang, N.K., 2012. Minocycline prevents paraquat-induced cell death through attenuating endoplasmic reticulum stress and mitochondrial dysfunction. Toxicol. Lett. 209 (3), 203–210.

Huang, P., Yang, J., Song, Q., 2014. Atrazine affects phosphoprotein and protein expression in MCF-10A human breast epithelial cells. Int. J. Mol. Sci. 15 (10), 17806–17826.

Huculeci, R., Dinu, D., Staicu, A.C., Munteanu, M.C., Costache, M., Dinischiotu, A., 2009. Malathion-induced alteration of the antioxidant defence system in kidney, gill, and intestine of *Carassius auratus* gibelio. Environ. Toxicol. 24 (6), 523–530.

Husak, V.V., Mosiichuk, N.M., Maksymiv, I.V., Sluchyk, I.Y., Storey, J.M., Storey, K.B., Lushchak, V.I., 2014. Histopathological and biochemical changes in goldfish kidney due to exposure to the herbicide Sencor may be related to induction of oxidative stress. Aquat. Toxicol. 155, 181–189.

Issam, C., Samir, H., Zohra, H., Monia, Z., Hassen, B.C., 2009. Toxic responses to deltamethrin (DM) low doses on gonads, sex hormones and lipoperoxidation in male rats following subcutaneous treatments. J. Toxicol. Sci. 34 (6), 663–670.

Ivanović-Matić, S., Poznanović, G., Grigorov, I., Dinić, S., Mihailović, M., Grdović, N., Uskoković, A., Martinović, V., Arambasić, J., Petrović, M., Bogojević, D., 2008. The organophosphate-induced acute-phase response is characterized by synthesis of alpha 1-acid glycoprotein that exhibits an immunomodulatory effect. J. Appl. Toxicol. 28, 63–71.

Jett, D.A., 2012. Chemical toxins that cause seizures. Neurotoxicology 33 (6), 1473–1475.

Jin, J., Lao, A.J., Katsura, M., Caputo, A., Schweizer, F.E., Sokolow, S., 2014. Involvement of the sodium-calcium exchanger 3 (NCX3) in ziram-induced calcium dysregulation and toxicity. Neurotoxicology 45, 56–66.

Jones, G.M., Vale, J.A., 2000. Mechanisms of toxicity, clinical features, and management of diquat poisoning: a review. J. Toxicol. Clin. Toxicol. 38 (2), 123–128.

Jung, K.H., Kim, J.K., Kim, M.G., Noh, J.H., Eun, J.W., Bae, H.J., Chang, Y.G., Shen, Q., Park, W.S., Lee, J.Y., Nam, S.W., 2012. Characteristic molecular signature for early detection and prediction of persistent organic pollutants in rat liver. Environ. Sci. Technol. 46 (23), 12882–12889.

Kamboj, S.S., Kumar, V., Kamboj, A., Sandhir, R., 2008. Mitochondrial oxidative stress and dysfunction in rat brain induced by carbofuran exposure. Cell. Mol. Neurobiol. 28 (7), 961–969.

Kashyap, M.P., Singh, A.K., Siddiqui, M.A., Kumar, V., Tripathi, V.K., Khanna, V.K., Yadav, S., Jain, S.K., Pant, A.B., 2010. Caspase cascade regulated mitochondria mediated apoptosis in monocrotophos exposed PC12 cells. Chem. Res. Toxicol. 23 (11), 1663–1672.

Kazantseva, Y.A., Yarushkin, A.A., Pustylnyak, V.O., 2013. Dichlorodiphenyltrichloroethane technical mixture regulates cell cycle and apoptosis genes through the activation of CAR and ERα in mouse livers. Toxicol. Appl. Pharmacol. 271 (2), 137–143.

Kling, D.E., Aidlen, J.T., Fisher, J.C., Kinane, T.B., Donahoe, P.K., Schnitzer, J.J., 2005. Nitrofen induces a redox-dependent apoptosis associated with increased p38 activity in P19 teratocarcinoma cells. Toxicol. In Vitro 19, 1–10.

Klüver, N., Yang, L., Busch, W., Scheffler, K., Renner, P., Strähle, U., Scholz, S., 2011. Transcriptional response of zebrafish embryos exposed to neurotoxic compounds reveals a muscle activity dependent hspb11 expression. PLoS One 6 (12), e29063.

Korkaric, M., Xiao, M., Behra, R., Eggen, R.I., 2015. Acclimation of *Chlamydomonas reinhardtii* to ultraviolet radiation and its impact on chemical toxicity. Aquat. Toxicol. 167, 209–219.

Kubrak, O.I., Atamaniuk, T.M., Husak, V.V., Drohomyretska, I.Z., Storey, J.M., Storey, K.B., Lushchak, V.I., 2012. Oxidative stress responses in blood and gills of *Carassius auratus* exposed to the mancozeb-containing carbamate fungicide Tattoo. Ecotoxicol. Environ. Saf. 85, 37–43.

Kumar, S., Khodoun, M., Kettleson, E.M., McKnight, C., Reponen, T., Grinshpun, S.A., Adhikari, A., 2014. Glyphosate-rich air samples induce IL-33, TSLP and generate IL-13 dependent airway inflammation. Toxicology 325, 42–51.

Kwekel, J.C., Forgacs, A.L., Williams, K.J., Zacharewski, T.R., 2013. o-p'-DDT-mediated uterotrophy and gene expression in immature C57BL/6 mice and Sprague-Dawley rats. Toxicol. Appl. Pharmacol. 273 (3), 532–541.

Lasram, M.M., Dhouib, I.B., Annabi, A., El Fazaa, S., Gharbi, N., 2014. A review on the molecular mechanisms involved in insulin resistance induced by organophosphorus pesticides. Toxicology 322, 1–13.

Laville, N., Balaguer, P., Brion, F., Hinfray, N., Casellas, C., Porcher, J.M., Aït-Aïssa, S., 2006. Modulation of aromatase activity and mRNA by various selected pesticides in the human choriocarcinoma JEG-3 cell line. Toxicology 228, 98–108.

Lee, J.E., Kang, J.S., Shin, I.C., Lee, S.J., Hyun, D.H., Lee, K.S., Koh, H.C., 2011. Fluazinam induced apoptosis of SH-SY5Y cells is mediated by p53 and Bcl-2 family proteins. Neurotoxicology 32 (6), 702–710.

Lee, Y.S., Lewis, J.A., Ippolito, D.L., Hussainzada, N., Lein, P.J., Jackson, D.A., Stallings, J.D., 2016. Repeated exposure to neurotoxic levels of chlorpyrifos alters hippocampal expression of neurotrophins and neuropeptides. Toxicology 340, 53–62.

Leist, M., Volbracht, C., Fava, E., Nicotera, P., 1998. 1-Methyl-4-phenylpyridinium induces autocrine excitotoxicity, protease activation, and neuronal apoptosis. Mol. Pharmacol. 54 (5), 789–801.

Levin, E.D., Swain, H.A., Donerly, S., Linney, E., 2004. Developmental chlorpyrifos effects on hatchling zebrafish swimming behavior. Neurotoxicol. Teratol. 26 (6), 719–723.

L'Héritier, F., Marques, M., Fauteux, M., Gaudreau, L., 2014. Defining molecular sensors to assess long-term effects of pesticides on carcinogenesis. Int. J. Mol. Sci. 15 (9), 17148–17161.

Li, T., Zhao, H., Hung, G.C., Han, J., Tsai, S., Li, B., Zhang, J., Puri, R.K., Lo, S.C., 2012. Differentially expressed genes and pathways induced by organophosphates in human neuroblastoma cells. Exp. Biol. Med. 237 (12), 1413–1423.

Li, H., Wu, S., Chen, J., Wang, B., Shi, N., 2013. Effect of glutathione depletion on Nrf2/ARE activation by deltamethrin in PC12 Cells. Arh. Hig. Rada. Toksikol. 64 (1), 87–97.

Liang, Y.J., Wang, H.P., Long, D.X., Li, W., Wu, Y.J., 2013. A metabolonomic investigation of the effects of 60 days exposure of rats to two types of pyrethroid insecticides. Chem. Biol. Interact. 206 (2), 302–308.

Liu, H., Xu, L., Zhao, M., Liu, W., Zhang, C., Zhou, S., 2009. Enantiomer-specific, bifenthrin-induced apoptosis mediated by MAPK signalling pathway in Hep G2 cells. Toxicology 261 (3), 119–125.

Liu, H., Liu, J., Xu, L., Zhou, S., Li, L., Liu, W., 2010. Enantioselective cytotoxicity of isocarbophos is mediated by oxidative stress-induced JNK activation in human hepatocytes. Toxicology 276 (2), 115–121.

Liu, Y., Chen, T., Li, M.H., Xu, H.D., Jia, A.Q., Zhang, J.F., Wang, J.S., 2015a. (1)H NMR based metabolomics approach to study the toxic effects of dichlorvos on goldfish (*Carassius auratus*). Chemosphere 138, 537–545.

Liu, L., Xu, Y., Xu, L., Wang, J., Wu, W., Xu, L., Yan, Y., 2015b. Analysis of differentially expressed proteins in zebrafish (Danio rerio) embryos exposed to chlorpyrifos. Comp. Biochem. Physiol. C Toxicol. Pharmacol. 167, 183–189.

Lu, J.C., 2015. Related factors of sperm DNA damage: advances in studies. Zhonghua Nan Ke Xue 21 (8), 675–680.

Lu, X., Yu, C., 2014. Enantiomer-specific profenofos-induced cytotoxicity and DNA damage mediated by oxidative stress in rat adrenal pheochromocytoma (PC12) cells. J. Appl. Toxicol. 34 (2), 166–175.

Lu, X., Hu, F., Ma, Y., Wang, C., Zhang, Y., Zhao, M., 2011. The role of oxidative stress in enantiomer-specific, bifenthrin-induced cytotoxicity in PC12 cells. Environ. Toxicol. 26 (3), 271–278.

Luna-Acosta, A., Renault, T., Thomas-Guyon, H., Faury, N., Saulnier, D., Budzinski, H., Le Menach, K., Pardon, P., Fruitier-Arnaudin, I., Bustamante, P., 2012. Detection of early effects of a single herbicide (diuron) and a mix of herbicides and pharmaceuticals (diuron, isoproturon, ibuprofen) on immunological parameters of Pacific oyster (*Crassostrea gigas*) spat. Chemosphere 87 (11), 1335–1340.

Madhubabu, G., Yenugu, S., 2014. Allethrin induces oxidative stress, apoptosis and calcium release in rat testicular carcinoma cells (LC540). Toxicol. In Vitro 28 (8), 1386–1395.

Mangum, L.C., Borazjani, A., Stokes, J.V., Matthews, A.T., Lee, J.H., Chambers, J.E., Ross, M.K., 2015. Organochlorine insecticides induce NADPH oxidase-dependent reactive oxygen species in human monocytic cells via phospholipase A2/arachidonic acid. Chem. Res. Toxicol. 28 (4), 570–584.

Matsuya, Y., Ihara, D., Fukuchi, M., Honma, D., Itoh, K., Tabuchi, A., Nemoto, H., Tsuda, M., 2012. Synthesis and biological evaluation of pyrethroid insecticide-derivatives as a chemical inducer for BDNF mRNA expression in neurons. Bioorg. Med. Chem. 20 (8), 2564–2571.

Miller, G.W., Kirby, M.L., Levey, A.I., Bloomquist, J.R., 1999. Heptachlor alters expression and function of dopamine transporters. Neurotoxicology 20 (4), 631–637.

Milzani, A., Dalledonne, I., Vailati, G., Colombo, R., 1997. Paraquat induces actin assembly in depolymerizing conditions. FASEB J. 11 (4), 261–270.

Mitra, S., Chakrabarti, N., Bhattacharyya, A., 2011. Differential regional expression patterns of α-synuclein, TNF-α, and IL-1β; and variable status of dopaminergic neurotoxicity in mouse brain after Paraquat treatment. J. Neuroinflammation 8, 163.

Mohamed, A.H., 2011. Sublethal toxicity of Roundup to immunological and molecular aspects of Biomphalaria alexandrina to Schistosoma mansoni infection. Ecotoxicol. Environ. Saf. 74 (4), 754–760.

Mottier, A., Séguin, A., Devos, A., Pabic, C.L., Voiseux, C., Lebel, J.M., Serpentini, A., Fievet, B., Costil, K., 2015. Effects of subchronic exposure to glyphosate in juvenile oysters (*Crassostrea gigas*): from molecular to individual levels. Mar. Pollut. Bull. 95 (2), 665–677.

Narahashi, T., Ginsburg, K.S., Nagata, K., Song, J.H., Tatebayashi, H., 1998. Ion channels as targets for insecticides. Neurotoxicology 19 (4–5), 581–590.

Narasimhan, M., Riar, A.K., Rathinam, M.L., Vedpathak, D., Henderson, G., Mahimainathan, L., 2014. Hydrogen peroxide responsive miR153 targets Nrf2/ARE cytoprotection in paraquat induced dopaminergic neurotoxicity. Toxicol. Lett. 228 (3), 179–191.

Newhouse, K., Hsuan, S.L., Chang, S.H., Cai, B., Wang, Y., Xia, Z., 2004. Rotenone-induced apoptosis is mediated by p38 and JNK MAP kinases in human dopaminergic SH-SY5Y cells. Toxicol. Sci. 79, 137–146.

Novais, S.C., De Coen, W., Amorim, M.J., 2012. Gene expression responses linked to reproduction effect concentrations (EC 10,20,50,90) of dimethoate, atrazine and carbendazim, in *Enchytraeus albidus*. PLoS One 7 (4), e36068.

Olivero-Verbel, J., Guerrero-Castilla, A., Ramos, N.R., 2011. Biochemical effects induced by the hexachlorocyclohexanes. Rev. Environ. Contam. Toxicol. 212, 1–28.

Paganelli, A., Gnazzo, V., Acosta, H., López, S.L., Carrasco, A.E., 2010. Glyphosate-based herbicides produce teratogenic effects on vertebrates by impairing retinoic acid signaling. Chem. Res. Toxicol. 23 (10), 1586–1595.

Pancetti, F., Olmos, C., Dagnino-Subiabre, A., Rozas, C., Morales, B., 2007. Noncholinesterase effects induced by organophosphate pesticides and their relationship to cognitive processes: implication for the action of acylpeptide hydrolase. J. Toxicol. Environ. Health B Crit. Rev. 10 (8), 623–630.

Pesonen, M., Pasanen, M., Loikkanen, J., Naukkarinen, A., Hemmilä, M., Seulanto, H., Kuitunen, T., Vähäkangas, K., 2012. Chloropicrin induces endoplasmic reticulum stress in human retinal pigment epithelial cells. Toxicol. Lett. 211 (3), 239–245.

Peyre, L., Zucchini-Pascal, N., de Sousa, G., Rahmani, R., 2012. Effects of endosulfan on hepatoma cell adhesion: epithelial-mesenchymal transition and anoikis resistance. Toxicology 300 (1–2), 19–30.

Pomeroy-Black, M., Ehrich, M., 2012. Organophosphorus compound effects on neurotrophin receptors and intracellular signaling. Toxicol. In Vitro 26 (5), 759–765.

Proskocil, B.J., Bruun, D.A., Thompson, C.M., Fryer, A.D., Lein, P.J., 2010. Organophosphorus pesticides decrease M2 muscarinic receptor function in guinea pig airway nerves via indirect mechanisms. PLoS One 5 (5), e10562.

Raisuddin, S., Kwok, K.W., Leung, K.M., Schlenk, D., Lee, J.S., 2007. The copepod Tigriopus: a promising marine model organism for ecotoxicology and environmental genomics. Aquat. Toxicol. 83 (3), 161–173.

Rankin, G.O., Hong, S.K., Anestis, D.K., Lash, L.H., Miles, S.L., 2001. In vitro nephrotoxicity induced by N-(3,5-dichlorophenyl)succinimide (NDPS) metabolites in isolated renal cortical cells from male and female Fischer 344 rats: evidence for a nephrotoxic sulfate conjugate metabolite. Toxicology 163 (2–3), 73–82.

Richendrfer, H., Pelkowski, S.D., Colwill, R.M., Créton, R., 2012. Developmental sub-chronic exposure to chlorpyrifos reduces anxiety-related behavior in zebrafish larvae. Neurotoxicol. Teratol. 34 (4), 458–465.

Rodríguez-Serrano, M., Pazmiño, D.M., Sparkes, I., Rochetti, A., Hawes, C., Romero-Puertas, M.C., Sandalio, L.M., 2014. 2,4-Dichlorophenoxyacetic acid promotes S-nitrosylation and oxidation of actin affecting cytoskeleton and peroxisomal dynamics. J. Exp. Bot. 65 (17), 4783–4793.

Sai, L., Liu, Y., Qu, B., Yu, G., Guo, Q., Bo, C., Xie, L., Jia, Q., Li, Y., Li, X., Ng, J.C., Peng, C., 2015. The effects of simazine, a chlorotriazine herbicide, on the expression of genes in developing male *Xenopus laevis*. Bull. Environ. Contam. Toxicol. 95 (2), 157–163.

Salazar, Z., Ducolomb, Y., Betancourt, M., Bonilla, E., Cortés, L., Hernández-Hernández, F., González-Márquez, H., 2007. Gene expression analysis on the early development of pig embryos exposed to malathion. Int. J. Toxicol. 26 (2), 143–149.

Salazar, K.D., Ustyugova, I.V., Brundage, K.M., Barnett, J.B., Schafer, R., 2008. A review of the immunotoxicity of the pesticide 3,4-dichloropropionanalide. J. Toxicol. Environ. Health B Crit. Rev. 11 (8), 630–645.

Serra, A.A., Couée, I., Renault, D., Gouesbet, G., Sulmon, C., 2015. Metabolic profiling of *Lolium perenne* shows functional integration of metabolic responses to diverse subtoxic conditions of chemical stress. J. Exp. Bot. 66 (7), 1801–1816.

Sipes, N.S., Martin, M.T., Reif, D.M., Kleinstreuer, N.C., Judson, R.S., Singh, A.V., Chandler, K.J., Dix, D.J., Kavlock, R.J., Knudsen, T.B., 2011. Predictive models of prenatal developmental toxicity from toxcast high-throughput screening data. Toxicol. Sci. 124, 109–127.

Sledge, D., Yen, J., Morton, T., Dishaw, L., Petro, A., Donerly, S., Linney, E., Levin, E.D., 2011. Critical duration of exposure for developmental chlorpyrifos-induced neurobehavioral toxicity. Neurotoxicol. Teratol. 33 (6), 742–751.

Slotkin, T.A., 2004. Guidelines for developmental neurotoxicity and their impact on organophosphate pesticides: a personal view from an academic perspective. Neurotoxicology 25 (4), 631–640.

Soetaert, A., van der Ven, K., Moens, L.N., Vandenbrouck, T., van Remortel, P., De Coen, W.M., 2007. *Daphnia magna* and ecotoxicogenomics: gene expression profiles of the anti-ecdysteroidal fungicide fenarimol using energy-, molting- and life stage-related cDNA libraries. Chemosphere 67, 60–71.

Song, X.Y., Li, J.N., Wu, Y.P., Zhang, B., Li, B.X., 2015. Atrazine causes autophagy- and apoptosis-related neurodegenerative effects in dopaminergic neurons in the rat nigrostriatal dopaminergic system. Int. J. Mol. Sci. 16 (6), 13490–13506.

Svendsen, C., Siang, P., Lister, L.J., Rice, A., Spurgeon, D.J., 2010. Similarity, independence, or interaction for binary mixture effects of nerve toxicants for the nematode *Caenorhabditis elegans*. Environ. Toxicol. Chem. 29 (5), 1182–1191.

Swedenborg, E., Pongratz, I., Gustafsson, J.A., 2010. Endocrine disruptors targeting ERbeta function. Int. J. Androl. 33 (2), 288–297.

Tao, Y., Pan, L., Zhang, H., Liu, N., 2013. Identification of genes differentially expressed in clams *Ruditapes philippinarum* in response to endosulfan after different exposure time. Ecotoxicol. Environ. Saf. 89, 108–116.

Taylor, J.S., Thomson, B.M., Lang, C.N., Sin, F.Y., Podivinsky, E., 2010. Estrogenic pyrethroid pesticides regulate expression of estrogen receptor transcripts in mouse Sertoli cells differently from 17beta-estradiol. J. Toxicol. Environ. Health A 73 (16), 1075–1089.

Timofeeva, O.A., Roegge, C.S., Seidler, F.J., Slotkin, T.A., Levin, E.D., 2008. Persistent cognitive alterations in rats after early postnatal exposure to low doses of the organophosphate pesticide, diazinon. Neurotoxicol. Teratol. 30, 38–45.

Uren Webster, T.M., Santos, E.M., 2015. Global transcriptomic profiling demonstrates induction of oxidative stress and of compensatory cellular stress responses in brown trout exposed to glyphosate and Roundup. BMC Genom. 16, 32.

Vaithinathan, S., Saradha, B., Mathur, P.P., 2009. Methoxychlor-induced alteration in the levels of HSP70 and clusterin is accompanied with oxidative stress in adult rat testis. J. Biochem. Mol. Toxicol. 23, 29–35.

Vaithinathan, S., Saradha, B., Mathur, P.P., 2010. Methoxychlor induces apoptosis via mitochondria- and FasL-mediated pathways in adult rat testis. Chem. Biol. Interact. 185 (2), 110–118.

Valentine, W.M., Amarnath, V., Amarnath, K., Graham, D.G., 1995. Characterization of protein adducts produced by N-methyldithiocarbamate and N-methyldithiocarbamate esters. Chem. Res. Toxicol. 8 (2), 254–261.

Valmas, N., Ebert, P.R., 2006. Comparative toxicity of fumigants and a phosphine synergist using a novel containment chamber for the safe generation of concentrated phosphine gas. PLoS One 1, e130.

Ventura, C., Venturino, A., Miret, N., Randi, A., Rivera, E., Núñez, M., Cocca, C., 2015. Chlorpyrifos inhibits cell proliferation through ERK1/2 phosphorylation in breast cancer cell lines. Chemosphere 120, 343–350.

Viviani, B., Bartesaghi, S., Binaglia, M., Corsini, E., Boraso, M., Grazi, E., Galli, C.L., Marinovich, M., 2008. Dithiocarbamate propineb induces acetylcholine release through cytoskeletal actin depolymerization in PC12 cells. Toxicol. Lett. 182 (1–3), 63–68.

Walker, C.H., 1995. Biochemical biomarkers in ecotoxicology—some recent developments. Sci. Total Environ. 171 (1–3), 189–195.

Walsh, L.P., McCormick, C., Martin, C., Stocco, D.M., 2000. Roundup inhibits steroidogenesis by disrupting steroidogenic acute regulatory (StAR) protein expression. Environ. Health Perspect. 108 (8), 769–776.

Wang, X., Qin, Z.H., Leng, Y., Wang, Y., Jin, X., Chase, T.N., Bennett, M.C., 2002. Prostaglandin A1 inhibits rotenone-induced apoptosis in SH-SY5Y cells. J. Neurochem. 83 (5), 1094–1102.

Wang, C., Zhang, N., Li, L., Zhang, Q., Zhao, M., Liu, W., 2010. Enantioselective interaction with acetylcholinesterase of an organophosphate insecticide fenamiphos. Chirality 22 (6), 612–617.

Weber, G.J., Sepúlveda, M.S., Peterson, S.M., Lewis, S.S., Freeman, J.L., 2013. Transcriptome alterations following developmental atrazine exposure in zebrafish are associated with disruption of neuroendocrine and reproductive system function, cell cycle, and carcinogenesis. Toxicol. Sci. 132 (2), 458–466.

Wills, J., Credle, J., Oaks, A.W., Duka, V., Lee, J.H., Jones, J., Sidhu, A., 2012. Paraquat, but not maneb, induces synucleinopathy and tauopathy in striata of mice through inhibition of proteasomal and autophagic pathways. PLoS One 7 (1), e30745.

Wirbisky, S.E., Weber, G.J., Sepúlveda, M.S., Xiao, C., Cannon, J.R., Freeman, J.L., 2015. Developmental origins of neurotransmitter and transcriptome alterations in adult female zebrafish exposed to atrazine during embryogenesis. Toxicology 333, 156–167.

Wu, F., Wang, Z., Gu, J.H., Ge, J.B., Liang, Z.Q., Qin, Z.H., 2013. p38(MAPK)/p53-mediated Bax induction contributes to neurons degeneration in rotenone-induced cellular and rat models of Parkinson's disease. Neurochem. Int. 63 (3), 133–140.

Xie, F., Fang, C., Schnittke, N., Schwob, J.E., Ding, X., 2013. Mechanisms of permanent loss of olfactory receptor neurons induced by the herbicide 2,6-dichlorobenzonitrile: effects on stem cells and noninvolvement of acute induction of the inflammatory cytokine IL-6. Toxicol. Appl. Pharmacol. 272 (3), 598–607.

Xu, L.C., Liu, L., Ren, X.M., Zhang, M.R., Cong, N., Xu, A.Q., Shao, J.H., 2008. Evaluation of androgen receptor transcriptional activities of some pesticides in vitro. Toxicology 243 (1–2), 59–65.

Xu, H.D., Wang, J.S., Li, M.H., Liu, Y., Chen, T., Jia, A.Q., 2015. (1)H NMR based metabolomics approach to study the toxic effects of herbicide butachlor on goldfish (*Carassius auratus*). Aquat. Toxicol. 159, 69–80.

Yamada, A., Aki, T., Unuma, K., Funakoshi, T., Uemura, K., 2015. Paraquat induces epithelial-mesenchymal transition-like cellular response resulting in fibrogenesis and the prevention of apoptosis in human pulmonary epithelial cells. PLoS One 10 (3), e0120192.

Yan, D., Jiang, X., Yu, G., Zhao, Z., Bian, Y., Wang, F., 2006. Quantitative structure-toxicity relationships of organophosphorous pesticides to fish (*Cyprinus carpio*). Chemosphere 63 (5), 744–750.

Yavuz, T., Delibas, N., Yildirim, B., Altuntas, I., Candir, O., Cora, A., Karahan, N., Ibrisim, E., Kutsal, A., 2005. Vascular wall damage in rats induced by organophosphorus insecticide methidathion. Toxicol. Lett. 155, 59–64.

Zerin, T., Song, H.Y., Kim, Y.S., 2015. Extracellular signal-regulated kinase pathway play distinct role in acetochlor-mediated toxicity and intrinsic apoptosis in A549 cells. Toxicol. In Vitro 29 (1), 85–92.

Zhang, X., Jones, D., Gonzalez-Lima, F., 2006. Neurodegeneration produced by rotenone in the mouse retina: a potential model to investigate environmental pesticide contributions to neurodegenerative diseases. J. Toxicol. Environ. Health A 69 (18), 1681–1697.

Zhang, X., Wallace, A.D., Du, P., Lin, S., Baccarelli, A.A., Jiang, H., Jafari, N., Zheng, Y., Xie, H., Soares, M.B., Kibbe, W.A., Hou, L., 2012a. Genome-wide study of DNA methylation alterations in response to diazinon exposure in vitro. Environ. Toxicol. Pharmacol. 34 (3), 959–968.

Zhang, Q., Wang, C., Zhang, X., Jin, D., Huang, C., Zhao, M., 2012b. Enantioselective aquatic toxicity of current chiral pesticides. J. Environ. Monit. 14 (2), 465–472.

Zhao, L., Huang, Y., Hu, J., Zhou, H., Adeleye, A.S., Keller, A.A., 2016. (1)H NMR and GC-MS based metabolomics reveal defense and detoxification mechanism of cucumber plant under nano-Cu stress. Environ. Sci. Technol. 50 (4), 2000–2010.

Zhuang, S., Zhang, J., Wen, Y., Zhang, C., Liu, W., 2012. Distinct mechanisms of endocrine disruption of DDT-related pesticides toward estrogen receptor α and estrogen-related receptor γ. Environ. Toxicol. Chem. 31 (11), 2597–2605.

Zucchini-Pascal, N., de Sousa, G., Pizzol, J., Rahmani, R., 2011. Molecular investigation of the effects of lindane in rat hepatocytes: microarray and mechanistic studies. Food. Chem. Toxicol. 49 (12), 3128–3135.

Zuryn, S., Kuang, J., Ebert, P., 2008. Mitochondrial modulation of phosphine toxicity and resistance in *Caenorhabditis elegans*. Toxicol. Sci. 102, 179–186.

12

A SIMPLE WHOLE CELL MICROBIAL BIOSENSORS TO MONITOR SOIL POLLUTION

Prabhakaran Rajkumar*, Tharmarajan Ramprasath*,, Govindan Sadasivam Selvam***

**Madurai Kamaraj University, Department of Biochemistry, School of Biological Sciences, Madurai, Tamil Nadu, India; **Georgia State University, Center for Molecular and Translational Medicine, Atlanta, GA, United States*

1 Introduction

Human life and the life of other organisms are predominantly dependent on soil. Soil is made up of decaying or decayed living organisms, natural resources, and humus (partly decayed plant material). Soil provides nutrients, raw materials, water, and microorganisms (rhizobacteria) that promote plant growth and renew the soil (Chiou et al., 1985). Soil acts as an essential part in human survival and is intrinsically linked to public health. For example, most essential trace elements necessary for human beings are derived from soil (Chahal et al., 2014). Soil contamination is caused by the occurrence of anthropogenic (human-made) chemicals (Darnley et al., 1995; Hudson et al., 2014; Gerbersdorf et al., 2015) or other modifications in the usual soil environs. Soil contamination can include a number of undesirable disease-causing bacteria; heavy metal accumulation [arsenic (As), cadmium (Cd), chromium (Cr), cobalt (Co), copper (Cu), mercury (Hg), manganese (Mn), nickel (Ni), lead (Pb), and zinc (Zn)] (Pinto et al., 2015; Maisto et al., 2011); industrial waste; pesticides such as organophosphate (OPP) and organochlorine (OCPs), including dichloro-diphenyl-trichloroethane and hexachlorocyclohexane (Sagarkar et al., 2014; Feng et al., 2003); herbicides (Kanissery and Sims, 2011); and polycyclic aromatic hydrocarbons from industrial processes, such as naphthalene, phenanthrene or benzo[a]pyrene (Weissenfels et al., 1992). These contaminants enter the soil environment posing an enormous risk to human health and the natural ecosystem (Pinto et al., 2015; Chen et al., 2015). In addition,

New Pesticides and Soil Sensors. http://dx.doi.org/10.1016/B978-0-12-804299-1.00013-8

soil pollution leads to changes in the natural water by accumulating chemicals leaching into groundwater. Eventually, this process contaminates drinking water and the ocean itself, resulting in dramatic environmental contamination (Guerin, 2001; Maisto et al., 2011; Sakrabani et al., 2012). In this chapter, we briefly review the process of pesticide, heavy metal, and anthropogenic waste accumulation in soil and the ways to monitor these contaminants using conventional methods, such as gas chromatography, high performance liquid chromatography, atomic absorption spectroscopy, and inductively coupled plasma-atomic emission/mass spectroscopy (ICP-AE/MS), along with their advantages and limitations. This is followed by a discussion on the use of simple, quantifiable, and cost-effective microbial biosensors to monitor soil pollution more effectively. Design and recognition elements, such as enzymes, antibodies, aptamers, and DNA, are introduced briefly, followed by transducer operations, such as electrochemical (amperometric, potentiometric, conductometric, and voltammetric) and optical (fluorescent, luminescent, colorimetric) methods. Finally, this chapter concludes by discussing various successful experimentations with microbial biosensors for detecting soil contaminants (Fig. 12.1).

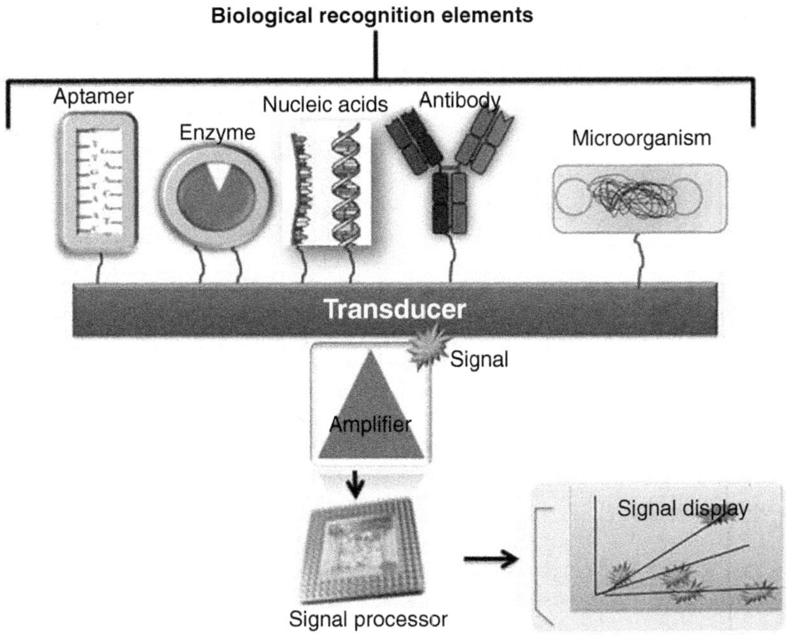

Figure 12.1. Schematic diagram represents summary of this chapter.

2 Soil Contamination Around the World

Anthropogenic waste accumulation is the prime factor in soil contamination. Major categories of xenobiotic waste include pesticides and heavy metals. Apart from these, the pathogenic bacteria population in soil is yet another factor that poses a severe threat to health. In general, we can classify the contaminants into three major types, namely pesticides, heavy metals, and pathogenic bacteria.

2.1 Pesticide Contamination

An increase in population leads to a huge demand for food; in order to meet urgent need for increased food production, treatment with pesticides in agriculture and the food industry has been increased worldwide (Bai et al., 2006). Pesticides are used in agriculture because of their ability to reduce crop loss, but the entry of pesticides into the soil is highly toxic and creates an environmental hazard by modifying the treated soil biochemically and altering its innate microbial community (Dailey, 2004; Gonzalaez et al., 2010; Oyekunle et al., 2011; Van Geest et al., 2014). Accumulation of pesticides in food becomes a serious public health issue as well since the recent discovery that many pesticides play a significant role in the epigenetic alteration of genetic material of higher organisms, including humans (Sancho et al., 2010; Zhu et al., 2009). In Asian countries, organophosphate and OCPs hexachlorocyclohexane and dichloro-diphenyl-trichloroethane (Dibenzofurans, 2003; Zhang et al., 2006; Torres Padrón et al., 2006; Huang et al., 2010) were produced and used for the control of diseases such as malaria, typhus, and cholera (Loganathan, 1994). Dichloro-diphenyl-trichloroethane is a persistent organic pollutant, as well as the α,β,γ-hexachlorocyclohexanes. These organochlorine pesticide compounds cannot be simply degraded by physiochemical or biological methods within a short period of time. In addition, the lipophilic property of these pesticides allows them to be absorbed and accumulated in animal lipids and their cellular toxicity increases the risk of cancer (Megharaj et al., 1999; Connell et al., 2003; Wong et al., 2005; Hao et al., 2008). For these reasons, identification of soil contamination by pesticides has generated considerable research interest. The Gong et al. (2004) study revealed that where ρ,ρ'-dichlorodiphenyldichloroethane accumulated in China's surface soil, the concentration range of these contaminants was 27.5 and 18.8 ng/g, respectively.

2.2 Heavy Metal Contamination

Heavy metals are found by nature in the Earth's crust. They occur naturally in soil and rocks with a subsequent range of background concentrations in soils, sediment, water, and organisms. Examples of heavy metals are cadmium, chromium, copper, mercury, lead, zinc, arsenic, boron (B), and the platinum (Pt) group metals, including platinum, palladium, rhodium, ruthenium, osmium, and iridium.

The most significant natural source of heavy metal is geologic parent material or rock outcropping. Inorganic and organic fertilizers are the major source of heavy metals in agricultural soil. Industrial sources include mining and refinement. Activities such as mining and refinement, smelting operations, and agriculture have contaminated extensive areas around world, including Japan, Indonesia and China, most heavily impacted by heavy metals, such as cadmium, copper, and zinc.

Heavy metal is an extremely toxic and hazardous element to the environment and human health (Shi et al., 2007). Although the toxicity of heavy metal is well established, the involvement is increasing every day. The major reason for the large increase of heavy metal in the last few years is the usage of phosphate fertilizers in developing and underdeveloped countries and the revolution of electronic products (Gimeno-García et al., 1996). Domestic, industrial, and stream water are liberating heavy metals into the environment primarily due to the advent of urbanization and industrialization. Because of their persistent nature, heavy metals are one of the major contributors to environmental pollution. Heavy metals have specific gravity $>5\ g/cm^3$ (Valdman et al., 2001). Heavy metal pollution can originate from both natural and anthropogenic sources (Aleem et al., 2003). It becomes toxic when they are accumulated in the soft tissues of animal cells (Wang et al., 2012; Yin et al., 2012). For example, heavy metal such as Pb has a soil retention time of 150–5000 years and its average biological half-life in the human body is estimated to be 18 years (Gisbert et al., 2003; Mani and Kumar, 2014). Yuswir et al. (2015) stated that oil terminal and metal industries commonly release Co into the soil (Lihan et al., 2006). Increasing use of the Cu alloy in the manufacturing of corrosion resistant mechanical parts and the subsequent release of Cu into the environment has influenced soil pH (Hussain, 1990; Shamshuddin et al., 2011). Cd, Pb, Co, Cu, and Cr may have their origin in the electronics and semiconductor industry, and vehicular emissions (Shazili et al., 2006; Debnárová and Weissmannová, 2011; Garba et al., 2014). Some nonessential elements (e.g., arsenic, cadmium, mercury, and lead) are extremely toxic to biota even at very low concentrations.

In most countries, including India, electronic waste is accumulating a great rate, because there is no proper channel to dispose of it (Ravenscroft et al., 2009). Heavy metals liberated from this toxic waste can enter the human body through soil, food, water, air, or absorption through the skin, as a form of occupational exposure (Adams et al., 2012; Bernhoft, 2013).

Heavy metal toxicity exceeding the critical concentration in animal/human cells alters cellular function, leading to number of diseases. For example, cadmium stress in cells may cause oxidative stress (Cuypers et al., 2010) and the accumulation of arsenic, lead, and other heavy metals in animal bodies can affect the lung and brain, create kidney dysfunction, and increase the risk of cancer (Coen et al., 2001; Cope, 2004; Karri et al., 2008). Bones are softened by reason of metal exposure (Duruibe et al., 2007). Long-term exposure to cadmium can cause Itai–Itai disease; mercury poisoning in the Japanese population can cause Minamata disease (Cope, 2004); copper accumulation can cause anemia, insomnia, stuttering, and mental disorders; and the uptake of chromium can cause organ damage in human populations (Lakherwal, 2014).

Similarly, soil pollution has an impact on plant growth and yield. For example, heavy-metal-polluted water on soil can affect the yield of wheat grain (Saha et al., 2014). Consequently, regulatory compliance monitoring is essential, as is determining the source of heavy metal contamination for framing remediation and awareness programs. The physiochemical techniques used for the analysis of heavy metal are highly sensitive. The commonly employed methods are atomic absorption spectroscopy (AAS) (Halloran et al., 1997; Hauser et al., 1972) and ICP-AE/MS, which are expensive and time consuming, and the process of testing is extremely complex. In particular, the sample preparation for ICP-MS requires additional care and specially trained personnel (Clement et al., 1997; Kim et al., 2015).

2.3 Pathogens

Pathogens are microbes that have the ability to cause illness and are a major cause of death among children and young adults. About 13 million deaths are reported every year (Singh et al., 2014). Microbes are disseminated in soil, marine sediments, and the intestinal tract of animals. Some pathogens are soil-borne microorganisms (i.e., bacteria, fungi, and viruses) which in conjunction with a number of parasites, are capable of communicating a disease to humans (Park et al., 2002). Foodborne pathogens, such as *Salmonella* sp., *Escherichia coli, Staphylococcus aureus, Campylobacter jejuni, Campylobacter coli, Bacillus cereus* (Swaminathan and Feng, 1994), *S. aureus, B. cereus, Shigella* sp., *Salmonella* sp.,

Fusarium oxysporum f. sp. *Lycopersici, Rhizoctonia solani,* and *Vibrio* spp., are the most important disease-causing agents for plants, wildlife, and humans (Sneh et al., 1983; Santamaría and Toranzos, 2003).

To clarify the connection between soil–disease–plants–humans, diseases linked with soil are classified based on the origin of the etiological agent. They are described as follows:

1. *Ordinary soil microbiota:* soil-associated diseases produced by way of opportunistic or emerging pathogens (e.g., lung infection through the inhalation of *Aspergillus fumigatus,* a very common fungus occurring in soil as spores).
2. *Soil-related diseases:* caused by the ingestion of food contaminated with entero- or neurotoxins (e.g., *Clostridium botulinum, Clostridium perfrigens,* and *B. cereus*).
3. *Soil-based diseases:* caused by indigenous soil pathogens (e.g., *Clostridium tetani, Bacillus anthracis, and Clostridium perfringens*).
4. *Soil-borne diseases:* caused by enteric pathogens that are introduced into soil by means of human or animal excreta (e.g., *Rhizoctoniasolani, Fusarium* sp., *Pythium* sp.).

3 Conventional Methods for Assessing Soil Pollutants

Several types of traditional and conventional methods can be used for monitoring pesticides, pathogens, and heavy metals in soil and the biological environment. However, all these methods have their own advantages and limitations with respect to the others.

3.1 Pesticides Detection

Organophosphates (OP) are dual-use compounds that have been employed both as chemical warfare agents (nerve gases) or weapons of mass destruction as well as pesticides that have been able to increase agricultural production around the globe, helping to feed the increasing global population. Because of the widespread use and consequent accumulation of these extremely toxic compounds as pesticides and insecticides in the rural and urban theater, trace amounts of these extremely toxic compounds have been seen in ground and surface waters and biological compounds (such as fresh and treated fruits and vegetables). These compounds undergo many transformations (chemical, biological, and photochemical) to form new compounds which are more toxic than the original. One promising technique is the advanced oxidation process, capable of converting toxic compounds (pesticides) into "biologically" harmless derivative products. To better understand these compounds (originating from both initial products and degradation ones) that cause environmental problems, it is significant to identify and determine their ecological lifespan and evaluate their toxicity. Pesticide accumulation in the environment can cause vomiting, faintness, respiratory paralysis, and death in humans and other living organisms (Abu-Qare et al., 2001; Edwards and Tchounwou, 2005; Wu et al., 2007; Pirvutoiu et al., 2008; Man et al., 2011). Consequently, there is an urgent need to detect these compounds for the protection of humans and animals.

Several analytical techniques have been used for monitoring pesticides, including the nonaqueous titration method, spectrophotometric methods (Dreassi et al., 1995; Bonazzi et al., 1995; El-Didamony, 2008), gas or liquid chromatography with different detectors, tandem mass spectrometry (GC–MS/MS), nuclear magnetic resonance spectrometry (Hooijschuur et al., 2002), capillary electrophoresis (Chen and Fung, 2010), and high performance liquid chromatography (Benson and McElnay, 1987; Nishitani et al., 1991). OCP γ-hexachlorocyclohexane (γ-HCH) detection techniques include the colorimetric measurement of chloride ions, the phenol red based colorimetric measurement method, and the determination of complete mineralization to $^{14}CO_2$ (Anu Prathap et al., 2012).

The existing drawback of these techniques is that the methods/tools are not appropriate for field measurement and also that the instrumentation is expensive (Köhler et al., 2000). Moreover, they require a large infrastructure, backup, and a highly qualified expert technician for operation. Recently, there has been an intense research effort to develop biosensor devices for the determination of organophosphorus pesticides (Laschi et al., 2007).

3.2 Heavy Metal Detection

Commonly available techniques for removing heavy metals from aqueous streams, include chemical precipitation, reverse osmosis, ultrafiltration, and electrodialysis. In chemical precipitation, coagulants such as alum, lime, iron salts, and other organic polymers are used to precipitate the metals (Lakherwal, 2014). Reverse osmosis is accomplished using a semipermeable membrane at a pressure higher than the osmotic pressure in wastewater due to dissolved solids (Malik, 2004; Kalam and Latifah, 2014). Ultrafiltration is a method in which heavy metals are removed by filtration through a porous membrane under pressure

(Lakherwal, 2014). In electrodialysis, semipermeable ion-selective membranes are used to separate heavy metals: the electrical potential between electrodes leads to the migration of ions to the desired electrodes (Lakherwal, 2014). The drawback of these processes is that they are ineffective and expensive when the heavy metal concentration is at 1–100 mg/L (Samarth et al., 2012).

Recently, the occurrence or availability of heavy metals in the soil and biological environment has been monitored by AAS (Manutsewee et al., 2007), anodic stripping voltammetry (Brainina et al., 2004), inductively coupled plasma mass spectrometry (ICP-MS) (Batista et al., 2008), flow injection atomic absorption (Corbisier et al., 1999), inductively coupled plasma atomic emission spectroscopy (ICP-AES) (Bettinelli et al., 2000; Rahmi et al., 2007; Tuzen et al., 2008; van Wezel et al., 2010), gaseous hydride atomic absorption spectrometry, and graphite furnace atomic absorption spectrometry (Roberto et al., 2002). Even though ICP techniques have low detection limits [ranges from parts per billion (ppb) to parts per trillion (ppt)] (Berezhetskyy et al. 2008), these methods consist of sample manipulations, extraction operations, and derivatization reactions that are liable to various interferences; they are also not applicable to colored and turbid solutions. These methods are expensive because they require a large infrastructure, backup, and skilled operators, and they are unsuitable for in-situ analysis (Woutersen et al., 2011).

3.3 Pathogen Detection

The commonly used microorganism identification methods are microscopy, culture, and serology. The simplest, easiest, and most versatile technique is microscopy. The culture technique is a famous benchmark for diagnosis for many microorganisms in the environment. For example, *Mycobacterium tuberculosis* has been identified by using this technique. Serology forms the backbone of identification in some of the diseases, such as syphilis. Note these additional points and methodologies:

- Conventional bacterial identification methods usually include a morphological evaluation of the microorganism, as well as tests for the organism's ability to grow in various media under a variety of conditions. Although standard microbiological techniques allow the detection of single cell bacteria, amplification of the signal is required through growth of a single cell into a colony. This process is relatively time-consuming.
- Traditional methods for the detection of bacteria involve following basic steps: preenrichment, selective enrichment, biochemical screening, and serological confirmation. Generally,

no single test is responsible for a conclusive identification of an unknown bacterium.

- Some new technologies are very sensitive; nevertheless, the analysis time is lengthy. For example, the polymerase chain reaction (PCR) can be used to amplify small quantities of genetic material to determine the presence of bacteria. The PCR method is extremely sensitive, but requires pure samples and hours of processing and expertise in molecular biology (Sperveslage et al., 1996; Meng et al., 1996).
- Microbial culture-based tests and molecular assays (immunological or nucleic acid technologies) are the most common methodologies currently used (Lazcka et al., 2007).
- Culture-based tests, biochemical assays, antibody-based methods including agglutination and enzyme-linked assays, molecular methods, and microscopic study for cell counting (Vollenhofer-Schrumpf et al., 2005; Lazcka et al., 2007).
- Flow cytometry (Delagrave et al., 1995; Heim and Tsien, 1996; Cormack et al., 1996; Errampalli et al., 1999) measuring physical parameters by piezocrystals, impedimetry, redox reactions, optical methods, ultrasound techniques, calorimetry, and detecting cellular compounds, such as ATP, DNA, protein and lipid derivatives, and radioactive isotopes.
- The primary physicochemical methods include the detection of some naturally occurring components of the bacterium. For example, GC and infrared (IR) are used for bacterial identification. In gas chromatography, the microorganism's fatty acid profile was analyzed for microorganism identification (Swaminathan and Feng, 1994). In IR, bacteria are smeared onto an IR cell and an IR absorbance spectra is acquired using conventional instrumentation. The IR method used to evaluate the chemical composition of bacteria is equal to molecular level.

These traditional, conventional, and instrumental methods are extremely precise; however, they have the disadvantage of high costing, large stationary laboratories because of complex instrumentation, not easily amenable, and require routine screening and highly qualified expertise (Jokerst et al., 2012).

Flow cytometry has a number of advantages, such as information on cell size, shape and structure, cell mass, and bacterial growth (Lloyd, 1993). Flow cytometry has been used almost exclusively for measurements of mammalian or at least eukaryotic cells, remaining a rarity in microbiology, including bacteriology. The main experimental difficulty in analyzing bacteria using flow cytometry is that many of the biological characteristics (including size, shape, and DNA content) vary depending upon the growth conditions used, or the source from which the organism was obtained (Allman et al., 1993). The lack of progress in microbiological applications of flow cytometry is the result of several problems encountered when analyzing bacteria. The small size of bacteria and the low number of DNA molecules present to be stained (typically three orders of magnitude less than a mammalian cell), require instruments with high sensitivity and sophistication. Strict reproducibility of conditions is also required in order to produce consistent data. Finally, the capital cost involved in flow cytometry analyses is hig, further restricting its use.

According to available literature, microbial biosensors are an outstanding tool to assess the bioavailability of heavy metal in soil and water (Kalam and Latifah, 2014; Kim et al., 2015), and the rapid detection of pathogens (Venugopal, 2002; Lazcka et al., 2007; Torres-Chavolla and Alocilja, 2009; Sharma and Mutharasan, 2013; Singh et al., 2014; Zhao et al., 2014a) and pesticides (Su et al., 2011; López Rodriguez et al., 2015). Microbial biosensors have several advantages when compared to chemical and existing ecotoxicity testing methods. Microbial biosensor based assays are quick and economical and exhibit easy reproducibility, with the ability to detect trace amounts of pollutants.

4 Microbial Biosensor

In 1996, Turner first introduced the microbial biosensor. Microbes are present ubiquitously and can easily metabolize a wide range of chemical compounds, pesticides, polyaromatic hydrocarbons, and heavy metals. Microorganisms have a great capacity to adapt to adverse conditions and to develop the ability to degrade new molecules over time. Microbes are also amenable to genetic modifications through mutation or through recombinant DNA technology and serve as an economical source of intracellular enzymes (Kumar et al., 2006; Odaci et al., 2009; Reshetilov et al., 2010; Zhang and Keasling, 2011).

Biosensors are devices that use specific biochemical reactions, mediated by isolated enzymes, immunosystems, tissues, organelles, or whole cells, to detect chemical compounds—usually by electrical, thermal, or optical signals (IUPAC definition). From another aspect, a biosensor is an analytical device that consists of immobilized biological material in intimate contact with a compatible transducer, which converts the biochemical signal into a quantifiable electrical signal. Microorganisms, especially bacteria, proliferate very rapidly under aerobic or anaerobic condition in relatively inexpensive media. Green fluorescent protein (GFP)-expressing (Delvigne et al., 2011b) bacterial biosensors can be used as an alternative method for detecting environmental pollution. The flexibility of the chemical, physical, and metabolic features of microorganisms makes this possible. These microbial biosensors are simple and efficient in determining the toxicity levels of contaminants, making biosensors capable tools in detecting changes associated with the bioremediation process. Biosensors have wide-ranging applicability because of these factors: accurate, rapid real-time response(s), sensitive, reproducible, easy to calibrate, user friendly, robust, no sample pretreatment needed, no interference expected from the culture or conditions, no added reagents, large dynamic range, low instrumentation and operator cost, ability to detect viable microorganisms, minimal operator skill required, and online capability (Tkac et al., 2002; Yagi 2007; Su et al., 2011; Hasan et al., 2014; Hobson et al., 1996; Yu Lei et al., 2005). Biosensor classification is dependent on its biorecognition element [e.g., enzyme, DNA, antibody, or whole-cell biosensor (WCB)] or on its transduction principle (e.g., electrochemical, optical, piezoelectrical, or thermal biosensor) (Wang et al., 2014).

4.1 Biosensor Design

A biosensor system is composed of two components: a sensitive receptor, which is a biological component (responsible for the selectivity of the device), and a detection system, capable of measuring the reaction of the biological component with the analyte being monitored (Su et al., 2011; Kaur et al., 2015). Generally, biosensors are made up of a biological sensing element, transducer, and signal receiving processor (Fig. 12.2) (Yang et al., 2013). The biological receptor can be a specific cellular component [e.g., enzyme (Prodromidis and Karayannis, 2002), antibody (Conroy et al., 2009; Bromage et al., 2007; Perumal and Hashim, 2014), nucleic acids (Singh et al., 2010; Torres-Chavolla and Alocilja, 2009; Singh et al., 2014), or whole cells (Yagi 2007;

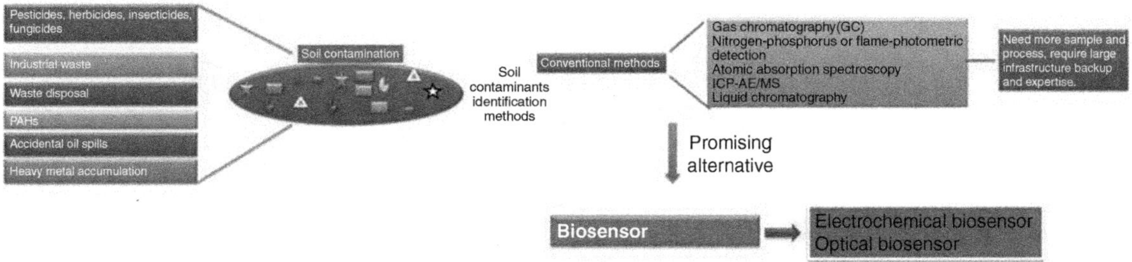

Figure 12.2. Schematic representation for the construction of biosensor.

Verma et al., 2011; Wu et al., 2009; Lim et al., 2012; Wong et al., 2013; Taylor et al., 2014)]. The biological reaction detected can be of any metabolic process (e.g., an enzymatic activity, a gene expression) or even cellular toxicity (Selifonova and Burlage, 1993). The biosensors can be constructed with intact organisms or with isolated biological components. There are several advantages of WCBs over biosensors composed of isolated biological components (D'Souza and Souza, 2001; Strosnider, 2003; Paitan et al., 2004; Rogers 2006; Gutierrez et al., 2015). Microorganisms are cheaper to produce than specific biological components because they do not need to be isolated. They also have different types of defense mechanisms against environmental pollution (Yagi, 2007) and can be cultivated easily, meaning that large quantities can be prepared relatively inexpensively (Ramanathan et al., 1997). Growth conditions when using WCBs, however, must be closely controlled to ensure reproducibility (Gu et al., 2004). Age, temperature, cell density, and aeration of the culture during the period in which the selected biosensor is exposed to the inducer substance can affect the biosensor response (Selifonova and Burlage, 1993). Consider this example of a microbial biosensor: a sulfur-oxidizing bacteria (SOB) biosensor/sulfur-oxidizing bacterial biosensor, used for the detection of toxic chemicals present in the environment (Hassan et al., 2012). SOB, in the presence of oxygen, oxidizes the sulfur, producing sulfuric acid, which leads to a change in pH and electrical conductivity. In the presence of a toxic chemical, such as hexavalent chromium, the bacteria is also be affected, impacting the pH and electrical conductivity changes. These changes can be monitored by simple EC and pH meters (Oh et al., 2011).

4.1.1 Biological Sensing Element

As the biorecognition element determines the degree of selectivity and specificity of the biosensor, the transducer method has a large impact on the sensitivity, speed, efficacy, and simplicity of the device (Reshetilov et al., 2010; Guo, 2012). Electrochemical impedance is considered an effective, cheap, and nondestructive transducer technique for sensing the biorecognition event. The metabolic activity of microorganisms can be evaluated by measuring the impedance change caused by modifications in the medium resistance and in the interface reactance.

4.1.2 Reporter Gene

The chief component in the WCB design is the reporter gene. Based on its substrate dependency, the reporter gene can be divided into two types (Robbens et al., 2005): substrate dependent (e.g., luciferase, β-galactosidase, and alkaline phosphatase) and substrate independent (e.g., fluorescent protein). Some of the reporter gene functions and characteristics are summarized in Table 12.1.

Bacterial enzyme β-galactosidase is encoded by the *lacZ* gene of *E. coli*; luciferases is encoded by *luxA* (luciferase alpha chain) and *luxB* (luciferase beta chain) of the *lux* operon of *Vibrio fischeri* and *Vibrio harveyi* respectively (King et al., 1990); β-*Lactamase* is encoded by the *bla* gene of *E. coli* (West et al., 1994); and firefly luciferase is encoded by the *luc* gene (Szittner and Meighen, 1990). Hydrolase enzyme alkaline phosphatase (ALP or ALKP) is responsible for eliminating phosphate groups from many types of macromolecules and small molecules (Köhler et al., 2000). GFP does not have any enzymatic catalysis reaction and GFP production does not require any exogenous substrate or adenosine triphosphate (Stiner and Halverson, 2002; Delvigne et al., 2011a).

Reporter genes are either readily detectable, such as GFP, or have easily measurable activity. The choice of reporter gene depends on the specificity of the biosensor construction and environmental conditions. Monitoring success depends predominantly on the accurate selection of the reporter (Köhler et al., 2000; Yagi, 2007).

4.2 Specificity-Based Types of Whole Cell Biosensors

1. *Effect-specific biosensors* are stimulated by modifications to physiological and chemical conditions, such as pH, temperature, or osmotic changes, or pollutants that give rise to a specific type of toxicity (e.g., oxidative stress or protein damage) (Gutierrez et al., 2015).
2. *Compound-specific biosensors* respond to only one type of pollutant or compounds with similar chemical features (e.g., any heavy metal) (Wu et al., 2009; Verma et al., 2011).
3. Other specificity-based classifications of WCBs are:
    a. Class-I biosensors—respond to a specific or exclusive pollutant.
    b. Class-II biosensors—respond to a specific cellular stress.
    c. Class-III biosensors—respond unspecifically to different pollutants or stress conditions. These are also classified as constitutive WCBs (Magrisso et al., 2008).

Table 12.1 Characteristics of Commonly Used Reporter Genes for Whole Cell Biosensors Design

Substrate Dependent Reporter Gene					
Gene	**Protein**	**Advantages**	**Defects**	**Reaction With Substrate**	**References**
lux	Bacterial luciferase Luminescent bacteria (*V. fischeri, V. harvey*)	Ease of measurement rapid response	Heat lability	Aldehydes (C9–C14)	Billard and DuBow (1998); Gu et al. (2004); Gutierrez et al. 2015)
luc	Firefly luciferase (*Photinus pyralis*)	High sensitivity No heat lability	Exogenous substrate Oxygen requirement	Luciferin	Gu et al. (2004); Greer and Szalay (2002); Gutierrez et al. (2015)
lacZ	β-Galactosidase (*E. coli*)	Detection by naked eye Wide variety of detection methods	Exogenous substrate requirement Complicated colorimetric operation	Lactose (galactose + glucose) O-nitro-phenol β-D-galactopyranoside methyllumbelliferyl-β-D-galactopyranoside (MUG) or fluorescein-di-β-D-galactopyranoside (FDG)	Gu et al. (2004)
bla	β-Lactamase (*E. coli*)	High sensitivity	Complicated colorimetric operation	Lactamides	Yoon et al. (1991); Moore et al. (1997)
crtA	Spheroidenone (*Rhodovulum sulfidophilum*)	High sensitivity	Complicated colorimetric operation	Demethylspheroidene	Yagi (2007)
phoA	Alkaline phosphatase (various origin)	High sensitivity	Colorimetric, chemiluminescence	Phosporylated organics	Bronstein et al. (1994); Beck and Burtscher (1994)
uidA (*gusA, gurA*)	β-Glucuronidase (*E. coli*)	High sensitivity	Colorimetric, fluorescence, luminescence	β-Glucuronides	Togo et al. (2007)
Substrate Independent Reporter Gene					
gfp	Green fluorescent protein (Pacific jellyfish *Aequoria Victoria*)	Autofluorescence No substrate requirement	Low sensitivity Lag time before expression	No catalysis reaction	Gutierrez et al. (2015); Billard and DuBow (1998); Hakkila et al. (2002)

In the construction of WCBs, eukaryotic microorganisms are also frequently used. The reasons for this are:

- Eukaryotic microorganisms give satisfactorily quantifiable signals.
- Biomass is reached in a short period of time because of their growth speed and quick generation time.
- Microorganisms are easily employable, occurring all over the world.
- Microbial genetic analysis methodology and an increase in genomic sequencing make the experimental modifications needed for introducing transduction capacity during WCB design easier.
- Similar metabolism, genomes, and cellular organization exist as compared with other eukaryotic organisms, such as humans.
- In WCB construction, three different taxonomic groups have been used: fungi, microalgae, and protozoa.

4.2.1 Constitutive Systems

In normal conditions the gene promoter is highly expressed. As a consequence, the reporter gene basal expression level is also notably high (Belkin, 2003). However, in the presence of toxic conditions this gene promoter expression decreases. For this reason, the gene promoter has been used in constitutive expression systems. Turn-off bioassays are based on constitutive WCBs, because in the presence of toxic pollutants the basal expression level is decreased. This reduction in this parameter is correlated and inversely proportional to the environmental sample toxicity (Gutierrez et al., 2015).

4.2.2 Inducible Systems

The inducible promoter is fused with the reporter gene in an inducible promoter system. This construct is classified under turn-on assays (Meer and Belkin, 2010; Magrisso et al., 2008). In the presence of chemical or environmental pollutants, the specific gene promoter is induced to express the reporter gene (Wu et al., 2009).

4.3 Types of Sensing Techniques in Biosensors

Biosensors can be categorized into different types, based on their sensing techniques or the transducer components, as defined further in Fig. 12.3. These include:

Electrochemical microbial biosensors

- Amperometric microbial biosensors
- Potentiometric transducers

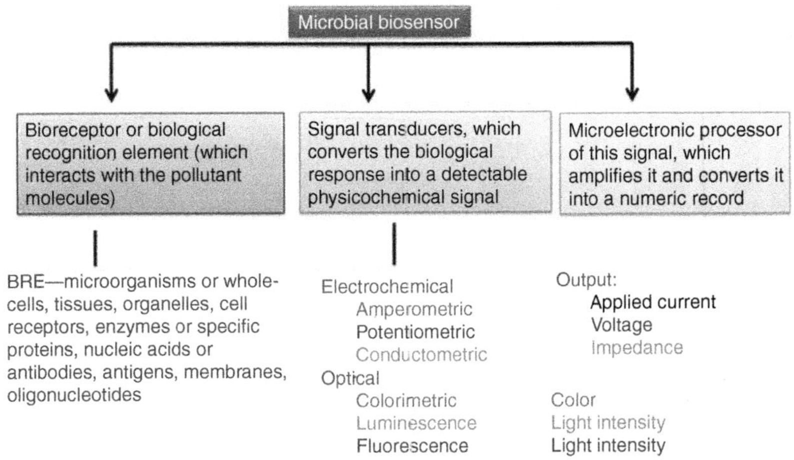

Figure 12.3. Schematic diagram represents components of microbial biosensor.

- Conductometric sensors
- Voltammetry

Optical microbial biosensors

- Fluorescent microbial biosensors
- Bioluminescent microbial biosensors
- Colorimetric microbial biosensors

4.3.1 Electrochemical Techniques

The first electrochemical biosensor was developed by Clark and Lyons (1962). Electrochemical biosensors are commonly based on the enzymatic catalysis of a reaction that produces or puts away electrons (such enzymes are rightly called redox enzymes) (Hasan et al., 2014). In electrochemical biosensors, the reporter signal is monitored by the production of electrochemical reactions (Ron, 2007; Su et al., 2011; Grieshaber et al., 2008). The Clark and Lyons biosensor has the enzyme glucose oxidase (GOD) and an amperometric electrode for the electrochemical signal production. This enzyme and electrode have been incorporated to produce a signal that is directly proportional to the amount of oxygen present in blood. At present, transducers based on semiconductors and screen-printed electrodes form a typical platform for the construction of biosensors. Electrochemical biosensors are predominantly used for the detection of hybridized DNA and glucose concentration (Hasan et al., 2014).

The electrochemical biosensor creates a new strategy for detecting pesticides, such as the OCP lindane, in the soil and environment. *Streptomyces* strain M7 (SM7) is capable of growing in the presence of OCPs as the carbon source. Based on this valuable ability, the SM7 spore becomes a platform to detect and quantify lindane with electrochemical impedance spectroscopy as the transduction method. Using this technique, the metabolic bacterial action is evaluated by a set of electrical parameters calculated by fitting the measured impedance spectra through an equivalent electrical circuit. The advantage of this OCP biosensor is that it does not call for a sample pretreatment for pesticide extraction of the supernatants, as regularly used in chromatographic methods of analysis (López Rodriguez et al., 2015).

In recent years, the nucleic acid biosensor has become a well-known device for the clinical monitoring of life-threatening pathogens (Tallury et al., 2010; Syam et al., 2012; Singh et al., 2014). Voltammetry of nucleic acids produced the finding of an anodic peak specific for guanine: a significant breakthrough in the monitoring of double- and denatured single-stranded DNA. Monitoring modification in the DNA redox reaction (oxidation of guanine) gives an exclusive perspective on the hybridization process (Cagnin et al., 2009). The electrochemical DNA biosensors are predominantly based on the redox indicators. These are methylene blue (MB) (Singh et al., 2012a; Singh et al., 2012b); daunomycin (Chandra et al., 2011); and metal complexes such as ruthenium (Ru) complex (Pieper et al., 2008) and cobalt complex (Li et al., 2008). These have been found to be beneficial by reason of the reusability of the electrode.

For the detection of toxic metals (toluene, Ni^{2+}, or Cu^{2+}) in the environment in areas such as soil, electrochemical biosensors play a vital role. As an example, *Chlamydomonas reinhardtii* were used for the development of a biosensing system, with this biosensor dependent on its unicellular flagellate motility and negative gravitaxis changes (Shitanda et al., 2005). In this system, *C. reinhardtii* flagellar movement changes were examined in the redox currents for a coexisting redox marker (i.e., oxidation of ferrocyanide as the redox marker).

Electrochemical biosensors do not have need of a supplementary labeling step. They can also be effortlessly incorporated with electronics for the construction of smaller devices for the detection of pathogenic microorganisms of environmental and clinical concern. As a consequence, electrochemical biosensor technology is at the frontline of clinical diagnosis and measurement of heavy metal contamination and pesticide accumulation in soil, all of which commonly rely on measuring techniques. These measuring systems are classified into three types according to the operating principle governing their method of measurement: amperometric, potentiometric, or conductometric microbial biosensors (Fig. 12.4) (Kumar and D'Souza, 2011; Su et al., 2011).

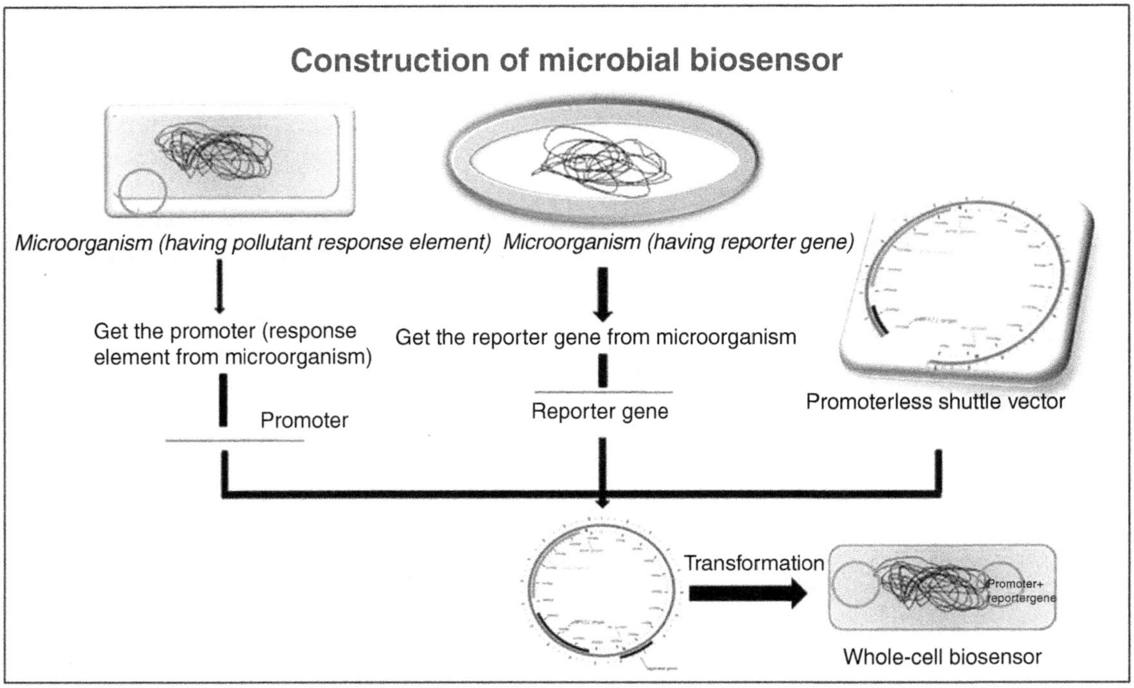

Figure 12.4. Schematic diagram representation of electrochemical biosensor.

4.3.1.1 Amperometric Microbial Biosensors

Amperometry is the term representing all electrochemical techniques in which a current is measured as a function of an independent variable: that is, typically, time or electrode potential (Perumal and Hashim, 2014). The amperometric biosensor contains three electrodes: one is the working electrode, the second is the reference electrode, and the third electrode is a counter or auxiliary. The working electrode is normally made of gold (Au), carbon (C), altered forms of carbon, or platinum (Pt); silver or silver chloride (Ag/AgCl) is mainly used as a reference electrode; and, finally, the third electrode is a counter or auxiliary involved, on occasion, to help measure the current flow (Ivnitski et al., 1999; Wang et al., 2008; Perumal and Hashim, 2014). In these electrochemical amperometric biosensors the redox reaction (certain molecules get oxidized or reduced) takes place in an inert metal electrode; as a result, the working electrode is driven to a positive potential or negative potential. If it is positive, the oxidation reaction may possibly take place; if it is negative, the reduction reaction may possibly take place. In these reactions electrons are transferred through electroactive species (analyte) to working electrode or electrode to electroactive species (Parkinson and Pejcic, 2005).

Amperometric biosensors produce a current relative to the concentration of the component to be detected. The best common amperometric biosensors use the Clark oxygen electrode. In the glucose amperometric biosensor, the Clark oxygen electrode is separated from glucose by a membrane, which is permeable to oxygen. A biocatalyst GOD is housed between this membrane and another membrane that separates it from the glucose. The membrane that separates GOD and glucose is permeable to both oxygen and glucose. In effect, the enzyme GOD is immobilized between two membranes, one being permeable only to oxygen and the other to both oxygen and glucose.

The amperometric microbial biosensors for organophosphate pesticides are classified into two groups: inhibition-based (Lei et al., 2005) and catalytic-based. One example is the genetically engineered *Pseudomonas putida* JS444, which is immobilized on the carbon paste electrode to express organophosphorus hydrolase (OPH). OPH catalyzes the hydrolysis of paraoxon, parathion, and methyl parathion, such as the *p*-nitrophenyl substituent organophosphorus pesticides, to release *p*-nitrophenol (PNP). In this enzyme conversion process the intermediates produce the electrooxidation current. The current production depends on the concentration of organophosphorus pesticides (Yu Lei et al., 2005). Similarly, *p*-nitrophenyl-substituted organophosphate nerve agent detecting amperometric biosensors are highly sensitive and selective in nature.

The amperometric biosensor for pathogenic microorganism detection mainly depends mainly on the measurement of current signal production by way of enzyme catalyzed redox reactions (Sharma and Mutharasan, 2013). The immobilization of target-specific antibodies on the working electrode surface produces the current signal caused by the binding of target with immobilized specific antibodies; it shows the detection response. Signal amplification can also be done by using a second enzyme–antibody complex that would bind to the target on the electrode. The enzyme would then catalyze a redox reaction to generate an electroactive product leading to an enhanced current signal. For example, a horseradish peroxidase enzyme was immobilized on the working electrode for the detection of cyanide (Ghanavati et al., 2014).

For monitoring heavy metals such as Ni^{2+} or Cu^{2+} in water supplies and reservoirs, flagellate microalga *Chlamydomonas reinhardtii* has been used on the basis of mobility (Shitanda et al., 2005). Moyo et al. (2014) immobilized horseradish peroxidase (HRP) onto a maize tassel multiwalled carbon nanotube (MT-MWCNT/GC) electrode through adsorption to build an amperometric biosensor used to detect Pb^{2+} and Cu^{2+}. The detection is based on the enzyme horseradish peroxidase catalytic activity inhibition to reduce hydrogen peroxide (H_2O_2). Subsequently, the current change is detected and it relates to the analyte concentration.

Microbes having highest sensitivity to heavy metals, for example, *Psychrobacter* sp., have a greater sensitivity to environmental pollutants (Cd^{2+}, Pb^{2+}, Hg^{2+}, Zn^{2+}, and Cu^{2+}). By measuring the growth in between logarithmic to stationary phase, making use of this sensitivity, the ρ-benzoquinone-mediated amperometric biosensor (ToxTell) was developed by Wang et al. (2013). Babkina and Ulakhovich (2004), studied the heavy metal occurrence in milk and blood serum using an immobilized single-stranded DNA (ssIDNA)-based amperometric biosensor technique. Megharaj et al. (1999) and Mohammadi et al. (2005) have demonstrated a three-enzyme system (invertase, mutarotase, and glucose oxidase) based on amperometric biosensors for heavy metal analysis.

4.3.1.2 Potentiometric Microbial Biosensors

Potentiometric transduction is a widely used electrochemical detection method which has been well utilized in environmental pollution detection. Potentiometric biosensors make use of ion-selective electrodes (ISEs) in order to transduce the biological reaction into an electrical signal. The working and reference electrode potential difference measurement is used in potentiometric biosensors; this difference being equal to the amount of analytes. The transducers are an ion-selective or gas-sensing electrode (Su et al., 2011). The first potentiometric biosensor was developed for detection of urea in the year 1969. The urea detecting potentiometric biosensor is an enzyme based biosensor (Saxena and Malhotra, 2003). In the simplest terms, a potentiometric biosensor consists of an immobilized enzyme membrane surrounding the probe from a pH-meter, where the catalyzed reaction generates or absorbs hydrogen ions. The reaction occurring next to the thin sensing glass membrane causes a change in pH which may be read directly from the pH-meter's display. Analytical methods based on potentiometric detection with ISEs can be considered good alternatives because of their attractable characteristics, such as simple design, ease of construction, reasonable selectivity, rapid response time, and applicability to colored and turbid solutions, providing possible interfacing with automated and computerized systems. One example is the sensor for rapid determination of benzydamine [(1-benzyl-3-(3-dimethylamino-propoxy)-1H-indazole hydrochloride (Benz)] in pure and dosage forms. Both polyvinyl chloride and coated-wire sensors were fabricated and subjected to a series of tests to select sensors possessing the most favorable analytical characteristics. The sensors developed were applied in the potentiometric determination of benzydamine in batch analysis using standard addition and potentiometric titration (Khalil et al., 2015). Recently, Khalil et al. (2015) have developed potentiometric biosensors for the determination of benzydamine (1-benzyl-3-(3-dimethylamino-propoxy)-1H-indazole hydrochloride), a tertiary amine, with a nonsteroidal drug using polyvinyl chloride membrane, pharmaceutical compounds, biological fluids, and coated wire sensors. In the Khalil et al. (2015) study, determination of Benz was from pharmaceutical formulation, pure and biological fluids (plasma and urine), and using two kinds of sensors. These were PVC sensors (sensor 1, 2, and 3) and silver coated-wire sensors (sensor 4, 5, and 6). The sensors showed satisfactory performance features with tiny response times (~5 s), a wide pH range in the middle of 3–8 and 2–8 for PVC membrane and coated-wire sensors—in that order, low detection limits of 7.0×10^{-6} mol/L and 7.2×10^{-6} mol/L over the concentration range from 7.0×10^{-6} to 1.0×10^{-2} mol/L and 1.0×10^{-6}–1.0×10^{-2} mol/L, for PVC membrane and coated-wire sensors respectively.

Mulchandani et al. (1998) have used the recombinant *E. coli* cells to determine organophosphate. This recombinant *E. coli* carried plasmid pJK33 that expressed the OPH enzyme intracellularly. The cells were immobilized behind a microporus membrane prepared on the surface of a pH electrode. Attributable to the enzyme catalysis reaction of organophosphorus pesticides to release protons, these protons can sense by glass membrane pH electrode. The signal is proportional to the presence of organophosphorus concentration which is directly proportional to the amount of hydrolyzed substrate. Zhang et al. (2009) established a potentiometric biosensor for detection of organophosphorus pesticides using immobilization of acetylcholinesterase enzyme.

Guilbault and Montalvo (1969) reported the first enzyme-based potentiometric biosensor. Zelada-Guillén et al. (2010) demonstrated the detection of pathogenic living bacteria in real samples, such as milk and apple juice. In this potentiometric aptamer-based biosensor pathogenic *E. coli* O157:H7 used as a test, *E. coli* CECT 675 cells used as nonpathogenic bacteria immobilized aptamers as biorecognition elements and single-walled carbon nanotubes as excellent ion-to-electron transducers. The interaction between aptamer and target pointedly changes the electrical potential, which results in instant identification and detection of the target.

Pathogenic bacteria *Listeria monocytogenes* (LM) have internalin A protein in their surface. Ding et al. (2014) has developed a rapid, sensitive potentiometric aptasensor for *L. monocytogenes*. The aptasensor has a biological sensing element as an aptamer with a transducer as a polycation-sensitive electrode. Protamine used as an indicator for the transduction bind to the *L. monocytogenes* and the produced potential signal was sensed and detected down to 10 colony-forming units per milliliter through a protamine-sensitive membrane electrode. Byrne et al. (2009) proposed potentiometric sensor [light-addressable potentiometric sensor (LAPS)] for the detection of pathogens. Potentiometric sensor [immune-ligand assay (ILA) in conjunction with LAPS] for the rapid detection of *E. coli* O157:H7 has been reported by Gehring et al. (1998).

To date, an enzyme inhibiting activity method serves as a very sensitive monitoring technique for environmental heavy metals assessment. For instance, the enzyme [ultrathin polypyrrole–GOD (PP_y–GO_x)] activity inhibition was used in potentiometric biosensors for the detection of trace metals, such as Cu^{2+}, Hg^{2+}, Cd^{2+}, and Pb^{2+} ions (Ayenimo and Adeloju, 2015). In addition, an ammonia oxidizing bacterial potentiometric microbial biosensor has also been used to detect toxicity in the environment because of its sensitivity and robust identification (Zhang et al., 2013).

4.3.1.3 Conductometric Microbial Biosensors

The transducer for this conductometric biosensor is a conductometric electrode (Soldatkin et al., 1998). The first conductometric transducer was introduced by Watson et al. (1987). Habitually, an enzyme-based conductometric microbial biosensor has been aimed at the determination and identification of environmental contamination (Jaffrezic-renault and Dzyadevych, 2008). Soldatkin et al. (1994) has reported an enzyme cholinesterase based conductometric biosensor for the detection of pesticides. Dzyadevych et al. (2002) described a conductometric biosensor technique for the detection of the toxicity of organophosphate pesticides. In order to identify the pesticides associated with an inhibition of cholinesterase activity, the inhibition mechanism operates by phosphorylating the active site serine OH group by reason of pesticide toxicity. The methyl parathion (O,O-dimethyl O-4-nitrophenyl phosphorothioate) pesticide was identified through this conductometric biosensor.

In some conductometric biosensors, three enzymes (such as urease, acetylcholinesterase, and butyrylcholinesterase) have been used. These three enzymes have the highest sensitivity to toxic substances. In this multiset biosensor, thin-films interdigitated electrodes and potentiometric pH-sensitive field-effect transistors have been used for pesticide and heavy metal detection (Arkhypova et al., 2001). Enzymes alkaline phosphatase and acetylcholinesterase were used for the bi-enzymatic conductometric biosensor development. This enzyme combination was used for the assessment of pesticides and heavy metal contamination. These two enzymes can produce conductivity variations for contaminant detection. Alkaline phosphatase can generate the conductometric change in the presence of Cd^{2+} and Zn^{2+} and the acetylcholinesterase can generate the conductometric change in the presence of carbamates and OP pesticides (Chouteau et al., 2005).

The determination of heavy-metal ions using the urease-immobilized biosensor is based on the measurement of the urease enzymatic activity, which is inhibited by heavy-metal ions. It is well known that inhibition of urease by these ions results from the reaction with sulfhydryl groups at the active site of the enzyme (Zhylyak et al., 1995). A conductometric biosensor is based on sol–gel-immobilized-urease on a screen-printed interdigitated array electrode (a configuration of electrodes used for measuring either an electric current or voltage) for the determination of heavy metal ions, such as cadmium, copper, and lead in synthetic effluents. The sol–gel silicate matrix possesses chemical inertness, physical rigidity, negligible swelling in aqueous solution, and high thermal stability (Ilangovan et al., 2006).

Enzyme-based sensors are extremely selective systems for the detection of toxic compounds because of their high specificity of groups of inhibitors toward a particular enzyme. The enzyme alkaline phosphatase activity has been changed or inhibited by the presence of heavy metals (Durrieu et al., 2003). By using this enzymatic activity change Chouteau et al. (2004) have configured an enzyme–based whole cell conductometric biosensor for monitoring the heavy metal—especially cadmium—existence in an environment. Immobilized *Chlorella vulgaris* microalgae have been used as a bioreceptor for this whole cell conductometric biosensor. Zhylyak et al. (1995) proposed a conductometric biosensor for monitoring trace metals. Their biosensor's sensitive element is an immobilized urease because urease is highly affected or inactivated by heavy metal ions (Krajewska, 1991; Hiromitsu et al., 1991) and the transducer is an interdigitated thin-film gold electrode. This urease conductometric biosensor has numerous benefits including: being smaller in size, having the highest sensitivity for heavy metals, and requiring low power for pollution detection. In recent times, Soldatkin et al. (2012) reported a three enzyme (invertase, mutarotase, and glucose oxidase) conductometric system for the assessment of heavy metal ions (Hg^{2+} and Ag^{+}); this enzyme system was immobilized on the thin-film interdigitated electrodes transducer surface. Conductometric biosensors have numerous advantages, being relatively cost-effective and easy to operate, of simple construction, and demonstrating the highest sensitivity and greatest specificity toward heavy metal ions and toxic substances (Stepurska et al., 2015).

4.3.1.4 Voltammetric Microbial Biosensors

The other universally used biosensor is voltammetry. It is the most adaptable technique in electrochemical biosensors (Su et al., 2011). The changes of current and potential are detected and recorded in this technique. In addition, voltammetry has low noise and high sensitivity (Wang, 1985). Recently, Xue et al. (2014) developed a cyclic voltammetric biosensor for OP pesticide (methyl parathion) analysis. Alpat et al. (2008) have reported a voltammetric microbial biosensor for the determination of Cu^{2+}. Modified carbon paste electrode and *Circinella* sp. was used in this biosensor. The electrode contains preconcentrated Cu^{2+} and is monitored by cyclic voltammetry (CV). The detection limit of this CV could be as low as 54 nM Cu^{2+}. Enzyme acetylcholinesterase has been used for pesticide detection. The inhibition of the enzyme by pesticides, such as monocrotophos, dimethoaten, carbaryl, and malathion, creates the electrochemical behavioral change that was monitored. The enzyme activity was regenerated by pralidoxime iodide (Du et al., 2007). The enzyme inhibition was related to the pesticide concentration and inhibition rates varied for different pesticides. Du et al. (2008) illustrated the electrodeposition of AuNPs (gold nanoparticles) onto the gold electrode to generate a surface for enzyme acetylcholinesterase attachment. Finally, the enzyme catalyzes the substrate acetylthiocholine chloride to form the product thiocholine. The thiocholine produced gets chemisorbed/desorbed on interface. A simple approach for the determination of pesticides was developed based on this process. Viswanathan et al. (2009) also described an acetylcholine enzyme-based electrochemical biosensor for methyl parathion and chlorpyrifos pesticide detection in vegetable crops. For improving acetylcholinesterase voltammetric biosensor redox peak current, the exfoliated graphite nanoplatelets (xGnPs) were used. These exfoliated graphite nanoplatelets using biosensors have outstanding sensitivity and stability in the detection of pesticides (Ion et al., 2010). An enzyme OPH which converts methyl parathion into PNP and dimethyl thiophosphoric acid products was used for the development of biosensors. Using glutaraldehyde, the OPH containing recombinant *E. coli* were immobilized onto screen printed carbon electrodes (SPCEs). The cell immobilized

SPCE was connected with cyclic voltammetry and cyclic voltammograms and finally, with the presence of methyl parathion, the microbial biosensor can produce the signal (Kumar and D'Souza, 2011).

Liao et al. (2007) devised an advanced electrochemical voltammetric DNA biosensor for pathogenic bacteria detection. Target Bacterial 16S rRNA was hybridized with fluorescein-modified detector probes and biotin-modified capture probes fixed to the sensor surface. As a result, signal was produced through oxidation reduction current by means of the conjugation between anti-fluorescein monoclonal Fab (fragment, antigen-binding) with an enzyme horseradish peroxidase. In this way, the uriopathogenic strains, such as *Klebsiella pneumonia* strain Kp295, *Enterococcus faecalis, E. coli* strain Ec103, *Proteus mirabilis* strain Pm278, and *Pseudomonas aeruginosa* strains Pa3 were identified.

The protein based biosensor developed by Bontidean et al. (1998), used the metal binding proteins SmtA (Metallothioneins) and MerR (Regulator protein) to assess the heavy metals. Since metallothionein SmtA is a metal binding protein, it has the highest response against raised concentrations of Cd^{2+} or Zn^{2+}, with a better affinity for Zn^{2+} than equine metallothionein, but the lowest affinity for Cd^{2+} and Cu^{2+}. MerR is a metal regulatory protein in *P. aeruginosa* that offers better selectivity and specificity for Hg^{2+} metal binds with the metal binding to produce a conformational change detected by a capacitive transducer with immobilized antibodies. These principles were used in a protein-based biosensor to detect heavy metal ions (Bontidean et al., 1998).

Corbisier et al. (1999) have used two types of strategies to assess heavy metals. The copper, mercury, lead, and chromate ions are detected by a luminescent and fluorescent biosensor system. A second type of sensor was a metal-binding protein based cyclic voltammetric biosensor. In this case the immobilized metal binding GST-SmtA fusion protein (as a synechoccocal metallothionein) and the MerR (mercury regulatory protein) have direct interaction between heavy metal ions. As a result, the capacitance variations of the proteins were measured by gold electrode in the presence of metal ions (copper, cadmium, mercury, and zinc ions). The results state that GST-SmtA protein has a wide-ranging selectivity to heavy metals. Another capacitance biosensor for heavy metals is described by Bontidean et al. (2003). This biosensor has the highest sensitivity for Zn^{2+} ion and is used for the sensing of all heavy metal ions. Synthetic phytochelatins (PCs) are cysteine-rich peptides, used as a sensing element for the capacitance biosensor. These protein based cyclic voltammetric biosensors have the highest selectivity and sensitivity for heavy metals.

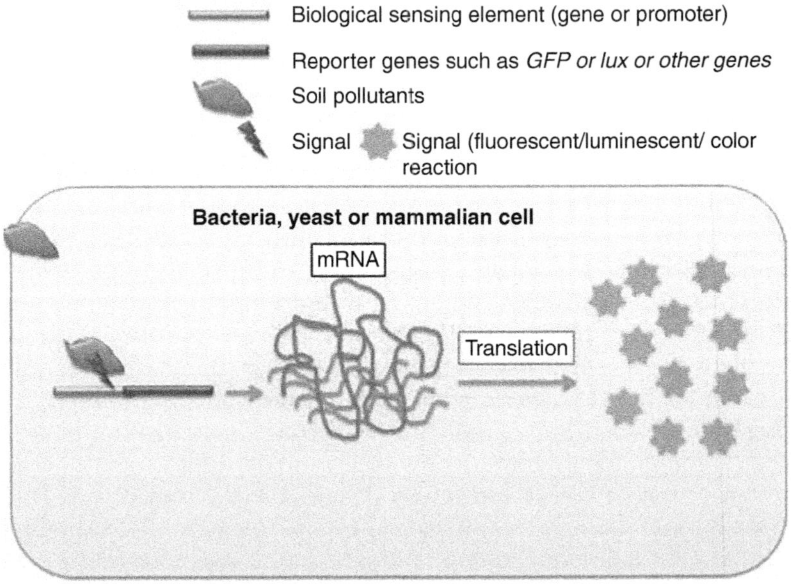

Figure 12.5. Schematic diagram represents the mechanism of optical biosensor.

4.3.2 Optical Microbial Biosensors

Another significant category of biosensor that is widely used in soil and environmental pollution analysis is an optical biosensor (Sharma and Mutharasan, 2013; Wang et al., 2014). Optical biosensors have had tremendous growth in the last few decades by reason of their simple, disposable, cost-effective, no need for sample processing, low amount of sample requirements, and single step, label-free environmental pollution detection, plus high reproducibility (Kumar et al., 2006; Sharma et al., 2013; Orazio, 2011). An optical biosensor is a device that makes use of an optical transducer to produce alterations in diverse optical properties, such as absorption, fluorescence, luminescence, or refractive index, which are relative to the analyte concentration (Fig. 12.5) (Wang et al., 2014; Watts et al., 1994; Kumar et al., 2006; Wong et al., 2013). In optical microbial biosensors the reporter genes are functional biorecognition materials (e.g., enzymes, aptamers, deoxyribozymes/catalytic DNA/DNA enzymes, antibodies, and whole cells) that facilitate the increasing application of optical biosensors (Long et al., 2013b; Rogers, 2006). In the presence of the analyte, the microorganism which has the ability to sense analyte can produce the optical signals which correlate with analyte concentration. Colorimetric, luminescent, and fluorescent signals are widely used optical signals in optical biosensors. Other optical signals also have been used in some microbial biosensors (Su et al., 2011).

The optical microbial biosensor plays a vital role in the detection of pathogenic organisms, such as *Campylobacter* spp. (Rowe-Taitt et al., 2000; Yang et al., 2013). It has advantages in the detection of pesticide (metaphos/methyl parathion) (Kumar et al., 2006). Long et al. (2013a) developed an onsite mercury ions detecting optical biosensor. The mechanism of this biosensor is the fluorescence labeled DNAs that contains thymine–thymine (T–T), which has the capacity for selectively capturing mercury ions. The presence of mercury in the environmental sample binds with fluorescence labeled DNAs to produce the T-Hg^{2+}-T, which leads to the hybridization and hairpin formation due to this effect. The fluorescent signal production also affects these changes that are monitored and confirm the occurrence of mercury (Hg) in the environment.

In some whole-cell microbial biosensors, the immobilization system was used and designed with two things in mind: the geometry of the apparatus and the need for control of genetically modified bacteria that is the fallout of the bioavailability of the environmental contamination to the biosensor (Philp et al., 2003). Whole-cell immobilized microbial biosensors as well have some supplementary advantages including biological stability and plasmid stability.

4.3.2.1 Fluorescent Microbial Biosensors

Fluorescent microbial biosensors can give out fluorescent light that is proportional to the analytes concentration at a low level. The toxicity stress responsive genes or promoters couple with the GFP coding sequence with the intention of allow easy monitoring of the fluorescent signal (Delvigne et al., 2011a). The GFP has an ability to stablize at high temperatures of about 60°C, pH values about 6–10, and in the presence of many denaturants and proteases (Ward Willium et al., 1980), with no need of exogenous substrate or cofactor (Futra et al., 2015). Many studies have been carried out by using GFP as a marker for the detection of pathogens and pollution in environment (Zhao et al., 2014b; Errampalli et al., 1999).

The basis of the fluorescent microbial biosensor is to fuse an inducible promoter to a reporter gene to encode a fluorescent protein, which can emit detectable fluorescence in a genetically modified microorganism (Su et al., 2011). Fluorescent microbial biosensors are widely used in analytical chemistry because of their advantages, such as easy to handle, time required, and no need for the sample preparation process. Commonly two types of fluorescent microbial biosensors occur, that is, in vivo or in vitro types. An in vivo fluorescent biosensor does not need any exogenous stimulation or fluorescent element; it in itself can produce fluorescent protein.

Nowadays, anthropogenic activities create contamination in soil and the environment, leading to the decline of an essential element, such as ferric iron. The ferric iron element is essential for plant and bacterial growth (Lindsay and Schwab, 1982). Accordingly, ferric iron prediction in soil is an important ecological concern. This was resolved by the development of a whole-cell GFP-based bacterial biosensor (Joyner and Lindow, 2000).

These optical fluorescent biosensors used for the detection of toxic metals, such as Cu(II), Ag(I) Cd(II), Co(II), Zn(II), Cr(VI), Pb(II), Ni(II), and Fe(III), evaluate metal toxicity by single and combined form (Futra et al., 2015).

For heavy metals detection metal resistance bacteria were used for the most part; for example, the *P. aeruginosa* BC15 used in microbial biosensor development. Because *P. aeruginosa* BC15 has the highest heavy metal resistance capacity it can resist 6 mM of cadmium (Edward Raja et al., 2008). This resistance capacity was obtained by the *cadR* [Cd(II)/Pb(II)-responsive transcriptional regulator] (Raja and Selvam, 2012) and *CadA* genes (cadmium-translocating P-type ATPase) (Yoon et al., 1991). The metalloprotein *cadR* is a cadmium-sensing regulatory protein, and has been used as a biological cadmium sensing element (Ivask et al., 2009; Wu et al., 2009) in whole-cell bacterial biosensors (Raja and Selvam, 2011; Hu-Chun Tao et al., 2013), and reporter gene as a reporter gene GFP. Corbisier et al. (1999) developed WCB using fluorescent protein as a reporter gene in this biosensor, with the sensing element as a promoter, that is, *cop*SRA promoter region used for copper detection and *mer* promoter used for mercury detection.

4.3.2.2 Bioluminescent Microbial Biosensors

Bioluminescence is a visible light emitted from a living organism, for instance, the glow of a firefly or jellyfish. The recombinant bacteria used as bioremedial treatment agents are single-celled organisms that don't glow naturally, but are modified by scientists to do so. The altered bacteria carry a reporter protein (Luciferin) and a sensor (Stocker et al., 2003). The natural bioluminescent bacteria can be principally sensitive to some environmental contaminants (such as industrial heavy metal wastes, pesticides) and therefore their response to normal functioning conditions does not reflect the eminence of the microbial community responsible for treatment (Charrier et al., 2010). Moreover, the salt dependence of the marine bioluminescent bacteria, and the temperature sensitivity of some strains, further complicates their use in the construction of whole-cell genetically modified bioluminescent biosensors and their immobilization for use in monitoring the toxicity of a complex industrial wastewater containing phenolic materials (Girotti et al., 2008).

Detection of heavy metals in the environment is a health and economic issue (Charrier et al., 2010). In order to assess heavy metals in polluted soil and the environment, the luminescent dependent *E. coli* WCB has been used (Hou et al., 2015). In this category of luminescent biosensors biological sensing elements are commonly metal responding protein or promoter from microorganisms. For example, the *zntR* (zinc-responsive transcriptional regulator) gene has been used in the detection of zinc [MC1061(pzntRluc)]; similarly, the *chrB* gene was used for the detection of chromate [AE104(pchrBluc)] (Ivask et al., 2002). As mentioned earlier, luminescent sensors harboring the firefly luciferase gene as a reporter have been used, with this reporter gene under the control of metal-inducible regulatory unit from metal resistance *E. coli* or from *Ralstonia metallidurans* (Ivask et al., 2002). Some of the luminescent biosensors are constructed for the detection of cadmium, lead, and antimony in the environment (Tauriainen et al., 1998). Recently, Soangra et al. (2015) have developed whole-cell bioluminescent biosensors for the determination of bioavailable arsenic in environment pollution. With whole-cell bioluminescent biosensors, the biological recognizing element is a microorganism and the transducer is the microilluminator. In the presence of metal (arsenic), the promoter gene (arsenic sensible promoter) can be activated and transcribed. In a recombinant cell, a metal recognizing promoter gene was fused with the reporter gene (*lux* gene) to produce luminescent response; this luminescent response is related to metal concentration. In some whole-cell microbial biosensors, σ-^{54} promoters [*ChrA* (chromate transport protein) promoter used biological chromate detection] were used as a sensing element for assessing biologically available heavy metals and promoter specificity was determined by bioluminescent (*luxCDABE*) reporter systems (Corbisier et al., 1999).

4.3.2.3 Colorimetric Microbial Biosensor

Colorimetric microbial biosensors make use of the changes in the color of the special compound to determine the concentration of the target analytes. Methyl parathion can be hydrolyzed by bacterium into a chromophoric product, PNP, which can be measured by a colorimetric method. For example, *Sphingomonas* bacterium was immobilized onto a polystyrene microplate surface for the construction of colorimetric microbial biosensors, which have the same linear range to pesticides, such as methyl parathion.

In recent years, a colorimetric biosensor was considered one of the most attractive and compatible methods of assessing soil and water pollution compared with other existing methods. A number of trials have been carried out in this field, such as a colorimetric biosensor for glucose, based on peroxidase-likeprotein-Fe_3O_4 (Magnetite) and GOD nanocomposites (Liu et al., 2014). Development of this colorimetric biosensor can produce several advantages, including sensing glucose, simplicity due to one-step detection, reusable enzymes (peroxidase mimic and oxidase), and high sensitivity. It is a fantastic technique that can be employed in detection of bacterial contamination. Pires et al. (2011) developed a colorimetric biosensor for the detection of pathogenic bacterial contamination (*Staphylococcus aureus* and *E. coli*) in apple juice. In this biosensor, vesicles (10,12-pentacosadyinoic acid–TDER, *N*-[(2-tetradecanamide)-ethyl]-ribonamide PCDA) have been used for color development. These surfactant-functionalized PDA vesicles have given the colorimetric response in the presence of bacterial substrates/metabolites. In order to identify the pathogens, such as *E. coli* O157:H7, *Salmonella typhimurium,* and *Listeria monocytogenes,* a simple paper-based analytical device (μPAD) was developed by Jokerst et al. (2012). The μPAD colorimetric microspot assay was carried out in wax printing on filter paper, making use of the reaction between pathogenic species associated enzymes and chromogenic substrates, and finally to produce the color. This color change indicates the presence of pathogenic strains in samples.

In some biosensors, colorimetric indicators have been used for detection of soil heavy metal contamination. For instance, prussian blue (PB) was used as an indicator for the detection of 3,5-dichlorophenol (DCP), As^{3+}, Cr^{6+}. In the *E. coli* respiration process to produce electrons, these electrons have been accepted by ferricyanide and to form ferrocyanide, which consequently reacts with ferric ions to yield the blue color due to the production of PB. However, this reaction or prussian blue formation amount can be affected by the existence of toxicants, such as 3,5-dichlorophenol, As^{3+} and Cr^{6+}. These phenomena have been used in the Zhai et al. (2013) colorimetric biosensor. The color change was identified by naked eye, which is one of the main advantages of this colorimetric biosensor. An enzyme-based colorimetric paper biosensor for heavy metal assessment was described by Zakir Hossain and Brennan (2011). An enzyme β-galactosidase (B-GAL) was fabricated by inkjet printing of solgel based bioinks that provide heavy metal ions detection, such as Hg(II), Ag(I), Cu(II), Cd(II), Pb(II), Cr(VI), and Ni(II).

5 Conclusions

A review of various monitoring techniques for heavy metals, pesticides, and pathogenic microorganism assessment shows that microbial biosensors have great potential for the monitoring of ecological toxicity in soil conditions. These microbial biosensors provide high sensitivity, economical use, relatively good accuracy, short experimental periods, as well as ease of use. Routine screening models for detection of metals and pesticides are time-consuming, require exhaustive sample preparation, are expensive, and can have poor selectivity. Advanced methods, such as antibody-based ELISA and DNA-based PCR techniques overcome these disadvantages but they require trained personnel and expensive instruments. Low detection limit and long-term stability are key factors for successful biosensing applications. Another challenge is that complex a environment matrix can produce strong interferences when detection of target analytes by biosensors.

Biosensors are devices that are easy to use without training, yield results in nearly real time with sensitivity and selectivity, comparable to the culture-based methods for microorganism detection. These microbial biosensor devices work with moderately complex target samples without the need for sample enrichment and without a major compromise on either sensitivity or selectivity. Most sensors for pathogen detection are dependent on the binding affinity of the antibodies to their specific antigens, which either deteriorate or change with time. Microbial biosensors should be used to minimize cost and time, and maximize monitoring soil conditions. In the future, more studies should be carried out utilizing smaller, low-cost biosensors, and more flexible biosensor techniques to promote large scale use in assessing soil conditions.

References

Abu-Qare, A.W., Abdel-Rahman, A.A., Ahmad, H., Kishk, A.M., Abou-Donia, M.B., 2001. Absorption, distribution, metabolism and excretion of daily oral doses of [^{14}C]methyl parathion in hens. Toxicol. Lett. 125, 1–10.

Adams, S.V., Newcomb, P.A., White, E., 2012. Dietary cadmium and risk of invasive postmenopausal breast cancer in the VITAL cohort. Cancer Causes Control 23, 845–854.

Aleem, A., Isar, J., Malik, A., 2003. Impact of long-term application of industrial wastewater on the emergence of resistance traits in Azotobacter chroococcum isolated from rhizospheric soil. Bioresour. Technol. 86, 7–13.

Allman, R., Manchee, R., Lloyd, D., 1993. Flow cytometric analysis of heterogeneous bacterial populations. In: Lloyd, D. (Ed.), Flow Cytometry in Microbiology. Springer Verlag, London, pp. 27–47.

Alpat, S,., Alpat, S.K., Çadirci, B.H., Yaşa, I., Telefoncu, A., 2008. A novel microbial biosensor based on Circinella sp. modified carbon paste electrode and its voltammetric application. Sens. Actuat. 134, 175–181.

Anu Prathap, M.U., Chaurasia, A.K., Sawant, S.N., Apte, S.K., 2012. Polyaniline-based highly sensitive microbial biosensor for selective detection of lindane. Anal. Chem. 84, 6672–6678.

Arkhypova, V.N., Dzyadevych, S.V., Soldatkin, A.P., El'skaya, A.V., Jaffrezic-Renault, N., Jaffrezic, H., Martelet, C., 2001. Multibiosensor based on enzyme inhibition analysis for determination of different toxic substances. Talanta 55, 919–927.

Ayenimo, J.G., Adeloju, S.B., 2015. Inhibitive potentiometric detection of trace metals with ultrathin polypyrrole glucose oxidase biosensor. Talanta 137, 62–70.

Babkina, S.S., Ulakhovich, N.A., 2004. Amperometric biosensor based on denatured DNA for the study of heavy metals complexing with DNA and their determination in biological, water and food samples. Bioelectrochemistry 63, 261–265.

Bai, Y., Zhou, L., Wang, J., 2006. Organophosphorus pesticide residues in market foods in foodchem. Food Chem. 98, 240–242.

Batista, B.L., Rodrigues, J.L., Nunes, J.A., Tormen, L., Curtius, A.J., Barbosa, Jr., F., 2008. Simultaneous determination of Cd, Cu, Mn, Ni, Pb and Zn in nail samples by inductively coupled plasma mass spectrometry (ICP-MS) after tetramethylammonium hydroxide solubilization at room temperature: comparison with ETAAS. Talanta 76 (3), 575–579.

Beck, R., Burtscher, H., 1994. Expression of human placental alkaline phosphatase in *Escherichia coli*. Protein Expr. Purif. 5, 192–197.

Belkin, S., 2003. Microbial whole-cell sensing systems of environmental pollutants. Curr. Opin. Microbiol. 6, 206–212.

Berezhetskyy, A.L., Sosovska, O.F., Durrieu, C., Chovelon, J.-M., Dzyadevych, S.V., TranMinh, C., 2008. Alkaline phosphotase conductometric biosensor for heavy metal ions determination. ITBM-RBM 29, 136–140.

Bernhoft, R.A., 2013. Cadmium toxicity and treatment. Sci. World J. 2013, 394652.

Bettinelli, M., Beone, G., Spezia, S., Baffi, C., 2000. Determination of heavy metals in soils and sediments by microwave-assisted digestion and inductively coupled plasma optical emission spectrometry analysis. Anal. Chim. Acta 424, 289–296.

Billard, P., DuBow, M.S., 1998. Bioluminescence-based assays for detection and characterization of bacteria and chemicals in clinical laboratories. Clin Biochem. 31, 1–14.

Benson, H.A., McElnay, J.C., 1987. High-performance liquid chromatography assay for the measurement of benzydamine hydrochloride in topical pharmaceutical preparations. J. Chromatogr 394 (2), 395–399.

Bonazzi, D., Andrisano, V., Gatti, R., Cavrini, V., 1995. Analysis of pharmaceutical creams: a useful approach based on solid-phase extraction (SPE) and UV spectrophotometry. J. Pharm. Biomed. Anal. 13, 1321–1329.

Bontidean, I., Berggren, C., Johansson, G., Csöregi, E., Mattiasson, B., Lloyd, J.R., Jakeman, K.J., Brown, N.L., 1998. Detection of heavy metal ions at femtomolar levels using protein-based biosensors. Anal. Chem. 70, 4162–4169.

Bontidean, I., Ahlqvist, J., Mulchandani, A., Chen, W., Bae, W., Mehra, R.K., Mortari, A., Csöregi, E., 2003. Novel synthetic phytochelatin-based capacitive biosensor for heavy metal ion detection. Biosens. Bioelectron. 18, 547–553.

Brainina, Kh., Stozhko, N.Yu., Belysheva, G.M., Inzhevatova, O.V., Kolyadina, L.I., Carlo Cremisini, 2004. Determination of heavy metals in wines by anodic stripping voltammetry with thick-film modified electrode. Anal. Chim. Acta 514 (2), 227–234.

Bronstein, I., Fortin, J.J., Voyta, J.C., Juo, R.R., Edwards, B., Olesen, C.E., 1994. Chemiluminescent reporter gene assays: sensitive detection of the GUS and SEAP gene products. Biotechniques 17, 172–174.
Bromage, E.S., Vadas, G.G., Harvey, E., Unger, M.A., Kaattari, S.L., 2007. Validation of an antibody-based biosensor for rapid quantification contamination in ground water and river water. Environ. Sci. Technol 41 (20), 7067–7072.
Byrne, B., Stack, E., Gilmartin, N., Kennedy, R.O., 2009. Antibody-Based Sensors: principles, problems and potential for detection of pathogens and associated toxins. Sensors 9, 4407–4445.
Cagnin, S., Caraballo, M., Guiducci, C., Martini, P., Ross, M., Santaana, M., Danley, D., West, T., Lanfranchi, G., 2009. Overview of electrochemical DNA biosensors: new approaches to detect the expression of life. Sensors 9, 3122–3148.
Chahal, V., Nagpal, a, Pakade, Y.B., Katnoria, J.K., 2014. Ecotoxicological studies of soil using analytical and biological methods: a review. Int. J. Biol. Agric. 8, 292–308.
Chandra, P.N., Noha, H.B., Wonb, M.S., Shim, Y.B., 2011. Bioelectrochemistry fundamentals, experimental techniques and applications. Biosens. Bioelectron. 26, 4442–4449.
Charrier, T., Durand, M.J., Affi, M., Jouanneau, S., 2010. Bacterial bioluminescent biosensor characterisation for on-line monitoring of heavy metals pollutions in waste water treatment plant effluents. Biosensors, 181–206.
Chen, Q., Fung, Y., 2010. Capillary electrophoresis with immobilized quantum dot fluorescence detection for rapid determination of organophosphorus pesticides in vegetables. Electrophoresis 31, 3107–3114.
Chen, M., Xu, P., Zeng, G., Yang, C., Huang, D., Zhang, J., 2015. Bioremediation of soils contaminated with polycyclic aromatic hydrocarbons, petroleum, pesticides, chlorophenols and heavy metals by composting: applications, microbes and future research needs. Biotechnol. Adv. 33, 745–755.
Chiou, C.T., Shoup, T.D., Porter, P.E., 1985. Mechanistic roles of soil humus and minerals in the sorption of nonionic organic compounds from aqueous and organic solutions. Org. Geochem. 8, 9–14.
Chouteau, C., Dzyadevych, S., Chovelon, J.-M., Durrieu, C., 2004. Development of novel conductometric biosensors based on immobilised whole cell Chlorella vulgaris microalgae. Biosens. Bioelectron. 19, 1089–1096.
Chouteau, C., Dzyadevych, S., Durrieu, C., Chovelon, J.M., 2005. A bi-enzymatic whole cell conductometric biosensor for heavy metal ions and pesticides detection in water samples. Biosens. Bioelectron. 21, 273–281.
Clark, L., Lyons, C., 1962. Electrode systems for continuous monitoring in cardiovascular surgery. Ann NY Acad Sci. 102, 29–45.
Clement, R.E., Yang, P.W., Koester, C.J., 1997. Environmental analysis. Anal. Chem. 69, 251R–287R.
Coen, N., Mothersill, C., Kadhim, M., Wright, E.G., 2001. Heavy metals of relevance to human health induce genomic instability. J. Pathol. 195, 293–299.
Connell, D.W., Fung, C.N., Minh, T.B., Tanabe, S., Lam, P.K.S., Wong, B.S.F., Lam, M.H.W., Wong, L.C., Wu, R.S.S., Richardson, B.J., 2003. Risk to breeding success of fish-eating Ardeids due to persistent organic contaminants in Hong Kong: evidence from organochlorine compounds in eggs. Water Res. 37, 459–467.
Conroy, P.J., Hearty, S., Leonard, P., O'Kennedy, R.J., 2009. Antibody production, design and use for biosensor-based applications. Semin. Cell Dev. Biol. 20, 10–26.
Cope, W.G., 2004. Exposure classes, toxicants in air, water, soil, domestic and occupational settings. A Textb. Mod. Toxicol., 31–48.

Corbisier, P., van der Lelie, D., Borremans, B., Provoost, A., de Lorenzo, V., Brown, N., Lloyd, J., Hobman, J., Csöregi, E., Johansson, G., Mattiasson, B., 1999. Whole cell- and proteine-based biosensor for the detection of bioavailable heavy metals in environmental samples. Anal. Chim. Acta 387, 235–244.

Cormack, B.P., Valdivia, R.H., Falkow, S., 1996. FACS-optimized mutants of the green fluorescent protein (GFP). Gene 173, 33–38.

Cuypers, A., Plusquin, M., Remans, T., Jozefczak, M., Keunen, E., Gielen, H., Opdenakker, K., Nair, A.R., Munters, E., Artois, T.J., Nawrot, T., Vangronsveld, J., Smeets, K., 2010. Cadmium stress: an oxidative challenge. BioMetals 23, 927–940.

D'Souza, S.F., Souza, S.F.D., 2001. Microbial biosensors. Biosens. Bioelectron. 16, 337–353.

Dailey, O.D., 2004. Volatilization of alachlor from polymeric formulations. J. Agric. Food Chem. 52, 6742–6746.

Darnley, A.G., Björklund, A., Bølviken, B., Gustavsson, N., Koval, P.V., Plant, J.A., Steenfelt, A., Tauchid, M., Xie, Xuejing., 1995. A global geochemical database for environmental and resource management. Recommendations for International Geochemical Mapping. Final report of IGCP project 259, UNESCO Publishing.

Debnárová, A., Weissmannová, H.D., 2011. Assessment of heavy metal pollution (Cd, Cu, Pb, Hg) in urban soils of roadsides in brno. Trans. Transp. Sci. 3, 147–156.

Delagrave, S., Hawtin, R.E., Silva, C.M., Yang, M.M., Youvan, D.C., 1995. Red-shifted excitation mutants of the green fluorescent protein. Biotechnology 13, 151–154.

Delvigne, F., Brognaux, A., Francis, F., Twizere, J.C., Gorret, N., Sorensen, S.J., Thonart, P., 2011a. Green fluorescent protein (GFP) leakage from microbial biosensors provides useful information for the evaluation of the scale-down effect. Biotechnol. J. 6, 968–978.

Delvigne, F., Brognaux, A., Gorret, N., Neubauer, P., Delafosse, A., Collignon, M.L., Toye, D., Crine, M., Boxus, M., Thonart, P., 2011b. Characterization of the response of GFP microbial biosensors sensitive to substrate limitation in scale-down bioreactors. Biochem. Eng. J. 55, 131–139.

Dibenzofurans, P., 2003. Open dumping site in Asian developing countries: a potential source of polychlorinated dibenzo-p-dioxins and polychlorinated dibenzofurans. Environ. Sci. Technol. 37 (8), 1493–1502.

Ding, J., Lei, J., Gong, J., Qin, W., 2014. Potentiometric aptasensing of *Listeria monocytogenes* using protamine as an indicator. Anal Chem. 86, 9412–9416.

Dreassi, E., Ceramelli, G., Corti, P., Massacesi, M., Perruccio, P.L., 1995. Quantitative Fourier transform near-infrared spectroscopy in the quality control of solid pharmaceutical formulations. Analyst 120, 2361.

Du, D., Huang, X., Cai, J., Zhang, A., 2007. Comparison of pesticide sensitivity by electrochemical test based on acetylcholinesterase biosensor. Biosens. Bioelectron. 23, 285–289.

Du, D., Ding, J., Tao, Y., Chen, X., 2008. Application of chemisorption/desorption process of thiocholine for pesticide detection based on acetylcholinesterase biosensor. Sens. Actuat. 134, 908–912.

Durrieu, C., Badreddine, I., Daix, C., 2003. A dialysis system with phytoplankton for monitoring chemical pollution in freshwater ecosystems by alkaline phosphatase assay. J. Appl. Phycol. 15, 289–295.

Duruibe, J.O., Ogwuegbu, M.O.C., Egwurugwu, J.N., 2007. Heavy metal pollution and human biotoxic effects. Int. J. Phys. Sci. 5, 112–118.

Dzyadevych, S.V., Soldatkin, A.P., Chovelon, J.M., 2002. Assessment of the toxicity of methyl parathion and its photodegradation products in water samples using conductometric enzyme biosensors. Anal. Chim. Acta 459, 33–41.

Edward Raja, C., Sasikumar, S., Selvam, G.S., 2008. Adaptive and cross resistance to cadmium (II) and zinc (II) by *Pseudomonas aeruginosa* BC15. Biologia 63, 461–465.

Edwards, F.L., Tchounwou, P.B., 2005. Environmental research and public health environmental toxicology and health effects associated with methyl parathion exposure—a scientific review. Environ. Toxicol. 2, 430–441.

El-Didamony, A.M., 2008. Spectrophotometric determination of benzydamine HCl, levamisole HCl and mebeverine HCl through ion-pair complex formation with methyl orange. Spectrochim. Acta—Part A 69, 770–775.

Errampalli, D., Leung, K., Cassidy, M.B., Kostrzynska, M., Blears, M., Lee, H., 1999. Applications of the green fluorescent protein as a molecular marker in environmental microorganisms. J. Microbiol. Methods 35 (3), 187–199.

Feng, K., Yu, B.Y., Ge, D.M., Wong, M.H., Wang, X.C., Cao, Z.H., 2003. Organo-chlorine pesticide (DDT and HCH) residues in the Taihu Lake Region and its movement in soil—water system I. Field survey of DDT and HCH residues in ecosystem of the region 50, 683–687.

Futra, D., Heng, L.Y., Ahmad, A., Surif, S., Ling, T.L., 2015. An optical biosensor from green fluorescent *Escherichia coli* for the evaluation of single and combined heavy metal toxicities. Sensors 15 (6), 12668–12681.

Garba, S.T., Ahmed, I., Akan, J.C., Dauda, B.A., 2014. Distribution pattern of the heavy metals: Pb, Zn, Cd, and Cu in roadside soils of Maiduguri Metropolis, Borno State Nigeria. Int Res J Pure Appl Chem. 4 (5), 486.

Gehring, A.G., Patterson, D.L., Tu, S., 1998. Use of a Light-Addressable Potentiometric Sensor for the Detection of *Escherichia coli* O157: H7 1. Anal. Biochem. 298, 293–298.

Gerbersdorf, S.U., Cimatoribus, C., Class, H., Engesser, K.-H., Helbich, S., Hollert, H., Lange, C., Kranert, M., Metzger, J., Nowak, W., Seiler, T.-B., Steger, K., Steinmetz, H., Wieprecht, S., 2015. Anthropogenic Trace Compounds (ATCs) in aquatic habitats—research needs on sources, fate, detection and toxicity to ensure timely elimination strategies and risk management. Environ. Int. 79, 85–105.

Ghanavati, M., Azad, R.R., Mousavi, S.A., 2014. Amperometric inhibition biosensor for the determination of cyanide. Sensors Actuators 190, 858–864.

Gimeno-García, E., Andreu, V., Boluda, R., 1996. Heavy metals incidence in the application of inorganic fertilizers and pesticides to rice farming soils. Environ. Pollut. 92, 19–25.

Girotti, S., Ferri, E.N., Fumo, M.G., Maiolini, E., 2008. Monitoring of environmental pollutants by bioluminescent bacteria. Anal. Chim. Acta 608, 2–29.

Gisbert, C., Ros, R., De Haro, A., Walker, D.J., Bernal, M.P., Serrano, R., Navarro-Aviñó, J., 2003. A plant genetically modified that accumulates Pb is especially promising for phytoremediation. Biochem. Biophys. Res. Commun. 303, 440–445.

Gong, Z.M., Tao, S., Xu, F.L., Dawson, R., Liu, W.X., Cui, Y.H., Cao, J., Wang, X.J., Shen, W.R., Zhang, W.J., Qing, B.P., Sun, R., 2004. Level and distribution of DDT in surface soils from Tianjin. China Chemosphere 54, 1247–1253.

Gonzalaez, M., Miglioranza, K.S., Aizpun, J.E., Isla, F.I., Pena, A., 2010. Assessing pesticide leachate and desorption in soils with different agricultural activities from Argentina (Pampa and Patagonia). Chemosphere 81, 351–358.

Greer, L.F., Szalay, A.A., 2002. Imaging of light emission from the expression of luciferases in living cells and organisms: a review. Luminescence 17, 43–74.

Grieshaber, D., MacKenzie, R., Vörös, J., Reimhult, E., 2008. Electrochemical biosensors—sensor principles and architectures. Sensors 8, 1400–1458.

Gu, M.B., Mitchell, R.J., Kim, B.C., 2004. Whole-cell-based biosensors for environmental biomonitoring and application. Adv. Biochem. Eng. Biotechnol. 87, 269–305.

Guerin, T.F., 2001. Environmental monitoring in soil contamination and remediation programs: how practitioners are using the Internet to share knowledge. J. Environ. Monit. 3, 267–273.
Guilbault, G.G., Montalvo, J.G., 1969. A Urea-specific enzyme electrode. J. Am. Chem. Soc. 91, 2164.
Guo, X., 2012. Surface plasmon resonance based biosensor technique: a review. J. Biophotonics 5, 483–501.
Gutierrez, J.C., Amaro, F., Martin-Gonzalez, A., 2015. Heavy metal whole-cell biosensors using eukaryotic microorganisms: an updated critical review. Front. Microbiol., 6.
Hakkila, K., Maksimow, M., Karp, M., Virta, M., 2002. Reporter genes lucFF, luxCDABE, gfp, and dsred have different characteristics in whole-cell bacterial sensors. Anal. Biochem. 301, 235–242.
Halloran, J.O., Walsh, A.R., Fitzpatrick, P.J., 1997. The determination of trace elements in biological and environmental samples using atomic absorption spectroscopy. Sheehan, D. (Ed.), Methods in Biotechnology, Bioremediation Protocols, vol. 2, Humana Press, New Jersey, pp. 201–211.
Hao, H., Sun, B., Zhao, Z., 2008. Effect of land use change from paddy to vegetable field on the residues of organochlorine pesticides in soils. Environ. Pollut. 156, 1046–1052.
Hasan, A., Morshed, M., Paul, A., Polini, A., Kuila, T., Hariri, M.Al, Lee, Y., Jaffa, A.A., 2014. Recent advances in application of biosensors in tissue engineering. Biomed. Res. Int. 2014, 307519.
Hassan, S.H.A., Ginkel, S.W. Van, Oh, S., 2012. Detection of Cr^{6+} by the sulfur oxidizing bacteria biosensor: effect of different physical factors. Environ. Sci. Technol. 46 (14), 7844–7848.
Hauser, T.R., Hinners, T.A., Kent, J.L., 1972. Atomic absorption determination of cadmium and lead in whole blood by a reagent-free method. Anal. Chem. 44 (11), 1819–1821.
Heim, R., Tsien, R.Y., 1996. Engineering green fluorescent protein for improved brightness, longer wavelengths and fluorescence resonance energy transfer. Curr. Biol. 6, 178–182.
Hiromitsu, S., Noriaki, K., Hirotoshi, T., Hiroshi, H., 1991. Determination of heavy metal ions by urea sensor using ISFET. Sens. Mater. 2, 217–227.
Hobson, N.S., Tothill, I., Turner, A.P.F., 1996. Microbial detection. Biosens. Bioelectron. 11, 455–477.
Hooijschuur, E.W.J., Hulst, A.G., De Jong, A.L., De Reuver, L.P., Van Krimpen, S.H., Van Baar, B.L.M., Wils, E.R.J., Kientz, C.E., Brinkman, U.A.T., 2002. Identification of chemicals related to the chemical weapons convention during an interlaboratory proficiency test. Trends Anal. Chem. 21, 116–130.
Hou, Q., Ma, A., Wang, T., Lin, J., Wang, H., Du, B., Zhuang, X., Zhuang, G., 2015. Detection of bioavailable cadmium, lead, and arsenic in polluted soil by tailored multiple *Escherichia coli* whole-cell sensor set. Anal. Bioanal. Chem. 407, 6865–6871.
Huang, W., Gao, L., Gong, A., Li, C., Wang, P., Fu, S., Xiao, K., Zhang, B., Liu, W., 2010. Determination of trace organochlorine pesticides in soil using isotope dilution-high resolution gas chromatography. Se Pu. 28, 460–464.
Hu-Chun Tao., Peng, Z., Li, P., Yu, T., Su, J., 2013. Optimizing cadmium and mercury specificity of CadR-based *E. coli* biosensors by redesign of CadR. Biotechnol. Lett. 8, 1253–1258.
Hudson, L.N., Newbold, T., Contu, S., Hill, S.L.L., Lysenko, I., Palma, D., Phillips, H.R.P., Senior, R.A., Bennett, D.J., Booth, H., Garon, M., Michelle, L., Correia, D.L.P., Day, J., Echeverr, S., Harrison, K., Ingram, D.J., Jung, M., Kemp, V., Kirkpatrick, L., Callum, D., Pan, Y., White, H.J., Aben, J., Abrahamczyk, S.,

Adum, G.B., Armbrecht, I., Azhar, B., Bates, A.J., Bayne, E.M., Beja, P., Banks, E., Barlow, J., Buczkowski, G., Buscardo, E., Cabra-garc, J., Cameron, S.A., Cancello, E.M., Carrijo, T.F., Carvalho, A.L., Castro-luna, A.A., Cerda, R., Cerezo, A., Chauvat, M., Darvill, B., Dauber, J., Dejean, A., Diek, T., Giordani, P., Giordano, S., Gottschalk, M.S., Goulson, D., Aaron, D., Grogan, J., Hanley, M.E., Hanson, T., Hashim, N.R., Joseph, E., Helden, A.J., Hern, L., Herzog, F., Higuera-diaz, D., Hilje, B., Horgan, F.G., Horv, R., Hylander, K., Isaacs-cubides, P., Ishitani, M., Jacobs, C.T., J., V., Jauker, B., Jonsell, M., Jung, T.S., Kapoor, V., Kati, V., Lantschner, V., F., V. Le, Lebuhn, G., Jean-philippe, L., Louhaichi, M., Mallari, A., Marin-spiotta, E., Marshall, E.J.P., Mart, E., Muchane, M.N., Muchane, M., Naidoo, R., Nakamura, A., Naoe, S., Fernando, A.B., 2014. The PREDICTS database: a global database of how local terrestrial biodiversity responds to human impacts. Ecol. Envol. 4 (24), 4701–4735.

Hashimah Bt Hussain, 1990. Determination of lead, chromium and mercury in industrial effluents (waste water). Inst. Teknol. Mara, Malaysia.

Ilangovan, R., Daniel, D., Krastanov, A., Zachariah, C., Elizabeth, R., 2006. Enzyme based biosensor for heavy metal ions determination. Biotechnol. Biotechnol. 20 (1), 184–189.

Ion, A.C., Ion, I., Culetu, A., Gherase, D., Moldovan, C.A., Iosub, R., Dinescu, A., 2010. Acetylcholinesterase voltammetric biosensors based on carbon nanostructure—chitosan composite material for organophosphate pesticides. Mater. Sci. Eng. 30, 817–821.

Ivask, A., Virta, M., Kahru, A., 2002. Construction and use of specific luminescent recombinant bacterial sensors for the assessment of bioavailable fraction of cadmium, zinc , mercury, and chromium in the soil. Soil Biol. Biochem. 34, 1439–1447.

Ivask, A., Rõlova, T., Kahru, A., 2009. A suite of recombinant luminescent bacterial strains for the quantification of bioavailable heavy metals and toxicity testing. BMC Biotechnol. 9, 41.

Ivnitski, D., Abdel-Hamid, I., Atanasov, P., Wilkins, E., 1999. Biosensors for detection of pathogenic bacteria. Biosens. Bioelectron. 14, 599–624.

Jaffrezic-renault, N., Dzyadevych, S.V., 2008. Conductometric microbiosensors for environmental monitoring. Sensors 8 (4), 2569–2588.

Jokerst, J.C., Adkins, J.A., Bisha, B., Mentele, M.M., Goodridge, L.D., Henry, C.S., 2012. Development of a paper-based analytical device for colorimetric detection of select foodborne pathogens. Anal. Chem. 84 (6), 2900–2907.

Joyner, D.C., Lindow, S.E., 2000. Heterogeneity of iron bioavailability on plants assessed with a whole-cell GFP-based bacterial biosensor. Microbiology 146, 2435–2445.

Kalam, A., Latifah, A., 2014. Genetically engineered organisms for bioremediation of pollutants in contaminated sites. Chin. Sci. Bull. 59, 703–714.

Kanissery, R.G., Sims, G.K., 2011. Biostimulation for the enhanced degradation of herbicides in soil. Appl. Environ. Soil Sci. 2011, 1–10.

Karri, S.K., Saper, R.B., Kales, S.N., 2008. Lead encephalopathy due to traditional medicines. Curr. Drug Saf. 3, 54–59.

Kaur, H., Kumar, R., Babu, J.N., Mittal, S., 2015. Advances in arsenic biosensor development—a comprehensive review. Biosens. Bioelectron. 63, 533–545.

Khalil, M.M., Issa, Y.M., Korany, M.A., 2015. Potentiometric determination of Benzydamine hydrochloride using PVC membrane and coated wire sensors in pure form, pharmaceutical compounds and biological fluids. Int. J. Eng. Res. General Sci. 3 (1), 2091–2730.

Kim, M., Lim, J.W., Kim, H.J., Lee, S.K., Lee, S.J., Kim, T., 2015. Chemostat-like microfluidic platform for highly sensitive detection of heavy metal ions using microbial biosensors. Biosens. Bioelectron. 65, 257–264.

King, J.M., Digrazia, P.M., Applegate, B., Burlage, R., Sanseverino, J., Dunbar, P., Larimer, F., Sayler, G.S., 1990. Rapid, sensitive bioluminescent reporter technology for naphthalene exposure and biodegradation. Science 249, 778–781.

Köhler, S., Belkin, S., Schmid, R.D., 2000. Reporter gene bioassays in environmental analysis. Fresenius J. Anal. Chem. 366, 769–779.

Krajewska, B., 1991. Urease immobilized on chitosan membrane. Inactivation by heavy metal ions. J. Chem. Technol. Biotechnol. 52, 157–162.

Kumar, J., D'Souza, S.F., 2011. Microbial biosensor for detection of methyl parathion using screen printed carbon electrode and cyclic voltammetry. Biosens. Bioelectron. 26, 4289–4293.

Kumar, J., Jha, S.K., D'Souza, S.F., 2006. Optical microbial biosensor for detection of methyl parathion pesticide using Flavobacterium sp. whole cells adsorbed on glass fiber filters as disposable biocomponent. Biosens. Bioelectron. 21, 2100–2105.

Lakherwal, D., 2014. Adsorption of Heavy Metals: a review. Int. J. Environ. Res. Dev. 4, 41–48.

Laschi, S., Ogon´czyk, D., Palchetti, I., Mascini, M., 2007. Evaluation of pesticide-induced acetylcholinesterase inhibition by means of disposable carbon-modified electrochemical biosensors. Enzyme Microb. Technol. 40, 485–489.

Lazcka, O., Campo, F.J.Del, Muñoz, F.X., 2007. Pathogen detection: a perspective of traditional methods and biosensors. Biosens. Bioelectron. 22, 1205–1217.

Lei, Y., Mulchandani, P., Wang, J., Chen, W., Mulchandani, A., 2005. Highly sensitive and selective amperometric microbial biosensor for direct determination of *p*-nitrophenyl-substituted organophosphate nerve agents. Environ. Sci. Technol. 39, 8853–8857.

Li, G., Liu, N., Liu, S., Zhang, S., 2008. Electrochemical biosensor based on the interaction between copper(II) complex with 4,5-diazafluorene-9-one and bromine ligands and deoxyribonucleic acid. Electrochim. Acta 53, 2870–2876.

Liao, J.C., Mastali, M., Li, Y., Gau, V., Suchard, M.A., Babbitt, J., Gornbein, J., Landaw, E.M., McCabe, E.R.B., Churchill, B.M., Haake, D.A., 2007. Development of an advanced electrochemical DNA biosensor for bacterial pathogen detection. J. Mol. Diagn. 9, 158–168.

Lihan, T., Rahim, S.A., Kadir, A.A., 2006. Physico-chemical characteristics of soil at Western part of Pulau Indah, Klang, Selangor. Sains Malays 35, 23–30.

Lim, M.J.K.L.S., Kim, D., Joe, M.-H., Lee, K.-H., Lim, S.-Y., Im, S.-H., Song, H.-P., Lee, I.S., Kim, D., 2012. Pigment-based whole-cell biosensor system for cadmium detection using genetically engineered *Deinococcus radiodurans*. Bioprocess. Biosyst. Eng. 35, 265–272.

Lindsay, W.L., Schwab, A.P., 1982. The chemistry of iron in soils and its availability to plants. J. Plant Nutr. 5, 821–840.

Liu, Y., Yuan, M., Qiao, L., Guo, R., 2014. An efficient colorimetric biosensor for glucose based on peroxidase-like protein-Fe_3O_4 and glucose oxidase nanocomposites. Biosens. Bioelectron. 52, 391–396.

Lloyd, D., 1993. Flow Cytometry in Microbiology. Springer-Verlag London Limited, Germany, pp. 188.

Loganathan BG, K.K., 1994. Global organochlorine contamination trends: an overview. Ambio 23, 187–191.

Long, F., Zhu, A., Shi, H., Wang, H., Liu, J., 2013a. Rapid on-site/in-situ detection of heavy metal ions in environmental water using a structure-switching DNA optical biosensor. Sci. Rep. 3, 2308.

Long, F., Zhu, A., Shi, H., 2013b. Recent advances in optical biosensors for environmental monitoring and early warning. Sensors 13 (10), 13928–13948.

López Rodriguez, M.L., Benimeli, C., Madrid, R.E., Giacomelli, C.E., 2015. A simple Streptomyces spore-based impedimetric biosensor to detect lindane pesticide. Sens. Actuat. 207, 447–454.

Magrisso, S., Erel, Y., Belkin, S., 2008. Microbial reporters of metal bioavailability. Microb. Biotechnol. 1, 320–330.

Maisto, G., Manzo, S., De Nicola, F., Carotenuto, R., Rocco, A., Alfani, A., 2011. Assessment of the effects of Cr, Cu, Ni, and Pb soil contamination by ecotoxicological tests. J. Environ. Monit. 13, 3049.

Malik, A., 2004. Metal bioremediation through growing cells. Environ. Int. 30, 261–278.

Man, Y.B., Chow, K.L., Wang, H.S., Lau, K.Y., Sun, X.L., Wu, S.C., Cheung, K.C., Chung, S.S., Wong, M.H., 2011. Health risk assessment of organochlorine pesticides with emphasis on DDTs and HCHs in abandoned agricultural soils. J. Environ. Monit. 13, 2250–2259.

Mani, D., Kumar, C., 2014. Biotechnological advances in bioremediation of heavy metals contaminated ecosystems: an overview with special reference to phytoremediation. Int. J. Environ. Sci. Technol. 11, 843–872.

Manutsewee, N., Aeungmaitrepirom, W., Varanusupakul, P., Imyim, A., 2007. Determination of Cd, Cu, and Zn in fish and mussel by AAS after ultrasound-assisted acid leaching extraction. Food Chem. 101, 817–824.

Meer, J.R.Van Der, Belkin, S., 2010. Where microbiology meets microengineering: design and applications of reporter bacteria. Nat. Publ. Gr. 8, 511–522.

Megharaj, M., Boul, H.L., Thiele, J.H., 1999. Effects of DDT and its metabolites on soil algae and enzymatic activity. Biol. Fertil. Soils 29, 130–134.

Meng, J.H., Zhao, S.H., Doyle, M.P., Kresovich, S., 1996. Polymerase chain-reaction for detecting *E. coli* 0157:H7. Intl. J. Food Microbiol. 32 (1–2), 103–113.

Mohammadi, H., Amine, A., Cosnier, S., Mousty, C., 2005. Mercury-enzyme inhibition assays with an amperometric sucrose biosensor based on a trienzymatic-clay matrix. Anal. Chim. Acta 543, 143–149.

Moore, J.T., Davis, S.T., Dev, I.K., 1997. The development of [beta]-Lactamase as a highly versatile genetic reporter for eukaryotic cells. Anal. Biochem. 247, 203–209.

Moyo, M., Okonkwo, J.O., Agyei, N.M., 2014. An amperometric biosensor based on horseradish peroxidase immobilized onto maize tassel-multi-walled carbon nanotubes modified glassy carbon electrode for determination of heavy metal ions in aqueous solution. Enzyme Microb. Technol. 56, 28–34.

Mulchandani, A., Mulchandani, P., Chauhan, S., Kaneva, I., Chen, W., 1998. A potentiometric microbial biosensor for direct determination of organophosphate nerve agents. Electroanalysis 10, 733–737.

Nishitani, A., Tsukamoto, Y., Kanda, S., Imai, K., 1991. Determination of the fluorescent drugs dipyridamole and benzydamine in rat plasma by liquid chromatography with peroxyoxalate chemiluminescence detection. Anal. Chim. Acta 251, 247–253.

Odaci, D., Timur, S., Telefoncu, A., 2009. A microbial biosensor based on bacterial cells immobilized on chitosan matrix. Bioelectrochemistry 75, 77–82.

Oh, S.E., Hassan, S.H.A., Van Ginkel, S.W., 2011. A novel biosensor for detecting toxicity in water using sulfur-oxidizing bacteria. Sen. Actuat 154, 17–21.

Orazio, P.D., 2011. Clinica Chimica Acta Biosensors in clinical chemistry. Clin. Chim. Acta 412, 1749–1761.

Oyekunle, J.A.O., Ogunfowokan, A.O., Torto, N., Akanni, M.S., 2011. Determination of organochlorine pesticides in the agricultural soil of Oke-Osun farm settlement, Osogbo. Nigeria. Environ. Monit. Assess. 177, 51–61.

Paitan, Y., Biran, I., Shechter, N., Biran, D., Rishpon, J., Ron, E.Z., 2004. Monitoring aromatic hydrocarbons by whole cell electrochemical biosensors. Anal. Biochem. 335, 175–183.

Park, J.O., El-Tarabily, K.A., Ghisalberti, E.L., Sivasithamparam, K., 2002. Pathogenesis of Streptoverticillium albireticuli on *Caenorhabditis elegans* and its antagonism to soil-borne fungal pathogens. Lett. Appl. Microbiol. 35, 361–365.

Parkinson, G., Pejcic, B., 2005. Using Biosensors to Detect Emerging Infectious Diseases. Nanochemistry Research Institute, Curtin University of Technology Perth, Perth, Australia.

Perumal, V., Hashim, U., 2014. Advances in biosensors: principle, architecture and applications. J. Appl. Biomed. 12, 1–15.

Philp, J.C., Balmand, S., Hajto, E., Bailey, M.J., Wiles, S., Whiteley, A.S., Lilley, A.K., Hajto, J., Dunbar, S.A., 2003. Whole cell immobilised biosensors for toxicity assessment of a wastewater treatment plant treating phenolics-containing waste. Anal. Chim. Acta 487, 61–74.

Pieper, S.B., Mestas, S.P., Lear, K.L., Zhong, Z., Reardon, K.F., 2008. Phosphorescence characteristics of ruthenium complex as an optical transducer for biosensors. Appl. Phys. Lett. 92, 5–7.

Pinto, M.M.S.C., Ferreira, E., Silva, M.M.V.G., Melo-gonçalves, P., 2015. Heavy metals of Santiago Island (Cape Verde) top soils: estimated background value maps and environmental risk assessment. J. African Earth Sci. 101, 162–176.

Pires, A.C.D.S., Soares, N.D.F.F., da Silva, L.H.M., da Silva, M.D.C.H., De Almeida, M.V., Le Hyaric, M., Andrade, N.J.De, Soares, R.F., Mageste, A.B., Reis, S.G., 2011. A colorimetric biosensor for the detection of foodborne bacteria. Sens. Actuat. 153, 17–23.

Pirvutoiu, S., Ciucu, A., Magearu, V., Surugiu, I., Dey, E.S., Danielsson, B., Abu-Qare, A.W., Abdel-Rahman, A.A., Ahmad, H., Kishk, A.M., Abou-Donia, M.B., Mohammadi, H., Amine, A., Cosnier, S., Mousty, C., Edwards, F.L., Tchounwou, P.B., Wu, J., Lin, L., Luan, T., Chan Gilbert, Y.S., Lan, C., Pieper, S.B., Mestas, S.P., Lear, K.L., Zhong, Z., Reardon, K.F., Fan, H., Ju, P., Ai, S., Oyekunle, J.A.O., Ogunfowokan, A.O., Torto, N., Akanni, M.S., García-Martinez, G., Bustabad, E.A., Perrot, H., Gabrielli, C., Bucur, B., Lazerges, M., Rose, D., Rodriguez-Pardo, L., Fariña, J., Compère, C., Vives, A.A., Syam, R., Davis, K.J., Pratheesh, M.D., Anoopraj, R., Joseph, B.S., Singh, R., Matharu, Z., Srivastava, A.K., Sood, S., Gupta, R.K., Malhotra, B.D., Li, G., Liu, N., Liu, S., Zhang, S., Grieshaber, D., MacKenzie, R., Vörös, J., Reimhult, E., 2008. Determination of organochlorine pesticides in the agricultural soil of Oke-Osun farm settlement, Osogbo, Nigeria. Sensors 177, 98–104.

Prodromidis, M.I., Karayannis, M.I., 2002. Enzyme based amperometric biosensors for food analysis. Electroanalysis 14, 241–261.

Rahmi, D., Zhu, Y., Fujimori, E., Umemura, T., Haraguchi, H., 2007. Multielement determination of trace metals in seawater by ICP-MS with aid of down-sized chelating resin-packed minicolumn for preconcentration. Talanta 72, 600–606.

Raja, C.E., Selvam, G.S., 2011. Construction of green fluorescent protein based bacterial biosensor for heavy metal remediation. Int. J. Environ. Sci. Technol. 8, 793–798.

Raja, C.E., Selvam, G.S., 2012. Characterization of chromosomal mediated cadmium resistance in *Pseudomonas aeruginosa* strain BC15. J. Basic Microbiol. 52, 175–183.

Ramanathan, S., Ensor, M., Daunert, S., 1997. Bacterial biosensors for monitoring toxic metals. Trends Biotechnol. 15, 500–506.

Ravenscroft, P., Brammer, H., Richards, K., 2009. Arsenic pollution: a global synthesis. first ed. Royal Geographical Society, Wiley Blackwell, New York.

Reshetilov, A.N., Iliasov, P.V., Reshetilova, T.A., 2010. The Microbial Cell Based Biosensors. In: Somerset, V.S. (Ed.), Intelligent and Biosensors. InTech, New York.

Robbens, J., Maras, M., Laureyn, W., De Coen, W., 2005. Whole cell biosensors for (Eco) toxicity screening: alternatives for the future. Nanotech 1, 497–500.

Roberto, F.F., Barnes, J.M., Bruhn, D.F., 2002. Evaluation of a GFP reporter gene construct for environmental arsenic detection. Talanta 58, 181–188.

Rogers, K.R., 2006. Recent advances in biosensor techniques for environmental monitoring. Anal. Chim. Acta 568, 222–231.

Ron, E.Z., 2007. Biosensing environmental pollution. Curr. Opin. Biotechnol. 18, 252–256.

Rowe-Taitt, C.A., Golden, J.P., Feldstein, M.J., Cras, J.J., Hoffman, K.E., Ligler, F.S., 2000. Array biosensor for detection of biohazards. Biosens. Bioelectron. 14, 785–794.

Sagarkar, S., Nousiainen, A., Shaligram, S., Björklöf, K., Lindström, K., Jørgensen, K.S., Kapley, A., 2014. Soil mesocosm studies on atrazine bioremediation. J. Environ. Manage. 139, 208–216.

Saha, J.K., Sharma, A.K., Srivastava, A., 2014. Impact of different types of polluted irrigation water on soil fertility and wheat grain yield in clayey black soils of central India. Env. Monit. Assess 186, 2349–2356.

Sakrabani, R., Deeks, L.K., Kibblewhite, M.G., Ritz, K., 2012. Impacts of agriculture upon soil quality. Environ. Impacts Mod. Agric. 34, 35–56.

Samarth, D.P., Chandekar, C.J., Kaustubh, R., 2012. Biosorption of heavy metals from aqueous solution using *Bacillus licheniformis*. Int. J. Pure Appl. Sci. Technol. 10, 12–19.

Sancho, E., Villarroel, M.J., Fernández, C., Andreu, E., Ferrando, M.D., 2010. Short-term exposure to sublethal tebuconazole induces physiological impairment in male zebrafish (Danio rerio). Ecotoxicol. Environ. Saf. 73, 370–376.

Santamaría, J., Toranzos, G.A., 2003. Enteric pathogens and soil: a short review. Int. Microbiol. 6, 5–9.

Saxena, V., Malhotra, B.D., 2003. Electrochemical biosensors. In: Malhotra, B.D., Turner, A.P.F. (Eds.), Advances in Biosensors: Perspectives In Biosensor. JAI Press, Stamford, pp. 63–100.

Selifonova, O., Burlage R, B.T., 1993. Bioluminescent sensors for detection of bioavailable Hg(II) in the environment. Appl. Environ. Microbiol. 59, 3083–3090.

Shamshuddin, J., Fauziah, C.I., Anda, M., Kapok, J., Shazana, M.aR.S., 2011. Using ground basalt and/or organic fertilizer to enhance productivity of acid soils in Malaysia for crop production. Malaysian J. Soil Sci. 15, 127–146.

Sharma, H., Mutharasan, R., 2013. Review of biosensors for foodborne pathogens and toxins. Sensors Actuators 183, 535–549.

Sharma, H., Agarwal, M., Goswami, M., Sharma, A., Roy, S.K., Rai, R., Murugan, M.S., 2013. Biosensors: tool for food borne pathogen detection. Vet. World 6, 968–973.

Shazili, N.A.M., Yunus, K., Ahmad, A.S., Abdullah, N., Rashid, M.K.A., 2006. Heavy metal pollution status in the Malaysian aquatic environment. Aquat. Ecosyst. Health Manag. 9, 137–145.

Shi, J., Wang, H., Xu, J., Wu, J., Liu, X., Zhu, H., Yu, C., 2007. Spatial distribution of heavy metals in soils: a case study of Changxing, China. Environ. Geol. 52, 1–10.

Shitanda, I., Takada, K., Sakai, Y., Tatsuma, T., 2005. Amperometric biosensing systems based on motility and gravitaxis of flagellate algae for aquatic risk assessment. Anal. Chem. 77, 6715–6718.

Singh, R., Dhand, C., Sumana, G., Verma, R., 2010. Polyaniline/carbon nanotubes platform for sexually transmitted disease detection. J. Mol. Recognit. 23 (5), 472–479.

Singh, R., Matharu, Z., Srivastava, A.K., Sood, S., Gupta, R.K., Malhotra, B.D., 2012a. Nanostructured platform for the detection of Neisseria gonorrhoeae using electrochemical impedance spectroscopy and differential pulse voltammetry. Microchim. Acta 177, 201–210.

Singh, R., Verma, R., Sumana, G., Srivastava, A.K., Sood, S., Gupta, R.K., Malhotra, B.D., 2012b. Nanobiocomposite platform based on polyaniline-iron oxide-carbon nanotubes for bacterial detection. Bioelectrochemistry 86, 30–37.

Singh, R., Mukherjee, M.Das, Sumana, G., Gupta, R.K., Sood, S., Malhotra, B.D., 2014. Biosensors for pathogen detection: a smart approach towards clinical diagnosis. Sens. Actuat. 197, 385–404.

Sneh, B., Katan, J., Abdul-raziq, A., 1983. Chemical control of soil-borne pathogens in tuff medium for strawberry cultivation. Pest Manage. Sci. 14 (2), 119–122.

Soangra, R., Majumder, C.B., Roy, P., 2015. Whole Cell Arsenic Biosensor- A Cheap Technology for Bioavailable Arsenic (As) Determination. Eur. J. Advances Eng. Technol. 2, 52–61.

Soldatkin, A.P., Hendjz, A.M.N., Jaffrezic-renault, N., 1994. Conductometric biosensors based on cholinesterases for sensitive detection of pesticides. Electroanalysis 6 (9), 752–758.

Soldatkin, A.P., Dzyadevich, S.V., Korpan, Y.I., Arkhipova, V.N., Zhylyak, G.A., Piletsky, S.A., Sergeeva, T.A., Panasyuk, T.L., El'skaya, A.V., 1998. Biosensors based on conductometric detection. Biopolymers Cell. 14, 268–277.

Soldatkin, O.O., Kucherenko, I.S., Pyeshkova, V.M., Kukla, A.L., Jaffrezic-Renault, N., El'skaya, A.V., Dzyadevych, S.V., Soldatkin, A.P., 2012. Novel conductometric biosensor based on three-enzyme system for selective determination of heavy metal ions. Bioelectrochemistry 83, 25–30.

Sperveslage, J., Stackebrandt, E., Lembke, F.W., Koch, C., 1996. Detection of bacterial contamination, including Bacillus spores, in dry growth media and in milk by identification of their 16S rDNA by polymerase chain reaction. J. Microbiol. Methods 26, 219–224.

Stepurska, K.V., Kucherenko, I.S., Arkhypova, V.M., 2015. Feasibility of application of conductometric biosensor based on acetylcholinesterase for the inhibitory analysis of toxic compounds of different nature. Anal. Chim. Acta 854, 161–168.

Stiner, L., Halverson, L.J., 2002. Development and characterization of a green fluorescent protein-based bacterial biosensor for bioavailable toluene and related compounds. Appl. Environ. Microbiol. 68, 1962–1971.

Stocker, J., Balluch, D., Gsell, M., Harms, H., Feliciano, J., Daunert, S., Malik, K.A., Van der Meer, J.R., 2003. Development of a set of simple bacterial biosensors for quantitative and rapid measurements of arsenite and arsenate in potable water. Environ. Sci. Technol. 37, 4743–4750.

Strosnider, H., 2003. Whole-Cell Bacterial Biosensors and the Detection of Bioavailable Arsenic. U.S. Environmental Protection Agency, Washington, DC.

Su, L., Jia, W., Hou, C., Lei, Y., 2011. Microbial biosensors: a review. Biosens. Bioelectron. 26, 1788–1799.

Bala Swaminathan, Feng, P., 1994. Rapid detection of food-borne pathogenic bacteria. Annu. Rev. Microbiol. 48, 401–426.

Syam, R., Davis, K.J., Pratheesh, M.D., Anoopraj, R., Joseph, B.S., 2012. Biosensors: a novel approach for pathogen detection. Vetscan 7, 14–18.

Szittner, R., Meighen, E., 1990. Nucleotide sequence, expression, and properties of luciferase coded by lux genes from a terrestrial bacterium. J. Biol. Chem. 265, 16561–16587.

Tallury, P., Malhotra, A., Byrne, L.M., Santra, S., 2010. Nanobioimaging and sensing of infectious diseases. Adv. Drug Deliv. Rev. 62, 424–437.

Tauriainen, S., Karp, M., Chang, W., Virta, M., 1998. Luminescent bacterial sensor for cadmium and lead 13, 931–938.

Taylor, P., Goron, T.L., Raizada, M.N., 2014. Critical Reviews in Plant Sciences Current and Future Transgenic Whole-Cell Biosensors for Plant Macro—and Micronutrients. Crit. Rev. Plant Sci. 33, 393–413.

Tkac, J., Vostiar, I., Gemeiner, P., Sturdik, E., 2002. Monitoring of ethanol during fermentation using a microbial biosensor with enhanced selectivity. Bioelectrochemistry 56, 127–129.

Togo, C.A., Wutor, V.C., Limson, J.L., Pletschke, B.I., 2007. Novel detection of *Escherichia coli* beta-D-glucuronidase activity using a microbially-modified glassy carbon electrode and its potential for faecal pollution monitoring. Biotechnol. Lett. 29 (4), 531–537.

Torres-Chavolla, E., Alocilja, E.C., 2009. Aptasensors for detection of microbial and viral pathogens. Biosens. Bioelectron. 24, 3175–3182.

Torres Padrón, M.E., Sosa Ferrera, Z., Santana Rodríguez, J.J., 2006. Optimisation of solid-phase microextraction coupled to HPLC-UV for the determination of organochlorine pesticides and their metabolites in environmental liquid samples. Anal Bioanal 386 (2), 332–340.

Tuzen, M., Saygi, K.O., Soylak, M., 2008. Solid phase extraction of heavy metal ions in environmental samples on multiwalled carbon nanotubes. J. Hazard. Mater. 152, 632–639.

Valdman, E., Erijman, L., Pessoa, F.L.P., Leite, S.G.F., 2001. Continuous biosorption of Cu and Zn by immobilized waste biomass *Sargassum* sp. Process Biochem. 36, 869–873.

Van Geest, J.L., Burridge, L.E., Fife, F.J., Kidd, K.A., 2014. Feeding response in marine copepods as a measure of acute toxicity of four anti-sea lice pesticides. Mar. Environ. Res. 101, 145–152.

Van Wezel, A., Mons, M., van Delft, W., 2010. New methods to monitor emerging chemicals in the drinking water production chain. J. Environ. Monit. 12, 80–89.

Venugopal, V., 2002. Biosensors in fish production and quality control. Biosens. Bioelectron. 17, 147–157.

Verma, N., Kumar, S., Kaur, H., 2011. Whole cell based disposable biosensor for Cadmium detection in milk. Biotecnology 10, 259–266.

Viswanathan, S., Radecka, H., Radecki, J., 2009. Electrochemical biosensor for pesticides based on acetylcholinesterase immobilized on polyaniline deposited on vertically assembled carbon nanotubes wrapped with ssDNA. Biosens. Bioelectron. 24, 2772–2777.

Vollenhofer-Schrumpf, S., Buresch, R., Unger, G., Stahl, N., Frnzl, G., Schinkingfr, M., 2005. Detection of *Salmonella* spp., *Escherichia coli* O157, Listeria monocytogenes and *Campylobacter* spp. in chicken samples by multiplex polymerase chain reaction and hybridization using the GeneGen major food pathogens detection kit. J. Rapid Methods Autom. Microbiol 13, 148–176.

Wang, J., 1985. Stripping Analysis: Principles, Instrumentation and Applications. VCH Publishers Inc, Florida, pp. 1–160.

Wang, Y., Xu, H., Zhang, J., Li, G., 2008. Electrochemical sensors for clinic analysis. Sensors 8, 2043–2081.

Wang, S., Zhang, D., Pan, X., 2012. Effects of arsenic on growth and photosystem II (PSII) activity of *Microcystis aeruginosa*. Ecotoxicol. Environ. Saf. 84, 104–111.

Wang, X., Liu, M., Wang, X., Wu, Z., Yang, L., Xia, S., Chen, L., Zhao, J., 2013. P-benzoquinone-mediated amperometric biosensor developed with *Psychrobacter* sp. for toxicity testing of heavy metals. Biosens. Bioelectron. 41, 557–562.

Wang, X., Lu, X., Chen, J., 2014. Development of biosensor technologies for analysis of environmental contaminants. Trends Environ. Anal. Chem. 2, 25–32.

Ward Willium, W., Cody, C.W., Harv, Russell Hart, C., Milton, J.C., 1980. Research note spectrophotometric identity of the energy transfer chromophores in renilla and aeq uorea green-fluorescent proteins. Photochem. Photobiol 31.

Watson, L.D., Maynard, P., Cullen, D.C., Sethi, R.S., Lowe, J.B., C.R., 1987. A microelectronic conductimetric biosensor. Biosensors 3, 101–115.

Watts, H.J., Lowe, C.R., Pollard-Knight, D.V., 1994. Optical biosensor for monitoring microbial cells. Anal. Chem. 66, 2465–2470.

Weissenfels, W.D., Klewer, H., Langhoff, J., 1992. Applied microbiology biotechnology adsorption of polycyclic aromatic hydrocarbons (PAHs) by soil particles: influence on biodegradability and biotoxicity. Appl. Microbiol. Biotechnol., 689–696.

West, S.E.H., Schweizer, H.P., Dall, C., Sample, A.K., Runyen-Janecky, L.J., 1994. Construction of improved *Escherichia-Pseudomonas* shuttle vectors derived from pUC18/19 and sequence of the region required for their replication in *Pseudomonas aeruginosa*. Gene 148, 81–86.

Wong, M.H., Leung, A.O.W., Chan, J.K.Y., Choi, M.P.K., 2005. A review on the usage of POP pesticides in China, with emphasis on DDT loadings in human milk. Chemosphere 60, 740–752.

Wong, L.S., Lee, Y.H., Surif, S., 2013. Whole cell biosensor using anabaena torulosa with optical transduction for environmental toxicity evaluation. J. Sensors 2013, 1–8.

Woutersen, M., Belkin, S., Brouwer, B., Van Wezel, A.P., Heringa, M.B., 2011. Are luminescent bacteria suitable for online detection and monitoring of toxic compounds in drinking water and its sources? Anal. Bioanal. Chem. 400, 915–929.

Wu, J., Lin, L., Luan, T., Sing, Y., Gilbert, C., Lan, C., 2007. Effects of organophosphorus pesticides and their ozonation byproducts on gap junctional intercellular communication in rat liver cell line 45, 2057–2063.

Wu, C.H., Le, D., Mulchandani, A., Chen, W., 2009. Optimization of a whole-cell cadmium sensor with a toggle gene circuit. Biotechnol. Prog 25, 898–903.

Xue, X., Wei, Q., Wu, D., Li, H., Zhang, Y., Feng, R., Du, B., 2014. Determination of methyl parathion by a molecularly imprinted sensor based on nitrogen doped graphene sheets. Electrochim. Acta 116, 366–371.

Yagi, K., 2007. Application of whole-cell bacterial sensors in biotechnology and environmental science. Appl. Microbiol. Biotechnol. 73, 1251–1258.

Yang, X., Kirsch, J., Simonian, A., 2013. *Campylobacter* spp. detection in the 21st century: a review of the recent achievements in biosensor development. J. Microbiol. Methods 95, 48–56.

Yin, X.X., Wang, L.H., Bai, R., Huang, H., Sun, G.X., 2012. Accumulation and transformation of arsenic in the blue-green alga *Synechocysis* sp. PCC6803. Water Air Soil Pollut. 223, 1183–1190.

Yoon, K.P., Misra, T.K., Silver, S., 1991. Regulation of the cadA cadmium resistance determinant of *Staphylococcus aureus* plasmid pI258. J. Bacteriol. 173, 7643–7649.

Yu, L., Mulchandani, P., Wang, J., Chen, W., Mulchandani, A., 2005. Highly Sensitive and selective amperometric microbial biosensor for direct determination of p-nitrophenyl-substituted organophosphate nerve agents. Environ. Sci. Technol. 39, 8853–8857.

Nurul Syazani Yuswir, S.M.P., Aris, A.Z., Ismail, S.N.S., Hashim, Z., 2015. Health risk assessment of heavy metal in urban surface soil. Bull. Environ. Contam. Toxicol.

Zakir Hossain, S.M., Brennan, J.D., 2011. β-Galactosidase-based colorimetric paper sensor for determination of heavy metals. Anal. Chem 83 (22), 8772–8778.

Zelada-Guillén, G.A., Bhosale, S.V., Riu, J., Rius, F.X., 2010. Real-time potentiometric detection of bacteria in complex samples. Anal. Chem. 82, 9254–9260.

Zhai, J., Yong, D., Li, J., Dong, S., 2013. A novel colorimetric biosensor for monitoring and detecting acute toxicity in water. Analyst 138, 702–707.

Zhang, F., Keasling, J., 2011. Biosensors and their applications in microbial metabolic engineering. Trends Microbiol. 19, 323–329.

Zhang, H.B., Luo, Y.M., Zhao, Q.G., Wong, M.H., Zhang, G.L., 2006. Residues of organochlorine pesticides in Hong Kong soils. Chemosphere 63, 633–641.

Zhang, J., Luo, A., Liu, P., Wei, S., Wang, G., Wei, S., 2009. Detection of organophosphorus pesticides using potentiometric enzymatic membrane biosensor based on methylcellulose immobilization. Anal. Sci. 25, 511–515.

Zhang, Q., Ding, J., Kou, L., Qin, W., Remediation, E., 2013. A Potentiometric flow biosensor based on ammonia-oxidizing bacteria for the detection of toxicity in water. Sensors 13, 6936–6945.

Zhao, X., Lin, C.-W., Wang, J., Oh, D.H., 2014a. Advances in rapid detection methods for foodborne pathogens. J. Microbiol. Biotechnol. 24, 297–312.

Zhao, Y., Wang, C., Xia, S., Jiang, J., Hu, R., Yuan, G., Hu, J., 2014b. Biosensor medaka for monitoring intersex caused by estrogenic chemicals. Environ. Sci. Technol. 48 (4), 2413–2420.

Zhu, Y., An, X., Li, S., Yu, S., 2009. Nanoencapsulation of β-cypermethrin by complex coacervation in a microemulsion. J. Surfactants Deterg. 12, 305–311.

Zhylyak, G.A., Dzyadevich, S.V., Korpan, Y.I., Soldatkin, a.P., El'skaya, a.V., 1995. Application of urease conductometric biosensor for heavy-metal ion determination. Sensors Actuators 24, 145–148.

FLOW ANALYSIS AS AN ANALYTICAL TOOL FOR SOIL MONITORING: FROM WET CHEMISTRY ASSAYS TO NANOMATERIALS BASED SAMPLE PREPARATION

Hugo M. Oliveira, António J.M. Fonseca, Ana R.J. Cabrita
REQUIMTE, LAQV, ICBAS, Institute of Biomedical Sciences Abel Salazar, University of Porto, Rua Jorge Viterbo Ferreira, Porto, Portugal

1 Introduction

The determination of the chemical parameters in soil samples delivers fundamental information about different aspects of the soils, from nutrition to contamination. For this reason, chemical monitoring of soils has been an important research topic over the last decades, where the evolution of analytical chemistry conducted by modern instrumentation has lead to readily available and high quality analytical information. Among the different breakthroughs in the analytical field, flow analysis has been a relevant tool for monitoring chemical parameters in soil samples. Flow analysis comprises a group of techniques used for automation purposes in the analytical laboratory (Trojanowicz, 2008; Kolev and Mckelvie, 2008; Cerdà et al., 2014) that combines the handling of liquids into a network made of tubing with internal diameters at the low millimetre level. Since the seminal paper of Ruzicka and Hansen (1975) introducing flow injection analysis (FIA), the concept of flow analysis has assimilated the progresses in science and technology, contributing for the establishment of a new analytical discipline devoted to the laboratory automation. Since a vast majority of the applications of flow analysis deals with wet-chemistry based assays (Hansen, 2015), it can be considered

New Pesticides and Soil Sensors. http://dx.doi.org/10.1016/B978-0-12-804299-1.00014-X

that the major breakthrough of flow analysis is the possibility of bypassing chemical equilibrium to obtain the chemical specie(s) that will be detected and converted in an analytical signal. This concept is not different from the flow chemistry definition that is currently a key approach in industrial chemical processes, due to the strict control reaction conditions in a predefined time frame (Darvas et al., 2014).

Under the conceptual point of view, all flow analysis techniques are based on the combination of three principles: (1) reproducible sample injection in a carrier/reagent stream, (2) controlled dispersion of the sample zone, and (3) reproducible timing from the injection point to the detection system (Ruzicka and Hansen, 1988). The readers should take in mind that these principles essentially consider the existence of a chemical process into the manifold, which may be absent, as we will see throughout this chapter. Analytical chemists and soil scientists have been taking advantage of these "precision" principles to implement a plethora of laboratory operations in a fully automatic fashion.

In a very simplified view, it is possible to compare the most basic single channel FIA setup with a liquid chromatography system where the separation column is absent. The basic components of a flow analysis system can be divided into three major categories (Fig. 13.1): (1) propulsion unit(s) (a device or a group of devices that ensure the propulsion of the solutions along the

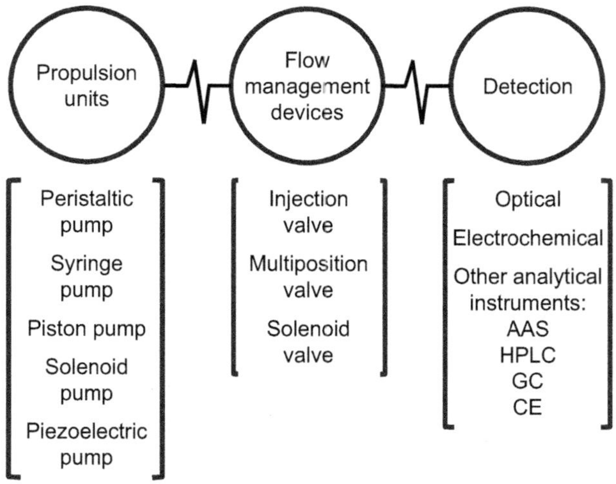

Figure 13.1. The typical components of a classic flow analysis manifold. Automatic systems usually comprise at least one item of each list connected by polymeric tubing. Other devices, such as solid-phase extraction columns, membrane holders (for gas-diffusion or pervaporation), mixing and/or dilution chambers may also be present.

manifold), (2) flow management device(s), which ensure the correct pathways of the liquids inside the manifold, and (3) a detection unit, able to provide the transduction into an analytical signal that can be further related with the concentration of an analyte under study. All these parts are connected by plastic [usually polytetrafluoroethylene (PTFE) or fluorinated ethylene propylene (FEP)] tubing with internal diameters up to 1.5 mm. Beyond this basic architecture, flow analysis manifolds can also include other devices necessary for the analytical operation [e.g., solid-phase extraction (SPE) columns, membrane separation devices, such as gas-diffusion, phase-separation, and dialysis units, filters]. Furthermore, the hyphenation of flow analysis with modern analytical instrumentation, such as atomic absorption spectrometry (AAS) (Gómez-Nieto et al., 2015) and inductively coupled plasma (ICP) (Rodriguez et al., 2015), or separation techniques, such as liquid (LC) (Oliveira et al., 2009) and gas-chromatography (GC) (Quintana et al., 2009), as well capillary electrophoresis (CE) (Horstkotte et al., 2008), has been described in the literature. More details about the coupling of flow analysis to modern analytical instrumentation can be found in reviews published elsewhere (Clavijo et al., 2015; Miró and Hansen, 2013; Miró et al., 2011)

From the chronological point of view, the evolution of flow analysis can be characterized by two major drivers: the downscale of analytical protocols (despite the original FIA concept can operate with very small sample volumes, commonly up to 500 μL), and the enhancement of the flexibility of the manifolds, which made possible the assembling of new devices capable to perform new unit operations that resulted in an expanded application scope of the techniques. The major developments in flow analysis are chronologically depicted in Fig. 13.2. It should be noted that the major differences among the techniques are essentially based on the introduction of new flow management strategies that could

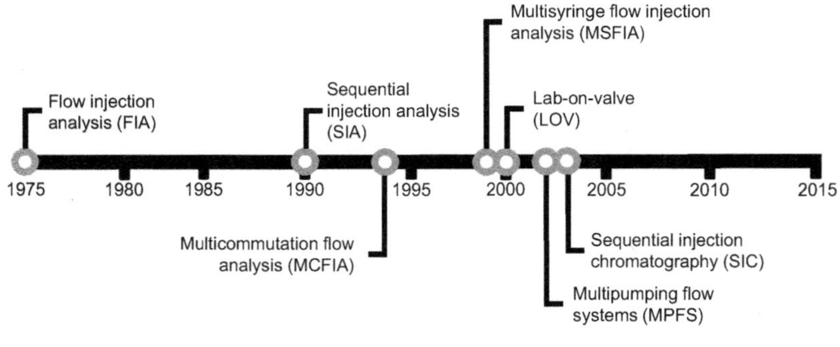

Figure 13.2. Timeline of the evolution flow analysis techniques.

have some advantages when compared with the previous ones. This fact essentially resulted from the use of new sample management devices and propulsion units. The exception to this evolution pattern was the sequential injection chromatography (SIC) (Šatínský et al., 2003) that introduced separation capabilities, typical from liquid chromatography, in a classic Sequential injection analysis (SIA) configuration.

The characterization of flow analysis techniques is essentially based on their ability to handle wet chemistry assays, which constitute the classic operation of these systems despite the same principles being also applied to other situations where chemical processes are absent.

FIA (Ruzicka and Hansen, 1975) is characterized by the use of multichannel peristaltic pumps that supply different unidirectional streams of reagents and carrier (Fig. 13.3A). The sample is inserted in the carrier stream and subsequently merged with reagents along the different sections of the manifold until the detector. For each method, the manifold has to be adjusted and reoptimized in order to comply with the chemistries that the user desires to implement. The original manifolds were manually operated (FIA is still the only flow technique that can be operated without computer control), but current commercially available instruments are fully computer controlled. This makes possible to apply different flow patterns, such as stopped flow or variable flow rates along the protocol sequence. In fact, FIA is currently one of workhorses for nutrient analysis in soils, regarding its compatibility with the classic chemistries of these assays, combined with the high sample throughput characteristic of these systems.

SIA (Ruzicka and Marshall, 1990) debuted the computer-controlled programmable flow and introduced two major features: bidirectional flow and an open architecture manifold. The basic configuration includes a syringe pump, a multiposition selection valve, and a detector. The flow management is ensured by a multiposition selector, which makes possible the introduction of small volumes (at the low microliter level) of solutions (and suspensions in some cases) and ensures the open architecture of SIA (Fig. 13.3B). The design of the valve makes the communication between the central channel and the different ports, where solutions or auxiliary devices can be placed, simple and straightforward. Sample and reagent(s) are sequentially aspirated into the holding coil [portion of tubing that connects the propulsion unit to the central channel of the valve (Fig. 13.3C, HC)]. After flow reversal, the previously stacked zones are directed to one of the lateral ports for additional processing or analyte detection. The sequential injection approach also introduced the widespread

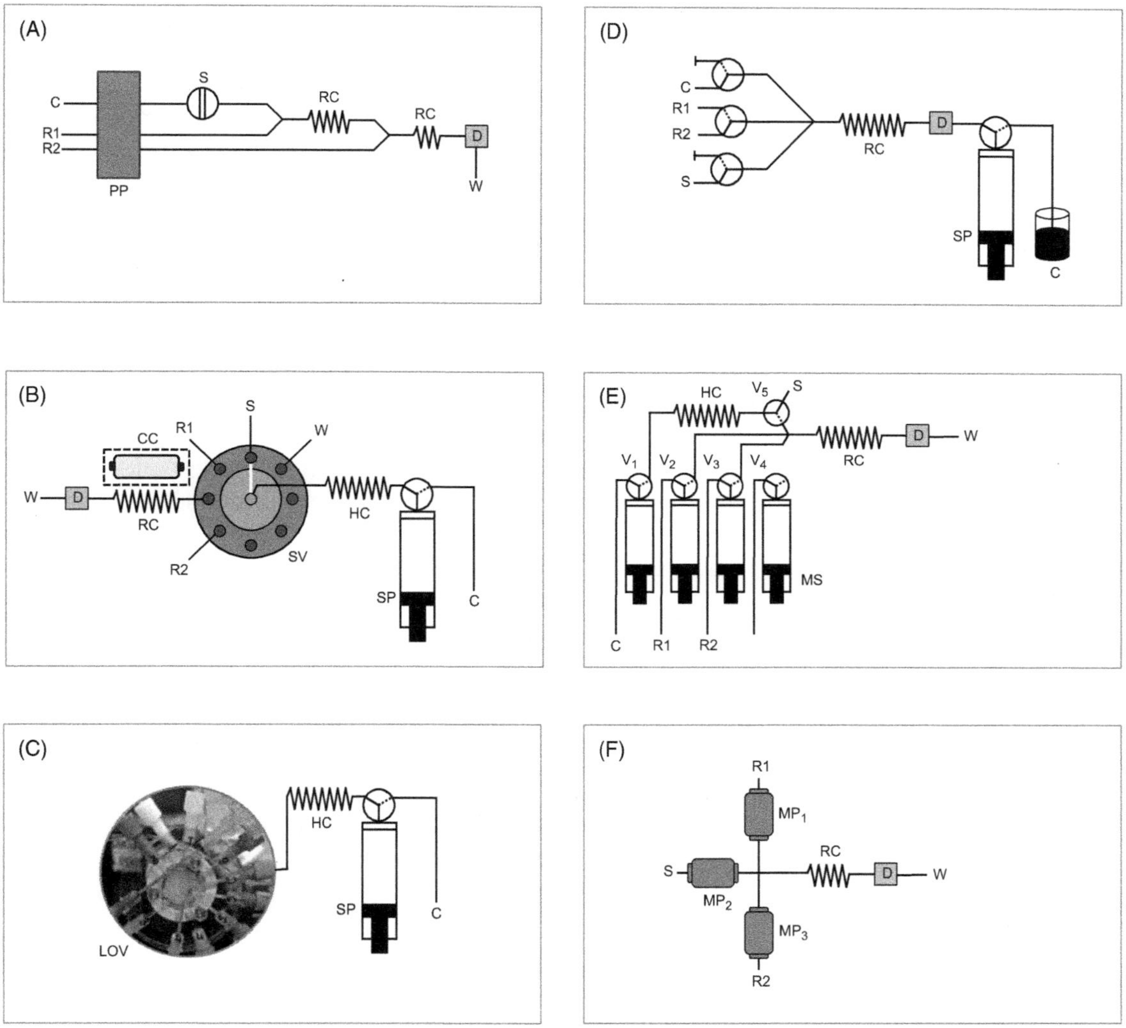

Figure 13.3. Typical configurations of the different flow analysis techniques and their respective acronyms. (A) Flow injection analysis (FIA), (B) sequential injection analysis (SIA) and sequential Injection chromatography (SIC), (C) microsequential injection lab-on-valve (μSI-LOV), (D) multicommutation flow injection analysis (MCFIA), (E) multisyringe flow injection analysis (MSFIA), and (F) multipumping flow system (MPFS). In scheme B, sequential injection chromatography *(SIC)* configuration corresponds to replacement of the reaction coil *(RC)* of sequential injection analysis *(SIA)* for a chromatographic column *(CC) (dashed line)*. C, carrier solution; R1, reagent 1; R2, reagent 2; S, sample; PP, peristaltic pump; RC, reaction coil; D, detector; W, waste; SP, syringe pump; HC, holding coil; SV, multiposition selection valve; CC, chromatographic column; LOV, lab-on-valve; V_i, three-way commutation valve; MS, multisyringe module; MP_i, micropump.

use of syringe pumps. This fact increased the robustness of the manifolds because these propulsion units avoid the use of flexible tubing that is present in peristaltic pumps and that are prone to fast deterioration under continuous operation of the instruments. Another key development introduced by SIA is the time-based injection. Flow rates and volumes are controlled by the software variables and not by the physical configuration of the manifold (e.g., in FIA the sample volume is controlled by the size of the loop placed at the injection valve and flow rate range is controlled not only by the pump rotation but also by the internal diameter of the flexible tubing of the peristaltic pump). In comparison with FIA, SIA commonly uses lower volumes of solutions, but also provides lower sample throughputs. Despite the single channel, SIA offers a very simple and flexible operation. However, it provides lower efficiency in the mixture of the different stacked zones, which can be troublesome when several plugs are involved in a chemical process.

The downscale of SIA lead to microsequential injection lab-on-valve (μSIA-LOV) concept (Ruzicka, 2000), which is a miniaturized version of SIA with important evolution features. The most relevant difference in this configuration is the existence of monolithic device containing a built-in detection unit mounted atop of the selection valve, the lab-on-valve (Fig. 13.3C). The LOV device is able to accommodate several configurations for different modes of optical detection (e.g., spectrophotometry (Lahdesmaki et al., 2009), fluorescence (Grand et al., 2011), and chemiluminescence (Oliveira et al., 2015)), and offer the possibility of handling solid suspensions at the microliter level, the so-called bead injection concept (Miró et al., 2008). Despite being originally developed to accommodate microscaled wet chemistry assays, the LOV has been showing unusual properties for the development of sample preparation protocols based on solid suspensions at the microliter level (Oliveira et al., 2011). Several examples of applications of these principles to sample preparation and hyphenation to modern analytical instrumentation can be found in recent review articles (Vidigal et al., 2013; Miró, 2014; Miró et al., 2011). Furthermore, the internal diameter of the channels (~1.6 mm) makes LOV a reliable and robust alternative to lab-on-chip microfluidics for the analysis of complex matrices (Miró and Hansen, 2007).

Beyond the abovementioned three generations of flow injection analysis (Hansen and Miró, 2007), other important evolutions of flow analysis were introduced, aiming a flexible and simple flow management. Two examples of this evolution are multicommutation flow analysis (MCFIA) (Reis et al., 1994) (Fig. 13.3D) and multisyringe flow injection analysis (MSFIA) (Cerdà et al., 1999) (Fig. 13.3E), which are based on the establishment of a "flow network." This flow network consists of an array of computer-controlled three-way commutation valves (V, Fig. 13.3D and E) connected to a propulsion unit. In the case of MCFIA, the propulsion unit is a syringe or peristaltic pump that ensure the unidirectional propulsion of the solutions to a detection system. Regarding MSFIA, the technique is based on a specific propulsion device, the multisyringe burette, which includes a set of four syringes driven by a single motor (Fig. 13.3E). At the top of each syringe, it is placed a three-way commutation valve. The multisyringe burette is also able to interface extra commutation valves in order to build the desired flow network. Due to its enhanced versatility (multichannel bidirectional flow) and enhanced chemical resistance (the syringe parts can easily handle organic solvents), MSFIA has been extensively used in protocols for sample preparation (Almeida et al., 2011; Segundo and Magalhães, 2006).

Multipumping flow systems (MPFS) (Lapa et al., 2002) are also under the umbrella of the "flow network" concept (Fig. 13.3F). Nevertheless, the configuration and manifold assembly of MPFS are substantially different from the other techniques. In this case, each solution has its own propelling device, a solenoid actuated micropump, which are combined in order to assemble the "flow network." In contrast to the laminar flow pattern found in other flow techniques, solenoid micropumps are able to produce a turbulent flow pattern (Fortes et al., 2009) that enhances mixing of the different solutions.

An important breakthrough in the development of flow analysis was the introduction of separation capabilities in the manifolds. SIC (Šatínský et al., 2003) (Fig. 13.3B) derived from advent of monolithic stationary phases for liquid chromatography (Guiochon, 2007), which made possible separation protocols where backpressure was compatible with the propulsion units commonly used in SIA. This added a novel selectivity dimension to flow analysis, with separation capabilities in some cases comparable with conventional liquid chromatography (Chocholouš et al., 2007). MSFIA also benefited from the same principles, leading to the introduction of multisyringe chromatography (Miguel et al., 2007). Additionally, the multichannel operation of the typical multisyringe manifolds also made possible to incorporate sample preparation (Maya et al., 2011; González et al., 2015) or postcolumn derivatization (Maya et al., 2011) steps. More recently, the introduction of core–shell columns increased the commercially available options for the development of high selective methodologies (Chocholouš et al., 2013).

This evolution of the flow techniques followed the evolution of technology, specially the computer control and the development of new software. It is difficult to consider one or other technique as the best one. Indeed, the recent developments have taken advantage of the combination among different techniques in order to minimize potential drawbacks and/or take full advantage of the main features. Flow techniques applied to the chemical monitoring of soil samples can be viewed in two complementary perspectives: as an analytical tool that can be applied in the routine analysis of different chemical parameters in soil matrices, or as a research tool able to expand our current view about soil analysis, especially by creating new possibilities in sample handling that may impact the further analytical determination, leading to an enhanced quality analytical information. In the latter case, the development of dynamic fractionation protocols is opening a complete new perspective for the concept of bioaccessibility of pollutants and it is creating a new panorama for pollutants monitoring regarding the timeframe of the analytical workflow when compared with the current batchwise methods (Rosende and Miró, 2013). Furthermore, the combination of nanostructured materials and flow analysis has been able to create new analytical methodologies with enhanced analytical performance.

In the analytical field, nanomaterials have been essentially applied to the enhancement of optical detection properties of some analytes (Frigerio et al., 2012), in the establishment of sensors (Valentini and Palleschi, 2008), and also in the development of new extraction protocols (Tian et al., 2013). Despite the widely reported use of nanomaterials with analytical purposes (Penn et al., 2003), their application in routine analysis is still scarce. This fact is motivated by the legal regulation that is behind the vast majority of these methods, and also due to the limited commercial-availability of some of these materials. Other important concern is also related with the toxicity of these materials and their global life cycles (Keller et al., 2013). In the particular case of soil analysis based on automated flow analysis methods, we observe a similar scenario. However, the mesofluidic scale and high precision flow control of flow analysis manifolds transform these techniques in versatile automation tools with high potential for handling nanomaterials with distinct physical and chemical properties (Passos et al., 2015).

Another relevant characteristic of flow analysis techniques is their potential to comply with green analytical chemistry principles (Gałuszka et al., 2013) Green analytical chemistry (Armenta et al., 2008) could be viewed as the application of the 12 green chemistry principles to the analytical field (Keith et al., 2007;

Anastas, 1999). These principles aim the reduction of the chemical risk through the minimization of hazards (Anastas, 1999). Nevertheless, flow analysis is able not only to downscale analytical procedures and thus minimizing chemicals consumption and waste disposal, but it is also able to operate in a closed circuit, minimizing risk to the analytical operator.

2 Monitoring of Soils Using Flow Analysis

The chemical information of soils is a key aspect to the knowledge of the correct level of nutrients as well of the contamination caused from anthropogenic and natural sources. Therefore, flow analysis techniques have been an important and widely used analytical tool for the chemical monitoring of soils in three complementary aspects: automation of wet chemistry assays, automation of sample preparation protocols, and automation of analytical protocols based on sensors.

Since the early times of FIA, a significant number of papers dealing with the analysis of soil samples, with a particular emphasis in the nutrients, can be found in the literature (Hansen, 2015). During the first decade of flow analysis, the new automated wet chemistry assays revolutionized all the protocols for the laboratorial analysis of soil extracts, with a particular impact in Brazil where a substantial part of these initial developments were performed (Batista et al., 2014). For example, the first generation of methodologies based on FIA made possible the generation of 120 measurements of available phosphate per hour using the molybdenum blue chemistry (Appelqvist et al., 1986). Flow injection analysis is currently a standard technique in soil laboratories due to the compliance with official methods and also due to its capacity of processing a high number of samples using reduced amounts of reagents per assay. After the establishment of these first generation of wet chemistry assays, the methodologies took advantage from the open architecture and miniaturization advances, moving toward more complexity through the addition of new sample preparation schemes (Fang, 1993).

In the present chapter, we intend to overview the recent developments of flow analysis based methodologies applied to the chemical analysis of soil samples (Fig. 13.4), with a particular emphasis on the actual and potential impact of nanotechnology in these determinations. Based on this background, we categorized our bibliography according to the main role of the assessed chemical species in the soil: nutrient or pollutant. In the latter case, we subdivided the section according to the organic or inorganic nature of the targeted analyte.

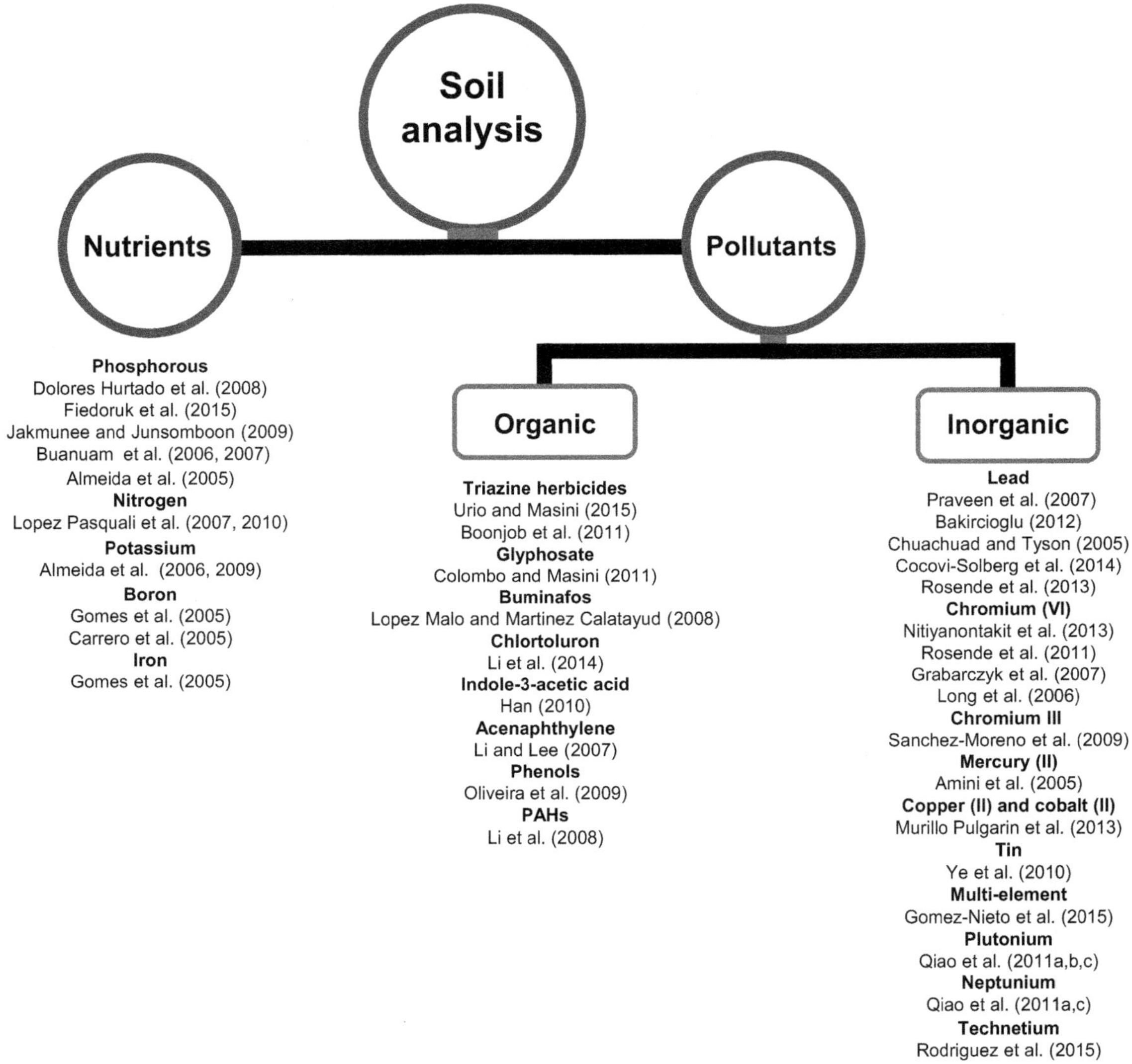

Figure 13.4. Selected applications of flow analysis for monitoring chemical species with nutritional and environmental interest reviewed in this chapter.

2.1 Nutrients

The monitoring of nutrients in soils is still a subject of interest for analytical chemists and soil scientists. In fact, to accurately supply the suitable amount of nutrients for crop growth it is important to have accurate estimations about the actual nutrient reserves of the soil. Therefore, monitoring soil nutrients is an essential component for developing an environmental management system, which comprises biophysical, economical, and socio-cultural aspects (Roy et al., 2003). Over the last decade, analytical methodologies based on flow analysis for the quantification of soil nutrients increased their degree of complexity, by incorporating innovative detection schemes and/or sample preparation features. Both macro and micronutrients for plants present in soils (White and Brown, 2010) were targeted by the recent developments, although macronutrients represent the most substantial part of the reports (Fig. 13.4).

Phosphorous (P), an essential macronutrient for plants that is present on soils (Jones, 2012) has still being one of the analytes targeted by the new methodologies developed during the last decade. All methodologies were essentially based on the reaction of molybdate and orthophosphate in acid solution that results in the formation of a yellow-colored phosphomolybdate complex (yellow chemistry). This complex can be further reduced by a reducing agent (e.g., ascorbic acid), which originates the final blue-colored product (blue chemistry) (Hansen and Miró, 2007). These compounds are detected by visible spectrophotometry at their maximum absorption wavelengths. Primary efforts were placed in the enhancement of the sensitivity of the assay, by using long optical path flow cells (40 mm) (Dolores Hurtado et al., 2008) or by adopting a fluorescence-based detection with a fluorometric paired emitter–detector diode (FPEDD) (Fiedoruk et al., 2015). The FPEDD detection principle required the use of two light emitting diodes (LED) as fluorescence inductors and one as detector of LED-induced fluorescence. In this latter case, the original molybdate blue chemistry was replaced by a fluorometric detection strategy based on the ion-pair formation between the yellow heteropolyacid and a fluorophore (rhodamine B) (Li et al., 2005). Based on the same chemical principles, amperometric detection based on the reduction of 12-molybdophosphate was also successfully used for the quantification of phosphate in soil extracts (Jakmunee and Junsomboon, 2009). This approach has some important advantages over the spectrophotometric methods since it worked in a broad concentration range, it avoided interferences from colored substances and colloids, and it also bypassed potential problems with the Schilieren effect that arises from the differences in the refractive index caused by the different composition of the zones delivered to the detector (Worsfold et al., 2005). Nevertheless, optical methods are still the most popular detection approach due to their widespread availability and easiness of use.

The other driver of the evolution of methodologies for the analysis of ortophosphate is sample preparation, including the direct handling of solid samples. The introduction of the dynamic sequential extraction, which is based on the consecutive addition of aliquots of extracting solution into the solid sample, could be considered the major breakthrough in flow-based soil analysis of the last decade. The hearth of this approach is the use of an extraction column that contains the sample under study. The biconical column has been playing a fundamental role in managing solid samples because it keeps the sample in a fluidized bed mode, which minimizes potential excessive backpressure during the extraction process (Chomchoei et al., 2004). This extraction column approach has been used for the simultaneous fractionation and determination of bioaccessible ortophosphate in soil samples (Buanuam et al., 2006, 2007; Fiedoruk et al., 2015). All developed methodologies adopted the Hieltjes–Lijklema (HL) scheme (Hieltjes and Lijklema, 1980), comprising the sequential use of 1.0 mol L^{-1} NH_4Cl, 0.1 mol L^{-1} NaOH and 0.5 mol L^{-1} HCl as leaching reagents. The HL scheme was also compared with the SMT (Standards, Measurements and Testing Program of the European Commission) scheme (Rauret et al., 1999), and showed enhanced phase resolution for the readily mobilizable elements (Buanuam et al., 2006). The same authors (Buanuam et al., 2007) also reported a critical comparison between HL and SMT extraction schemes. They showed that regarding the use of more aggressive leachants by the SMT method, it was not possible to determine the fraction of the labile inorganic phosphorous, which is the primary source for plant uptake. In any case, automation leads to a substantial reduction in the amount of reagent consumption and waste disposal when these assays were compared with similar batch and continuous-flow protocols (Table 13.1). MSFIA was also applied to the quantification of the available phosphorous by the molybdenum chemistry in soil extracts (Almeida et al., 2005). Comparing with previous reports, this methodology has an enhanced linear range of determination. Furthermore, the molybdenum blue dye adsorption to the tubing walls could be minimized by the addition of NaOH to the washing carrier solution.

Managing nitrogen (N) levels is another important aspect for the correct soil nutrition and fertilization. For this reason, new analytical methods dealing with N-nutrients (inorganic nitrogen species) have been introduced (López Pasquali et al., 2007, 2010). The most common approach for this determination is the classic Griess reaction (Tsikas, 2007) that produces an azo-dye that can be measured by visible spectrophotometry (543 nm). These two manifolds provided multiparametric determination of the various inorganic N-species using a copperized cadmium column or strong oxidant solutions (KBr and NaClO) to ensure the redox conversion of the target analytes (nitrite and nitrate) before chemical

Table 13.1 Comparison of the Extraction/Determination Parameters for the HL Scheme in SRM 2711 for Three Different Procedures Applied to Phosphorus Fractionation and Extract Analysis

	MSFIA (this work)		SI-MCE/FIA[a]		Batch[b]	
Parameters	Amount (mg)	Volume (μL)	Amount (mg)	Volume (μL)	Amount (mg)	Volume (μL)
1. Reagent consumption per extract analysis						
Ammonium molybdate	0.5	80	7.2	600	6.0	150
Reducing agent[c]	0.02	120	0.2	600	5.3	300
Masking agent[d]	0.1	80	2.4	1000	0.1	300
2. Extractant volume (mL)						
NH_4Cl fraction	4.5		25		2 × 50	
NaOH fraction	6		30		50	
HCl fraction	11		30		50	
3. Analysis time per extract (min)	0.77		0.74		20	
4. Operational time for overall fractionation and extract analysis per sample (h)	2.8		2.7		45.3	

[a] J. Buanuam, M. Miró, E.H. Hansen, J. Shiowatana, Anal. Chim. Acta 570 (2006) 224.
[b] A.H.M. Hieltjes, L. Lijklema, Journal of Environmental Quality 3 (1980) 405. More details about the extraction protocols can be found in the text.
[c] Tin(II) chloride was used as a reducing reagent for MSFIA and SI-MCE/FIA, while ascorbic acid was employed for batchwise analysis.
[d] Oxalic acid was employed as a masking agent for MSFIA, and tartaric acid for the SI-MCE/FIA and batch approaches.
Source: Reproduced and reprinted from Buanuam et al. (2007) with permission from Elsevier.

derivatization and photometric detection, with a linear range comprised between 0.02 and 1.60 mg L^{-1} (Fig. 13.5).

Potassium (K), other major soil nutrient, also benefited from the recent advances of flow analysis (Almeida et al., 2006; Almeida et al., 2009). The flow network based on MSFIA allowed the implementation of a fast method for soil extracts including in-line filtration and ionic strength adjustment followed by electrochemical detection by a potassium selective electrode (Almeida et al., 2006). The same authors also proposed an automated system using

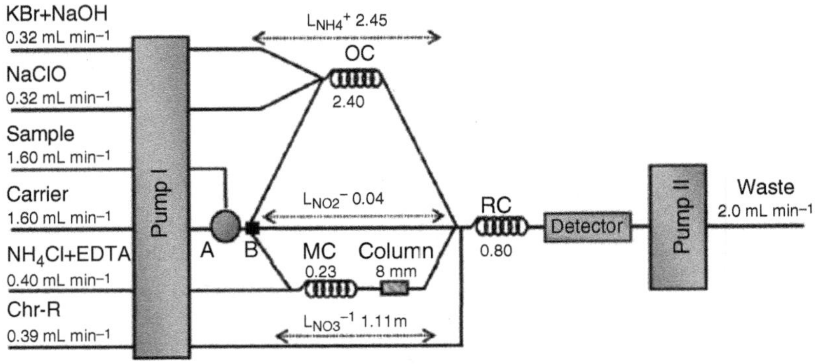

Figure 13.5. Schematic illustration of the flow injection manifold used for simultaneous determination of nitrite, nitrate, and ammonium. A, Injection valve; B, Hoffman key; OC, oxidation coil; RC, reaction coil; MC, mixing coil; Chr-R, chromogenic reagent. Reprinted from López Pasquali et al. (2007) with permission from Elsevier.

atomic emission spectrometry (AES) for the analysis of the same analyte (Almeida et al., 2009). This system hyphenated MSFIA with flame AES and included a feedback algorithm that automatically adjusted the dilution necessary to fit the concentration of the sample within the calibration range of the instrument. This is a good example of the development of smart analyzers that can create a dynamic linear working range for detection, which minimizes or even bypasses sample dilution.

Micronutrients (White and Brown, 2010) were also targeted by the recent development of flow analysis, such as boron (Gomes et al., 2005; Carrero et al., 2005) and iron (Gomes et al., 2005). For boron, the chemistry based on the formation of the complex boron-azomethine-H (Lobinski and Marczenko, 1996) has been adopted for its quantification with very different strategies. For example, Carrero et al. (2005) focused on the methyl borate separation from the sample prior to the complexation with azomethine. To this end, methyl borate was generated by the classic acidic esterification reaction using methanol and sulfuric acid (Blau and King, 1978). The methyl borate was then separated from the solution and the complex was hydrolyzed using an ammonium buffer solution with a pH of 6.8. The analytical cycle ends when the stripped boron reacted with azomethine-H and the complex is detected at 420 nm. This approach minimized the simultaneous detection of potential interferent species. However, the protocol is very complex, which makes the manifold difficult to adopt in a routine basis. On the other hand, Gomes et al. (2005) took advantage of the binary sampling (Reis et al., 1994) to maximize the mixture between labeling agent and sample, and also from the stopped flow to control the reaction time before detection. The same flow manifold was also used for the analysis of iron in the same samples. In this case binary sampling bypassed the differences in the refractive index of the solutions used.

2.2 Pollutants

Another important group of compounds targeted by flow analysis based methodologies are soil pollutants. The widespread introduction of xenobiotics from anthropogenic sources can disturb the regular nutrient cycles or contribute for the introduction of toxic species in the food chain (Mirsal, 2004). For these reasons, soil contamination monitoring has been a research topic of interest for both analytical and soil scientists. The identification and quantification of pollutants in soils is commonly based on multistep analytical methodologies, comprising sample preparation followed by identification and quantification using modern analytical instrumentation. Sample preparation is usually necessary to transfer the target compounds from the solid to a liquid phase that is usually mandatory for its identification and/or quantification. In the case of pollutants the analytical strategies based on flow analysis may handle directly the quantification of the target compounds through a wet chemistry assay or an assembled sensor or, alternatively, may act as front end to other analytical instrumentation. In the latter case, separation techniques are the most common choice for organic compounds, whereas atomic spectroscopy is commonly preferred for inorganic analytes. In order to simplify our overview of the literature, we subdivided the recent analytical developments based on flow analysis for soil monitoring according to chemical nature of the targeted pollutants: organic and inorganic.

2.2.1 Organic Pollutants

Different organic compounds have been analyzed by flow analysis methods, reflecting the chemical diversity of structures that are most currently contaminating the soils. The latest advances have been essentially focused on the analysis of herbicides (Urio and Masini, 2015; Boonjob et al., 2011; Colombo and Masini, 2011), pesticides (López Malo and Martinez Calatayud, 2008; Li et al., 2014; Wong and Taboada Sotomayor, 2014), and other molecules that can be originated either by natural or anthropogenic sources, such as phenols (Dolatto et al., 2012; Oliveira et al., 2009) and polycyclic aromatic hydrocarbons (PAHs) (Li and Lee, 2007; Li et al., 2008). In this particular case, it is possible to subdivide the methodologies in two distinct groups according to the number of chemical species targeted by the developed methodology: (1) single analyte determination, comprising the direct analysis of a soil extract by a wet chemistry assay with optical detection and (2) multi analyte determination, comprising automatic sample preparation protocols hyphenated to separation techniques.

In the former case, and conversely to the quantification of macronutrients, the targeted levels for the quantification of pollutants are at the low microgram per liter. This fact implied the use of more sensitive optical detection techniques, such as chemiluminescence (López Malo and Martinez Calatayud, 2008; Han, 2010; Li et al., 2014; Li and Lee, 2007) and fluorescence (Colombo and Masini, 2011), although UV-Vis spectrophotometry could also be used (Dolatto et al., 2012).

Chemiluminescence detection was adopted for the wet chemistry based determination of different organic compounds, such as buminafos (López Malo and Martinez Calatayud, 2008), chlortoluron (Li et al., 2014), indole-3-acetic acid (IAA) (Han, 2010), and acenaphthylene (ACY) (Li and Lee, 2007) from soil extracts. The reaction of these molecules with different chemiluminogenic agents, such as potassium permanganate (López Malo and Martinez Calatayud, 2008; Han, 2010), luminol-chitosan (Li et al., 2014) or tris(2,2′-bipyridine)ruthenium(II) (Li and Lee, 2007) allowed the determination of the target analytes at the microgram per liter level. In fact, flow analysis manifolds (particularly in a multichannel configuration) are particularly suited for chemiluminescence detection due to the reproducible timing of sample injection combined with a precise residence timing inside the tubing, which is a fundamental aspect for fast chemiluminogenic reactions (Zagatto et al., 2012). Nevertheless, these methodologies commonly show severe selectivity issues, due to the different components present in the sample matrix that may interact with the chemiluminogenic agent and modify the total amounts of photons emitted. This is the major reason why their application in routine analytical protocols is avoided.

Fluorescence detection was also reported. The quantification of glyphosate based on its oxidation to glycine followed by the reaction with *o*-phtaldialdehyde was used to study the adsorption behavior of this herbicide in a soil sample (Colombo and Masini, 2011). The authors calculated the adsorption parameters for the classic Langmuir and Freundlich models and discussed the potential adsorption mechanisms that can drive the retention of this compound in different soils. This work is a good example of the use of flow analysis as a research tool for in vitro testing of the behavior of some compounds in different environmental scenarios.

In order to circumvent some of the aforementioned selectivity issues it is necessary the use of chromatographic techniques. In this context, sample preparation is an essential step because it is necessary to extract the analytes from the soil sample to a liquid phase, and also because the concentration levels of the target compounds present in the soil extracts are commonly below the detection levels of the instrumentation, thus requiring a preconcentration step. The most recent advances are related with the development of automatic sample preparation protocols based on solid-phase extraction for the determination of phenolic compounds (Oliveira et al., 2009), triazine herbicides (Boonjob et al., 2011), and PAHs (Li et al., 2008) at trace levels using liquid chromatography (LC) coupled to optical detection. Online hyphenation between SPE-based flow analysis and LC can be operated in two distinct modes: (1) by inserting a plug of eluent through the sample loop of an injection valve (hearth-cut mode) (Oliveira et al., 2009; Boonjob et al., 2011) or (2) by eluting the analytes with the mobile phase from the extraction column that replaced the sample loop in the injection valve (column-switching mode) (Li et al., 2008).

In any case, all steps of a typical SPE protocol (conditioning, loading, washing, and elution) are performed in a fully automatic fashion. The sorbent is placed in a packed column and all the solutions (sample and solvents) necessary for the protocol are percolated through it. Polymeric or silica-based sorbents are the most commonly used materials to this end (Oliveira et al., 2011). Nevertheless, the evolution of the protocols for sample preparation is the application area where nanomaterials have been showing a greater impact due to their physical and chemical properties (Lucena et al., 2011). Among nanomaterials, carbon-based nanostructures are already widely established materials for the extraction and quantification of organic compounds in several matrices (Perez-López and Merkoci, 2012). However, flow analysis manifolds still have some problems in handling such structures due to their reduced dimensions and aggregation during fluidic manipulation. This is the most common cause of excessive back pressures into the manifold that cannot be properly handled by the flow management and propulsion devices. Promoting the fluidization of nanoparticles circumvented this problem, which resulted from the assembling of customized stirred flow chambers to the flow manifold (Boonjob et al., 2011; Rosende et al., 2011). This fluidization allows a convection movement of the particles when solutions are propelled to the chamber, which minimizes aggregation and deposition of the particles into the filters that confine the particles inside the device. This strategy was successfully applied to

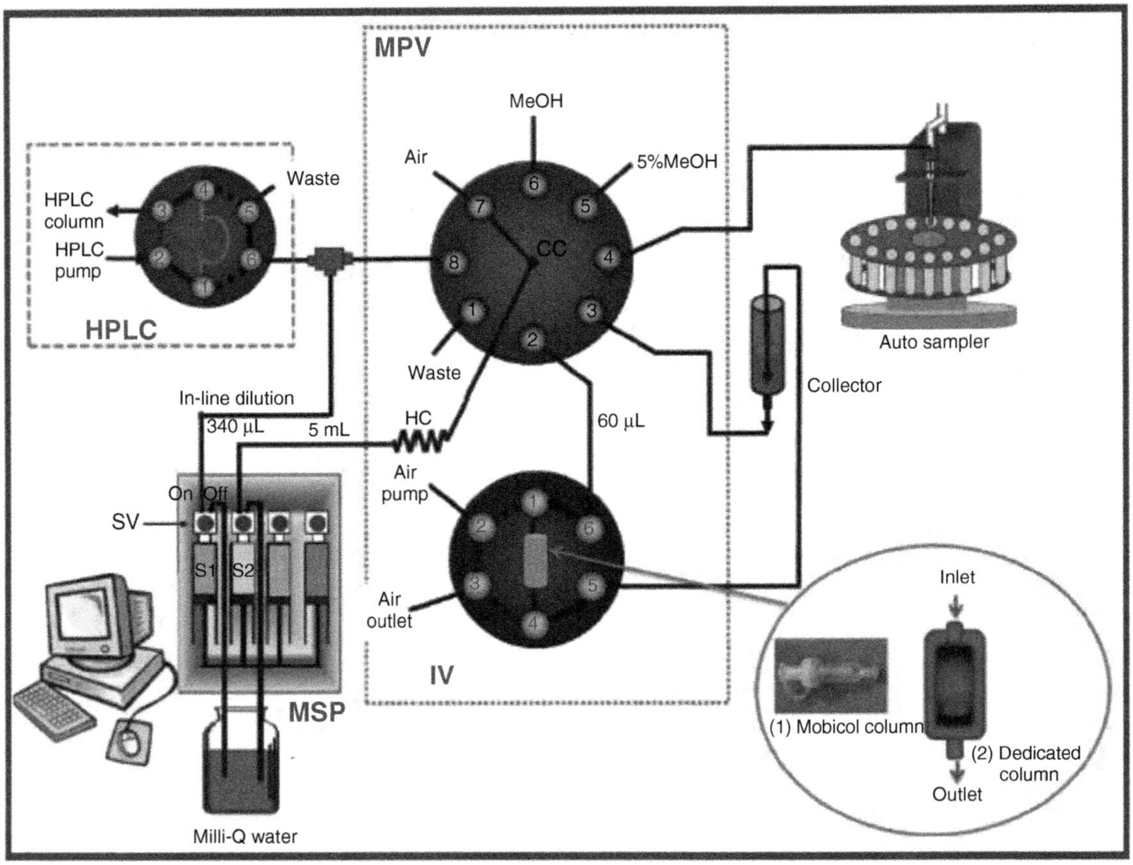

Figure 13.6. Schematic illustration of the SI-LC hyphenated setup for automated CNF-based microextraction and determination of trace level concentrations of triazine herbicides in environmental matrixes. MPV, Multiposition valve; IV, injection valve; MSP, multisyringe pump; HPLC, high performance liquid chromatograph; HC, holding coil; CC, communication channel. The inset illustrates two designs of stirred-flow chambers for micro-SPE. Reprinted with permission from Boonjob et al. (2011). Copyright (2011) American Chemical Society.

the analysis of triazine herbicides and dealkylated metabolites in soil extracts (Fig. 13.6) (Boonjob et al., 2011). In this case, a mass of 10 mg of different nanomaterials, such as multiwalled carbon nanotubes (MWCNT), carboxyl functionalized multiwalled carbon nanotubes (MWCNT-COOH), and carbon nanofibers (CNF) were compared. Carbon nanofibers were able to quantitatively retain all analytes with a higher extraction yield than the other materials tested. This enhanced performance is related with the large chemically surface available for adsorption, as a result of the cup-stacked arrangement of the carbon structures of the material. The mechanism of sorption of these analytes with the sorbent is related with the strong π–π interaction between the aromatic structure of triazines and the surface of the nanocarbon structure, which was able to process more than 120 mL of sample without observable deterioration of the extractive surface. This strategy made possible to analyze these compounds at the microgram per liter level with high precision and accuracy. The major drawback of this methodology is related with the complexity of the manifold, which requires a complex configuration with a selection and injection valve to accommodate the CNFs stirred chamber. Additionally, there are also some steps that may difficult to implement in routine analysis, such as a 10 min air-drying of the sorbent material before elution.

Urio and Masini (2015) recently described an alternative method for the quantification of the same triazine herbicides based on SIC. In this case, soil extracts were directly injected into the chromatographic column without any prior enrichment step. For this reason, the linear range of quantification was in the milligram per liter range instead of the microgram per liter reported in the aforementioned method (Boonjob et al., 2011). The authors compared different stationary phases, namely monolithic and core–shell columns, for the same analytical protocol, and concluded that monolithic columns provided faster and less sensitive separations than core–shell columns. The adjustment of the separation performance by fine-tuning the chemistry of the chromatographic stationary phase to the physical–chemical properties of the analytes is a recent topic in flow analysis-based chromatography (Batista et al., 2015). This fact results from the introduction of new stationary phases that create working backpressures compatible with the propulsion units commonly used. However, stationary phases containing nanostructures (Svec and Lv, 2015) are still an unknown territory at the low-pressure flow analysis based separation field.

2.2.2 Inorganic Pollutants

The recent advances in flow analysis have also targeted inorganic pollutants (Fig. 13.4). The increasing anthropogenic inputs of several inorganic species with potential impact into the environment and the human health has been creating a continuous quest for reliable, accurate, and precise automated methods for the quantification of several inorganic species in soil.

The biggest group of methodologies assessed metal species that can play a toxicological role in the food chain. In this particular topic, a high number of publications dealt with two specific analytes that fulfil these criteria: lead (Pb) and chromium (Cr). Different methods based on FIA (Praveen et al., 2007; Bakircioglu, 2012; Chuachuad and Tyson, 2005), SIA (Cocovi-Solberg et al., 2014), and a customized setup that combined batch and flow conditions

(Rosende et al., 2013) have been applied to the determination of Pb in soil samples. Atomic absorption spectrometry was the instrumental analytical approach for detection adopted in all methodologies. Automation of sample preparation was also present in all cases, but in different formats. For the quantification of total Pb in soils, SPE has been the preferred approach due to the possibility of modifying the sorbent surface to enhance the extractive performance. For example, Praveen et al. (2007) developed a sorbent material functionalized with dithiocarbamate. Dithiocarbamate was chemically bonded to the chloromethylated styrene-divinyl benzene polymer, resulting in a chelating resin able to preconcentrate lead from the soil extracts (Yebra-Biurrun et al., 1991). The manifold was directly coupled to the AAS instrument. The adjustment between the flow rates of the FIA system and the nebulizer favored the hyphenation. The lower eluent flow rate of the FIA system in comparison with the free uptake rate of the nebulizer resulted in smaller droplets, which minimized vaporization interferences. Solid-phase extraction was also used in anion exchange-mode for hydride generation and the quantification of Pb (Chuachuad and Tyson, 2005). Although this protocol is complex, with a high number of reagents and steps involved, it demonstrates the high flexibility of these systems to handle different chemistries and complex unit operations, such as gas–liquid separation.

Another relevant achievement of flow analysis applied to soil science is the possibility to evaluate the bioaccessbility and bioavailability of metal species that may be present in soil samples. Two reports dealing with bioaccessibility and bioavailability of Pb in soil samples have been recently published (Cocovi-Solberg et al., 2014; Rosende et al., 2013). In both cases, microdialysis was the strategy adopted for the measurement of the fractions of interest. The implementation of microdialysis in a fluidic format is a complex task due to need to reproduce the transport of the metal species between the different compartments. For this reason, it was crucial a detailed study about the different probe materials and fluidic conditions for an accurate evaluation of bioaccessibility of Pb from different soil samples using a hyphenated microdialysis-SIA approach (Cocovi-Solberg et al., 2014). The results obtained with this novel approach were compared with the in-line microfiltration method batchwise leaching test endorsed by SMT. The authors found that the dialysis profiles were the most interesting way to study bioaccessibility due to the differences observed between the nature of the samples and their respective chemical profiles. Furthermore, it was demonstrated that the current 16 h steady assay recommended by the SMT might not be sufficient for the evaluation of maximum bioaccessible fractions in some samples.

A similar strategy was adopted for the in vitro evaluation of the gastric and gastrointestinal (GI) bioavailability of Pb from soil samples under physiologically based conditions (Rosende et al., 2013). After an evaluation of the different membranes and dialysis probe designs, the manifold was applied to the in vitro studies, being possible to calculate the bioaccessible and bioavailable fractions of Pb present in the samples. A key finding of this contribution is the possibility to reduce the time necessary for evaluation of GI bioavailability due to the fast immobilization of the leached Pb, which is caused by the complexation and precipitation that results from the simultaneous presence of phosphates and neutral pH values. For more detailed information about these methodologies and their principles, the readers are referred to a recent review of the same authors (Rosende and Miró, 2013).

The speciation of metals in soils is other research topic where fast and accurate analytical methods have a pivotal role (Roberts et al., 2005), with a majority of the most recent developments focused on the analysis of chromium (Cr). Chromium is present in the environment in two different oxidation states [Cr (III) and Cr (VI)], with distinct chemical properties (Unceta et al., 2010). Cr (III) is a micronutrient with a key role in the regulation of metabolism (Vincent, 2000), whereas Cr (VI) has toxic effects (Unceta et al., 2010). Additionally, these two species can interchange their oxidation species in soils due to the ubiquitous presence other species with redox properties. For this reason, methods for the analysis of Cr (VI) (Nitiyanontakit et al., 2013; Rosende et al., 2011; Grabarczyk et al., 2007; Long et al., 2006) and Cr (III) (Sánchez-Moreno et al., 2009) have been developed. One of the most popular strategies for the analysis of Cr (VI) in soils is the chelate formation between 1,5-diphenylcarbazide (DPC) and Cr (VI) in acidic milieu (Pflaum and Howick, 1956), which can be detected by visible spectrophotometry (Rosende et al., 2011; Nitiyanontakit et al., 2013). Rosende et al. (2011) reported the preconcentration of this complex using different kinds of carbon nanostructures: CNF, MWCNT, MWCNT-COOH, and amino multiwalled carbon nanotubes (MWCNT-NH_2). All materials revealed adequate sorption characteristics and the recovery values were below 90% only for the MWCNT-COOH. The mechanism of retention of the complex Cr-DPC is based on the π–π interactions between the aromatic rings of the Cr-DPC complex (acting as electron acceptor), and the polarizable carbon sheets of the sorbent (acting as electrodonor). This mechanism explains why the sorbents used had a similar performance in the retention of the complex. Moreover, this method included the direct handling of the solid sample combined with Cr (VI) derivatization and detection, which minimized the risk of interconversion between oxidation states of Cr. Another important note about this method is the incorporation of carbon nanomaterials in a packed column into the manifold, which lead to excessive backpressures during the percolation of liquids throughout the sorbent bed. For this reason, the authors mixed the 7 mg of CNTs with 40 mg PTFE chunks in order to create sections in the column. This strategy overcame the excessive backpressure and made possible the extraction of the Cr-DPC complex from the reaction milieu using flow rates of 1.00 mL min^{-1}. By combining the dynamic extraction of the soil sample with the fluidic strategy for Cr-DPC complex enrichment and quantification with a first-order leaching model, it was also possible to reduce the assay time from 24 [in the reference batch method (DIN, 1984)] to approximately 6 h. Solid-phase extraction in renewable mode based on μSI-LOV was also combined with ET-AAS for the analysis of Cr (VI) (Long et al., 2006). In this case, the soil sample was also in-line extracted using the same dynamic strategy previously described (Miró and Hansen, 2006). Nevertheless, the extracted Cr (VI) was preconcentrated using a micro-SPE anion-exchange column prior to the ET-AAS analysis at the nanogram per liter level. Although based on the same extraction principles for handling the soil extraction, the sensitivity and limit of detection of the two aforementioned approaches for Cr (VI) were significantly different due to the flexibility of the manifold and the different detection strategies used. For example, the hybrid flow system with visible spectrophotometric detection (Rosende et al., 2011) provided a linear range between 5 and 500 μg L^{-1}, whereas in the case of the μSI-LOV strategy coupled to atomic absorption spectrometry (Long et al., 2006), this range was established between 0.011 and 0.33 μg L^{-1}.

Another exploited extraction technique for Cr (VI) based on the sequential injection technique was the hollow fiber liquid-phase membrane extraction (LPME) (Nitiyanontakit et al., 2013). The system includes a hollow fiber impregnated with an ionic liquid (methyltrioctyl ammonium chloride) that is automatically regenerated at the end of each cycle. This membrane regeneration impacted on the accuracy and the precision of the methodology when compared with previous approaches that were unable to incorporate this step. Furthermore, the automation of LPME completely modified the time-scale of the extraction, from the hour scale in batchwise format to minute scale in fluidic format. The extraction yield also benefited from the flow reversal cycle that was automatically performed by the system, providing a LOD of 4.6 μg L^{-1}. The fragility of the membrane may be considered the most relevant pitfall of this extraction approach.

An alternative strategy for Cr (VI) enrichment prior to its detection is the use of electrochemical methods. For example, the catalytic stripping voltammetry detection lead to a high sensitive and selective methodology, based on the deposition of the Cr (VI) during 30 s onto the Hg drop electrode (Grabarczyk et al., 2007) followed by the measurement of the respective peak current. The addition of diethylenetriaminepentaacetic acid (DTPA) masked the potential interference of Cr (III). The method also proved to be capable of handling other potential interferent species of the determination, such as humic acids, fulvic acids, and surfactants without any deterioration in the analytical performance of the methodology.

Regarding Cr (III), potentiometry also showed a relevant role for the direct analysis of soil extracts either using a batchwise or flow injection analysis approach (Sánchez-Moreno et al., 2009). The reported sensor contained a solid-state membrane based on carbon paste modified with di(2-hydroxyphenylimino)ethane (DHPE). The authors also exploited the differences in the performance of the sensor in the batch and flow mode. When compared with the batch approach, the flow injection potentiometry method requires a smaller sample volume and showed shorter linear range and higher precision. Nevertheless, the most interesting change in flow injection mode was the enhanced selectivity. The enhancement in flow mode format was attributed to kinetic differences in the response of the analyte versus interferent species, which is one of the most interesting and unique features of flow analysis (Pacey et al., 1986).

Another important method of sample preparation in flow analysis is gas diffusion (Kolev and Mckelvie, 2008). This membrane-based separation technique consists in the mass transfer of volatile species from a donor stream to an acceptor stream driven by the respective pressure differences (Kolev and Mckelvie, 2008). It was applied to the analysis of mercury using amperometric detection in soil extracts (Amini et al., 2005) at microgram per liter level. Mercury (II) from the liquid extracts was reduced to metallic Hg by mixing the sample with a reducing agent ($SnCl_2$) in acidic milieu. The volatile species were then transferred to the acceptor phase and then directed to the amperometric flow cell, where detection occurred using a gold working electrode with a potential of +600 mV versus the Ag/AgCl reference electrode. The addition of hydrazine sulfate (4.0 mg L^{-1}) and potassium iodide (30.0 mg L^{-1}) minimized the interferences from selenium (IV), silver (I), and copper (I). An important detail of this method is related with the worse performance observed when low flow rates were applied to the acceptor stream. A possible reason to this fact is related to the aggregation of atomic mercury into particulate form and/or its oxidation by dissolved oxygen.

Other metals were also targeted by the recent developments of the flow analysis with optical detection applied to soil monitoring. Due to its high sensitivity, chemiluminescence was applied to the determination of copper (II) (Murillo Pulgarin et al., 2013), cobalt (II) (Murillo Pulgarín et al., 2013), and tin (Ye et al., 2010). Nevertheless, chemiluminescence methods commonly have the same selectivity issues already present in the analysis of organic compounds, and for this reason their use as direct wet chemistry assays may arise in important accuracy issues. Therefore, chemiluminescence is preferably associated with some selective analytical step that can minimize these issues. This was the strategy adopted by Murillo Pulgarín et al. (2013) that combined ion chromatography with the luminol/perborate chemiluminescent system for the determination of copper (II) and cobalt (II) at the microgram per liter level after microwave digestion of the soil sample with aqua regia. Another example of chemiluminescence application to soil analysis is the determination of tin using flow injection hydride generation and cryotrapping (Ye et al., 2010). This is an unconventional analytical strategy due to the combination of gas and liquid phase chemistry in a single manifold. In brief, tin was reduced to stannane that was cryotrapped using liquid nitrogen. The stannane is then vaporized and directed to the flow cell, where suffers oxidation from ozone, producing photons that will be then collected by the chemiluminescence detector. Despite the very unique features of this method, the complexity of the manifold associated with the use of gases and liquid nitrogen make it unfeasible for routine analysis.

Flow injection analysis was also recently hyphenated to High Resolution–Atomic Absorption Spectrometry (HR-AAS) for the determination of different elements present in soil extracts (Gómez-Nieto et al., 2015). This method showed how the combination between a reproducible sample injection system based on FIA and the use of different spectral lines and pixel registration was able to modulate the analytical response of the HR-AAS instrument, leading to a broader linear working range (Table 13.2). This improvement on linear range operation bypassed the common dilution step necessary to adjust the sample concentration to the linear range of the instrument, and made possible a fast and sequential determination of all target species. Furthermore, this methodology also reduced the sample consumption approximately 8–9 times and improved LOD and LOQ values.

Another recent group of pollutants targeted by flow analysis based methodologies are radionuclides. Taking into account

Table 13.2 Figures of Merit for the Automatic Determination of Different Species by High Resolution–Atomic Absorption Spectroscopy

Element	Wave-length (nm)	Slope ($sLmg^{-1}$)	r	Upper Limit of Linear Range (mgL^{-1})	LOD (mgL^{-1})	LOQ (mgL^{-1})	Repeat-ability (RSD, %)	Repro-ducibility (RSD, %)
Cd	228.802	0.2843	0.9966	2.6	0.011	0.037	0.3–3.3	1.5–8.0
Ni	232.003	0.0780	0.9990	7.5	0.020	0.067	0.8–4.0	2.5–8.5
Pb	217.001	0.0427	0.9994	7.8	0.062	0.21	0.7–4.2	4.6–8.2
Cu	324.754	0.1664	0.9987	5.0	0.007	0.023	0.6–3.5	5.0–8.0
Zn	213.857	0.3912	0.9963	2.2	0.014	0.046	0.2–2.7	2.3–8.7
Mn	279.482	0.2442	0.9998	1.8	0.008	0.027	1.1–2.5	2.4–8.5
Mn	279.827	01660	0.9996	8.4	0.014	0.047	0.1–3.5	4.5–8.2
Mg	202.582	0.0545	0.9995	23	0.13	0.42	0.8–2.7	3.9–7.5
Fe	248.327	0.0862	0.9998	1.6	0.030	0.10	1.4–4.9	3.8–8.3
Fe	248.814	0.0413	0.9998	7.2	0.075	0.25	0.7–2.5	2.0–4.8
Fe	302.064	0.0191	0.9997	15	0.085	0.28	0.4–3.4	4.1–8.6
Fe	302.107	0.0057	0.9996	110	0.24	0.80	1.2–6.0	6.0–10.0
Ca	422.673	0.0511	0.9994	26	0.099	0.33	0.2–5.2	1.5–6.9
Ca	239.856	0.0007	0.9983	95	1.2	4.0	1.5–6.1	4.6–9.1
Na	589.592	0.2273	0.9998	11	0.014	0.047	0.1–2.3	4.7–8.1
Na	330.237	0.0042	0.9983	85	0.91	3.0	0.4–4.2	3.0–8.2
K	769.897	0.1540	0.9999	16	0.032	0.11	0.4–3.4	3.0–9.5
K	404.414	0.0016	0.9995	160	0.72	2.4	1.2–5.4	2.1–10.5

Source: Reprinted from Gómez-Nieto et al. (2015) with permission from Elsevier.

the very low levels and in some cases the short lifetime of these radioactive species, the bottleneck of radionuclides determination is sample preparation. For this reason, flow analysis manifolds have been performing automatic solid-phase extraction of the radionuclides, acting as online or offline front end to ICP-MS detection. Flow systems are extremely interesting tools for these kind of samples by considering two aspects: (1) enhanced flexibility, which make possible to handle a broad range (from the low μL to the high milliliter levels) of volumes of sample and other solvents necessary for the extraction and (2) closed-circuit operation, which minimizes the potential hazards of the analytical operator. Although FIA could also be used for this kind of determination (Godoy et al., 2006), the major developments are based on sequential injection technique that was successfully applied to the extraction of Plutonium (Pu) (Qiao et al., 2011a; Qiao et al., 2011b) (Qiao et al., 2011c), Neptunium (Np) (Qiao et al., 2011a; Qiao et al., 2011c), and Technetium (Tc) (Rodríguez et al., 2015) prior to ICP coupled to mass spectrometry (MS) analysis. Despite the need of an extensive sample preparation protocol of soil samples, including digestion, filtration, and oxidation, the SPE procedure is a fundamental step of the quantification of the radioactive species due to the coexistence of other elements with the same mass that may compromise the accuracy of the analysis. For this reason, these authors assessed different sorbents aiming the most suitable conditions for the separation of the target analyte(s). For example, a macroporous anion exchanger (AGMP1M) showed high chemical yields than a gel-type with similar anion exchange properties (AG-1X4) (Qiao et al., 2011a). The same authors also found that the cross-linking degree (percentage of divinylbenzene in the resin reaction mixture that affects the resin internal structure and consequently its swelling/shrinking properties) and the particle size are also crucial aspects to achieve high extraction yields with the desired mass selectivity (Qiao et al., 2011b). The use of flow-based SPE systems also allowed the use of renewable micro-SPE for the analysis of Tc using TEVA resin, another anion-exchange sorbent (Rodríguez et al., 2015). The use of programmable flow approaches for these analytical procedures increased the precision of the method due to the high precision of the propulsion units used, which impacts the methodologies at two different levels. The first one is related with the analytical and environmental performance of the methods, which results in enhanced reproducibility and minimum cross contamination between samples, as well fast separations. The time required for the analysis was drastically reduced in these methods (e.g., from 2 to 3 days in manual batch protocols to 2.5 h in flow mode (Qiao et al., 2011b)) and the reagent consumption and waste disposal were also minimized in several orders of magnitude. The second level is related with the particular chemistry behavior of these species. The repeatable and dynamic flow conditions made possible the use of tracers to improve the accuracy of the methods (Qiao et al., 2011a; Qiao et al., 2011c), and also opened the gate for the use of short-lived species that cannot be measured under nondynamic extraction conditions (Qiao et al., 2011c).

3 Conclusions and Future Perspectives

From the literature overviewed by this chapter, it is possible to conclude that the analytical partnership between flow analysis and nanomaterials applied to the chemical monitoring of soils is clearly an unexploited research topic that will certainly receive more attention in the next years.

A fundamental question about this topic is what will be the next analytical evolution step. Although flow analysis is clearly able to accommodate further nanoanalytical developments (Passos et al., 2015), the fast evolution in material science and electronics is accelerating the development of alternative platforms, such as microfluidics (Temiz et al., 2015), paper-based sensors (Hossain and Brennan, 2011), and other miniaturized discrete analyzers (Madou et al., 2006), which can be applied into the development of new protocols for direct sensing (Duford et al., 2013) or sample preparation (Xi et al., 2010). Furthermore, a significant group of flow analysis-based methodologies currently in use for routine determination of soil nutrients rely on well established classic wet chemistry assays and are often under the scope of a regulatory framework. This scenario contributes for a slower assimilation of the whole potential of nanotechnology for these particular methodologies.

On the other hand, chemical sensors based on nanomaterials are another emerging area (Perez-López and Merkoci, 2012; Bai and Zhou, 2014). The chemical kinetic features of flow analysis manifolds have excellent features for analyte discrimination that may contribute for the development and application of these sensors. To date, the most relevant application field of nanomaterials-based sensors is the biomedical (Penn et al., 2003; Perez-López and Merkoci, 2012), and for this reason significant advances in other analytical areas are expectable in the forthcoming years. Moreover, the emergence of precision agriculture (Lowenberg-Deboer, 2015) is also creating a quest for advanced chemical sensors for soil analysis capable to operate in network conditions (Srbinovska et al., 2015; Adamchuk et al., 2004).

Finally, the automation of sample preparation protocols for soil analysis is the area where flow analysis has been introducing the most relevant advances. The previously described dynamic extraction of soils and the determination of the bioaccessibility and bioavailability levels of chemical species represent a clear breakthrough that still lacks application in a large routine basis. The direct handling of the soil sample instead of a soil extract is also paving the ground for faster and reliable in vitro assays. Additionally, the use of nanomaterials for SPE purposes is other relevant topic that is also unexploited. However, this latter path has been slower because it is difficult to handle the nanoparticles into the flow channels without relevant backpressures problems. This is the reason why the reports that dealt with the use of carbon nanostructured sorbents used special devices to avoid excessive backpressures during the analytical cycles (Boonjob et al., 2011; Rosende et al., 2011). A possible way to minimize these backpressure issues (that are also present in other fluidic approaches, such as microfluidics) is the use a support material with micrometer dimensions that can be coated by the nanomaterials through physical or chemical interactions, though in this case the it may be not possible to take full advantage of the higher surface to mass ratio of these materials. This immobilization strategy for nanomaterials has been already used in stationary phases for liquid chromatography (Svec and Lv, 2015), which will certainly create new separation opportunities for sequential injection and multisyringe chromatography.

Acknowledgments

Hugo M. Oliveira thanks Fundação para a Ciência e a Tecnologia (FCT) and POPH (Programa Operacional Potencial Humano) for the postdoctoral grant SFRH/BPD/75065/2010. This work received financial support from the European Union (FEDER funds POCI/01/0145/FEDER/007265) and National Funds (FCT/MEC, Fundação para a Ciência e Tecnologia and Ministério da Educação e Ciência) under the Partnership Agreement PT2020 UID/QUI/50006/2013. To all financing sources the authors are greatly indebted.

References

Adamchuk, V.I., Hummel, J.W., Morgan, M.T., Upadhyaya, S.K., 2004. On-the-go soil sensors for precision agriculture. Comput. Electron. Agric. 44, 71–91.

Almeida, M.I.G.S., Estela, J.M., Cerdà, V., 2011. Multisyringe flow injection potentialities for hyphenation with different types of separation techniques. Anal. Lett. 44, 360–373.

Almeida, M.I.G.S., Segundo, M.A., Lima, J.L.F.C., Rangel, A.O.S.S., 2005. Multi-syringe flow injection system for the determination of available phosphorus in soil samples. Int. J. Environ. Anal. Chem. 85, 51–62.

Almeida, M.I.G.S., Segundo, M.A., Lima, J.L.F.C., Rangel, A.O.S.S., 2006. Potentiometric multi-syringe flow injection system for determination of exchangeable potassium in soils with in-line extraction. Microchem. J. 83, 75–80.

Almeida, M.I.G.S., Segundo, M.A., Lima, J.L.F.C., Rangel, A.O.S.S., 2009. Interfacing multisyringe flow injection analysis to flame atomic emission spectrometry: an intelligent system for automatic sample dilution and determination of potassium. J. Anal. At. Spectrom. 24, 340–346.

Amini, N., Cardwell, T.J., Cattrall, R.W., Kolev, S., 2005. Determination of mercury(II) at trace levels by gas-diffusion flow injection analysis with amperometric detection. Anal. Chim. Acta 539, 203–207.

Anastas, P.T., 1999. Green chemistry and the role of analytical methodology development. Crit. Rev. Anal. Chem. 29, 167–175.

Appelqvist, R., Beecher, G.R., Bergamin F, H., Den Boef, G., Emnéus, J., Fang, Z., Gorton, L., Hansen, E.H., Hare, P.E., Harris, J.M., Harrow, J.J., Ishibashi, N., Janata, J., Johansson, G., Karlberg, B., Krug, F.J., Van Der Linden, W.E., Luque De Castro, M.D., Markovarga, G., Miller, J.N., Mottola, H.A., Müller, H., Pacey, G.E., Riley, C., Ruzicka, J., Schothorst, R.C., Stewart, K.K., Townshend, A., Tyson, J.F., Ueno, K., Valcárcel, M., Vanderslice, J., Worsfold, P.J., Yoza, N., Zagatto, E.A.G., 1986. Flow injection analysis (FIA)—a personal view. Anal. Chim. Acta 180, 1–67.

Armenta, S., Garrigues, S., De La Guardia, M., 2008. Green analytical chemistry. Trends Anal. Chem. 27, 497–511.

Bai, J., Zhou, B.X., 2014. Titanium dioxide nanomaterials for sensor applications. Chem. Rev. 114, 10131–10176.

Bakircioglu, D., 2012. Cloud point extraction for the preconcentration of palladium and lead in environmental samples and determination by flow injection flame atomic absorption spectrometry. Environ. Sci. Pollut. Res. 19, 2428–2437.

Batista, A.D., Chocholouš, P., Šatínský, D., Solich, P., Rocha, F.R.P., 2015. On-line hyphenation of solid-phase extraction to chromatographic separation of sulfonamides with fused-core columns in sequential injection chromatography. Talanta 133, 142–149.

Batista, A.D., Sasaki, M.K., Rocha, F.R.P., Zagatto, E.A.G., 2014. Flow analysis in Brazil: contributions over the last four decades. Analyst 139, 3666–3682.

Blau, K., King, G.S., 1978. Handbook of Derivatives of Chromatography. Heyden & Son, Spectrum House, London, UK.

Boonjob, W., Miró, M., Segundo, M.A., Cerdà, V., 2011. Flow-through dispersed carbon nanofiber-based microsolid-phase extraction coupled to liquid chromatography for automatic determination of trace levels of priority environmental pollutants. Anal. Chem. 83, 5237–5244.

Buanuam, J., Miró, M., Hansen, E.H., Shiowatana, J., 2006. On-line dynamic fractionation and automatic determination of inorganic phosphorus in environmental solid substrates exploiting sequential injection microcolumn extraction and flow injection analysis. Anal. Chim. Acta 570, 224–231.

Buanuam, J., Miró, M., Hansen, E.H., Shiowatana, J., Estela, J.M., Cerdà, V., 2007. A multisyringe flow-through sequential extraction system for on-line monitoring of orthophosphate in soils and sediments. Talanta 71, 1710–1719.

Carrero, P., Malave, A., Rojas, E., Rondon, C., De Pena, Y.P., Burguera, J.L., Burguera, M., 2005. On-line generation and hydrolysis of methyl borate for the spectrophotometric determination of boron in soil and plants with azomethine-H. Talanta 68, 374–381.

Cerdà, V., Estela, J.M., Forteza, R., Cladera, A., Becerra, E., Altimira, P., Sitjar, P., 1999. Flow techniques in water analysis. Talanta 50, 695–705.

Cerdà, V., Ferrer, L., Avivar, J., Cerdà, A., 2014. Flow Analysis. A Practical Guide. Elsevier, Amsterdan.

Chocholouš, P., Solich, P., Šatínský, D., 2007. An overview of sequential injection chromatography. Anal. Chim. Acta 600, 129–135.

Chocholouš, P., Vackova, J., Sramkova, I., Šatínský, D., Solich, P., 2013. Advantages of core–shell particle columns in sequential injection chromatography for determination of phenolic acids. Talanta 103, 221–227.

Chomchoei, R., Hansen, E.H., Shiowatana, J., 2004. Utilizing a sequential injection system furnished with an extraction microcolumn as a novel approach for executing sequential extractions of metal species in solid samples. Anal. Chim. Acta 526, 177–184.

Chuachuad, W., Tyson, J.F., 2005. Determination of lead by flow injection hydride generation atomic absorption spectrometry with tetrahydroborate immobilized on an anion-exchange resin. J. Anal. At. Spectrom. 20, 282–288.

Clavijo, S., Avivar, J., Suárez, R., Cerdà, V., 2015. Analytical strategies for coupling separation and flow-injection techniques. Trends Anal. Chem. 67, 26–33.

Cocovi-Solberg, D.J., Rosende, M., Miró, M., 2014. Automatic kinetic bioaccessibility assay of lead in soil environments using flow-through microdialysis as a front end to electrothermal atomic absorption spectrometry. Environ. Sci. Technol. 48, 6282–6290.

Colombo, S.D.M., Masini, J.C., 2011. Developing a fluorimetric sequential injection methodology to study adsorption/desorption of glyphosate on soil and sediment samples. Microchem. J. 98, 260–266.

Darvas, F., Hessel, V., Dorman, G. 2014. Flow Chemistry Volume 1 Fundamentals.

DIN, 1984. German standard methods for the examination of water, waste water and sludge. Group S (sludge and sediments). Determination of leachability by water (S4). In: Normung, D.I.F.R. (Ed.) DIN 38414-S4. Berlin.

Dolatto, R.G., Messerschmidt, I., Pereira, B.F., Silveira, C.A.P., Abate, G., 2012. Determination of phenol and o-cresol in soil extracts by flow injection analysis with spectrophotometric detection. J. Braz. Chem. Soc. 23, 970–976.

Dolores Hurtado, M., Carmona, S., Delgado, A., 2008. Automated modification of the molybdenum blue colorimetric method for phosphorus determination in soil extracts. Commun. Soil Sci. Plant Anal. 39, 2250–2257.

Duford, D.A., Xi, Y., Salin, E.D., 2013. Enzyme inhibition-based determination of pesticide residues in vegetable and soil in centrifugal microfluidic devices. Anal. Chem. 85, 7834–7841.

Fang, Z., 1993. Flow Injection Separation and Preconcentration. VCH, Weinheim.

Fiedoruk, M., Cocovi-Solberg, D.J., Tymecki, L., Koncki, R., Miró, M., 2015. Hybrid flow system integrating a miniaturized optoelectronic detector for on-line dynamic fractionation and fluorometric determination of bioaccessible orthophosphate in soils. Talanta 133, 59–65.

Fortes, P.R., Feres, M.A., Sasaki, M.K., Alves, E.R., Zagatto, E.A.G., Prior, J.A.V., Santos, J.L.M., Lima, J.L.F.C., 2009. Evidences of turbulent mixing in multi-pumping flow systems. Talanta 79, 978–983.

Frigerio, C., Ribeiro, D.S.M., Rodrigues, S.S.M., Abreu, V.L.R.G., Barbosa, J.A.C., Prior, J.A.V., Marques, K.L., Santos, J.L.M., 2012. Application of quantum dots as analytical tools in automated chemical analysis: a review. Anal. Chim. Acta 735, 9–22.

Gałuszka, A., Migaszewski, Z., Namiesnik, J., 2013. The 12 principles of green analytical chemistry and the SIGNIFICANCE mnemonic of green analytical practices. Trac-Trends Anal. Chem. 50, 78–84.

Godoy, M.L.D.P., Godoy, J.M., Kowsmann, R., Dos Santos, G.M., Da Cruz, R.P., 2006. (234)U and (230)Th determination by FIA-ICP-MS and application to uranium-series disequilibrium in marine samples. J. Environ. Radioact. 88, 109–117.

Gomes, D.M.C., Segundo, M.A., Lima, J.L.C., Rangel, A.O.S.S., 2005. Spectrophotometric determination of iron and boron in soil extracts using a multi-syringe flow injection system. Talanta 66, 703–711.

Gomez-Nieto, B., Jesus Gismera, M., Teresa Sevilla, M., Procopio, J.R., 2015. Fast sequential multi-element determination of major and minor elements in environmental samples and drinking waters by high-resolution continuum source flame atomic absorption spectrometry. Anal. Chim. Acta 854, 13–19.

González, A., Avivar, J., Cerdà, V., 2015. Determination of priority phenolic pollutants exploiting an in-syringe dispersive liquid-liquid microextraction-multisyringe chromatography system. Anal. Bioanal. Chem. 407, 2013–2022.

Grabarczyk, M., Kaczmarek, L., Korolczuk, M., 2007. Determination of Cr(VI) in the presence of complexing agents and humic substances by catalytic stripping voltammetry. Electroanalysis 19, 1183–1188.

Grand, M., Oliveira, H.M., Ruzicka, J., Measures, C., 2011. Determination of dissolved zinc in seawater using micro-Sequential Injection lab-on-valve with fluorescence detection. Analyst 136, 2747–2755.

Guiochon, G., 2007. Monolithic columns in high-performance liquid chromatography. J. Chromatogr. A 1168, 101–168.

Han, S., 2010. Chemiluminescence determination of indole derivatives in human body fluids and soil by flow injection analysis using potassium permanganate. Microchim. Acta 168, 169–175.

Hansen, E.H. 2015. Flow injection analysis—bibliography database. Available from: www.flowinjectiontutorial.com

Hansen, E.H., Miró, M., 2007. How flow-injection analysis (FIA) over the past 25 years has changed our way of performing chemical analyses. Trends Anal. Chem. 26, 18–26.

Hieltjes, A.H.M., Lijklema, L., 1980. Fractionation of inorganic phosphates in calcareous sediments. J. Environ. Qual. 9, 405–407.

Horstkotte, B., Elsholz, O., Martin, V.C., 2008. Multisyringe flow injection analysis coupled to capillary electrophoresis (MSFIA-CE) as a novel analytical tool applied to the pre-concentration, separation and determination of nitrophenols. Talanta 76, 72–79.

Hossain, S.M.Z., Brennan, J.D., 2011. beta-galactosidase-based colorimetric paper sensor for determination of heavy metals. Anal. Chem. 83, 8772–8778.

Jakmunee, J., Junsomboon, J., 2009. Determination of available phosphorus in soils by using a new extraction procedure and a flow injection amperometric system. Talanta 79, 1076–1080.

Jones, Jr., J.B., 2012. Plant Nutrition and Soil Fertility Manual. CRC Press, Taylor & Francis Group, Boca Raton, FL.

Keith, L.H., Gron, L.U., Young, J.L., 2007. Green analytical methodologies. Chem. Rev. 107, 2695–2708.

Keller, A.A., Mcferran, S., Lazareva, A., Suh, S., 2013. Global life cycle releases of engineered nanomaterials. J. Nanopart. Res. 15.

Kolev, S., Mckelvie, I., 2008. Advances in Flow Injection Analysis and Related Techniques. Elsevier, Amsterdam.

Lahdesmaki, I., Chocholouš, P., Carroll, A.D., Anderson, J., Rabinovitch, P.S., Ruzicka, J., 2009. Two-parameter monitoring in a lab-on-valve manifold, applied to intracellular H(2)O(2) measurements. Analyst 134, 1498–1504.

Lapa, R.A.S., Lima, J.L.F.C., Reis, B.F., Santos, J.L.M., Zagatto, E.A.G., 2002. Multi-pumping in flow analysis: concepts, instrumentation, potentialities. Anal. Chim. Acta 466, 125–132.

Li, C.F., Wong, J.W.C., Huie, C.W., Choi, M.M.F., 2008. On-line flow injection-cloud point preconcentration of polycyclic aromatic hydrocarbons coupled with high-performance liquid chromatography. J. Chromatogr. A 1214, 11–16.

Li, M., Lee, S.H., 2007. Selective determination of acenaphthylene by flow injection analysis with tris(2,2′-bipyridine)ruthenium(II) chemiluminescence detection. Talanta 74, 265–270.

Li, Y., Zhang, J., Xiong, X., Luo, K., Guo, J., Shen, M., Wang, J., Song, Z., 2014. Determination of picogram quantities of chlortoluron in soil samples by luminol-chitosan chemiluminescence system. Environ. Sci. Pollut. Res. 21, 7204–7210.

Li, Z., Oshima, M., Sabarudin, A., Motomizu, S., 2005. Trace and ultratrace analysis of purified water samples and hydrogen peroxide solutions for phosphorus by flow-injection method. Anal. Sci. 21, 263–268.

Lobinski, R., Marczenko, Z., 1996. Spectrochemical Trace Analysis for Metals and Metalloids. Elsevier, Amsterdan, Netherlands.

Long, X.B., Miró, M., Hansen, E.H., 2006. On-line dynamic extraction and automated determination of readily bioavailable hexavalent chromium in solid substrates using micro-sequential injection bead-injection lab-on-valve hyphenated with electrothermal atomic absorption spectrometry. Analyst 131, 132–140.

López Malo, D., Martinez Calatayud, J., 2008. Photo-induced chemiluminescence determination of the pesticide Buminafos by a Multicommutation flow-analysis assembly. Talanta 77, 561–565.

López Pasquali, C.E., Fernández Hernando, P., Durand Alegría, J.S., 2007. Spectrophotometric simultaneous determination of nitrite, nitrate and ammonium in soils by flow injection analysis. Anal. Chim. Acta 600, 177–182.

López Pasquali, C.E., Gallego-Picó, A., Fernández Hernando, P., Velasco, M., Durand Alegria, J.S., 2010. Two rapid and sensitive automated methods for the determination of nitrite and nitrate in soil samples. Microchem. J. 94, 79–82.

Lowenberg-Deboer, J., 2015. The precision agriculture revolution making the modern farmer. Foreign Aff. 94, 105–112.

Lucena, R., Simonet, B.M., Cárdenas, S., Valcárcel, M., 2011. Potential of nanoparticles in sample preparation. J. Chromatogr. A 1218, 620–637.

Madou, M., Zoval, J., Jia, G., Kido, H., Kim, J., Kim, N., 2006. Lab on a CD. Annu. Rev. Biomed. Eng. 8, 601–628.

Maya, F., Estela, J.M., Cerdà, V., 2011. Multisyringe ion chromatography with chemiluminescence detection for the determination of oxalate in beer and urine samples. Microchim. Acta 173, 33–41.

Miguel, H.M.G.S., Alpizar-Lorenzo, J.M., Cerdà, V., 2007. Simultaneous determination of beta-lactamic antibiotics by a new high-performance low-pressure chromatographic system using a multisyringe burette coupled to a monolithic column (MSC). Anal. Bioanal. Chem. 387, 663–671.

Miró, M., 2014. On-chip microsolid-phase extraction in a disposable sorbent format using mesofluidic platforms. Trac-Trends Anal. Chem. 62, 154–161.

Miró, M., Hansen, E.H., 2006. Solid reactors in sequential injection analysis: recent trends in the environmental field. Trends Anal. Chem. 25, 267–281.

Miró, M., Hansen, E.H., 2007. Miniaturization of environmental chemical assays in flowing systems: The lab-on-a-valve approach vis-a-vis lab-on-a-chip microfluidic devices. Anal. Chim. Acta 600, 46–57.

Miró, M., Hansen, E.H., 2013. On-line sample processing involving microextraction techniques as a front-end to atomic spectrometric detection for trace metal assays: a review. Anal. Chim. Acta 782, 1–11.

Miró, M., Hartwell, S.K., Jakmunee, J., Grudpan, K., Hansen, E.H., 2008. Recent developments in automatic solid-phase extraction with renewable surfaces exploiting flow-based approaches. Trends Anal. Chem. 27, 749–761.

Miró, M., Oliveira, H.M., Segundo, M.A., 2011. Analytical potential of mesofluidic lab-on-a-valve as a front end to column-separation systems. Trends Anal. Chem. 30, 153–164.

Mirsal, I.A., 2004. Soil Pollution—Origin, Monitoring & Remediation. Springer-Verlag, Berlin, Germany.

Murillo Pulgarin, J.A., Garcia Bermejo, L.F., Carrasquero Duran, A., 2013. Fast simultaneous determination of traces of Cu(II) and Co(II) in soils and sediments with the luminol/perborate chemiluminescent system. Environ. Monit. Assess. 185, 573–580.

Nitiyanontakit, S., Varanusupakul, P., Miró, M., 2013. Hybrid flow analyzer for automatic hollow-fiber-assisted ionic liquid-based liquid-phase microextraction with in-line membrane regeneration. Anal. Bioanal. Chem. 405, 3279–3288.

Oliveira, H.M., Grand, M.M., Ruzicka, J., Measures, C.I., 2015. Towards chemiluminescence detection in micro-sequential injection lab-on-valve format: a proof of concept based on the reaction between Fe(II) and luminol in seawater. Talanta 133, 107–111.

Oliveira, H.M., Miró, M., Segundo, M.A., Lima, J.L.F.C., 2011. Universal approach for mesofluidic handling of bead suspensions in lab-on-valve format. Talanta 84, 846–852.

Oliveira, H.M., Segundo, M.A., Lima, J.L.F.C., Cerdà, V., 2009. Multisyringe flow injection system for solid-phase extraction coupled to liquid chromatography using monolithic column for screening of phenolic pollutants. Talanta 77, 1466–1472.

Pacey, G.E., Hollowell, D.A., Miller, K.G., Straka, M.R., Gordon, G., 1986. Selectivity enhancement by flow injection analysis. Anal. Chim. Acta 179, 259–267.

Passos, M.L.C., Pinto, P.C.A.G., Santos, J.L.M., Saraiva, M.L.M.F.S., Araújo, A.R.T.S., 2015. Nanoparticle-based assays in automated flow systems: a review. Anal. Chim. Acta 889, 22–34.

Penn, S.G., He, L., Natan, M.J., 2003. Nanoparticles for bioanalysis. Curr. Opin. Chem. Biol. 7, 609–615.

Perez-López, B., Merkoci, A., 2012. Carbon nanotubes and graphene in analytical sciences. Microchim. Acta 179, 1–16.

Pflaum, R.T., Howick, L.C., 1956. The Chromium-Diphenylcarbazide Reaction1. J. Am. Chem. Soc. 78, 4862–4866.

Praveen, R.S., Naidu, G.R.K., Rao, T.P., Inorganic Mat, G., 2007. Dithiocarbamate functionalized or surface sorbed Merrifield resin beads as column materials for on line flow injection-flame atomic absorption spectrometry determination of lead. Anal. Chim. Acta 600, 205–213.

Qiao, J., Hou, X., Roos, P., Miró, M., 2011a. High-throughput sequential injection method for simultaneous determination of plutonium and neptunium in environmental solids using macroporous anion-exchange chromatography, followed by inductively coupled plasma mass spectrometric detection. Anal. Chem. 83, 374–381.

Qiao, J., Hou, X., Roos, P., Miró, M., 2011b. Rapid isolation of plutonium in environmental solid samples using sequential injection anion exchange chromatography followed by detection with inductively coupled plasma mass spectrometry. Anal. Chim. Acta 685, 111–119.

Qiao, J., Hou, X., Roos, P., Miró, M., 2011c. Reliable determination of Np-237 in environmental solid samples using Pu-242 as a potential tracer. Talanta 84, 494–500.

Quintana, J.B., Boonjob, W., Miró, M., Cerdà, V., 2009. Online coupling of bead injection lab-on-valve analysis to gas chromatography: application to the determination of trace levels of polychlorinated biphenyls in solid waste leachates. Anal. Chem. 81, 4822–4830.

Rauret, G., López-Sanchez, J.F., Sahuquillo, A., Rubio, R., Davidson, C., Ure, A., Quevauviller, P., 1999. Improvement of the BCR three step sequential extraction procedure prior to the certification of new sediment and soil reference materials. J. Environ. Monit. 1, 57–61.

Reis, B.F., Giné, M.F., Zagatto, E.A.G., Lima, J.L.F.C., Lapa, R.A., 1994. Multicommutation in flow analysis. Part 1. Binary sampling: concepts, instrumentation and spectrophotometric determination of iron in plant digests. Anal. Chim. Acta 293.

Roberts, D., Nachtegall, M., Sparks, D.L., 2005. Speciation of Metals in Soils. Soil Sciency Society of America, Madison, WI, USA.

Rodríguez, R., Leal, L., Miranda, S., Ferrer, L., Avivar, J., García, A., Cerdà, V., 2015. Automation of Tc-99 extraction by LOV prior ICP-MS detection: application to environmental samples. Talanta 133, 88–93.

Rosende, M., Magalhaes, L.M., Segundo, M.A., Miró, M., 2013. Automated microdialysis-based system for in situ microsampling and investigation of lead bioavailability in terrestrial environments under physiologically based extraction conditions. Environ. Sci. Technol. 47, 11668–11675.

Rosende, M., Miró, M., 2013. Recent trends in automatic dynamic leaching tests for assessing bioaccessible forms of trace elements in solid substrates. Trends Anal. Chem. 45, 67–78.

Rosende, M., Miró, M., Segundo, M.A., Lima, J.L.F.C., Cerdà, V., 2011. Highly integrated flow assembly for automated dynamic extraction and determination of readily bioaccessible chromium(VI) in soils exploiting carbon nanoparticle-based solid-phase extraction. Anal. Bioanal. Chem. 400, 2217–2227.

Roy, R.N., Misra, R.V., Lesschen, J.P., Smaling, E.M., 2003. Assessment of Soil Nutrient Balance. Food and Agriculture Organization of the United Nations (FAO), Rome.

Ruzicka, J., 2000. Lab-on-valve: universal microflow analyzer based on sequential and bead injection. Analyst 125, 1053–1060.

Ruzicka, J., Hansen, E.H., 1975. Flow injection analysis. Part I. A new concept of fast continuous flow analyses. Anal. Chim. Acta 78, 145–157.

Ruzicka, J., Hansen, E.H., 1988. Flow Injection Analysis. Jonh Wiley & Sons, New York.

Ruzicka, J., Marshall, G.D., 1990. Sequential Injection—a new concept for chemical sensors, process analysis and laboratory assays. Anal. Chim. Acta 237, 329–343.

Sánchez-Moreno, R.A., Jesús Gismera, M., Teresa Sevilla, M., Procopio, J.R., 2009. Chromium(III) determination without sample treatment by batch and flow injection potentiometry. Anal. Chim. Acta 634, 68–74.

Šatínský, D., Solich, P., Chocholouš, P., Karlicek, R., 2003. Monolithic columns—a new concept of separation in the sequential injection technique. Anal. Chim. Acta 499, 205–214.

Segundo, M.A., Magalhães, L.M., 2006. Multisyringe flow injection analysis: state-of-the-art and perspectives. Anal. Sci. 22, 3–8.

Srbinovska, M., Gavrovski, C., Dimcev, V., Krkoleva, A., Borozan, V., 2015. Environmental parameters monitoring in precision agriculture using wireless sensor networks. J. Clean Prod. 88, 297–307.

Svec, F., Lv, Y.Q., 2015. Advances and recent trends in the field of monolithic columns for chromatography. Anal. Chem. 87, 250–273.

Temiz, Y., Lovchik, R.D., Kaigala, G.V., Delamarche, E., 2015. Lab-on-a-chip devices: how to close and plug the lab? Microelectron. Eng. 132, 156–175.

Tian, J.Y., Xu, J.Q., Zhu, F., Lu, T.B., Su, C.Y., Ouyang, G.F., 2013. Application of nanomaterials in sample preparation. J. Chromatogr. A 1300, 2–16.

Trojanowicz, M., 2008. Advances in Flow Analysis. Wiley-VCH, Weinheim.

Tsikas, D., 2007. Analysis of nitrite and nitrate in biological fluids by assays based on the Griess reaction: appraisal of the Griess reaction in the l-arginine/nitric oxide area of research. J. Chromatogr. B 851, 51–70.

Unceta, N., Séby, F., Malherbe, J., Donard, O.F.X., 2010. Chromium speciation in solid matrices and regulation: a review. Anal. Bioanal. Chem. 397, 1097–1111.

Urio, R.D.P., Masini, J.C., 2015. Evaluation of sequential injection chromatography for reversed phase separation of triazine herbicides exploiting monolithic and core–shell columns. Talanta 131, 528–534.

Valentini, F., Palleschi, G., 2008. Nanomaterials and analytical chemistry. Anal. Lett. 41, 479–520.

Vidigal, S.S.M.P., Toth, I.V., Rangel, A.O.S.S., 2013. Sequential injection lab-on-valve platform as a miniaturisation tool for solid phase extraction. Anal. Methods 5, 585–597.

Vincent, J.B., 2000. The biochemistry of chromium. J. Nutr. 130, 715–718.
White, P.J., Brown, P.H., 2010. Plant nutrition for sustainable development and global health. Ann. Bot. 105, 1073–1080.
Wong, A., Taboada Sotomayor, M.D.P., 2014. Determination of carbofuran and diuron in FIA system using electrochemical sensor modified with organometallic complexes and graphene oxide. J. Electroanal. Chem. 731, 163–171.
Worsfold, P.J., Townshend, A., Poole, C., 2005. Encyclopedia of Analytical Sciences. Elsevier, Amsterdam.
Xi, Y., Duford, D.A., Salin, E.D., 2010. Automated liquid-solid extraction of pyrene from soil on centrifugal microfluidic devices. Talanta 82, 1072–1076.
Ye, Y., Sang, J., Ma, H., Tao, G., 2010. Gas-phase chemiluminescence with ozone oxidation for the determination of total tin in environmental samples using flow injection hydride generation and cryotrapping. Anal. Chim. Acta 677, 149–155.
Yebra-Biurrun, M.C., Bermejo-Barrera, A., Bermejo-Barrera, M.P., 1991. Application of a poly(dithiocarbamate) resin with macroreticular support to the determination of trace amounts of cadmium and lead in non-saline waters. Analyst 116, 1033–1035.
Zagatto, E.A.G., Oliveira, C., Townshend, A., Worsfold, P., 2012. Flow Analysis with Spectrophotometric and Luminometric Detection. Elsevier, Amsterdam.

14

SMART NANOSENSORS FOR PESTICIDE DETECTION

Rajesh Kumar Saini, Laxmi P. Bagri, Anil Kumar Bajpai
Government Model Science College, Bose Memorial Research Laboratory, Department of Chemistry, Jabalpur, Madhya Pradesh, India

1 Introduction

Agrochemicals have become the most widely encountered class of compounds that are frequently found worldwide on earth surfaces and water bodies, as a result of their heavy applications in agricultural fields and other domestic areas. Apart from being inherently carcinogenic, toxic, and mutagenic in nature, these compounds show characteristic properties, such as persistence in the environment and movement to different areas. They have a potential to target the endocrine systems of living organisms, including humans (Armas et al., 2007). A survey has shown that agricultural producers use different types of agrochemicals, including pesticides, for the enhanced production and protection of crops. Among the surveyed farms, 55% used insecticides, 25% used fungicides, and 20% used herbicides. Pesticides used during agricultural production have increasingly been causing concerns due to their adverse effects on human health. Pesticides are toxic chemicals used in preventing, destroying, repelling, or mitigating pests. Their residues in or on plants may be unavoidable even when pesticides are used in accordance with good and recommended agricultural practices. Laboratory studies have shown that insecticides cause health problems, such as birth defects, nerve damage, cancer, and other effects depending on how toxic the pesticide is and how much is consumed. Some pesticides also pose unique health risks to children but at the same time they are one of the vital ingredients of crop production and enhance agricultural productivity. Thus, it is a challenge for the scientific and technological communities to maintain a balance between the utility of the agrochemical compounds in agricultural sectors, domestic uses, edible commodities, and so forth, and the health risks emerging from their uses. Whereas on one hand, their application to agricultural

New Pesticides and Soil Sensors. http://dx.doi.org/10.1016/B978-0-12-804299-1.00015-1

fields protects the crops and results in enhanced production, the compounds eventually percolate into underground water systems or other water bodies, creating various kinds of diseases, allergies, and other physiological disorders.

Paraquat (1-1′-dimethyl-4-4′-bipiridyl) is a well-known herbicide compound synthesized chemically as an ammonium-based dichloride salt. Introduced in the 1960s, the compound, at present, has crossed borders into more than 100 countries and is being widely employed in plantations of sugar cane, tobacco, rice, beans, and related crops (Almeida et al., 2007). Apart from these applications, this herbicide is widely used for direct sowing, either with other herbicides or alone. Moreover, it is also employed for weed control, particularly in uncultivated areas, preharvest drying, and pasture renewal (Marchi et al., 2008). As far as the acceptable limit of this herbicide in drinking water is concerned, the US Environmental Protection Agency has limited it to 0.030 mg L^{-1}, while its toxicity limit has been set as 15 mg L^{-1} in reference to aquatic organisms (USEPA, 2010). Furthermore, it has been classified as II for Environmental Danger Potential, while its toxicological classification is type II, which stands for highly toxic. There are no recognized lethal doses of paraquat for animals. However, the average lethal doses (LD_{50}) for oral administration have been reported to be 35 mg/kg^{-1} for cats, 25–50 mg/kg^{-1} for dogs and pigs, 50–75 mg/kg^{-1} for sheep, and 35–50 mg/kg^{-1} for cattle (Almeida et al., 2007). In a developing country like India, human life has also been threatened by various diseases, which endanger biological systems and cause permanent disability in the body.

The recent past has witnessed a growing interest in agricultural nanotechnology, which encompasses the use of nanostructures in agricultural areas. It is known that particles with dimensions between 1 and 100 nm are coined as nanoparticles (NPs), and they have a great potential to accommodate bioactive entities via absorption or dispersion within the NP matrix. Very often the host matrix of nanomaterials has been chosen as polymers of either synthetic or natural origin (Bogdansky, 1990), dendrimers (Kono, 2002), organic nanocarriers (Soppimath et al., 2001), cyclodextrins (de Jesus et al., 2006), and natural biodegradable polymers (Langer and Karel, 1981; Fernández-Pérez et al., 2000). The advanced studies concerning these materials justify the advantages they offer because of their small dimensions, which permit them to reach the targets with enhanced contact, which in general are not accessible. Another specialty is that these nanosystems may be easily optimized with respect to the kinetics of the release process and dosages of the encapsulated agents (Letchford and Burt, 2007; Schaffazick et al., 2003).

To fight against their aforementioned disadvantages, it is of foremost importance that suitable high-performance material–based nanosensors must be designed, which can not only function to detect pesticides in crops, but also be priced within reach of the majority of farmers.

2 The Need for Biomonitoring

Biomonitoring is a scientific technique for assessing the environment, including human exposures to natural and synthetic chemicals, based on sampling and analysis of an individual organism's tissues and fluids. The results of these measurements provide information about the amounts of natural and man-made chemicals that have entered and remained in the organisms and induce the corresponding effects. Due to consistency between the selected organisms and the corresponding living space, biomonitoring can directly offer data on the potential effects and actual integrated toxicities of pollutants, reflecting their corresponding deleterious degree in the environment (Zhoua et al., 2008).

An important approach toward the assessment of risks from the environmental and occupational exposures is biomonitoring, which provides an estimate of the total dose absorbed and gives indirect access to determine target site concentrations. To reveal the presence of pollutants and to measure their toxic effects, biological indicators can be used. Active and passive monitoring are two general approaches to assess the pollutants and their toxic effects at different levels from the species to the community level of any ecosystem. In passive monitoring, degradation of the ecosystem, elimination of sensitive species, and reduction of biodiversity can be revealed as adverse consequences of pollution at the level of populations, while at the level of the individual, accumulation of toxic substances in specimens, organs, and tissues, indicative of pollution in the environment, can be traced. In active monitoring, the response of artificial or modified populations; behavioral patterns of specimens; specific functions of organs, such as movement, feeding, respiration, reproduction, and the neural regulation; as well as cellular and subcellular events are studied under the effect of toxic substances (Vander Oost et al., 2003).

In biomonitoring surveys, the toxic elements, such as arsenic, cadmium, chromium, cobalt, lead, nickel, and so forth, are used as examples to illustrate the disturbing factors in the interpretation of biomonitoring results (Christensen, 1995). The accumulation of trace elements in aquatic consumers is of interest to environmental scientists concerned with the fate and effect of contaminants, as well as to ecologists interested in food web dynamics

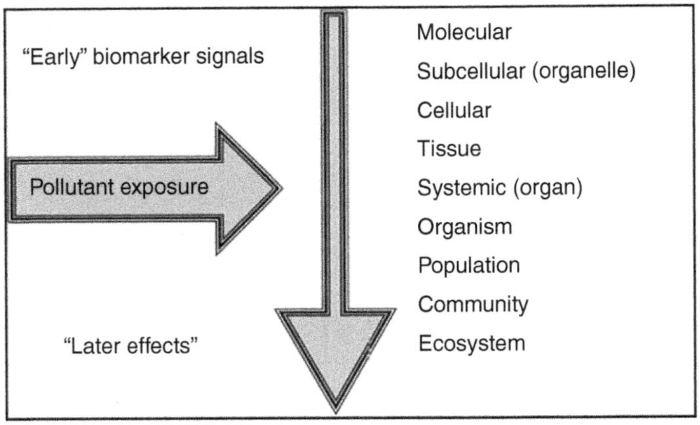

Figure 14.1. The schematic representation of the sequential order of responses to pollutant stress within a biological system.

and trace metal biogeochemical cycles to assess the toxic impact or distribution of contaminants (Nguyen et al., 2005). In the field, the ecotoxicological approach is very difficult for the evaluation of the impact of heavy metals in an aquatic environment due to the complexity of interrelationships between organisms and the ecosystems. However, field studies can enable assessment of the long-term effect of heavy metals on organisms (Gupta and Singh, 2011). The schematic representation of the sequential order of responses to pollutant stress within a biological system is shown in Fig. 14.1.

3 Nanomaterials

The field of nanotechnology involves understanding and controlling matter at the molecular or atomic level where materials, due to their small scale, exhibit unique properties and behaviors when compared to the same material in the bulk form (e.g., silver, copper, and iron) (USEPA, 2007). The nanoscale has been defined approximately as 1–100 nm, which is equal to one-billionth of a meter. For comparison, an average bacteria cell is approximately 1000 nm in diameter, there are 10 million nanometers in a centimeter, and there are 25.4 million nanometers in an inch (Davies, 2009; Zhang, 2003). However, the British Standards Institution, the American Society for Testing Materials, and the Scientific Committee on Emerging and Newly Identified Health Risks have adopted the definition to be any material with one dimension under 100 nm (Klaine et al., 2008). Within this group of materials are NPs, which are defined by the International Organization for Standardization (ISO, 2008) as materials with at least three dimensions between 1 and 100 nm.

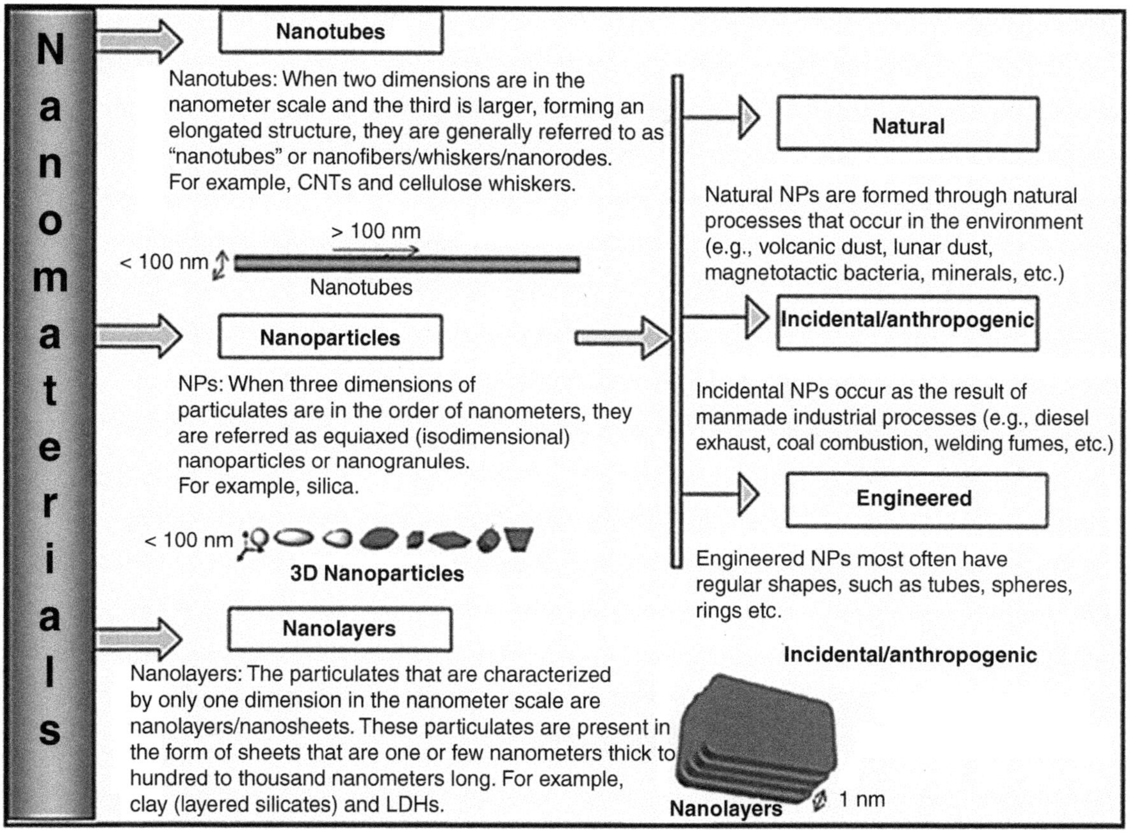

Figure 14.2. Schematic classification of nanomaterials. *CNTs,* Carbon nanotubes; *LDH,* layered double hydroxides; *NPs,* nanoparticles.

NPs as shown in Fig.14.2 are classified into three categories depending on their dimensions as follows:

- natural
- incidental
- engineered

There are many naturally occurring NPs, such as clays, weathered minerals, organic matter, and metal oxides (Watlington, 2005; NNI, 2009). Incidental NPs are generated in a relatively uncontrolled manner and can occur as a by-product of fuel combustion, manufacturing, agricultural practices, vaporization, and weathering, and are released into the environment from NP production facilities (DHHS, 2009; Klaine et al., 2008) (Table 14.1).

Engineered NPs are intentionally designed and manufactured with specific properties or compositions (e.g., shape, size, surface properties, and chemistry), and may be released into the

Table 14.1 Different Types of Nanomaterials

NPs	Description	Recent Applications
Nanocapsules	Vesicular systems in which the drug is surrounded by a polymeric membrane	Stability of the cisplatin nanocapsules has been optimized by varying the lipid composition of the bilayer coat (Xie et al., 2007).
Nanospheres	Matrix systems in which the drug is physically and uniformly dispersed	BSA nanospheres containing 5-fluorouracil show higher tumor inhibition than the free drug (Cao et al., 2004)
Micelles	Amphiphilic block copolymers that can self-associate in an aqueous solution	Micelle delivery of doxorubicin increases cytotoxicity to prostate carcinoma cells (He et al., 2007)
Ceramic NPs	NPs fabricated using inorganic compounds including silica, titania, etc.	Ultrafine silica–based NPs release water-insoluble anticancer drug (Phenrat et al., 2009)
Liposomes	Artificial spherical vesicles produced from natural phospholipids and cholesterol	Radiation-guided drug delivery of liposomal cisplatin to tumor blood vessels results in improved tumor growth delay (Saleh et al., 2007).
Dendrimers	Macromolecular compounds that comprise a series of branches around an inner core	Targeted delivery within dendrimers improves the cytotoxic response of the cells to methotrexate 100-fold over free drug (Zhang and Elliott, 2006)
SLN particles	NPs made from solid lipids	SLN powder formulation of all-*trans* retinoic acid may have the potential in cancer chemoprevention and therapeutics (Saleh et al., 2008).

BSA, Bovine serum albumin; SLN, solid-lipid nanoparticles.

environment through industrial or environmental applications (DHHS, 2009; NNI, 2009).

At present, engineered nanoparticles (e.g., silicon dioxide, titanium dioxide, cerium oxide, and iron oxides) have emerged as materials of major economic interest (Nowack and Bucheli, 2007). They have already been widely used in pharmacy, the electronic and cosmetic industry, and in consumer products, such as sunscreens, scratch-resistant paints, and semiconductors (Colvin, 2003).

Several studies have been undertaken to explore the inter- relationship between sensors and nanotechnology over the past several years (Ballesteros-Gomez and Rubio, 2009; Zhang et al., 2009; Singh, 2011). Researchers have put intensive efforts into designing nanomaterial-based biosensors that can offer high sensitivity and stability in terms of performance. Sensing devices interfaced with nanostructure assemblies have opened up new strategies to ensure sensitive optical and electrochemical detection of analyses. For instance, recently electrochemical enzyme biosensors have been designed that are fully based on nanostructures whose greater conductivity is said to augment the process of electron transfer between the enzyme redox center and the electrode surfaces (Sassolas et al., 2012). The nanomaterials part of the biosensor tends to lower the overpotential associated with electroactive compounds that minimize the interference present in the sample. In exceptional cases the nanomaterials function as labels for amplifying the measured signals.

The combination of nanotechnology with modern electrochemical techniques allows the introduction of powerful, reliable electrical devices for effective process and pollution control. Although the NPs in general play different roles in different electrochemical sensors, electroanalysis using a NP-modified electrode has several advantages:

1. effective catalysis
2. fast-mass transport
3. large effective sensor surface area, and
4. good control over electrode microenvironment (Hanrahan et al., 2004).

3.1 Types of Nanomaterials

Biosensors are important tools for personalized medicine, point-of care devices, and cheaper diagnostic tools, and have gained an important position in biomedical research. In the past decade, large number of nanomaterials, such as NPs, quantum dots (QDs), nanowires, graphene, graphene quantum dots (GQDs), or carbon nanotubes (CNTs) have been developed as highly sensitive and selective biosensors because they possess unique physical and chemical properties due to their nanosize.

3.1.1 Carbon Nanotubes

Among the different kinds of nanomaterials, CNTs have attracted much interest as promising building blocks for biosensor design because of their unique physical and chemical properties. CNTs are composed of sp^2-hybridized carbon atoms, and can be prepared by chemical vapor deposition, carbon arc discharge, and laser ablation. They can also be classified as single-walled carbon nanotubes (SWCNT) and multiwalled carbon nanotubes (MWCNT) on the basis of rolled-up cylinder (Strano et al., 2013).

3.1.2 Graphenes

Recently, various emerging nanomaterials have been developed for efficient biosensing. Out of these, carbon-based nanomaterials have been considered as promising materials due to their cost effectiveness, and with a high-surface area and energy capacity, especially in terms of the ratio of energy/weight cost. It has been observed that a two-dimensional (2D), single-atomic carbon sheet of graphene can be used as a building block for synthesizing. Zero-dimensional buckyball (consisting of graphene balled into a sphere through the introduction of some pentagons and hexagons into the lattice), 1D nanotube (rolled sheets of graphene), and 3D graphite (stack of graphene layers) can be used for effective energy conversion and energy storage applications (Singh et al., 2011; Pumera, 2011).

Graphene also called as "super carbon," is a one-atom thick, 2D honeycomb lattice network of sp^2-hybridized carbons (carbon–carbon distance of 0.142 nm), which makes it the "mother" of all carbon-based systems. It can be derived from naturally abundant, low-cost graphite via different synthetic techniques, such as liquid-phase exfoliation of graphite, chemical vapor deposition, self-assembly approach, and chemical reduction of graphite oxide. It was discovered in 2004, and since then has received tremendous attraction owing to its novel electrical performances and unique superior properties, such as good chemical stability, high surface area (2630 $m^2\ g^{-1}$) and mechanical strength, good thermal (~5000 $W\ m^{-1}\ K^{-1}$) and electrical conductivity (106 $S\ cm^{-1}$), high-charge mobility (200,000 $cm^2\ V^{-1}\ s^{-1}$), optical transmittance (~97.7%), and low price (Kim et al., 2011; Chen et al., 2012).

Graphene consists of a 2D hexagonal lattice of highly ordered carbon atoms with over 100-fold anisotropy of heat flow between the in-plane and out-of-plane directions in which each carbon atom is covalently bonded to three others, leaving one valence electron unoccupied that is responsible for the conduction of electricity. The thermal conductivity of graphene is due to strong and anisotropic bonding (covalent sp^2 bonding between carbon atoms) and low mass. However, weak van der Waals coupling reduces the out-of-plane heat flow (Pop et al., 2012).

3.1.3 Multiaptasensor

Aptamers are an emerging class of nucleic acid molecules. They can bind to numerous targets (large targets, such as proteins and cells or small targets, such as nucleotides, amino acids, and metal ions) with high specificity and affinity due to their properties, such as easy modification, smaller size (~1–2 nm, 10 kDa); higher surface density; decreased steric hindrance; performance under nonphysiological conditions, including extremely high or low temperatures or pHs; ease of labeling; cost effectiveness; and ability to be incorporated into 1D, 2D, or 3D DNA-based nanostructures. Aptamers can be synthesized by a process called systematic evolution of ligands by exponential enrichment (SELEX) in vitro. Although aptamers are excellent candidates as diagnostic and drug-delivery agents, they suffer from two major problems: nuclease degradation in cells or in blood, and decreased stability of RNA molecules due to hydrolysis in biological fluids (Lu et al., 2010). These problems can be overcome by the conjugation of aptamers with nanomaterials, such as QDs or semiconductor NPs.

3.1.4 Molecular Imprinted Polymer Nanoparticles

Multifunctional NPs are among the most exciting nanomaterials and have gained much attention for their applications in biosensing, bioassays, catalysis, and separations. During the past years, molecular imprinted polymer (MIP) nanostructured materials have attracted increasing scientific interest for their highly selective recognition of numerous molecules in different fields of analytical chemistry (drug delivery, biosensing, antibiotic substitutes, and capillary electrophoresis) due to some remarkable properties, such as high surface-to-volume ratio; stability at low and high pH, pressures, and temperatures (<180°C); and low-cost and straightforward preparation and handling. Molecular imprinting is a well-established method to introduce functional groups with specified stereochemical properties. They can be used for creating complementary cavities containing tailor-made polymeric materials that have advantages, such as excellent mechanical and chemical stability; easy preparation; and low cost and reusability for the specific target molecules, such as drugs, pesticides, peptides, and sugars, as well as larger organic compounds via complementary noncovalent binding sites, based on, for example, ionic, hydrophobic, or hydrogen bond interactions (Guo et al., 2015). The approach involves polymerization of functional monomers and a cross-linker to create a 3D polymeric matrix around a print or template molecule. After the matrix is removed, receptor sites are present in the material with function and shape complementary to the template (Poma et al., 2010). MIP NPs can be synthesized by precipitation polymerization, mini- and micro-emulsion polymerization, core–shell approaches (with subsequent grafting), and living radical polymerization processes, such as atom transfer radical polymerization (ATRP) and reversible addition fragmentation chain transfer polymerization (RAFT). Wang et al. (2015) synthesized molecularly imprinted NPs by in situ coating of cytochrome c to the surface of the carboxyl-modified upconversion NPs through sol–gel technique; characterized them by transmission electron microscopy (TEM), power X-ray diffraction (XRD), energy-dispersive X-ray analysis (EDXA), and X-ray photoelectron spectroscopic (XPS); and used them for the selective recognition of cytochrome C among other proteins, such as bovine serum albumin (BSA) and lysozyme.

3.1.5 Multifunctional Nanoparticles

Over the past few decades, a large number of NPs with various conformations, such as spheres, nanotubes, nanohorns, and nanocages, made of different materials with specific physical, chemical, and biological properties have been fabricated for biomedical applications. However, their properties can be tailored and improved by functionalization of their surface because multifunctional NPs are able to achieve a mixed effect using one system, that is, they have improved mechanical and chemical properties; enhanced NP solubilization in various solvents, which extends their application capabilities; reduced toxicity; modified electronic, optical, spectroscopic, and chemical properties; and the ability to target desired chemical, physical, or biological environments so that they can be applied in bioimaging, biosensing, cancer biomarking, and so forth (Díaz-García and de Dios, 2010).

3.1.6 Graphene Quantum Dots

Recently, GQDs have attracted tremendous attention as a novel kind of photoluminescent (PL) carbon dots (CDs). GQDs are a new type of small zero-dimensional PL carbon-based nanomaterial with characteristics derived from both graphene and CDs. They have lateral dimensions less than 100 nm in a single layer, double layers, and a few layers, and consist of very thin (typically 3–20 nm) graphene sheets with unique superior properties, such as chemical inertness, large-surface area, large diameter, fine-surface grafting using the p–p conjugated network or surface groups, ease of production, resistance to photobleaching, excellent water solubility and suitability for successive functionalization, low cytotoxicity, and excellent biocompatibility in comparison to conventional semiconductor QDs, which makes them attractive tools for research in various fields (photovoltaic devices, cellular imaging, and drug delivery). They show excellent optical and electrical properties due to their quantum confinement and edge effects. GQDs can be prepared by both a “top–down” approach (which includes cutting down large graphene sheets, carbon fibers, or graphite into small pieces using high-resolution electron beam lithography, acidic oxidation, reoxidation, hydrothermal, or solvothermal, microwave assisted, sonication assisted, electrochemical route, photo-Fenton reaction, selective plasma oxidation, and chemical exfoliation, or cage opening the fullerene on ruthenium surfaces), and a "bottom–up" approach (which includes use of small molecules, such as benzene derivatives to build GQDs, and carbonizing some special organic precursors, such as fullerenes, unsubstituted hexaperihexabenzocoronene by thermal treatment, oxidation, surface functionalization, reduction, or through ruthenium-catalyzed cage opening). "Bottom–up" strategies are more precise than "top–down" to control the morphology and size of nanomaterials (Dong et al., 2012).

GQDs have circular, elliptical, triangular, quadrate, and hexagonal dot shape but mainly contain less than five layers of graphene sheets (c. 2.5 nm). They contain similar functional groups (carbonyl, carboxyl, hydroxyl, and epoxy groups) on the surface, as well as a crystalline structure as graphene. GQDs have a nonzero band gap that can be altered by changing their size and surface properties, which is responsible for their PL activity. Presently, GQDs so prepared can emit blue, green, yellow, and red color, and this PL depends on the size, shape, excitation wavelength, pH, concentration, surface oxidation degree, surface functionalization, N-doping, and S-doping. Presently, GQDs are used in single-electron transistor (SET)–based charge sensors (switching device that uses controlled electron tunneling to amplify a current) as sensors for the detection of humidity and pressure.

4 Nanosensors

Nanotechnology can be defined as the science that involves synthesis, characterization, and application of nanomaterials in various medical fields. Nanomaterials used in sensing are called nanosensors that are built at an atomic scale to collect data and transfer them into data that can be analyzed for many applications, such as (1) monitoring physical and chemical phenomena in regions that are difficult to reach, (2) detecting biochemicals in cellular organelles, and (3) measuring nanoscopic particles in the industry and environment. They are highly sensitive chemical or physical sensors that can detect a single virus, as well as a low concentration of substance that could be potentially harmful. A nanosensor consists of a biosensitive layer (biological recognition element, i.e., antibody (Ab), enzyme, protein, DNA, etc., covalently attached to the transducer, at least one of their sensing dimensions being not greater than 100 nm) that produces a physiochemical change when the target analyst interacts with the bioreceptor and converts this change into an electrical signal.

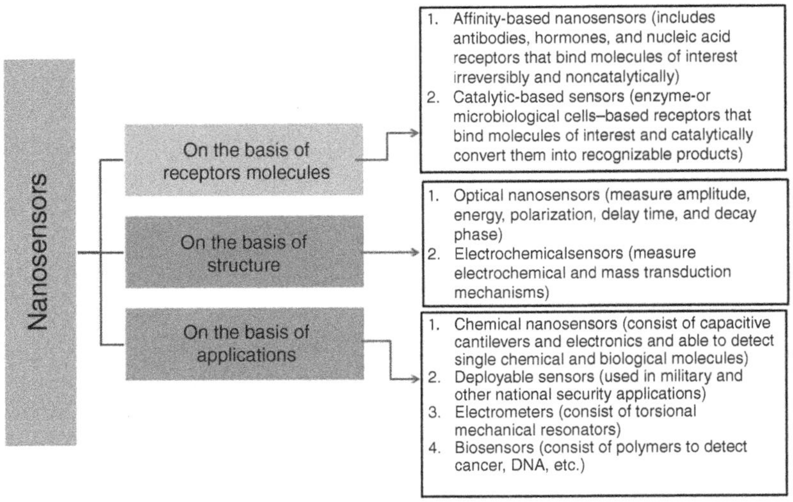

Figure 14.3. Schematic representation of classification of nanosensors.

Nanosensors can be classified on the basis of receptors molecules, structure, and applications (Fig. 14.3).

The ideal sensor should possess the following characteristics (Campbell and Compton, 2010):

1. specificity for the target species,
2. sensitivity to changes in target species concentrations,
3. fast response time,
4. extended lifetime of at least several months, and
5. small size (miniaturization) with the possibility of low-cost manufacture.

5 Nanobiosensors

The past several decades have given rise to significant advancements in nanotechnology, which were eventually transformed into fabrication of functional nanostructure-based biosensors. The so-designed devices have replaced the conventional technology-based sensing systems and offered not only improved sensitivity, but also selectivity and multiplexing capacity. Biosensors have an important impact on basic scientific research and healthcare. In this area, scientific breakthroughs are often facilitated by new sensing technologies that enable investigation of unstudied biological phenomena. Nowadays biosensors are very helpful tools in our everyday life, being used for the detection of allergens in food, toxicants in water, in chronic diseases control, pregnancy tests, and other diagnostic applications. Certainly, it can be anticipated that biosensors are going to become part of our lives in the future, so it is a research field looking for new and improved easy-to-use device technologies (Roy and Gao, 2009; Quesada-González and Merkoçi, 2015). The progress in nanofabrication techniques and tools coupled with improved nanomaterials with novel properties has provided great momentum to technologies used for designing functional nanomaterial-based biosensors. Due to the huge quantum availability of nanofabrication techniques and nanomaterials, the field of biosensors has acquired new dimensions. At present scientists are globally putting their efforts to develop nanomaterial-based ultrasensitive biosensors for advanced applications (Kruss et al., 2013).

The advancements in science and technology in the area of nanomaterials have opened up new avenues for great achievements in the development of biosensors. As materials science has shown remarkable progress in synthesizing inorganic–organic–based hybrid materials, it has also led to the possibility of designing biosensors that are competent enough to deliver on-site results of analyses without seeking expertise from skilled persons or using sophisticated modern instruments. Structurally a biosensor is a reagent-less device composed of biological sensing components (bioreceptor) linked to a detector or transducer. The function of the bioreceptor is to detect analytes, such as Abs, enzymes, aptamers, or single-stranded DNA, and microorganisms, and transform this detection into a recognizable signal that could be sensitively detected (Fig. 14.4). Biosensors generally produce an electronic or optical signal proportional to the specific interaction between the target and the recognition molecule immobilized on the biosensor. They also transform biological interactions into electronic signals that can be properly measured and recorded. A biosensor may be categorized on the basis of the type of bioreceptor, such as enzymatic, immune, and genobiosensors. Furthermore, depending on the kind of transduction process, they

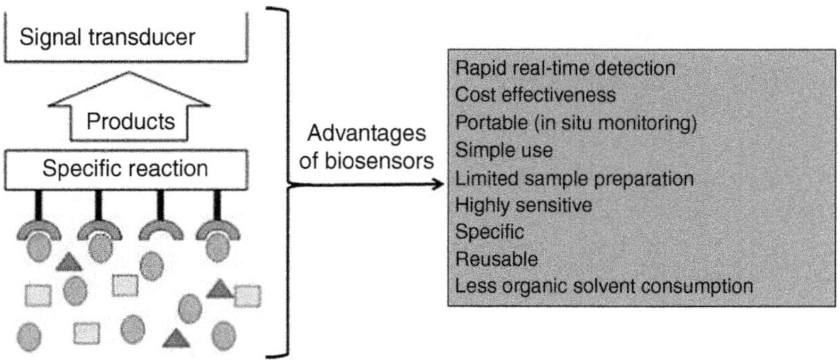

Figure 14.4. Schematic representation of the detection mechanisms of biosensors.

may also be named as piezoelectric, optical, electrochemical, and thermometric biosensors. Catalytic biosensors employ enzymes and microorganisms as the biorecognition molecules that catalyze a reaction involving the analyte to yield a product. Affinity biosensors are characterized by a binding event between the biorecognition molecule and the analyte (the affinity reaction), often with no further reaction occurring (Justin, 2006).

Among the various kinds of biosensors, electrochemical biosensors have been successfully commercialized because of their characteristics, such as prevalence, suitability for on-site analysis, and capability to be miniaturized for convenient handling. They further fall into potentiometric, impedimetric, and amperometric sensors. The history of biosensors dates back to 1962 when Leland C. Clark fabricated enzyme-sensitive electrodes. The field of biosensors prospered further when the scientists from different disciplines joined their hands to design more advanced, sophisticated, and reliable biosensors, which were efficient enough to detect small molecules precisely and rapidly. The so-developed biosensors found vast applications in areas, such as diagnostics, drug discovery, and allied biomedical and pharmaceutical fields (Kumar et al., 2015; Dzyadevych et al., 2008).

Commercial biosensors generally consist of a detector, sample application, and delivery system. Apart from these biosensors, there are immunochromatographic devices, which do not use any of the transducers mentioned earlier. These devices are based on lateral flow strips and they are ultrasensitive tests, which enable on-site visual detection of target molecules (Bahadır and Sezginturk, 2015; Baird and Myszka, 2001).

6 Types of Nanobiosensors

Environmental pollution is expeditiously increasing owing to global economic expansion and industrial development. Synthetic chemicals, pesticides, and heavy metals are major contaminants in environmental pollution. It is important for regulatory agencies, regulated community, and the general public to monitor the presence of pollutants by using fast and cost-effective analytical techniques. In this context, biosensors appear as suitable alternative or complementary analytical tools to measure pollutants in environmental samples, and for diverse environmental monitoring area. There are many biosensors under development and also an extensive literature in this area. The biosensors offer advantages over other sensors: they are specific in response and may work effectively even when the environments are not clean. However, only a small fraction of all biosensors developed are commercially available (Chee, 2013) (Table 14.2).

Table 14.2 Advantages and Limitations of Recognition Elements in Chemical Sensors and Biosensors

Recognition Elements	Sensor Designation	Advantages	Limitations
Enzymes	Enzymatic biosensor	Specificity and simplicity of apparatus and procedures	Purification is costly and time consuming, poor stability, efficiency only at optimum pH and temperature
Antibodies	Immunosensor	High affinity and specificity	Limited target (protein), laborious production, production requires use of animals, and lack of stability
Nucleic acids	Genosensor	Stability	Limited target (complementary nucleic acid)
Whole cells	Whole cell biosensor	Low-cost preparation and reduced purification requirements	—
Phages	Phage biosensor	Specificity, sensitivity, and stability	—
Aptamers (DNA, RNA, or peptides)	Aptasensor (particularly, DNA sensor or RNA sensor) and peptide sensor	Easy to modify, possibility to design structure, possibility to denaturalize and to rehybridize, possibility to distinguish targets with different functional groups, thermally stable, and in vitro synthesis	—
MIPs	MIP sensor	High thermal, chemical, and mechanical tolerance, reusability, and low cost	Complex fabrication methodology, time-consuming process, incompatibility with aqueous media, and leakage of template molecules
Affibodies	Affibody sensor	Lack of disulfide bonds that enable intracellular applications and long shelf life	—

MIP, Molecularly imprinted polymer.

6.1 Enzyme-Based Biosensors

A wide range of biomolecular recognition elements has been used for biosensors with potential environmental applications. One important step in biosensor development is the immobilization of the biological recognition element to the sensor surface. A number of innovative immobilization techniques have been

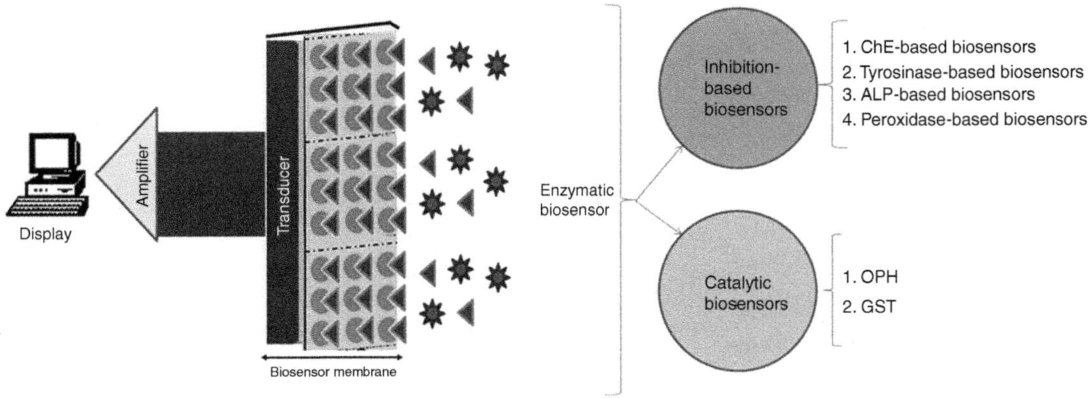

Figure 14.5. Types of enzyme-based biosensors. *ALP,* Alkaline phosphatase; *ChE,* choline esterase; *GST,* glutathione-S-transferase; *OPH,* organophosphorus hydrolase.

reported using enzymes. In principle, the detection of pesticides by enzyme biosensors rest upon either the measurement of enzyme inhibition or detection of the compounds, which are involved in the enzymatic reaction as shown in Fig. 14.5. Enzyme biosensors show sensitivity, stability, and excellent shelf life and improved electrochemical interfaces and mediate a more efficient operation. Their response can be increased by the modulation of the enzyme activity with respect to the target analyses.

In enzymatic biosensors, the enzyme (recognition element) reacts selectively with its substrate (target analyte). Enzymatic biosensors can measure the catalysis or the inhibition of enzymes by the target analyses by either of the two ways, that is:

1. The enzyme can metabolize the analyte, so that the concentration of the analyte is determined by measuring the catalytic transformation of the analyte by the enzyme.
2. The enzyme can be inhibited by the analyte, so that the concentration of the analyte is associated with a decreased enzymatic product formation (Wang et al., 2014).

However, they suffer from many problems, such as the limited number of substrates for which enzymes have evolved; the limited interaction between environmental pollutants and specific enzymes; and in the case of inhibitor formats, the lack of specificity in differentiating among compounds of similar classes, such as nerve agents, as well as organophosphates (OP) [synthetic compounds developed during World War II that are used as pesticides and nerve agents and exhibit severe toxicity on the human nervous system by inhibiting acetylcholinesterase (AChE) activity] and carbamate pesticides. The use of enzymes as recognition elements in biosensors has been increasing, also due to the combination of enzymes with nanomaterials such as NPs, nanorods, and CNTs (Tasca et al., 2010; Zheng et al., 2011; Ibupoto et al., 2011; Chauhan and Pundir, 2012; Ibupoto et al., 2012; Yan et al., 2013) (Fig. 14.6).

OP and carbamate pesticides are the main cholinesterase (ChE) inhibitors. Therefore, they are detected by ChE-based biosensors. Two types of natural ChE enzymes are known—AChE and butyrylcholinesterase (BChE)—and have been widely used for many years for the detection of these neurotoxic compounds, which irreversibly inhibit normal enzyme function. In turn, AChE is an enzyme commonly used in biosensors for the detection of OP pesticides, as its catalytic activity (hydrolysis of acetylcholine

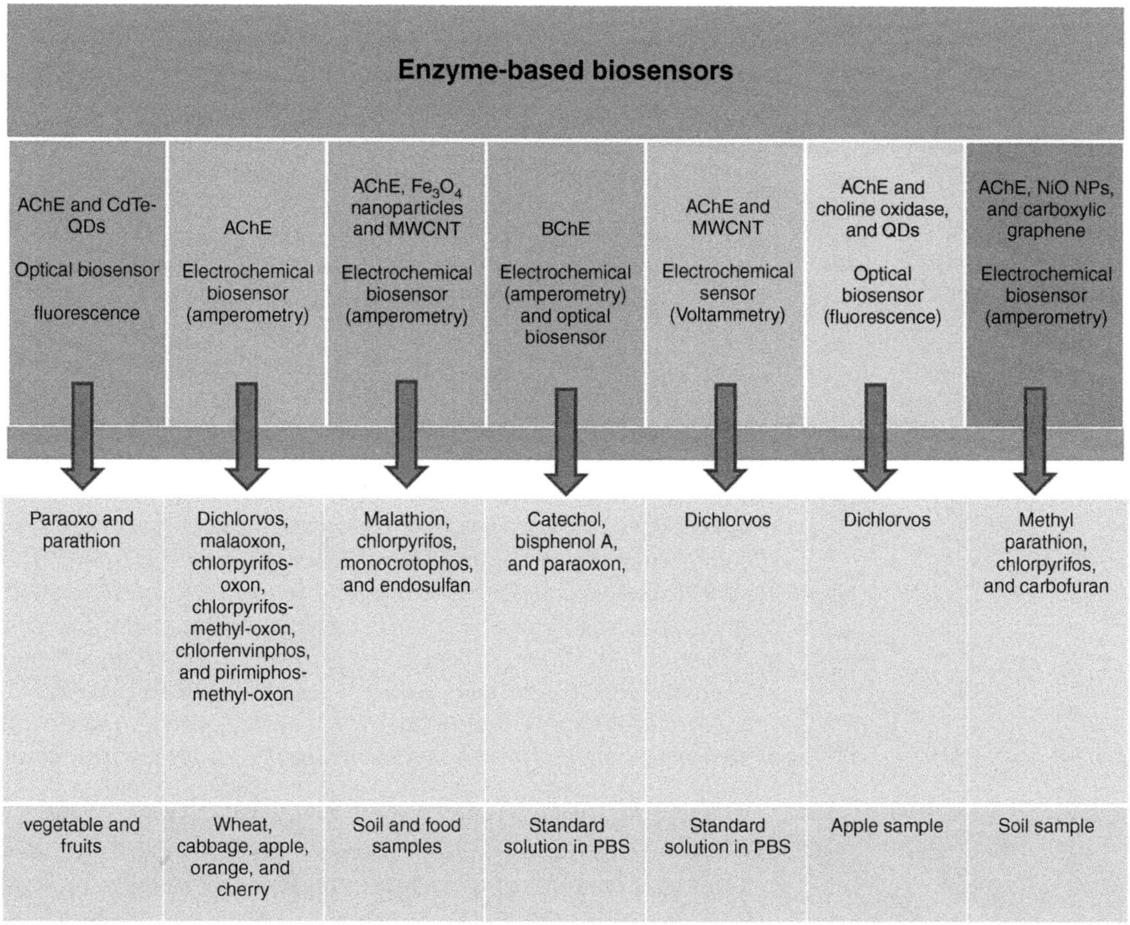

Figure 14.6. Commercially used enzyme-based biosensors for pesticide detection. *AChE,* Acetylcholinesterase; *BChE,* butyrylcholinesterase; *CdTe-QDs,* CdTe quantum dots; *MWCNT,* multiwalled carbon nanotubes; *PBS,* phosphate buffer saline.

to thiocholine) is inhibited by trace amounts of such compounds. Thus, such inhibition is monitored by the change of oxidation current of thiocholine at a certain potential in amperometric biosensors. These enzymes have different substrates: AChE preferentially hydrolyzes acetyl esters, such as acetylcholine, whereas BChE hydrolyzes butyrylcholine:

$$\text{Acetylcholine} + H_2O \xrightarrow{\text{AChE}} \text{Choline} + \text{Acetic acid}$$

$$\text{Butyrylcholine} + H_2O \xrightarrow{\text{BChE}} \text{Choline} + \text{Butyric acid}$$

Biosensors based on the inhibition of AChE have been widely used for many years for the detection of these neurotoxic compounds, which irreversibly inhibit normal enzyme function. The enzyme source has an important effect on the biosensor performance. The reactions that take place in an AChE-based biosensor are described in the following scheme:

$$\text{Acetylthiocholine} \xrightarrow{\text{AChE}} \text{Thiocholine} + CH_3COOH$$

$$\text{Thiocholine} + 2\text{Co-PC(ox)} \rightarrow \text{Thiocholine(ox)} + 2\text{Co-PC(red)}$$

$$\text{Co-PC(red)} \rightarrow \text{Co-PC(ox)} + 2e^-$$

The flow of electrons is proportional to the rate of acetylthiocholine hydrolysis, which decreases upon phosphorylation of a serine present in the enzyme active site by OP. There are different sources, such as human blood, horse serum, and bovine or human erythrocytes from which AChE enzymes may be isolated. However the ChE enzymes that are isolated from insects are more sensitive than those obtained from other sources. It is known that acetylthiocholine and butyrylthiocholine may also be used as artificial substrates for AChE and BChE enzymes, respectively. This biosensor has two advantages: (1) it is quite simple in design, and (2) its detection potential is low. The use of multiple enzymes in the same biosensor is of interest due to the versatility for detection of various analytes in biosensors. In this field, an electrochemical biosensor based on six AChE enzymes was fabricated (Crew et al., 2011) for the detection of six OP pesticides in food samples and water. The biosensor was portable for the advantageous in situ analysis of such samples, and incorporated a neural network program used for modeling the analytical response, leading to an efficient, accurate interpretation of the results. Similarly, a trienzymatic biosensor can be prepared by adding peroxidase to the bienzyme system.

Tyrosinase-based biosensors are synthesized to detect carbamate pesticides and atrazine. These biosensors are stable at high temperature, but they are not highly specific due to the short lifetime of the tyrosinase enzyme. Alkaline phosphatase (ALP)–based biosensors have been developed for the detection of pesticides. Detection of organochlorine pesticides, such as carbamate and fenitrothion, and heavy metal ions, such as cyanides, has been successfully detected by fluorescent ALP-based biosensors (Garcia Sanchez et al., 2003). ALP enzyme was found to catalyze the hydrolysis of 1-naphthyl phosphate to fluorescent 1-naphthol. Thiodicarb, a carbamate pesticide, can be detected by using peroxidase-based biosensors. There are some pesticides, which reversibly inhibit enzyme-like acid phosphatase, which have been used along with glucose oxidase to design a bienzymatic biosensor for detecting malathion, methyl parathion, and paraoxon (Mazzei et al., 1996).

Organophosphorus hydrolase (OPH)– and glutathione-S-transferase (GST)–based biosensors belong to catalytic biosensors that are used to detect parathion, methyl parathion (Du et al., 2010), or paraoxon (Lee et al., 2010; Pedrosa et al., 2010). These enzymes hydrolyze P—S, P—CN, and P—O bonds producing two protons, which may be detected electrochemically. Moreover, an alcohol is also generated, which is chromophoric and/or electroactive, and GST catalyzes the nucleophile attack of GSH on atrazine, releasing H^+. This pH variation is optically measured by color changes of bromocresol green.

Alonso et al. (2012) prepared a more selective, more efficient, one-step inhibition biosensor by screen-printed carbon electrodes and two different AChE enzymes that can be used to determine mixtures of three organophosphorus compounds, that is, chlorpyriphos-oxon, chlorfenvinphos, and azinphos methyl-oxon in water samples.

Recently, an enzymatic biosensor based on fluorescence was fabricated for the detection of OP pesticides using a complex of two enzymes (AChE and choline oxidase) and CdTe quantum dots (CdTe-QDs) as a recognition element, where a low limit of detection (LOD) (4.49 nM) was obtained, suggesting that the biosensor was suitable for detecting residues of OP pesticides in real samples (Meng et al., 2013). In another work, AChE and CdTe-QDs were combined to detect OP pesticides (paraoxon and parathion) using an optical biosensor (Table 14.2). The biosensor was based on enzyme inhibition mechanisms, obtaining LODs (1.05×10^{-11} M for paraoxon and 4.47×10^{-12} M for parathion) better than those obtained with GC–MS (5×10^{-8} M). However, the authors reported some limitations of the biosensors, such as the quenching of QDs, which was responsible for the recovery of only about 60% of the original fluorescence, and the sensor was designed for a one-time use (Zheng et al., 2011).

Electrochemical enzyme biosensors have been developed using various NPs, such as QDs, gold nanoparticles (AuNPs), etc. Using poly(*N*-vinyl-2-pyrrolidone) (PVP)–capped CDs QDs an enzyme biosensor was used for the amperometric detection of trichlorfon (Li et al., 2006). When the PVP-QD nanostructures are formed on the electrode surfaces, it provides a supportive microenvironment for the sensitive and stable electrochemical system with a detection limit of 4.8×10^{-3} M. Similarly, AuNPs are other potential NPs to constitute enzyme biosensors, which also provide a suitable microenvironment over the electrode surface so that the biomolecules may be favorably immobilized, maintaining their bioactivity. Mechanistically, a direct electron transfer is established by AuNPs between the electrode surface and immobilized redox proteins (Pingarron et al., 2008). The colloidal AuNPs-modified sol–gel interfaces were also utilized for the detection of monocrotophos, carbaryl, and methyl parathion (Du et al., 2008a). AuNPs are assembled on a sol–gel–derived silicate network that provides a conductive pathway for electron transfer and favors the enzymatic hydrolysis reaction, which augments the sensitivity of the technique, because AuNPs are easy to synthesize and manipulate, stable in time, size tunable, biocompatible, and have an intense red color that can easily be detected even by the naked eye or usually using color readers to achieve better detection limits. When the frequency of the incident photon and that of oscillation of conduction electron matches with each other, resonance occurs and an absorption band of AuNPs results, which is also termed the *localized surface plasmon resonance* (SPR), which can be used to develop a biosensor for the detection of paraoxon by immobilizing AChE onto AuNPs layer using a self-assembling technique. The so-designed biosensors offer good stability and even after a 30-day storage period, they retain 90% of the initial current. It was recently reported that a judicious combination of AuNPs and their QDs results in an efficient biosensor for the detection of monocrotophos. It was also found that the biosensor composed of a CdTe-QDs–AuNPs electrode system has more sensitivity than that based on QDs or AuNPs alone (Du et al., 2008b).

Another class of potential nanomaterials is CNTs, which are composed of cylindrical graphene sheets with nanometer diameters. Due to their unique optical, electrical, mechanical, physical, and chemical properties they could prove to be vital structural units of biosensors (Zhang et al., 2009). They can be chemically modified in such a way that biologically relevant molecules can be detected with high sensitivity and selectivity. Until the 1980s, only three carbon allotropes were known: graphite, amorphous carbon, and diamond. Since then, the discovery, characterization, and isolation of three additional carbon allotropes [fullerenes (Kroto et al., 1985), CNTs (Iijima, 1991), and graphene (Novoselov et al., 2004)] have fueled the advancement of a major field of science. CNTs include both single-walled and multiwalled structures composed of sp^2-hybridized carbon atoms and can be rationalized as rolled-up cylinders of graphene sheets. Since their discovery, they have found extensive applications in biomedical, nanoelectronics, biosensing, and bioanalysis fields. An important quality of CNT-based transducers is their tendency to promote electron transfer processes of species, which have been generated enzymatically, and this enables them to function as electrochemical biosensors (Wang, 2005). A recent work reports the use of CNTs as biosensors, which work on the basis of inhibition of AChE activity (Wang, 2005; Qu et al., 2010; Du et al., 2007; Oliveira and Mascaro, 2011; Firdoz et al., 2010). Based on the principle of layer-by-layer assembly, an amperometric biosensor was designed by the combination of SWCNT–poly(diallyldimethylammonium chloride) and AChE, which was used for the analysis of carbaryl. The biosensor was quite sensitive and stable and used for the monitoring of pesticides in water with a detection limit of 4.9×10^{-15} M. Other biosensors were also developed for the detection of pesticides by combining the properties of CNTs with those of NPs (Chen et al., 2011a,b).

Zhao and coworkers (Zhao et al., 2015) synthesized an ultrasensitive amperometric OP biosensor by immobilizing AChE on ERGO–AuNPs–β-CD/PBCS) nanocomposites film–modified GCE. The PBCS not only effectively catalyzed the oxidation of thiocholine, but also shifted its oxidation potential from 0.68 to 0.2 V, and accordingly the sensitivity of the biosensor was improved. The synergistic effect between ERGO and AuNPs significantly promoted the electron transfer between PBCS and GCE, and remarkably enhanced the electrochemical oxidation of thiocholine. Besides, β-CD could interact with substrate by reversible bonding, which contributed to increased enrichment of the substrate and improved the selectivity and sensitivity of the biosensor.

Another area of vital importance is optical biosensors where NPs have also been used and applied (Lin et al., 2006). With advancing nanotechnology, the QDs have successfully replaced conventional fluorescent markers, as in comparison to organic fluorophore the QDs have greater photostability. The QDs offer more sensitivity because they show higher fluorescence quantum yields in comparison to conventional organic fluorophores.

Making use of CdTe-QDs as fluorescence probes, an optical biosensor was recently designed for the detection of monocrotophos (Sun et al., 2011). Taking the advantage of the positive charge of chitosan and employing layer-by-layer technique, CdTe and AChE were assembled onto a quartz surface. It was found that the absence of pesticide led the biocatalytic hydrolysis of acetylcholine and acetic acid. The reaction brought about a fall in the pH due to release of acid, which was sensed by a pH indicator CdTe, which was immobilized on the quartz surface. The change in the fluorescence intensity was caused by the pesticide present, which was related to the pesticide concentration.

6.2 Antibody-Based Biosensors

Abs are the most popular affinity recognition elements used in biosensors and in a wide range of applications, such as food safety, environmental monitoring, clinical analysis, and medical diagnosis (Justino et al., 2010; Justino et al., 2013; Justino et al., 2014). The Abs can be polyclonal, if they are generated from a range of immune cells, or monoclonal, if they are generated from identical clones of a single-parent cell. Polyclonal Abs may bind to the antigen (Ag) at different locations or with different binding affinities, and monoclonal Abs bind to the same target region, named the epitope, with equivalent affinity, and are more selective than polyclonal Abs (Luo and Davis, 2013). Immunosensors are specific and able to evaluate total toxicity (Fig. 14.7). The underlying mechanism is based on the fact that on the surfaces of the transducers, the immobilized Ab or Ag and the specific analytes interact selectively and this gives rise to wide range of research areas, such as food safety, pharmaceutical chemistry, environmental monitoring, and clinical applications (Willander et al., 2014; Jiang et al., 2008; Mallat et al., 2001; Suri et al., 2009).

For pesticides detection, numerous immunosensors have also been designed that utilize transducers that work on optical, electrochemical, piezoelectric, and mechanical methods. Abs combined with nanomaterials are also used in biosensors (Fig. 14.8). Grennan et al. (2003) designed an amperometric immunosensor for the detection of the pesticide atrazine, which contained carbon paste solid polymer electrolyte comprised of polyaniline (PANI), a conducting polymer/poly(vinyl sulfonic acid) (PVS). Designing of several conductometric immunosensors has also been attempted for environmental analysis.

For detection of atrazine a method was designed by Valera et al. (2008, 2010a,b) that involves covalent immobilization of pesticide on interdigitated μ-electrodes (IDμE). An Ab was added into the

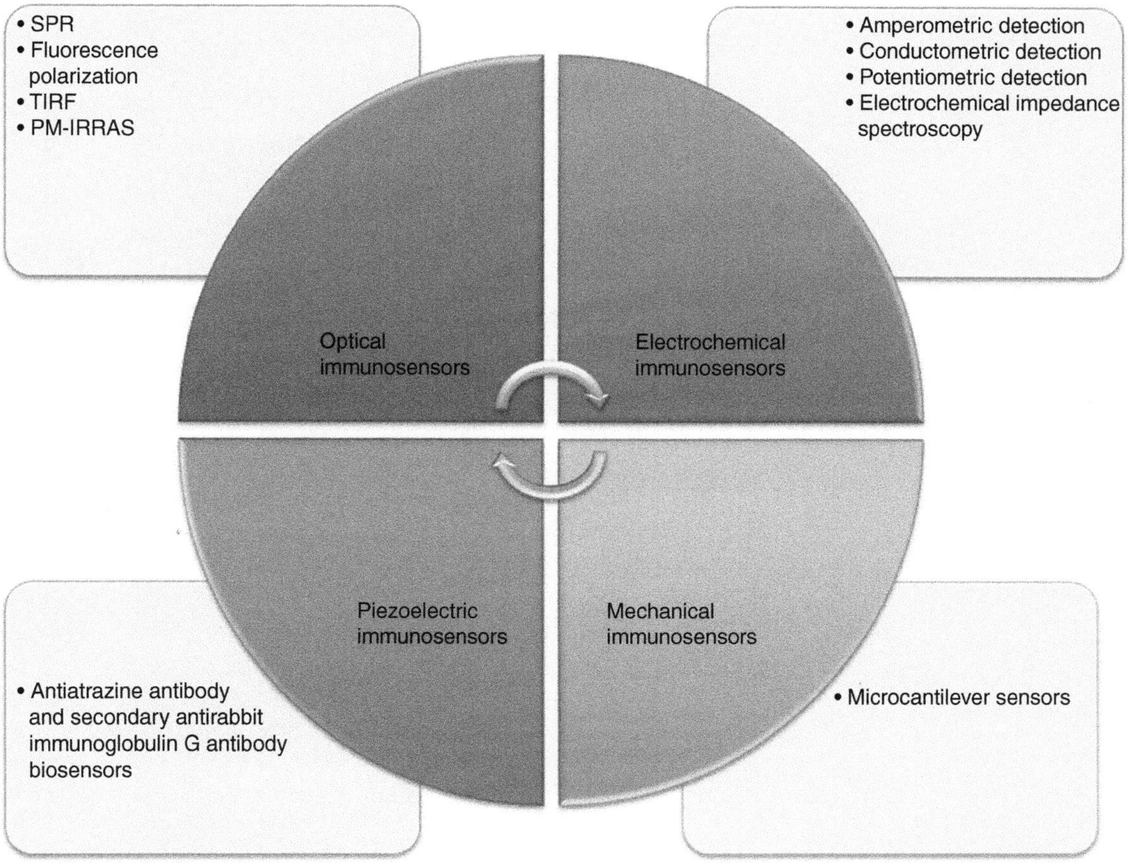

Figure 14.7. Types of immunosensors. *PM-IRRAS,* Polarization modulation infrared reflection–absorption spectroscopy; *SPR,* surface plasmon resonance; *TIRF,* Total internal reflection.

solution and free atrazine was detected through a competitive reaction with immobilized pesticide. It was shown by the authors that AuNPs amplify the conductive signal and permit assay of atrazine with the help of DC measurements. The method employed for detection was based on the fact that AuNPs were labeled to Abs and their presence augmented the conductivity signals. The designed biosensor was used to detect atrazine in red wines, as the matrix did not have any effect on the analysis.

In an attempt to design an electrochemical immunosensor for the detection of diuron, which is known to be a substituted phenyl urea–based herbicide (Sharma et al., 2011; Valera et al., 2008), economically viable electrodes of polystyrene were fabricated and modified with Prussian blue–AuNP film. It was found that due to the electrodeposition of Prussian blue–AuNP film, the electron

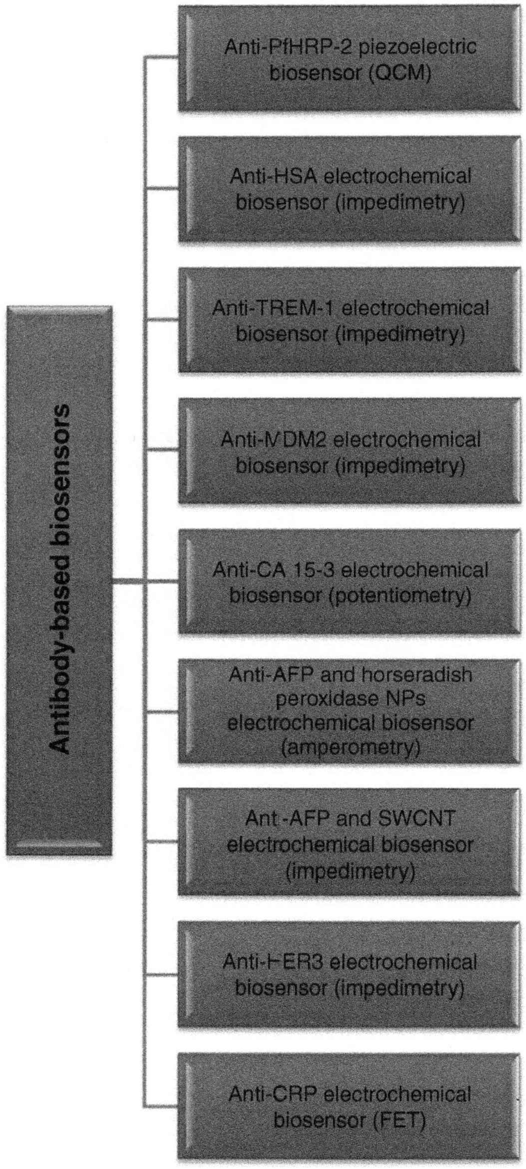

Figure 14.8. List of antibody-based biosensors. *SWCNT*, Single-walled carbon nanotubes.

transfer process was enhanced in the vicinity of the gold electrode, which eventually led to the enhanced sensitivity of the biosensor in comparison to unmodified gold electrodes.

For the detection of pesticides, electrochemical impedance spectroscopy is used as a cost-effective method, and it works on the principle that the binding of immobilized biomolecules to the analyte molecule results in a slight change in the electron transfer resistance at the interface between the electrode and the solution. The technique of impedance spectroscopy is advantageous in many ways: it offers ease of detection, higher signal-to-noise ratio, lower assay cost, faster assays, and shorter analysis times. The only drawbacks of this method are that the experimentation is quite time consuming and results are also not reproducible (Grieshaber et al., 2008).

Optical immunosensors are based on the principle that formation of Ab–Ag complexes induces the changes in the optical characteristics. Many optical immunosensors, such as SPR (allows real-time monitoring, shows good reproducibility, and does not require labeled molecules) (Homola et al., 1999), fluorescence polarization [consists of fluorescent labels (e.g., cyanine) and has photobleaching problems that can be overcome by the use of NPs as fluorescent reporters] (Cummins et al., 2003), total internal reflection fluorescence (TIRF) [called river analyzer (RIANA); used for water pollution control and to monitor the levels of atrazine, simazine, and alachlor] (Mallat et al., 2001), automated water analyzer computer supported system (AWACSS) (similar to RIANA immunosensor but able to detect multianalytes; unique design enables optical detection, fluidics that include compact integrated optics and microfluidics, and intelligent remote control for unattended continuous monitoring) (Tschmelak et al., 2005), and polarization modulation infrared reflection–absorption spectroscopy (PM-IRRAS) (developed to detect environmental pollutants; its sensor chips are coated with ovalbumine–atrazine derivatives) (Salmain et al., 2008; Boujday et al., 2009; Boujday et al., 2010).

Piezoelectric immunosensors are mass-sensitive devices that are fabricated by immobilization of Ab or Ag on the surfaces of quartz, and they are capable of measuring very small–mass changes (Kurosawa et al., 2006). However, only a few immunosensors were designed to detect pesticides, such as chlorpyrifos and triclopyr (March et al., 2009). Mechanical immunosensors, also called microcantilever sensors, are capable of measuring a surface stress change that arises as a result of an interaction between an analyte (e.g., an antigen) and an immobilized ligand (e.g., Ab). These immunosensors have benefits, such as high precision, reduced size, reliability, label-free detection, and easy fabrication of multielement sensor arrays (Sassolas et al., 2008).

6.3 Whole Cell Biosensors

Whole cell biosensors use living organisms, such as bacteria, fungi, yeast, algae, and tissue culture cells (from animals or plants) as recognition elements, and detect analytical signals by measuring the general metabolic status (growth inhibition, cell viability, cell respiration or bacterial bioluminescence, and substrate uptake) of such living organisms (Wang et al., 2014). Whole cells have several advantages over enzymes, such as high stability, reduced purification requirements, low cost of preparation, and efficient cofactor regeneration (de Carvalho 2011). They can be classified as microbial biosensors [which may be established by immobilizing microorganisms onto a transducer, adopting chemical and physical approaches, such as cross-linking and entrapment, respectively (Lei et al., 2006)], electrochemical microbial biosensors, and plant tissue– and photosynthesis-based biosensors [use plant tissue or whole cells (e.g., microalgae), chloroplasts or thylakoids, and photosystem II as an attractive alternative to enzymatic biosensors]. Microbial biosensors are able to metabolize a wide range of chemical compounds and avoid expensive protocols of enzyme purification, but they show a slow response in comparison to enzyme biosensors due to slow diffusion of substrate and products through the cell wall. However, this problem can be overcome by permeabilization of the cell (D'Souza, 2001).

Electrochemical microbial biosensors consist of a microbial film sandwiched between a porous cellulose membrane and a gas-permeable membrane, and are widely applied for the determination of biochemical oxygen demand of biodegradable organic pollutants in aqueous samples. They are based on the principle that organic waste diffuses via dialysis membranes, which are further assimilated by the immobilized microbial population, which consequently leads to an increase in the respiration rate of bacteria. Thus, the Clark oxygen electrode detects the sparingly soluble oxygen, which has diffused via an oxygen-permeable Teflon membrane (Liu and Mattiasson, 2002). Potentiometric microbial biosensors that are coated with an immobilized microbial layer make use of ion- or gas-selective electrodes, such as ammonium and pH, and pCO_2, respectively. These biosensors record the fluctuations in potential resulting from assimilation of substrates by microbes (Lei et al., 2006). Optical microbial biosensors are used for the detection of pollutants, such as phenols and heavy metals (Su et al., 2011; Lagarde and Jaffrezic-Renault, 2011). Plant tissue– and photosynthesis-based biosensors are low-cost, highly stable, and active lifetime biosensors with high reproducibility. Furthermore, the time-consuming and tedious steps, such as enzyme extraction and purification, are avoided and biosensors find applications in detecting pollutants found in water bodies and other aquatic ecosystems (Campas et al., 2008).

6.4 Phage Biosensors

Biosensors that use phages or bacteriophages as biorecognition elements are called phase biosensors, and are environmentally more robust than immunosensors, low in cost, easy to produce, and widely used to detect pathogens. They contain viruses that infect bacteria and display peptides or proteins on their surface, that is, bacterial host strains, through the specific receptor molecules present on the surface of the bacterial cell. Phage biosensors can be stored for longer times with minimal loss of binding affinity (Tawil et al., 2014; Chai et al., 2013).

6.5 Molecularly Imprinted Polymer–Based Biosensors

Recently, MIP-based biosensors have gained the attention of researchers in sensing applications in environmental, food, and pharmaceutical analysis due to their high selectivity, stability, short time of synthesis, high thermostability, and cost effectiveness. MIPs are synthetic cross-linked materials with molecularly imprinted cavities that have artificial recognition sites. Thus they mimick the biological activity of natural receptors, constitute a class of plastic Abs also known as artificial Abs, and are synthesized by electrochemical polymerization of functional monomers in a mixture with cross-linkers and in the presence of template molecules. It is worth mentioning that by excessive washing the interactions between the template and monomer molecules may be disrupted, which results in the removal of the template. Synthetic polymers that possess specific cavities that are complementary to the template in terms of their shape, size, and position of the functional group are obtained with binding specificity similar to that of typical Ab–Ag interactions, which are used as recognition elements for replacing biological Abs in nanosensors (Fig. 14.9) (Zhang et al., 2014; Volkert and Haes, 2014; Chen et al., 2011a,b; Luo and Davis, 2013). In the next step, the target analyte, mimicked by the template molecule, can selectively bind in molecular cavities due to the presence of the recognition sites (Mayes and Whitcombe, 2005; Pichon and Chapuis-Hugon, 2008). The main advantage of such biosensing systems is the direct, rapid determination of the interaction between the recognition element and the target analyte (identical to the template), compared to traditional bioassays (immunoanalytical systems) (Volkert and Haes, 2014). Jenkins et al. (2001) synthesized an optical sensor based on MIPs onto optical fibers using luminescent lanthanide (europium) as spectroscopic probe, which was incorporated into the polymer. It was used

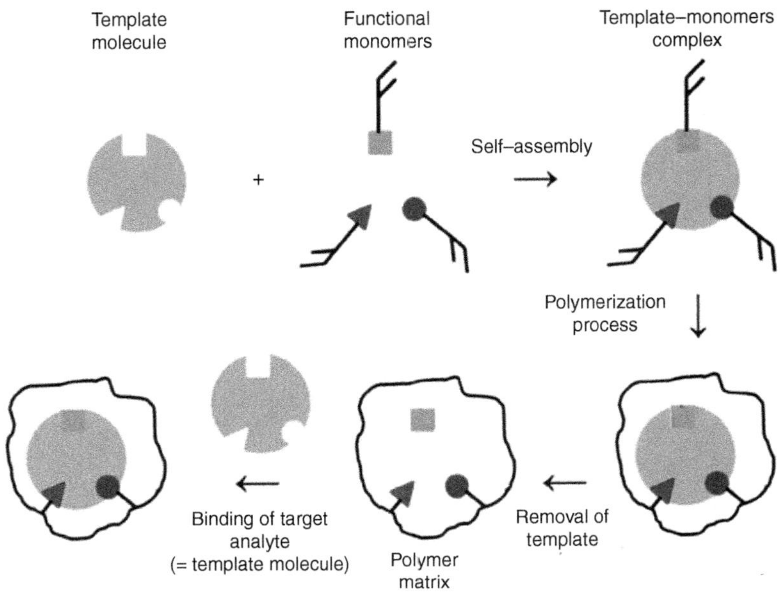

Figure 14.9. Schematic representation of the steps involved in the MIP process.

as an artificial recognition element in biosensors for the detection of pesticides, such as chloropyrifos, diazinon, and glyphosate, by observing changes that occur in the lanthanide spectrum.

Recent works with MIPs as recognition elements employed nanosized MIPs, which have an extremely high surface-area to volume ratio and possess notable advantages over normal MIPs, such as easier removal of template molecules, higher-binding capacity, faster-binding kinetics, and easier installation onto the surface of nanodevices (Li et al., 2015a,b). The incorporation of nanomaterials, such as noble metal NPs, into MIPs can enhance the sensitivity and the selectivity of sensors, in particular optical sensors. The introduction of noble metal NPs facilitates large changes of analytical signal, such as fluorescence (increases or decreases depending on the mechanisms of catalysis or inhibition), which leads to highly sensitive, selective sensors (Gültekin et al., 2012). According to Volkert and Haes (Volkert and Haes, 2014), there are three methods to incorporate nanomaterials into MIPs, that is:

1. suspending nanomaterials in the MIP matrix,
2. polymerizing NPs in the MIP matrix, and
3. polymerizing the MIPs onto the nanomaterials surface.

Li et al. (2015a,b) synthesized nanosized MIPs based on graphene as the recognition element on an electrochemical sensor but using CdSe–ZnS QDs (nanomaterials) and the enzyme AChE. The study suggested that nanocomposites of QDs, graphene, and

AChE can generate a stable photocurrent (because the hydrolysis of acetylthiolcholine to generate thiolcholine, which is an electron donor) that is inversely dependent on the concentration of the target analyte (OP pesticides paraoxon and dichlorvos).

6.6 Aptamer-Based Biosensors

In 1990, it was independently reported by Ellington and Szostak (1990), Gold's, and Robertson's group that they were successful in designing an in vitro selection technique that may discover binding between specific nucleic acid sequences and nonspecific nucleic acid targets with great specificity and affinity. The newly developed technique is called SELEX, while the resulting DNA or RNA oligonucleotides are termed *aptamers* (Famulok and Szostak, 1992; Stoltenburg et al., 2007; Hamula et al., 2011).

Aptamers can be considered as nucleic acid analogues of Abs; they can bind with high affinity and specificity to a broad range of targets, such as small molecules, proteins, viruses, or cells and they exhibit a great affinity for a great range of target analytes, which include metal ions, pathogenic microorganisms, and proteins. Another important property of aptamers is that they have numerous benefits over Abs, such as their reproducibility and accurate chemical production, greater stability than Abs, no requirement of immunization of animal hosts, ability to undergo reversible denaturation, easy modification with new functional groups without any effect on their activity for their immobilization by incorporating reporter molecules (e.g., fluorophores or enzymes) and functional groups, ability to bind to selected nucleic acids, and ability to work in extreme conditions, whereas Abs are only stable under physiological conditions and also have a higher-surface density of receptors (Jayasena, 1999). Due to their many advantages, numerous aptamer-based biosensors have been developed for the detection of a wide range of targets (Sassolas et al., 2011; Sassolas et al., 2009; Yuan et al., 2011; Radi, 2011; Xu et al., 2009). Currently, nucleic acid aptamers have been selected for more than 150 targets, including small molecules, such as cocaine, aspartame, growth factors, peptides, toxins, viral proteins, cells, and bacteria.

It is known that for the detection of pesticides a few apatamers have been chosen. A recent work describes a DNA aptamer specific for acetamiprid (He et al., 2011). Although direct detection of pesticide using aptamers has not been reported, biosensors based on aptamers may emerge as an excellent option over traditional methods for analysis of pesticides. Aptamers are short oligonucleotides (30–40 nucleobases) [RNA or single-stranded DNA (ssDNA)], synthesized in vitro with no need for animal or cell cultures (Barthelmebs et al., 2011; Song et al., 2012), and are able to bind to a specific target oligonucleotide analyte. Aptamers have a high affinity for their targets with values of dissociation constant (K_d) in the nanomolar to picomolar range (Yao et al., 2010). Also, aptamers typically fold into a unique 3D structure, which allows specific binding to target analytes; thus aptamers interact with their targets by complementary shape and not their sequence. The majority of research denominates aptamers as DNA or RNA aptamers, as previously identified, but some authors also associate aptamers to peptide aptamers (Song et al., 2012; Song and Park, 2011; Daprà et al., 2013). However, the term *affimer* is associated with peptide aptamers (Luo and Davis, 2013). Thus, in the present chapter, the term *aptamer* is associated with DNA, RNA, or peptide aptamers, with reference to their origin. Concerning peptide aptamers, they are monomeric and considered as non-Ab–recognition proteins, which are also used as recognition elements in biosensors (Luo and Davis, 2013; Johnson et al., 2012; Pavan and Berti, 2012). Peptides are conformationally constrained with the structure of a constant scaffold protein (Johnson et al., 2012).

Recently, aptamers were combined with nanomaterials to amplify the analytical signal of biosensors and to enhance affinity capture. For example, Zhang et al. (2013) synthesized an ultrahigh-sensitive fluorescent aptasensor (two DNA probes were added and hybridized with ochratoxin A aptamers) for the label-free detection of ochratoxin A (mycotoxin) in wheat samples. After the introduction of ochratoxin A, the probes were released, enhancing the emission of Tb^{3+} and increasing the fluorescence intensity. In this work, the authors observed an amplification of the fluorescence signal, leading to an excellent LOD (20 pg mL^{-1}), essentially due to the use of two DNA probes that allowed the combination of Tb^{3+} with more probes; the binding of ochratoxin A and aptamers occurred within 1 min, which allowed the analysis of a large number of individual samples.

Gu et al. (2015) developed and improved a new AuNP-based colorimetric multiaptasensor for the detection of two pesticides. It was found that for iprobenfos (IBF) and edifenphos (EDI) the binding affinities of the aptamer EIA2 were 1.67 mM and 38 nM, respectively, which was further confirmed by the isothermal calorimetry assay technique. It was also confirmed by AuNPs assays that the aptamer EIA2 was selective to IBF and EDI. The use of multiaptasensor enabled the detection of both the pesticides, IBF and EDI, in a range from 10 to 5 nM, respectively. Another significant application of this multiaptasensor was in the detection of spiked rice, and it was reported that this AuNP-based multiaptasensor offered an accuracy of nearly 80 and 90%, respectively. It is important to note that the aptamer EIA2 may not only be used to detect pesticides in real samples of agricultural fields, but may also find use as a bioreceptor for other aptasensors.

6.7 Affibody-Based Biosensors

Affibodies are a new class of engineered affinity proteins that can reach considerable affinity and specificity to any target protein or peptide after their isolation (Justino et al., 2015). Affibodies have a single domain and three-helical structures where 13 amino acid positions are present on the helices; 1 and 2 are randomized to create diversity (Nygren, 2008). The isolation of affibodies is based on nonimmunoglobulin scaffolds using synthetic combinatorial libraries and selection systems, mainly by the phage display technology (Justino et al., 2015). Although affibodies are well known for their use in imaging, diagnostics, and therapeutics, their role as recognition elements in biosensors is at a very early stage, as recently reviewed (Justino et al., 2015), but we anticipate their increased use due to their properties of affinity and specificity for target analytes.

Recently, a nanobead-based sandwich immunoassay was proposed (Lee et al., 2012), where affibodies combined with polystyrene nanobeads (85 nm) were used for the detection of fluorescent dye–labeled IgG and vascular endothelial growth factor A via a capture Ab. It is therefore expected that more applications will be developed due to the known high affinity and specificity of affibodies with target analytes, such as tumor antigens (Gu et al., 2015).

7 Conclusions and Future Challenges

There currently exists a clear and increasing need for environmental analytical methods that are fast, portable, and cost effective. The increasing number of potentially harmful pollutants in the environment calls for fast and cost-effective analytical techniques. Most of traditional analytical methods (e.g., chromatographic methods) are difficult and need expensive instrumentation and specialized personnel. In this context, biosensors appear to be suitable alternative or complementary analytical tools because they provide highly accurate results in the field and in the lab, with results that are quick and reliable. Furthermore, biosensors are easy to use; do not require expensive readers; and use optical, electrochemical, and acoustic signal transducers, which have been reported to measure a significant number of environmental pollutants.

Despite the extensive research performed in the past two decades and the clear demand for online measurement, biosensors have been used in only clinical, food, environmental, and biothreat/biowarfare applications. The use of biosensors for food analysis can provide a specific, sensitive, rapid, and cheap method for monitoring a range of target analytes. In the coming days the use of commercial biosensors is expected to spread in the food industry.

There are many biosensors, such as enzymes and Abs, and the recent recognition elements, such as MIPs and aptamers under development, and there is also extensive literature in this area. However, only a small number of biosensors are commercially available. Despite the use of classical recognition elements resulting in a wide range of useful chemical sensors and biosensors, the search for new elements is of constant interest in this scientific field to develop more robust, rapid, cost effective, and miniaturized chemical sensing and biosensing platforms. It is important that there exists a free flow of creative ideas concerning the use of diverse biological recognition elements, alternative operating formats, and innovative signal transducers. In the coming days research in biosensor technology is expected to focus on transducer technology and sensing element development. The use of nanostructures as recognition elements has also increased the development of efficient nanosensors, particularly for clinical diagnosis and environmental monitoring.

Another issue of great concern is how the scientific and technological expertise will be commercially realized with an effective, efficient, and economically viable outcome. Though the principle of the biosensor is sound, the fabrication of the device with required specificity and sensitivity is also a challenge.

The technical obstacles to the commercialization of biosensors for environmental applications are the broad number and class range of environmental pollutants; sample handling, including drinking water, surface water, ground water, soil, sludge, sediment, leachates, air, and biota; wide range of concentrations encountered in various applications; and the effect of chemically reactive cocontaminants that has a direct consequence on the monitoring tasks. These practical obstacles include:

- The requirement for a substantial operational or cost benefit over other existing or emerging field analytical methods.
- The lack of well-established expectations [i.e., data quality objectives (DQOs)] by the potential market for field analytical methods.
- The presence of a sufficient market (for any particular application or group of related applications) to offset the expense of moving a laboratory prototype to the market.

- The field testing, evaluation, and validation required by regulatory agencies for method approval for specific applications in specific media.
- The time required to move a new method and associated technology through the regulatory approval process.

References

Almeida, G.L., Schmitt, G.C., Bairros, A.V., Emanuelli, T., Garcia, S.C., 2007. Os riscos e danos nas intoxicac¸ões por paraquat em animais domésticos. Ciênc. Rural 37, 1506.

Alonso, G.A., Istamboulie, G., Noguer, T., Marty, J.L., Muñoz, R., 2012. Rapid determination of pesticide mixtures using disposable biosensors based on genetically modified enzymes and artificial neural networks. Sens. Actuat. B 164, 22–28.

Armas, E.D., Monteiro, R.T.R., Antunes, P.M., Santos, M.A.P.F., Camargo, P.B., 2007. Uso de agrotóxicos em cana-de açúcar na bacia do rio Corumbataí e o risco de poluição hídrica. Quim. Nova 30, 1119.

Bahadır, E.B., Sezginturk, M.K., 2015. Applications of commercial biosensors in clinical, food, environmental, and biothreat/biowarfare analyses. Anal. Biochem. 478, 107–120.

Baird, C.L., Myszka, D.G., 2001. Current and emerging commercial optical biosensors. J. Mol. Recognit. 14, 261–268.

Ballesteros-Gomez, A., Rubio, S., 2009. Recent advances in environmental analysis. Anal. Chem. 81 (12), 4601–4622.

Barthelmebs, L., Hayat, A., Limiadi, A.W., Marty, J.L., Noguer, T., 2011. Electrochemical DNA aptamer-based biosensor for OTA detection, using superparamagnetic nanoparticles. Sens. Actuat. B 156, 932–937.

Bogdansky, S., 1990. Natural polymers as drug delivery systems. In: Chasin, M., Langer, R. (Eds.), Biodegradable Polymers As Drug Delivery Systems. Marcel Dekker Inc., NY, USA.

Boujday, S., Gu, C., Girardot, M., Salmain, M., Pradier, C.M., 2009. Surface IR applied to rapid and direct immunosensing of environmental pollutants. Talanta 78 (1), 165–170.

Boujday, S., Nasri, S., Salmain, M., Pradier, C.M., 2010. Surface IR immunosensors for label-free detection of benzo[a]pyrene. Biosens. Bioelectron. 26 (4), 1750–1754.

Campas, M., Carpentier, R., Rouillon, R., 2008. Plant-tissue and photosynthesis-based biosensors. Biotech. Adv. 26 (4), 370–378.

Campbell, F.W., Compton, R.G., 2010. The use of nanoparticles in electroanalysis: an updated review. Anal. Bioanal. Chem. 396, 241–259.

Cao, J.Q., Wang, Y.X., Yu, J.F., Xia, J.Y., Zhang, C.F., Yin, D.Z., Hafeli, U.O., 2004. Preparation and radio-labeling of surface-modified magnetic nanoparticles with rhenium-188 for magnetic targeted radiotherapy. J. Magn. Magn. Mater. 277, 165–174.

Chai, Y., Horikawa, S., Simonian, A., Dyer, D., Chin, B.A., 2013. Wireless magnetoelastic biosensors for the detection of *Salmonella* on fresh produce. In: IEEE 174–177. Seventh International Conference on Sensing Technology.

Chauhan, N., Pundir, C.S., 2012. An amperometric acetylcholinesterase sensor based on Fe_3O_4 nanoparticle/multi-walled carbon nanotube-modified ITO-coated glass plate for the detection of pesticides. Electrochim. Acta 67, 79–86.

Chee, G., 2013. Development and characterization of microbial biosensors for evaluating low biochemical oxygen demand in rivers. Talanta 117, 366–370.

Chen, J., Mao, S., Pu, H., 2012. Graphene oxide and its reduction: modeling and experimental progress. RSC Adv. 2, 2643–2662.

Chen, L., Xu, S., Li, J., 2011a. Recent advances in molecular imprinting technology: current status, challenges and highlighted applications. Chem. Soc. Rev. 40, 2922–2942.

Chen, S., Huang, J., Du, D., Li, J., Tu, H., Liu, D., Zhang, A., 2011b. Methyl parathion hydrolase based nanocomposite biosensors for highly sensitive and selective de-termination of methyl parathion. Biosens. Bioelectron. 26 (11), 4320–4325.

Christensen, J.M., 1995. Human exposure to toxic metals: factors influencing interpretation of biomonitoring results. Sci. Tot. Environ. 166, 89–135.

Colvin, V.L., 2003. The potential environmental impact of engineered nanomaterials. Nat. Biotechnol. 10, 1166–1170.

Crew, A., Lonsdale, D., Byrd, N., Pittson, R., Hart, J.P., 2011. A screen-printed, amperometric biosensor array incorporated into a novel automated system for the simultaneous determination of organophosphate pesticides. Biosens. Bioelectron. 26, 2847–2851.

Cummins, C.M., Koivunen, M.E., Stephanian, A., Gee, S.J., Hammock, B.D., Kennedy, I.M., 2003. Application of europium(III) chelate-dyed nanoparticle labels in a competitive atrazine fluoroimmunoassay on an ITO wave-guide. Biosens. Bioelectron. 21 (7), 1077–1085.

D'Souza, S.F., 2001. Microbial biosensors. Biosens. Bioelectron. 16, 337–353.

Daprà, J., Lauridsen, L.H., Nielsen, A.T., Rozlosnik, N., 2013. Comparative study onaptamers as recognition elements for antibiotics in a label-free all-polymer biosensor. Biosens. Bioelectron. 43, 315–320.

Davies, C.J., 2009. Oversight of next generation nanotechnology. Project on Emerging Nanotechnologies at the Woodrow Wilson International Center for Scholars. Available from: http://www.nanotechproject.org/process/assets/files/7316/pen-18.pdf

de Carvalho, C.C.C.R., 2011. Enzymatic and whole cell catalysis: finding new strategies for old processes. Biotechnol. Adv. 29, 75–83.

de Jesus, M.B., Pinto, L.M.A., Fraceto, L.F., Takahata, Y., Lino, A.C.S., Jaime, C., de Paula, E., 2006. Theoretical and experimental study of a praziquantel and beta-cyclodextrin inclusion complex using molecular mechanic calculations and H1-nuclear magnetic resonance. J. Pharmaceut. Biomed. Anal. 41, 1428–1432.

DHHS, 2009. Department of Health and Human Services, Centers for Disease Control and Prevention and National Institute for Occupational Safety and Health. Approaches to safe nanotechnology: managing the health and safety concerns associated with engineered nanomaterials. Publication No. 2009-125. Available from: https://www.cdc.gov/niosh/docs/2009-125/pdfs/2009-125.pdf

Díaz-García, M.E., de Dios, A.S., 2010. Multifunctional nanoparticles: analytical prospects. Anal. Chim. Acta 666, 1–22.

Dong, Y., Shao, J., Chen, C., Li, H., Wang, R., Chi, Y., Lin, X., Chen, G., 2012. Blue luminescent graphene quantum dots and graphene oxide prepared by tuning the carbonization degreeof citric acid. Carbon 50, 4738–4743.

Du, D., Chen, S., Cai, J., Zhang, A., 2008a. Electrochemical pesticide sensitivity test using acetylcholinesterase bio-sensor based on colloidal gold nanoparticle modified sol-gel interface. Talanta 74 (4), 766–772.

Du, D., Chen, S., Song, D., Li, H., Chen, X., 2008b. Development of acetylcholinesterase biosensor based on CdTe quantum dots/gold nanoparticles modified chitosan microspheres interface. Biosens. Bioelectron. 24 (3), 475–479.

Du, D., Chen, W., Zhang, W., Liu, D., Li, H., Lin, Y., 2010. Covalent coupling of organophosphorus hydrolase loaded quantum dots to carbon nanotube. Au nano-composite for enhanced detection of methyl parathion. Biosens. Bioelectron. 25 (6), 1370–1375.

Du, D., Huang, X., Cai, J., Zhang, A., 2007. Comparison of pesticide sensitivity by electrochemical test based on acetylcholinesterase biosensor. Biosens. Bioelectron. 23 (2), 285–289.

Dzyadevych, S.V., Arkhypova, V.N., Soldatkin, A.P., Elskaya, A.V., Martelet, C., Jaffrezic-Renault, N., 2008. Amperometric enzyme biosensors: past, present and future. IRBM 29, 171–180.

Ellington, A.D., Szostak, J.W., 1990. In vitro selection of RNA molecules that bind specific ligands. Nature 346 (6287), 818–822.

Famulok, A., Szostak, J.W., 1992. In vitro selection of specific ligand binding nucleic acids. Angew. Chem. Int. Ed. 31 (8), 979–988.

Fernández-Pérez, M., Villafranca-Sánchez, E., González-Pradas, E., Martinez-López, F., Flores-Céspedes, F., 2000. Controlled release of carbofuran from an alginate–bentonite formulation: water release kinetics and soil mobility. J. Agric. Food. Chem. 48, 938–943.

Firdoz, S., Ma, F., Yue, X., Dai, Z., Kumar, A., Jiang, B., 2010. A novel amperometric biosensor based on single walled carbon nanotubes with acetylcholine esterase for the detection of carbaryl pesticide in water. Talanta 83 (1), 269–273.

Garcia Sanchez, F., Navas Diaz, A., Ramos Peinado, M.C., Belledone, C., 2003. Free and sol-gel immobilized alkaline phosphatase-based biosensor for the determination of pesticides and inorganic compounds. Anal. Chim. Acta 484 (1), 45–51.

Grennan, K., Strachan, G., Porter, A.J., Killard, A., Smyth, M.R., 2003. Atrazine analysis using an amperometric immunosensor based on single-chain antibody fragments and regeneration-free multi-calibrant measurement. Anal. Chim. Acta 500 (1–2), 287–298.

Grieshaber, D., MacKenzie, R., Vöros, J., Reimhult, E., 2008. Electrochemical biosensors—sensor principles and architectures. Sensors 8 (3), 1400–1458.

Gu, M.B., Kwon, Y.S., Nguyen, Y.T., Park, J.G., 2015. Detection of iprobenfos and edifenphos using a new multi-aptasensor. Anal. Chim. Acta 868, 60–66.

Gültekin, A., Ersöz, A., Denizli, A., Say, R., 2012. Preparation of new molecularly imprinted nanosensor for cholic acid determination. Sens. Actuat. B 162, 153–158.

Guo, J., Wang, Y., Liu, Y., Zhang, C., Zhou, Y., 2015. Magnetic-graphene based molecularly imprinted polymer nano-composite for the recognition of bovine hemoglobin. Talanta 144, 411–419.

Gupta, S.K., Singh, J., 2011. Trends in biohydrogen production: major challenges and state-of-the-art developments. IIOAB J. 2, 49–57.

Hamula, C.L.A., Guthrie, J.W., Zhang, H., Li, X.F., Le, X.C., 2011. Selection and analytical applications of aptamers. Trends Anal. Chem. 30 (10), 1587–1597.

Hanrahan, G., Patil, D.G., Wang, J., 2004. Electrochemical sensors for environmental monitoring: design, development and applications. J. Environ. Monit. 6, 657.

He, J., Liu, Y., Fan, M., Liu, X., 2011. Isolation and identification of the DNA aptamer target to acetamiprid. J. Agric. Food Chem. 59 (5), 1582–1586.

He, F., Zhao, D., Liu, J., Roberts, C.B., 2007. Stabilization of Fe–Pd nanoparticles with sodium carboxymethyl cellulose for enhanced transport and dechlorination of trichloroethylene in soil and groundwater. Ind. Eng. Chem. Res. 46, 29–34.

Homola, J., Yee, S.S., Gauglitz, G., 1999. Surface Plasmon resonance sensors: review. Sens. Actuat. B 54 (1–2), 3–15.

Ibupoto, Z.H., Ali, S.M.U., Khun, K., Chey, C.O., Nur, O., Willander, M., 2011. ZnO nanorods based enzymatic biosensor for selective determination of penicillin. Biosensors 1, 153–163.

Ibupoto, Z.H., Ali, S.M.U., Khun, K., Willander, M., 2012. Electrochemical l-lactic acid sensor based on immobilized ZnO nanorods with lactate oxidase. Sensors 12, 2456–2466.

Iijima, S., 1991. Helical microtubules of graphitic carbon. Nature 354 (6348), 56–58.

International Organization for Standardization, 2008. Nanotechnologies—terminology and definitions for nano-objects—nanoparticle, nanofibre and nanoplate. ISO/TS 27687 (2008-08-15).

Jayasena, S.D., 1999. Aptamers: an emerging class of molecules that rival antibodies in diagnostics. Clin. Chem. 45 (9), 1628–1650.

Jenkins, A.L., Yin, R., Jensen, J.L., 2001. Molecularly imprinted polymer sensors for pesticide and insecticide detection in water. Analyst 126, 798–802.

Jiang, X., Li, D., Xu, X., Ying, Y., Li, Y., Ye, Z, Wang, J., 2008. Immunosensors for detection of pesticides residues. Biosens. Bioelectron. 23 (11), 1577–1587.

Johnson, A., Song, Q.F., Ferrigno, P.K., Bueno, P.R., Davis, J.J., 2012. Sensitive affimer and antibody based impedimetric label-free assays for C-reactive protein. Anal. Chem. 84, 6553–6560.

Justin, J., 2006. Gooding biosensor technology for detecting biological warfare agents: recent progress and future trends. Anal. Chim. Acta 559, 137–151.

Justino, C.I.L., Duarte, K., Lucas, S., Chaves, P., Bettencourt, P., Freitas, A.C., et al., 2014. Assessment of cardiovascular disease risk using immunosensors for determination of C-reactive protein levels in serum and saliva: a pilot study. Bioanalysis 6, 1459–1470.

Justino, C.I.L., Duarte, A.C., Rocha-Santos, T.A.P., 2015. Analytical applications of affibodies. Trends Anal. Chem. 65, 73–82.

Justino, C.I.L., Freitas, A.C., Amaral, J.P., Rocha-Santos, T.A.P., Cardoso, S., Duarte, A.C., 2013. Disposable immunosensors for C-reactive protein based on carbon nanotubes field effect transistors. Talanta 108, 165–170.

Justino, C.I.L., Rocha-Santos, T.A., Duarte, A.C., 2010. Review of analytical figures of merit of sensors and biosensors in clinical applications. Trends Anal. Chem. 10, 1172–1183.

Kim, H., Kobayashi, S., AbdurRahim, M.A., Zhang, M.J., Khusainova, A., Hillmyer, M.A., Abdala, A.A., Macosko, C.W., 2011. Graphene/polyethylene nanocomposites: effect of polyethylene functionalization and blending methods. Polymer 52, 1837–1846.

Klaine, S.J., Alvarez, P.J., Batley, G.E., Fernandes, T.F., Hand, R.D., Lyon, D.Y., Mahendra, S., McLaughlin, M.J., Lead, J.R., 2008. Environ. Toxicol. Chem. 27, 1825–1851.

Kono, K., 2002. Application of dendrimers to drug delivery systems—from the view point of carrier design based on nanotechnology. Drug Deliv. Syst. 17, 462–470.

Kroto, H.W., Heath, J.R., O'Brien, S.C., Curl, R.F., Smalley, R.E., 1985. C60: buckminster fullerene. Nature 318 (6042), 162–163.

Kruss, S., Hilmer, A.J., Zhang, J., Reuel, N.F., Mu, B., Strano, M.S., 2013. Carbon nanotubes as optical biomedical sensors. Adv. Drug Deliv. Rev. 65, 1933–1950.

Kumar, S., Ahlawat, W., Kumar, R., Dilbaghi, N., 2015. Graphene, carbon nanotubes, zinc oxide and gold as elite nanomaterials for fabrication of biosensors for healthcare. Biosens. Bioelectron. 70, 498–503.

Kurosawa, S., Park, J.W., Aiwaza, H., Wakida, S.I., Tao, H., Ishihara, K., 2006. Quartz crystal microbalance immunosensor for environmental monitoring. Biosens. Bioelectron. 22 (4), 473–481.

Lagarde, F., Jaffrezic-Renault, N., 2011. Cell-based electrochemical biosensors for water quality assessment. Anal. Bioanal. Chem. 400 (4), 947–964.
Langer, R., Karel, M., 1981. Controlled release technology: polymers in medicine, food and agriculture. Poly News 7, 250–258.
Lee, J.H., Park, J.Y., Min, K., Cha, H.J., Choi, S.S., Yoo, Y.J., 2010. A novel organophosphorus hydrolase-based biosensor using mesoporous carbons and carbon black for the detection of organophosphate nerve agents. Biosens. Bioelectron. 25 (7), 1566–1570.
Lee, H.L., Weng, Y.P., Ku, W.Y., Huang, L.L.H., 2012. A nanobead based sandwich immunoassay. J. Taiwan Inst. Chem. Eng. 43, 9–14.
Lei, Y., Chen, W., Mulchandani, A., 2006. Microbial bio-sensors. Anal. Chim. Acta 568 (1–2), 200–210.
Letchford, K., Burt, H., 2007. A review of the formation and classification of amphiphilic block copolymer nanoparticulate structures: micelles, nanospheres, nanocapsules and polymersomes. Eur. J. Pharm. Sci. 65, 259–269.
Li, X., Zheng, Z., Liu, X., Zhao, S., Liu, S., 2015a. Nanostructured photoelectrochemical biosensor for highly sensitive detection of organophosphorus pesticides. Biosens. Bioelectron. 64, 1–5.
Li, X., Wang, X., Li, L., Duan, H., Luo, C., 2015b. Electrochemical sensor based on magnetic graphene oxide@gold nanoparticles-molecular imprinted polymers for determination of dibutyl phthalate. Talanta 131, 354–360.
Li, X.H., Xie, Z., Min, H., Li, C., Liu, M., Xian, Y.J., 2006. Development of quantum dots modified acetylcholinesterase biosensor for the detection of trichlorfon. Electroanalysis 18 (22), 2163–2167.
Lin, T.J., Huang, K.T., Liu, C.Y., 2006. Determination of organophosphorous pesticides by a novel biosensor based on localized surface plasmon resonance. Biosens. Bioelectron. 22 (4), 513–518.
Liu, J., Mattiasson, B., 2002. Microbial BOD sensors for wastewater analysis. Water Res. 36 (15), 3786–3802.
Lu, Y., Lee, J.H., Yigit, M.V., Mazumdar, D., 2010. Molecular diagnostic and drug delivery agents based on aptamer-nanomaterial conjugates. Adv. Drug Deliv. Rev. 62, 592–605.
Luo, X., Davis, J.J., 2013. Electrical biosensors and the label free detection of protein disease biomarkers. Chem. Soc. Rev. 42, 5944–5962.
Mallat, E., Barcelo, D., Barzen, C., Gauglitz, G., Abuknesha, R., 2001. Immunosensors for pesticide determination in natural waters. Trends Anal. Chem. 20 (3), 124–132.
March, C., Manclus, J.J., Jimenez, M., Arnau, A., Montoya, A., 2009. A Piezoelectric immunosensor for the determination of pesticide residues and metabolites in fruit juices. Talanta 78 (3), 827–833.
Marchi, G., Marchi, E.C.S., Guimarães, T.G., 2008. Herbicidas: Mecanismos de Ac¸ ão e Uso, first ed. Embrapa Cerrado, Planaltina.
Mayes, A.G., Whitcombe, M.J., 2005. Synthetic strategies for the generation of molecularly imprinted organic polymers. Adv. Drug Deliv. Rev. 57 (12), 1742–1778.
Mazzei, F., Botrè, F., Botrè, C., 1996. Acid phosphatase/glucose oxidase-based biosensors for the determination of pesticides. Anal. Chim. Acta 336 (1), 67–75.
Meng, X., Wei, J., Ren, X., Ren, J., Tang, F., 2013. A simple and sensitive fluorescence biosensor for detection of organophosphorus pesticides using H_2O_2-sensitive quantum dots/bi-enzyme. Biosens. Bioelectron. 47, 402–407.
Nguyen, H.L., Leermakers, M., Osan, J., Torok, S., Baeyens, W., 2005. Heavy metals in Lake Balaton: water column, suspended matter, sediment and biota. Sci. Tot. Environ. 340, 213–230.

NNI, 2009. National Nanotechnology Initiative. Leading to a revolution in technology and industry. Available from: http://www.nano.gov/about-nni

Novoselov, K.S., Geim, A.K., Morozov, S.V., Jiang, D., Zhang, Y., Dubonos, S.V., Grigorieva, I.V., Firsov, A.A., 2004. Electric field effect in atomically thin carbon films. Science 306 (5696), 666–669.

Nowack, B., Bucheli, T.D., 2007. Occurrence, behavior and effects of nanoparticles in the environment. Environ. Pollut. 150, 5–22.

Nygren, P.Å., 2008. Alternative binding proteins: affibody binding proteins developed from a small three-helix bundle scaffold. FEBS J. 275, 2668–2676.

Oliveira, A.C., Mascaro, L.H., 2011. Evaluation of acetylcholinesterase biosensor based on carbon nanotube paste in the determination of chlorphenvinphos. Int. J. Anal. Chem., Article ID 974216.

Pavan, S., Berti, F., 2012. Short peptides as biosensor transducers. Anal. Bioanal. Chem. 402, 3055–3070.

Pedrosa, V.A., Paliwal, S., Balasubramanian, S., Nepal, D., Davis, V., Wild, J., Ramanculov, E., Simonian, A., 2010. Enhanced Stability of enzyme organophosphate hydrolase interfaced on the carbon nanotubes. Colloids Surf. B 77 (1), 69–74.

Phenrat, T., Kim, H.-J., Fagerlund, F., Illangasekare, T., Tilton, R.D., Lowry, G.V., 2009. Particle size distribution, concentration, and magnetic attraction affect transport of polymer-modified Fe(0) nanoparticles in sand columns. Environ. Sci. Technol. 43, 5079–5085.

Pichon, V., Chapuis-Hugon, F., 2008. Role of molecularly imprinted polymers for selective determination of environmental pollutants—a review. Anal. Chim. Acta 622 (1–2), 48–61.

Pingarron, J., Yanez-Sedeno, P., Gonzalez-Cortes, A., 2008. Gold nanoparticles-based electrochemical biosensors. Electrochim. Acta 53 (19), 5848–5866.

Poma, A., Turner, A.P.F., Piletsky, S.A., 2010. Advances in the manufacture of MIP nanoparticles. Trends Biotech. 28 (12), 629–637.

Pop, E., Varshney, V., Roy, A.K., 2012. Thermal properties of graphene: fundamentals and applications. MRS Bull. 37, 1273–1281.

Pumera, M., 2011. Graphene-based nanomaterials for energy storage. Energy Environ. Sci. 4, 668–674.

Qu, Y., Sun, Q., Xiao, F., Shi, G., Jin, L., 2010. Layer-by-layer self-assembled acetylcholienesterase/PAMAM-Au on CNTs modified electrode for sensing pesticides. Bioelectrochemistry 77 (2), 139–144.

Quesada-González, D., Merkoçi, A., 2015. Nanoparticle-based lateral flow biosensors. Biosens. Bioelectron. 73, 47–63.

Radi, A.E., 2011. Electrochemical aptamer-based biosensors: recent advances and perspectives. Int. J. Electrochem., Article ID 863196.

Roy, S., Gao, Z., 2009. Nanostructure-based electrical biosensors. Nano Today 4, 318–334.

Saleh, N., Kim, H.J., Phenrat, T., Matyjaszewski, K., Tilton, R.D., Lowry, G.V., 2008. Ionic strength and composition affect the mobility of surface-modified Fe0 nanoparticles in water-saturated sand columns. Environ. Sci. Technol. 42, 3349–3355.

Saleh, N., Sirk, K., Liu, Y., Phenrat, T., Dufour, B., Matyjaszewski, K., Tilton, R.D., Lowry, G.V., 2007. Surface modifications enhance nanoiron transport and NAPL targeting in saturated porous media. Environ. Eng. Sci. 24, 45–57.

Salmain, M., Fischer-Durand, N., Pradier, C.M., 2008. Infrared optical immunosensors: application to the measurement of the herbicide atrazine. Anal. Biochem. 373 (1), 61–70.

Sassolas, A., Blum, L.J., Leca-Bouvier, B.D., 2009. Electrochemical aptasensors. Electroanalysis 21, 1237–1250.

Sassolas, A., Blum, L.J., Leca-Bouvier, B.D., 2011. Optical Detection systems using immobilized aptamers. Biosens. Bioelectron. 26 (9), 3725–3736.
Sassolas, A., Blum, L.J., Leca-Bouvier, B.D., 2012. Immobilization strategies to develop enzymatic biosensors. Biotech. Adv. 30 (3), 489–511.
Sassolas, A., Leca-Bouvier, B.D., Blum, L.J., 2008. DNA biosensors and microarrays. Chem. Rev. 108 (1), 109–139.
Schaffazick, S.R., Guterres, S.S., Freitas, L.L., Pohlmann, A.R., 2003. Aracterizacao e estabilidade físico-química de sistemas poliméricos nanoparticulados para administracao de fármacos. Quim. Nova 5, 726–737.
Sharma, P., Sablok, K., Bhalla, V., Suri, C.R., 2011. A novel disposable electrochemical immunosensor for phenyl urea herbicide diuron. Biosens. Bioelectron. 26 (10), 4209–4212.
Singh, R., 2011. Prospects of nanobiomaterials for biosensing. Int. J. Electrochem., Article ID 125487.
Singh, V., Joung, D., Zhai, L., Das, S., Khondaker, S.I., Seal, S., 2011. Graphene based materials: past, present and future. Prog. Mater. Sci. 56, 1178–1271.
Song, H.S., Park, T.H., 2011. Integration of biomolecules and nanomaterials: towards highly selective and sensitive. Biosens. Biotechnol. J. 6, 1310–1316.
Song, K.M., Lee, S., Ban, C., 2012. Aptamers and their biological applications. Sensors 12, 612–631.
Soppimath, K.S., Kulkarni, A.R., Aminabhavi, T.M., Bhaskar, C., 2001. Cellulose acetate microspheres prepared by O/W emulsification and solvent evaporation method. J. Microencapsul. 18, 811–817.
Stoltenburg, R., Reinemann, C., Strehlitz, B., 2007. SELEX—A (r)evolutionary method to generate high-affinity nucleic acid ligands. Biomol. Eng. 24 (4), 381–403.
Strano, M.S., Kruss, S., Hilmer, A.J., Zhang, J., Reuel, N.F., Mu, B., 2013. Carbon nanotubes as optical biomedical sensors. Adv. Drug Deliv. Rev. 65, 1933–1950.
Su, L., Jia, W., Hou, C., Lei, Y., 2011. Microbial biosensors: a review. Biosens. Bioelectron. 26 (5), 1788–1799.
Sun, X., Liu, B., Xia, K., 2011. A Sensitive and regenerable biosensor for organophosphate pesticide based on self-assembled multilayer film with CdTe as fluorescence probe. Luminescence 26 (6), 616–621.
Suri, C.R., Boro, R., Nangia, Y., Gandhi, S., Sharma, P., Wangoo, N., Rajesh, K., Shekhawat, G.S., 2009. Immunoanalytical techniques for analyzing pesticides in the environment. Trends Anal. Chem. 28, 29–39.
Tasca, F., Zafar, M.N., Harreither, W., Nöll, G., Ludwig, R., Gorton, L., 2010. A third generation glucose biosensor based on cellobiose dehydrogenase from *Corynascus thermophilus* and single-walled carbon nanotubes. Analyst 136, 2033–2036.
Tawil, N., Sacher, E., Mandeville, R., Meunier, M., 2014. Bacteriophages: biosensing tools for multi-drug resistant pathogens. Analyst 139, 1224–1236.
Tschmelak, J., Proll, G., Riedt, J., Kaiser, J., Kraemmer, P., Barzaga, L., Wilkinson, J.S., Hua, P., Hole, J.P., Nudd, R., Jackson, M., Abuknesha, R., Barcelo, D., Rodriguez-Mozaz, S., de Alda, M.J., Sacher, F., Stien, J., Slobodnik, J., Oswald, P., Kozmenko, H., Korenkova, E., Tothova, L., Krascsenits, Z., Gauglitz, G., 2005. Automated water analyser computer supported system (AWACSS) part I: project objectives, basic technology, immunoassay development, software design and networking. Biosens. Bioelectron. 20 (8), 1499–1508.
USEPA, 2007. Treatment technologies for site cleanup: annual status report, twelfth ed. Office of Solid Waste and Emergency Response. Report number: EPA-542-R-07-012. Available from: https://www.epa.gov/sites/production/files/2015-09/documents/asr12_full_document.pdf
USEPA, 2010. United State Environmental Protection Agency. Available from: http://www.epa.gov/

Valera, E., Muniz, D., Rodriguez, A., 2010a. Fabrication of Flexible interdigitated μ-electrodes (FIDμEs) for the development of a conductimetric immunosensor for atrazine detection based on antibodies labeled with gold nanoparticles. Microelectron. Eng. 87 (2), 167–173.

Valera, E., Ramon-Azcon, J., Barranco, A., Alfaro, B., Sanchez-Baeza, F., Marco, M.P., Rodriguez, A., 2010b. Determination of atrazine residues in red wine samples. A conductimetric solution. Food Chem. 122 (3), 888–894.

Valera, E., Ramon-Azcon, J., Sanchez, F.J., Marco, M.P., Rodriguez, A., 2008. Conductimetric immunosensor for atrazine detection based on antibodies labelled with gold nanoparticles. Sens. Actuat. B 134 (1), 95–103.

Vander Oost, R., Beyer, J., Vermeulen, N.P.E., 2003. Fish bioaccumulation and biomarkers in environmental risk assessment: a review. Environ. Toxicol. Pharmacol. 13, 57–149.

Volkert, A.A., Haes, A.J., 2014. Advancements in nanosensors using plastic antibodies. Analyst 139 (1), 21–31.

Wang, J., 2005. Carbon-nanotube based electrochemical biosensors: a review. Electroanalysis 17 (1), 7–14.

Wang, S., Guo, T., Deng, Q., Fang, G., Liu, C., Huang, X., 2015. Molecularly imprinted upconversion nanoparticles for highly selective and sensitive sensing of cytochrome c. Biosens. Bioelectron. 74, 498–503.

Wang, X., Lu, X., Chen, J., 2014. Development of biosensor technologies for analysis of environmental contaminants. Trends Environ. Anal. Chem. 2, 25–32.

Watlington K., 2005. Emerging nanotechnologies for site remediation and wastewater treatment. Environmental Protection Agency. Available from: https://clu-in.org/download/studentpapers/K_Watlington_Nanotech.pdf

Willander, M., Khun, K., Ibupoto, Z.H., 2014. Metal oxide nanosensors using polymeric membranes, enzymes and antibody receptors as ion and molecular recognition elements. Sensors 14, 8605–8632.

Xie, J., Xu, C., Kohler, N., Hou, Y., Sun, S., 2007. Controlled PEGylation of monodisperse Fe_3O_4 nanoparticles for reduced non-specific uptake by macrophage cells. Adv. Mater. 19, 3163–3166.

Xu, Y., Cheng, G., He, P., Fang, Y., 2009. A review: electrochemical aptasensors with various detection strategies. Electroanalysis 21 (11), 1251–1259.

Yan, J., Guan, H., Yu, J., Chi, D., 2013. Acetylcholinesterase biosensor based on assembly of multiwall carbon nanotubes onto liposome bioreactors for detection of organophosphates pesticides. Pestic. Biochem. Physiol. 105, 197–202.

Yao, C., Zhu, T., Qi, Y., Zhao, Y., Xia, H., Fu, W., 2010. Development of a quartz crystal microbalance biosensor with aptamers as bio-recognition element. Sensors 10, 5859–5871.

Yuan, T., Liu, Z.Y., Hu, L.Z., Xu, G.B., 2011. Electrochemical and electrochemiluminescent aptasensors. Chinese J. Anal. Chem. 39 (7), 972–977.

Zhang, W.X., 2003. Nanoscale iron particles for environmental remediation: an overview. J. Nanopart. Res. 5, 323–332.

Zhang, X.W., Elliott, D.W., 2006. Applications of iron nanoparticles for groundwater remediation. Remediation J. 16, 7–21.

Zhang, X., Guo, Q., Cui, D., 2009. Recent advances in nanotechnology applied to biosensors. Sensors 9 (2), 1033–1053.

Zhang, X., Peng, Y., Bai, J., Ning, B., Sun, S., Hong, X., et al., 2014. A novel electrochemical sensor based on electropolymerized molecularly imprinted polymer and gold nanomaterials amplification for estradiol detection. Sens. Actuat. B 200, 69–75.

Zhang, J., Zhang, X., Yang, G., Chen, J., Wang, S., 2013. A signal-on fluorescent aptasensor based on Tb^{3+} and structure-switching aptamer for label-free detection of ochratoxin A in wheat. Biosens. Bioelectron. 41, 704–709.

Zhao, H., Ji, X., Wang, B., Wang, N., Li, X., Ni, R., Ren, J., 2015. An ultra-sensitive acetylcholinesterase biosensor based on reduced graphene oxide-Au nanoparticles-β-cyclodextrin/Prussian blue-chitosan nanocomposites for organophosphorus pesticides detection. Biosens. Bioelectron. 65, 23–30.

Zheng, Z., Zhou, Y., Li, X., Liu, S., Tang, Z., 2011. Highly-sensitive organophosphorus pesticide biosensors based on nanostructured films of acetylcholinesterase and CdTe quantum dots. Biosens. Bioelectron. 26, 3081–3085.

Zhoua, Q., Zhanga, J., Fua, J., Shia, J., Jiang, G., 2008. Biomonitoring: an appealing tool for assessment of metal pollution in the aquatic. ecosystem. Ana. Chim. Acta. 606, 135–150.

SOIL SENSORS: DETAILED INSIGHT INTO RESEARCH UPDATES, SIGNIFICANCE, AND FUTURE PROSPECTS

Alka Dwevedi*, Promod Kumar*, Pravita Kumar*, Yogendra Kumar*, Yogesh K. Sharma, Arvind M. Kayastha**[†]

**University of Delhi, Sri Aurobindo College, South Campus, New Delhi, India; **University of Delhi, Swami Shraddhanand College, North Campus, New Delhi, India; [†]Banaras Hindu University, School of Biotechnology, Institute of Science, Varanasi, India*

1 Introduction

Soil plays an important role in providing water, nutrients, and an adequate environment for plant growth. It is responsible for the maintenance of biodiversity, crop yield, water partition, solute flow, filtering, and buffering, as well as nutrient cycling (Doran and Zeiss, 2000). The properties of soil are defined by parameters, such as texture, salinity, acidity, waterlogging, and compaction. They are not constant due to soil having spatiotemporal variations in very short time intervals (Ye et al., 2015); hence, obtaining their measurements is very difficult and complicated. A method is needed that is cost-effective, simple, and fast to measure physical properties of field soil. There are various external factors that are responsible for extensive spatiotemporal variations of soil. Most importantly, these factors include methods of cultivation (responsible for the mechanical mixing of soil compacts, aggregate shearing, filling of pore spaces, and exposure of organic matter to increase its rate of decay and oxidation) and irrigation (level of aggregation and disaggregation and effect percentage of exchangeable sodium, thus the salinity content of the soil). Various researchers across the world have focused on aspects of soil that have a maximum effect on the

New Pesticides and Soil Sensors. http://dx.doi.org/10.1016/B978-0-12-804299-1.00016-3

growth of plants. It has been found that soil moisture content is directly related to important soil properties like texture, organic matter content, and macroporosity. It directly regulates the type of vegetation cover, its density, and its uniformity (Barron-Gafford et al., 2011).

Variability in soil moisture content is strongly influenced by topographical (slope, aspect, curvature, and relative elevation), climatological, and meteorological factors (Zhao et al., 2011). With respect to topographical factors, slope influences infiltration, subsurface drainage, runoff, amount of solar irradiance received (responsible for the rate of evapotranspiration from the land surface), and the degree of orographic precipitation (Choi et al., 2007). Rainfall and precipitation patterns are the important components of climatological and meteorological factors responsible for variability in surface soil moisture content (Baier, 1965). Land use is another influential factor being studied for spatial variability of soil moisture content, as it directly regulates the rate of transpiration (Gao et al., 2014).

Gravimetric, nuclear-based, electromagnetic, tensiometer-based, and hygrometric methods have been developed for measuring soil moisture content in the field. Previously there were various conventional methods for estimating soil moisture content, but they could not achieve much significant data due to their nonapplicability under all circumstances. Techniques based on sensors have been developed recently, requiring extensive calibration, installation conditions (e.g., depth and wind direction), spatial resolution, geographical coverage, and representative measurements and reliability, as well as accuracy of the obtained data. There are several arguments across the world related to absolute accuracies of various sensors available in the market. Accuracy ranges from 5% to 8% (v/v), which is acceptable for almost all types of applications. However, intensive calibration of these sensors under laboratory conditions is needed before they can be used in the field. The regions having maximum spatiotemporal variability are being monitored using remote sensing to take simultaneous soil moisture content measurements over very large areas (Ye et al., 2015). Remote sensing has not reached across all the parts of the world, but is being used in few countries, such as the United States, Australia, Italy, France, and Spain. This chapter aims to provide an overview of the soil properties, their significance in plant growth, and methods of monitoring soil, especially its moisture content (a key factor in determining soil properties), as well as their advantages, disadvantages, cost, possible scale of operation, and response time.

2 Soil Types and Their Properties

Soil is the most important natural resource for sustaining all types of natural ecosystems (excluding aquatic ecosystems); it is a major source of nutrients to growing plants, and it provides anchorage support to plant roots. Soil, with its various types, takes several years to form, depending on type of rock, climate, vegetation (determines the amount and type of organic matter in the soil), landscape (maintenance of soil's integrity), and time (https://en.wikipedia.org/wiki/Pedogenesis). Healthy soil contains rich amounts of minerals, organic matter, and decomposers. Decomposers [bacteria (e.g., *Actinomyces*), fungi, earthworms, etc.] are the key factors in making soil well suited for plant growth by recycling all of the micro- and macronutrients, and are helpful in the formation of humus, making tunnels in the soil for proper aeration, excreting mucus for binding soil particles, etc. (Megías and Müller, 2010). There are three types of soil: sandy, loamy, and clay (Fig. 15.1). Sandy soil, containing minerals, is light brown in color; however, it is not suited for plant growth due to excessive drying and low water-holding capacity. Loamy soil is dark brown to black in color, containing a proportional amount of minerals as well as organic matter, making it well suited for plant growth. Clay is usually slippery when wet but becomes hard on drying. Its color

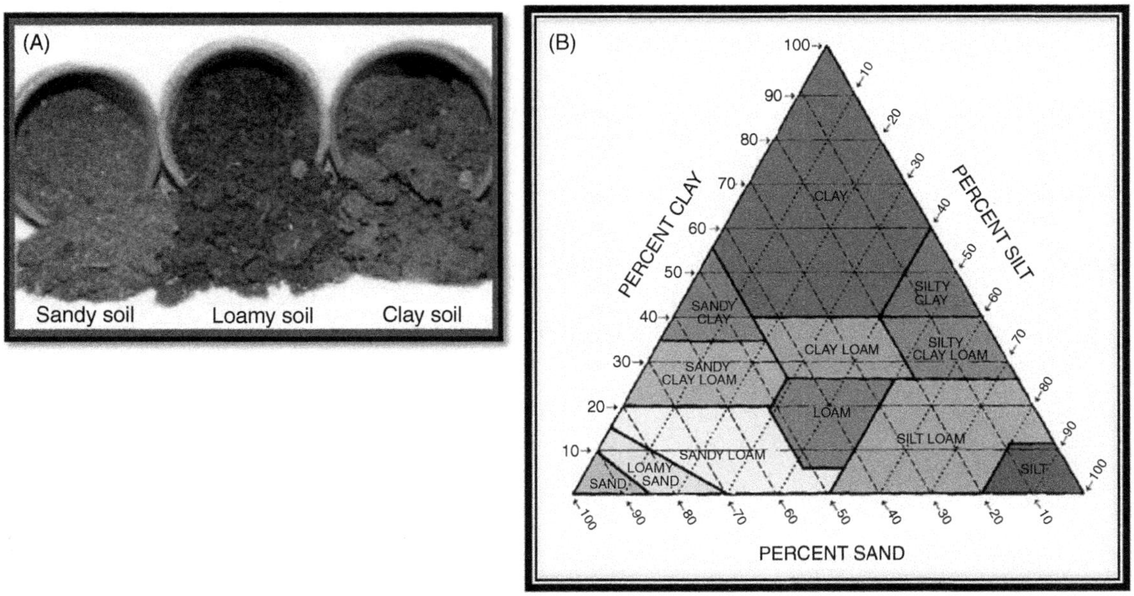

Figure 15.1. (A) Morphological outlook of soils (sandy, loamy, and clay). (B) Soil texture based on different composition (http://www.nrcs.usda.gov/).

is determined by the composition of minerals present. It has much less organic matter than loamy soil, although it promotes plant growth (Zandonadi et al., 2013). Different plants are adapted for different types of soils. Here, a brief is presented on different types of soil found with respect to their characteristics in an Indian context. Fig. 15.2 shows different soils and their localizations in India.

2.1 Black Soil

Black soil gets its name from its color, which is attributed to the presence of titaniferous magnetite, derived from trap lava. It has a large component of clay (60%) without gravel and coarse sand, and contains alumina (10%), iron oxide (10%), lime, magnesium carbonates (8–10%), and potash (<0.5%) with a very low phosphate, nitrogen, and humus content. It is highly resistant to wind and soil erosion and has a very high moisture-retentive capacity. It swells

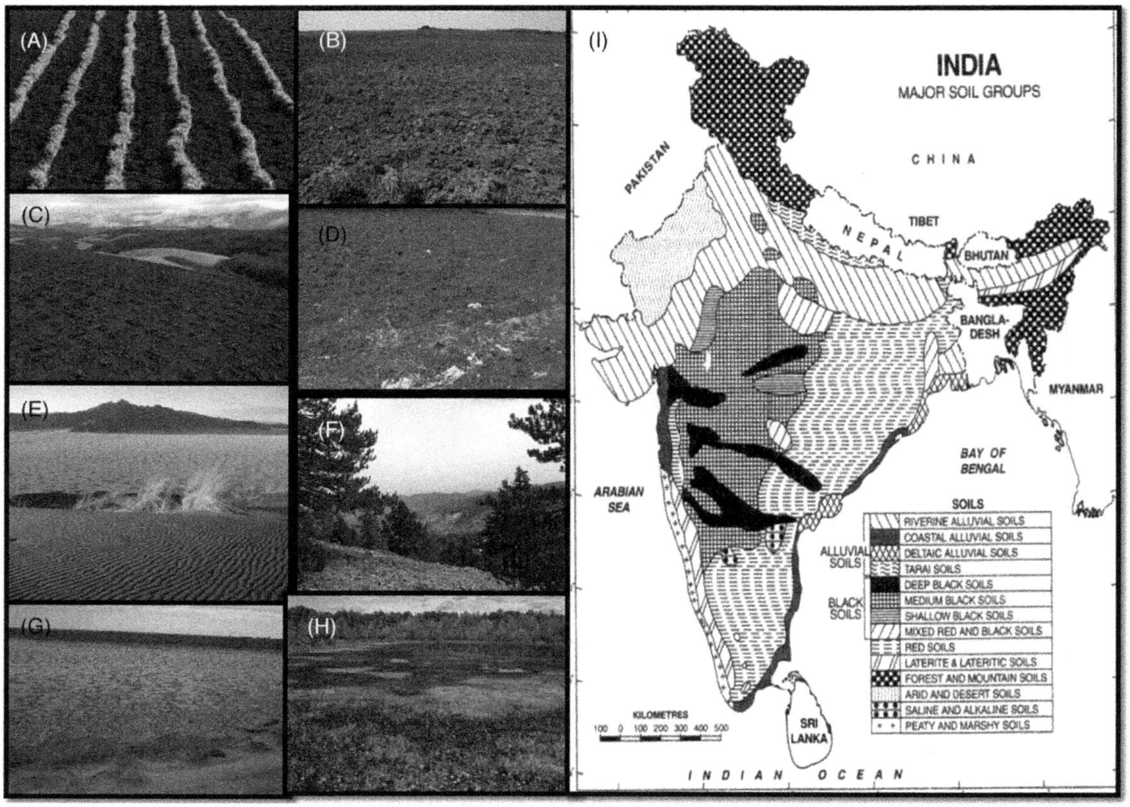

Figure 15.2. Different soils found in India: (A) black soil, (B) alluvial soil, (C) red soil, (D) laterite soil, (E) desert soil, (F) forest and mountain soil, (G) saline and alkaline soil, (H) peaty and marshy soil; and (I) their localizations (http://www.mapof.india.com/).

rapidly and becomes sticky during the rainy season due to its high moisture retention, which makes it impossible to plow. However, during the hot, dry season, the soil shrinks due to water evaporation, making broad and deep cracks, which permit oxygenation of the soil and thus impart extraordinary fertility. This soil is best suited for growing crops such as cotton, wheat, *jowar*, linseed, Virginia tobacco, castor, sunflowers, millets, vegetables, fruits, rice, and sugarcane even without fertilizers and manure. This soil usually occurs in regions having annual rainfalls ranging from 50 to 80 cm. India has black soil spread over 16.6% of the total geographical area, including Maharashtra, parts of Karnataka, Andhra Pradesh, Tamil Nadu, the interior of Gujarat, Madhya Pradesh, and on the Deccan lava plateau and the Malwa Plateau (Roy and Barde, 1962).

2.2 Alluvial Soil

Alluvial soil has the highest productivity with respect to other soils. It is present mostly along rivers and is carried by its streams during weathering of rocks. The soil is generally covered by tall grasses and forests, as well as a number of crops, such as rice, wheat, sugarcane, tobacco, maize, cotton, soybean, jute, oilseeds, fruits, vegetables, etc. This soil has very soft strata with the lowest proportion of nitrogen and humus but with an adequate amount of phosphate. There is a wide variation in the amount of iron oxide and lime in different regions. Alluvial soil is one of the best soils, requiring the least water due to its high porosity. The consistency of alluvial soil ranges from drift sand and rich, loamy soil to silt clays. India is one of the richest countries in the world in terms of alluvial soil, which covers more than 46% of its total land area. Most alluvial soils are derived from the sediment being deposited by the river Ganga in the Indo–Gangetic plain, ranging from Punjab in the west to West Bengal and Assam in the east, as well as in the coastal areas of northern parts of Gujarat, Narmada, and Tapi valleys, which are formed by sea waves. The alluvial soil found in India, particularly in the Indo–Gangetic plain, is of two types: *khaddar* (pale brown, sandy clays to loamy, less calcareous and carbonaceous soil, and found in the low areas of valley that are regularly flooded) and older *bhangar* soils (dark colored, mostly clayey, and containing lime nodules) (https://en.wikipedia.org/wiki/Alluvium).

2.3 Red Soil

The color of red soil ranges from red to brown, chocolate, yellow, gray, or sometimes even black. Red soil contains a high percentage of iron content, which is responsible for its color. This soil is deficient in nitrogen, humus, phosphoric acid, magnesium, and lime but fairly rich in potash, with its pH ranging from neutral to acidic. It is formed by the weathering of ancient crystalline and metamorphic rocks, particularly acid granites and gneisses, quartzitic rocks, and felspathic rocks. Chemically, red soil is siliceous and aluminous, with free quartz as sand, but is rich in potassium, ranging from sand to clay with the majority being loamy. The lowermost area of red soil is dark in color and very fertile, while the upper layer is sandy and porous. Thus, proper use of fertilizers and irrigation yields high production of cotton, wheat, rice, pulses, millets, tobacco, oil seeds, potatoes, and fruits. Approximately 10.6% of the total geographical area of India is covered by red soil, including Tamil Nadu, parts of Karnataka, southeastern Maharashtra, eastern Andhra Pradesh and Madhya Pradesh, Orissa, Chhattisgarh, Chota Nagpur (Jharkhand), south Bihar, West Bengal (Birbhum and Bankura), Uttar Pradesh (Mirzapur, Jhansi, Banda, and Hamirpur), Aravallis, eastern Rajasthan, Assam, Nagaland, Manipur, Mizoram, Tripura, and Meghalaya (http://www.importantindia.com/12596/red-soil-in-india/).

2.4 Laterite Soil

Laterite soil is reddish to yellow in color with a lower content of nitrogen, phosphorus, potassium, lime, and magnesia with 90–100% of iron, aluminum, titanium, and manganese oxides. The word laterite has been derived from the Latin word that means brick. The laterite soil is formed under conditions of high temperature and heavy rainfall with alternate wet and dry periods, which leads to leaching of soil, leaving only oxides of iron and aluminum. It lacks fertility due to a lower base-exchanging capacity and a lower content of nitrogen, phosphorus, and potassium. However, proper irrigation and use of fertilizers make it suitable for growing crops, such as tea, coffee, rubber, cinchona, coconut, etc. It also supports growth of paddy (rice) in low-lying areas. Laterite soil is one of the valuable sources for building material, as it can be easily cut with a spade but hardens like iron when exposed to air. In India, laterite soil is widespread, covering over 10% of the total geographical area, namely on the summits of the Western Ghats, Eastern Ghats (Rajamahal Hills, Vindhyas, Satpuras, and Malwa Plateau), southern parts of Maharashtra, parts of Karnataka, Andhra Pradesh, West Bengal Orissa, Jharkhand, Kerala, Assam, and Meghalaya (https://en.wikipedia.org/wiki/Laterite).

2.5 Desert Soil

Desert soil is mostly sandy soil (90–95%) found in low-rainfall regions. It has a low content of nitrogen and organic matter with very high calcium carbonate and phosphate, thus making it infertile. The amount of calcium is 10 times higher in the lower layer than in the topsoil. The availability of nitrogen in the form of nitrates, using fertilizer and proper irrigation, in addition to the already-present phosphates makes it useful in growing crops such as barley, rape, cotton, wheat, millets, maize, and pulses. For example, the Indira Gandhi canal command area is one of the best examples, showing maximum utility of the desert soils. This soil is susceptible to wind erosion and supports a low density of population. India has approximately 4% of total area covered with desert soil in the regions of Rajasthan, adjoining areas of Punjab and Haryana lying between the Indus and the Aravallis, the Rann of Kuchchh in Gujarat, and coastal regions of Orissa, Tamil Nadu, and Kerala (https://en.wikipedia.org/wiki/Desert).

2.6 Forest and Mountain Soils

Forest and mountain soils occur not only at higher elevations, but also at lower elevations that have sufficient rainfall. They are formed by the deposition of organic matter derived from forest growth and are heterogeneous in nature, depending on parent rocks, ground configuration, and climate. They are generally infertile for the production of field crops, but useful for supplying forest products, such as timber and fuel. They are rich in humus, but are deficient in potash, phosphorus, and lime; thus, they require a large amount of fertilizers for plantations of tea, coffee, spices, and tropical fruits. These soils occupy approximately 8.7% of the total land area of India, including the Himalayan region of Jammu and Kashmir, Himachal Pradesh, and Uttaranchal, and also some parts of the Western and Eastern Ghats and the Peninsular plateau. Some parts of Karnataka, Tamil Nadu, and Kerala also contain these soils (http://www.indianetzone.com/24/desert_soils_mountain_soil.htm).

2.7 Saline and Alkaline Soils

Saline and alkaline soils occur in the areas having little rainfall (more than areas of desert soils). They are known by various names, namely *reh*, *kallar*, *usar*, *thur*, *rakar*, *karl*, and *chopan*. They are formed by the weathering of rocks rich in minerals, like calcium, magnesium and sodium, and in acids like sulfurous acid. These minerals are transported by rivers to subsoils of plainer region. In the canal-irrigated and high-subsoil water table areas, salts accumulate in the lower layer and come to the surface by capillary action during dry seasons as a result of evaporation. These soils have poor drainage and the lowest fertility, rendering them unfit for agriculture. In

India, they are found in the drier areas of Uttar Pradesh, Punjab, Andhra Pradesh, Karnataka, Haryana, Rajasthan, Maharashtra, and Gujarat (Gulf of Khambhat and estuaries of Narmada, Tapi, Mahi, and Sabarmati) (http://www.biologydiscussion.com/essay/types-effects-and-management-of-saline-and-alkaline-soils/2431).

2.8 Peaty and Marshy Soils

Peaty and marshy soils are black colored, heavy, and highly acidic soils. They are deficient in potash and phosphate. These soils contain considerable amounts of soluble salts and 10–40% of organic matter contributed by the decomposition of growing vegetation over several hundred years. These soils are best suited for the growth of rice when properly drained and fertilized. They are found in Kerala (Kottayam and Alappuzha districts), Orissa and Tamil Nadu (coastal regions), West Bengal (Sunderbans), Bihar, and Uttaranchal (Almora district) (http://www.yourarticlelibrary.com/soil/soil-groups-8-major-soil-groups-available-in-india/13902/).

3 Important Parameters Determining Quality of Soil, as Well as Its Fertility

Soil contains physical and chemical compounds, including both organic and inorganic compounds. Important characteristic properties of soil are texture, structure, density, porosity, consistency, temperature, color, water-holding capacity, and pH. These properties are determining factors for the types of crops that can be grown in the particular soil and their productivity. Soil should have a very good water-holding capacity, as well as good nutrient-retentive ability, which are required for growing crops. It should have a high microbial diversity, providing suitable rhizosphere for roots of the plants, as well as avoiding the growth of various pests and weeds. Soils also sequester carbon from the atmosphere and thus help in the cleansing of groundwater (Harper et al., 2007). Soil health is very important for giving productive farming practices, giving sustainable productivity, maintenance of environmental quality, and promoting plant and animal health (www.sare.org). Fertile soil provides all the essential nutrients to plants, including macronutrients (e.g., nitrogen, phosphorus, and potassium) and micronutrients (e.g., boron and manganese). Good-quality soils have optimum amounts of the previously described elements taken by the plants for their growth, but the amounts are low enough to be leached into groundwater as they would be toxic for other growing living organisms. The physical characteristic of soil such as the formation of aggregates is helpful in infiltration of water and air, providing spacing for plant rooting and its expansion. Further, it also determines the population of active biota growing in the soil, which helps in decomposition and nutrients recycling (Ayres et al., 2006). The following sections describe soil properties and their significance.

3.1 Temperature

Soil temperature has a profound effect on plant growth, living biota, and composition of organic matter. The effect of temperature ranges from positive to negative. It has been found that major changes are seen at 40°C, as it is the temperature that directly controls water content present in the soil. There is an approximately 2% change in various parameters present in the soil with every degree change in the temperature (Frey et al., 2013). Therefore, measurement of soil temperature using various instruments helps in predicting soil conditions and suitability in growing different types of crops. A plant needs water to grow, while soil temperature directly affects the rate of water flow in the soil by controlling water viscosity, surface tension (via an inverse relation), and relative hydraulic conductivity (via a direct relation) (Marios, 2002). It has been found that dry soil freezes quicker (with several layers deeper inside) than wet soil, reflecting the higher thermal conductivity and heat capacity of wet soil as compared to dry soil. When experimentation to find the effect of soil temperature on the growth rate of maize seedlings was performed, it was found that the growth rate was a function of dry matter production. The water used by the plants is closely associated with dry matter production. It was found that maximum water was used at the soil temperature nearly optimum for plant growth (59°F), and that soil temperature also affected aging in plants. Lower soil temperature with higher variation of the optimum temperature leads to a higher rate of plant aging, as elucidated in the cases of barley, corn, and sugar beet. Therefore, accurate measurement of soil temperatures would help in modulating plant growth and increasing plant yield (Burkholder, 1920). Further, being cognizant of average active rhizosphere temperatures would help in the elucidation of accurate plant behavior with soil temperature variations. Therefore, there is an explicit need for intensive research on soil temperatures to aid in developing practices beneficial for plant growth. Soil temperature directly affects the activity of the soil biota (both microscopic and macroscopic organisms) by determining the rate of physiological activity (e.g., enzyme activity) and indirectly by affecting physicochemical properties, such as diffusion and solubility of nutrients, mineral weathering, and rate of evaporation (Dif and Bluemel, 1991). All organisms have a specific range of temperature corresponding to the operation of their biological activities. It has been found that most common soil organisms have an active range of temperature from 0 to 60°C. This temperature range is largely determined by their ability to produce several survival structures under adverse conditions. Further, each organism has its own optimum level of best performance with respect to biological functions. Beyond this temperature, cellular processes do not work efficiently, leading to irreversible changes at higher temperatures, subsequently causing death, whereas lower temperatures usually lead to dormancy or hibernation (Schipper et al., 2014).

Soil temperature directly affects the rate of decomposition of soil organic matter, and is critical in maintaining global carbon and nitrogen balance. The quality of soil organic matter and the sensitivity to temperature are determined by litter composition contributed by different types of forest cover. For example, decomposition of soil organic matter followed the trend in the forest (sugar maple, balsam fir, and black spruce) as highest in balsam fir while lowest in black spruce (Paré et al., 2006). The temperature dependencies of soil organic decomposition with respect to carbon and nitrogen were found to be highest at warmer temperatures. However, the process of decomposition at low temperatures is relatively higher than higher temperatures. The rate of soil organic matter decomposition directly affects the net primary productivity. It has been found that every 1°C increase in temperature could ultimately lead to a loss of about 10% of soil organic carbon and nitrogen in regions of the world. However, there is no equation for the temperature dependence of net primary productivity with respect to carbon and nitrogen content of soil organic matter (Alt et al., 2000; Maire et al., 2012).

3.2 Fire

Fire leads to the evaporation of soil moisture as the temperature reaches 100°C, bringing a number of physical and chemical changes in the soil. Further, an increment in temperature degrades lignin, hemicelluloses (between 130 and 190°C), and cellulose (at 280°C). As the temperature due to combustion reaches 500°C, soil organic matter is ignited and undergoes rapid charring in the soil (Gonzalez-Perez et al., 2004). Soil properties, particularly on or near the soil surface, are most likely to change due to direct exposure to fire, while inner layers are affected depending on the fuel load and burning conditions. This is due to the fact that volatilization of litter as well as the upper mineral layer of organic matter on the soil surface leads to the formation of a water-repellent layer, which impedes infiltration of temperature gradients deep into the soil. Further, the width of the water-repellent layer formed on the soil surface depends on the soil properties; for example, clayey soil is maximally unaffected due to the formation of a thickened layer of insulation on its surface (Campbell et al., 1997). Further, hydrology of the soil is severely affected by fire. There is a huge loss of various nutrients present in the soil organic matter, in the following order of importance: nitrogen > sulfur > potassium > phosphorus > magnesium > calcium > manganese. Detailed analyses on effects of fire on soil are described further in the following.

3.2.1 Nutrients

Most of the changes in the nutrients present in the soil are brought about by in situ changes and the translocation of organic substances downward into the soil. It has been found that there is very little change in different nutrients present more than about 4–5 cm below the soil surface, unless the fire is long-lasting (for several days). Nutrients such as nitrogen (N), phosphorus (P), and sulfur (S) have a very low threshold temperature and thus are easily volatilized (Fowells and Stephenson, 1934). The estimation of the amount of N is usually done to calculate the amount of nutrients loss due to fire, as it is the limiting factor with respect to other nutrients present in the soil. Further, the total amount of N volatilized during combustion is found to be directly proportional to the amount of organic matter combusted. However, P responds differently, as there is a loss of only about 60% of the total P during a fire. Thus, a substantial amount of P is found in the ash, as well as on the soil surface soon after a fire. As P does not translocate downward in the soil profile as readily as N compounds, it is mainly present on the soil surface. In the case of S, percentage loss is intermediate to N and P, that is, about 20–40% of the total S present in the aboveground biomass. The studies on the effect of fire on the amount of cations (Ca^{2+}, Mg^{2+}, and K^{+}) have not yet been done thoroughly. However, it has been elucidated that they have a crucial role in controlling soil pH regimes (Nduwumuremyi et al., 2013).

3.2.2 Soil Microorganisms

Soil microorganisms are most sensitive to soil heating during a fire, especially nitrifiers, endo- and ectomycorrhizae. Most of the ectomycorrhizae (namely vesicular–arbuscular mycorrhizae) are present in the organic matter on or near to the soil surface, and are thus mostly affected by fire. The decrease in vesicular–arbuscular mycorrhizae colonization leads to long-term loss in soil productivities (Marschener and Dell, 1994; Harrison and Buuren, 1995). The sensitivity of microorganisms to higher temperatures due to fire differs significantly depending on the presence of protective structures as discussed in Section 3.1. Soil heating affects microorganisms either directly by killing them or altering their reproductive capabilities or indirectly by altering the composition of organic matter present in the soil. There is a complex relationship between higher temperatures caused by fire and the response of microbial growth. It has been found that soil microorganisms are physiologically active in moist soil while dormant in dry soil (Yuste et al., 2007).

3.2.3 Organic Matter

Organic matter consists of six easily recognizable components: litter layer (consisting of plant litter), duff layer (composed of partially decomposed plant litter), humus layer (decayed and disintegrated organic matter), decayed wood (residual lignin matrix obtained from the decomposition of woody material), charcoal (charred wood), and underlying mineral soil. During a forest fire, it is the mineral layer that is least affected compared to other layers. Degradation of layers ahead of the duff layer affects the fertility of soil enormously (DeBano et al., 1976). Therefore, recurring fires at frequent intervals make soil completely infertile. However, fire has a long-term positive impact on nutrient cycling in the ecosystem. The rate of nutrient cycling is several times higher during a fire than by decomposition. It acts as a rapid mineralizing agent that releases nutrients more instantaneously than the natural decomposition processes, which require years or several decades (in some cases). It leads to increase availability of various nutrients, excluding N, P, and S contents. The loss of soil organic matter due to fire leads to a lowering of cation-exchange capacity, aggregation stability, infiltration, organic chelation, macropore spacing, and loss of various useful soil microorganisms (particularly decomposers) (Hosking, 1938).

3.3 Concentration of Dissolved Gases

The composition of gases found in the soil is entirely different from that found in the atmosphere. Earth's atmosphere contains two major gases, N_2 and O_2, while minor gases are CO_2 and argon (Ar). However, soil has a much higher concentration of CO_2 (~40%) due to plant root respiration and microbial breakdown of carbon-based organic compounds, with ~50% of O_2 accumulation due to photosynthesis and ~10% of N_2 due to nitrification and ammonification (Farrell et al., 2014). There is an inverse relation between the concentration of CO_2 and O_2 in the soil, with their concentrations varying with different seasons. The level of CO_2 is often higher at the bottom of the soil profile (i.e., root zone) than the soil surface due to a poor rate of O_2 aeration. Further, the high concentration of CO_2 at greater soil depths is also attributed to its higher molecular weight (44 g) with respect to other gases (nitrogen: 28 g, oxygen: 32 g, water: 16 g). High CO_2 content is found mostly in waterlogged regions and is thus responsible for creating anaerobic conditions inside the soil. In addition, it leads to increased alkalinity, which is responsible for increased weathering rates of primary minerals (Kuzyakov, 2006).

The movement of air inside the soil profile in the root zone depends on its solubility, pore size distribution, water-retention capacity, temperature, hydraulic conductivity, and pressure of gases. Air permeability, particularly porosity of 0.075 mm or larger, is effective for an equal distribution of various gases and their effect on various biological activities inside the soil. The previously defined parameters for air movement are greatly dependent on the texture of the soil and are thus responsible for varied activities, namely soil fertility, types of crops, population of microbial growth, etc. The air transport inside the soil is determined by mass flow and diffusive flow (Nielsen et al., 1997). Mass flow depends on temperature changes, barometric pressure fluctuations, wind velocity, and water infiltration, while diffusive flow is governed by concentration differences of different gases with indirect dependency on air pressure or temperature. There are almost negligible studies related to the effect of each parameter on various gases found in the soil. The difference in temperature between various parts of the soil (surface soil has a higher temperature than the subsoil) results in density and pressure gradients, allowing a flow of gases from the surface to the root zone. Similarly, an increase in barometric pressure in the atmosphere results in a flow of gases into the root zone. There are few studies on the effect of wind velocity on soil air movement. It has been found that irrigation and rainfall are quite helpful in carrying dissolved oxygen to the root zone (Abuarab et al., 2013). However, excess water leads to anaerobic conditions. Therefore, an optimum amount of water has to be maintained for healthy soil and its associated activities. Poor aeration, high moisture content, and low temperature and pH lead to a higher rate of iron chelation (greatly affecting soil fertility), which is caused by incorrect maintenance equipment and topdressing materials. Therefore, wise irrigation is critical in addition to good mechanical aerification; coring, slicing, spiking, and forking are to be done in proper time intervals for promoting good soil aeration and healthy levels of soil gases (Heiskanen, 1995).

3.4 Soil Structure and Texture

The structure and texture of the soil are the crucial determining factors for crop productivity, particularly the proportion of mineral particles and the size of the soil particles. The type of agricultural activities, such as addition of pesticides, insecticides, fungicides, and fertilizers, and their concentrations depend on the texture of the soil. Water-holding capacity of the soil is highly influenced by the soil texture, in addition to the amount of organic matter present in the soil. It has been found that soil texture regulates the movement of various contaminants from agricultural land into the groundwater table (Li and Shuman, 1996). The components of soil structure are soil particles, organic matter, and aggregates. The discussion will be restricted to soil particles and aggregates, while organic matter has been discussed in Sections 3.2.3 and 3.6. There are three main size fractions present in the soil, sand (0.05–2 mm), silt (>2 mm), and clay (<0.002 mm). Loamy soil is the mixture of sand, silt, and clay. Sand particles are generally round, while silt and clay particles are usually thinner and flatter. There are a large number of spaces present in the sand particles due to their round shape, thus the least water-holding capacity, making sandy soil prone to drought. However, sandy soil has good aeration due to its large particle size. Sandy soil is highly susceptible to wind erosion due to its loose structure. It has been recommended that practices like crop rotations, reduced tillage, cover cropping for residue enhancing, and shelterbelts should be implemented for the improvement of agricultural activities. It has been found that overfertilization of sandy soil with nitrogen may lead to contamination of groundwater due to its leaching, which poses a health risk to infants and immune-suppressed individuals. Silty soil is also highly susceptible to water erosion. The speed of erosion is highest at very high altitudes, contributed mostly by high-stream waterfalls. The recommended agricultural practices for reducing soil erosion are: cover and contour cropping, crop rotations, conservation tillage, grassed waterways and vegetated buffer strips. Clayey soil is very sticky, is difficult to cultivate, holds a lot of water, and becomes waterlogged (especially in winter). Some soils containing clay are layered which are often called sheets. These layered structures help in holding water and nutrients to provide to growing plants. Further, within these layered structures many "parking spaces" are found that act as reservoirs for nutrients. Research has elucidated that these spaces are negatively charged sites, while many of the nutrients are positively charged; thus they hold nutrients tightly and make them available for plants. Clayey soil is good for various agricultural activities, however the soil has serious risk of rapid contamination from various chemical based fertilizers, insecticides, fungicides etc. due to having very small particle size. Further, surface structure of the clayey soil is often degraded due to crust formation. As clayey soil is smallest in size of particles, it increases their time of settling in streams and lakes, and thus the cost of water treatment. Clayey soils may also be highly susceptible to wind erosion, especially under dry conditions in which the soil surface becomes pulverized. The recommended agricultural practices for reducing water erosion in the clayey soil include crop rotations, cover cropping, conservation tillage, contour cropping, vegetated buffer strips, and grassed waterways (Tilman et al., 2002).

It has been found that soil rich in organic matter has large aggregates rather than separate soil particles. These aggregates frequently occur in clayey soil, with their size ranging from a few millimeters (such as granules and crumbs) to several centimeters (such as columns and prisms). Aggregates are formed by various ways, *viz.* bacterial exudates, soil particles entanglement by fungal hyphae, and digestive products produced by earthworms (growing on organic matter). Soil aggregates are helpful in sustaining soil under extreme conditions. Soils having low aggregate-forming capability form surface crusts, which reduce the rate of water infiltration and air exchange, thus obstructing plant growth. Repeated soil tillage leads to a breakdown of stable soil aggregates and thus reduces soil productivity. Soil compaction is another important parameter which makes it less porous. It reduces the amount of air-filled pores and oxygen cannot reach the soil interior. Extreme compaction often restricts plant growth due to space constrains. Compacted soils have fewer and smaller roots. Soil compaction can be alleviated through the addition of organic matter, mechanical loosening, and by selecting a rotation, including crops with strong taproots (which penetrate and break down compacted soils) (West and Post, 2002).

3.5 Acidity and Alkalinity

Acidity and alkalinity define the amount of H^+ present in the soil. It is one of the most crucial determining factors in soil fertility, crop selection, fertilizer usage, microbial population, and their diversity. Generally, the pH in the soil lies between 3 and 8, with pH below 7.0 being acidic and above 7.0 being alkaline. Most of the world's soils have a pH between 5.5 and 7.5. Soil pH is measured using a variety of kits and devices (dyes, paper strips, and glass electrodes) after complete removal of all the moisture to minimize biological activities. It has been found that the texture of the soil determines the buffering capacity of the soil; namely, clay has more capacity to resist pH change than loamy soil has, followed by sand. There are various factors responsible for the change in soil pH. Fertilizers containing ammonium ions are responsible for soil acidification significantly with respect to other fertilizers due to rapid release of H^+ via conversion into nitrates when introduced into a field. Rainfall is another important contributing factor in the acidity of the soil, as water forms carbonic acid (a weak acid) by reacting with dissolved CO_2 present in the soil. H^+ released by carbonic acid replaces calcium ions present in soil colloids, subsequently making the soil more acidic. It has been found that regions having low rainfall conditions tend to be more basic, but there have been no intensive studies on the mechanism of alkalinity. Acidic soil is deficient in calcium, magnesium, nitrogen (nitrate), phosphorus, boron, and molybdenum, whereas aluminum and manganese are abundant (toxic to some plants). Alkaline soil is deficient in phosphorus, iron, copper, zinc, and boron (White and Zasoski, 1999; Loneragan and Webb, 1993). It has been found that bacterial populations are higher at neutral pH, while fungal populations grow at both acidic and alkaline pH. Low pH in the topsoil reduces activity of *Rhizobia* responsible for nitrogen fixation in plants, thus leading to nitrogen deficiency as indicated by necrosis and chlorosis in the leaves, with intensive redness in the stems and petioles of leguminous plants. It has been found that mineralization of organic matter slows down at both acidic and alkaline pH due to poor bacterial activities at pH beyond neutral pH. Soil pH is a determining factor in the formation of aggregates in the soil by effectuating cation availability, particularly calcium ions that act as the bridge between organic colloids and soil particles (Bronick and Lal, 2005). Many plant diseases perpetuate under acidic or alkaline pH; namely, take-all disease, caused by the fungus *Gaeumannomyces graminis*, is favored at alkaline pH infecting wheat, barley, rye, etc. Various cycles (C, N, S, and P) almost stop functioning at extreme pH and thus unbalance the whole ecosystem. The availability of various nutrients is also affected by soil pH. A pH level below 5.5 leads to a low availability of nitrogen, phosphorus, potassium, sulfur, calcium, manganese, and also the trace elements such as molybdenum, magnesium, and phosphorus. However, the solubility of aluminum, iron, and boron is higher at a low pH. High-pH soils have an inadequate availability of iron, manganese, copper, and zinc, as well as phosphorus and boron. It has been found that if the pH of the soil is outside the allowed range, the pesticides are ineffective due to their degradation or conversion to undesired states. Many heavy metals are more soluble under acidic conditions due to which they move downward, contaminating groundwater, as well as aquifers, surface streams, and lakes (McBride, 1989).

Acidic pH of the soil can be corrected using liming chemicals, such as limestone, calcitic lime, and dolomitic lime. Sometimes, two or more liming chemicals are mixed to increase their efficacy, namely fluid lime consisting of finely ground limestone suspended in water in a 1:1 ratio of water to limestone. In all cases, liming chemicals are finely ground to increase the rate of the reaction, with the amount of applicability depending on the amount of organic matter, soil texture, soil pH profile, lime quality, farming system, and rainfall. Further, the reaction rate of liming chemicals is increased by increasing soil temperature and moisture content. Liming has been found to be the most economical method to correct the soil pH of acidic soil (Haynes and Naidu, 1998). This technique, along with crop rotation, was found to be 5 times more effective than individual techniques. Generally, lime in all cases after fine grinding is passed through 100–200 sieves and applied directly into the field. The pH of alkaline soil can be corrected by applying ammonium-based fertilizers, urea, and sulfur/ferrous sulfate; irrigation with acidifying fertilizers; or usage of acidifying residues, such as acid moss, pine needles, and sawdust. Elemental sulfur is very helpful when there is a requirement of pH correction to precision. It takes almost 6 weeks for correcting soil pH, which occurs by the oxidation of sulfur using microbial activities. In this case too, finely grinded chemicals are used to increase the rate of reaction at optimum temperature and moisture content (Rajan, 1987).

3.6 Organic Matter

Organic matter constitutes about 6% of the total soil volume and consists of three components: living organisms (bacteria, fungi, protozoa, earthworms, and tiny insects), fresh residue, and well-decomposed residue. Living organisms are an important component, constituting about 15% of the total soil organic matter organisms. They help in the decomposition of plant and animal residues, as well as in nutrient and biological cycling. Organic matter has a crucial effect on the properties of the topsoil as compared to other layers. Further, topsoil structures are smaller than subsoil structures due to the presence of organic matter. It improves soil properties, including soil structure, tilth, aeration, water infiltration rate, water-holding capacity, cation-exchange capacity, pH stabilization (releasing H^+ in response to the addition of alkaline materials and adsorbing H^+ in response to the addition of acidic materials), and chelation of micronutrients and trace elements important for plant growth (Franzluebbers, 2002). Binding capacity of the soil to water is dependent on the pore size of the soil particles and amount of organic matter present in the soil. Water is held in the soil pores with different degrees of strength; namely, sandy soil has the least water-binding strength, making it highly prone to drought, whereas clayey soil has many small pores, and thus holds water very tightly and retains it for a very long duration. Soil organic matter influences chemical, biological, and physical properties of the soil, therefore directly controlling crop productivity (Schmidt et al., 2011).

The most common sources of organic matter are crop residues, cover crop residues, manures, and composts. However, the largest source of organic matter added to soil is the remaining residue following crop production. Manure also helps in increasing soil organic matter indirectly by increasing crop yields. It has been found that solid and semisolid manures have higher organic matter than liquid manure because of added bedding. The addition of manure affects nutrient cycling, soil microbial biomass and activity, and enzymatic processes. Manure-amended soil has a generally high concentration of nitrogen compared to nonmanured soil. However, manures with toxic trace metals should be avoided, as they have an adverse effect on the soil. Synthetic fertilizers have no contribution toward increasing the soil organic matter in any respect. Generally, soil organic matter has two fractions based on its color, that is, light and dark fractions. The light fraction of organic matter is a highly reactive pool of organic matter consisting of new and uncomplexed organic residues at various stages of decomposition, while the dark fraction of organic matter consists of highly decomposed, stable, and humic substances that form organomineral complexes with a large number of stable soil aggregates. Humus of soil organic matter is the most resistant portion, with a shelf life of several hundred years. It constitutes about 70% of the total organic matter present in the soils. It has a very high water-holding capacity, is important in enhancing soil nutrient holding (especially cations), improves soil structure and its tilth, and thus affects soil fertility significantly (Saxton and Rawls, 2005). Fresh crop residues undergo decaying immediately after humus addition into the soil and release CO_2 and water. However, release of minerals takes from a few months to several years. This process provides energy (e.g., via respiration) for soil microbes and mineral nutrients for both microbes and plants (e.g., crops). Growth of microbes leads to excretion of sticky substances, which hold the soil together and convert it into aggregates that further provide food to an entire web of other soil organisms. Microbes consumed by other microscopic organisms, such as worms and nematodes, are helpful in increasing nitrogen content by excreting ammonia in the soil, which is beneficial for plant growth. Soil microbial activity is important, as it is responsible for the decomposition of crop residues and mineralization of organic nutrients into inorganic forms for plant uptake (Fontaine et al., 2003). It is generally accepted that the larger the soil microbial community, the greater would be the diversity, and thus the greater the potential for nutrient mineralization. Manure has a significant effect on the diversity of microbial communities, as well as their enzymatic activities. Various enzymatic activities, particularly those of dehydrogenase, chitinase, urease, and glutaminase, are significantly affected; namely, the activity of urease (converting urea in manure or synthetic fertilizer to ammonium N) and phosphatase (mineralizing organic P) increases with the application of manure (Albiach et al., 2000).

4 Need for Soil Monitoring

The rational utilization and conservation of soil are crucial as they are important contributors to a country's economy and important constituents of our environment and agricultural sustainability. Major parameters that are monitored for the assessment of soil health are: carbonate and salinity/alkalinity status, hydrophysical properties, depth of the soil, amount of organic matter, depth of the humus horizon, depth of the groundwater table, soil type, and pH (Filip, 2002). Agricultural practices, such as cropping pattern, soil cultivation, use of fertilizers, and water conservation practices (irrigation and drainage), have major effects on the soil quality. Particularly, depth of the water table and the groundwater regime are critical (Swartjes, 1999). Following are the enlisted agrotechnologies being used these days for soil health monitoring and assessment (Karlen et al., 1995):

- Site-specific precision agrotechnologies for controlling soil moisture, water and nutrient supply, and soil and environmental pollution.
- Assessment of the agroecological potential of soil structure and texture (e.g., clay mineral associations and soil productivity index).
- Generation of a topographical map based on the parameters of surface waters, land use, infrastructure, and sequence of soil layers, as well as hydrophysical properties of soils (texture, saturation percentage, field capacity, wilting percentage, available moisture range, infiltration rate, saturated hydraulic conductivity, and unsaturated capillary conductivity).

- Status of soil erosion from strongly to slightly eroded lands, sedimentation areas, territories under the influence of wind erosion, and the quality of the parent material.
- Salt-affected soils, moisture and nutrient regime, and rate of soil degradation process.

Based on various soil-monitoring technologies, soil is characterized under various categories: sensitivity/susceptibility/vulnerability to various natural- and human-induced stresses, susceptibility to water and wind erosion, extent of acidification/salinization/alkalization/sodification, physical degradation (such as structure destruction, compaction, and surface sealing), and vulnerability to various pollutants (e.g., hazard of nitrate leaching). The scientifically based planning for sustainable land use and conservation of soil, in addition to water and the surrounding environment, requires adequate information on different soil types using territorial data; understanding temporal variability of various soil processes; soil-forming factors (geology, climate and weather conditions, surface and subsurface hydrology, natural vegetation, and human activities); relationship between soil with existing biota, vegetation, and cultivated crops; mechanism of pedotransfer and application of simulation models (validated and calibrated) based on the prediction of the potential consequences of various human activities; and selecting suitable alternative measures for maximal increase in soil efficiency. This will lead to rational land use, proper cropping pattern, and control of limiting factors responsible for soil fertility and its degradation processes, soil and water pollution, moisture and nutrient regimes, and biodiversity and landscape deterioration (Chantigny, 2003).

Various monitoring systems have been developed to combat soil degradation and its pollution, namely soil information and monitoring system (gives basic topographic information, such as characteristics of soil profiles and their different layers and diagnostic horizons, pedotransfer functions, soil processes, and soil–plant–environment relationships) and environmental information and monitoring system (particularly focuses on environmentally threatened "hot spot" regions, such as degraded soils, ameliorated soils, drinking water supply areas, and watersheds of important lakes and reservoirs; "hot spots" of industrial, agricultural, urban, and transport pollution, military fields; and areas affected by mining, wastewater disposal affected spots, etc.). The "representative" sampling sites are selected by regional soil experts based on the available soil information (profile descriptions, results of laboratory analysis, long-term field observations, maps, etc.) and on their local experiences. In the monitoring system, some soil parameters are measured every year, while others after every 3–6 years, depending on their stability. There is a wide range of practical use of soil databases and monitoring systems as follows (Johnson et al., 1990; Herrick, 2000):

- Establishment of potential conservative measures connections for regional, continental, and global actions of sustainable development.
- Proper organization of hierarchic soil database at global, continental, regional, national, subregional, local, farm, and field level.
- Identification of susceptibility factors of soils to various natural and anthropogenic impacts and environmental hazards.
- Well-validated simulated model based on the forecast of soil processes that help in an efficient control and prevention of undesirable changes (such as soil degradation processes, soil pollution, extreme moisture, and nutrient regime).
- Optimization and zonation of land use, including both agricultural and nonagricultural land, and their efficient amelioration and remediation strategies.
- Rural development, sustainable biomass production, and rational environment protection.
- Development and formulation of economically viable, socially acceptable, and environmentally sound land use policy and legislation measures.

5 Soil Monitoring Using Soil Sensors

Soil monitoring is generally done with respect to its moisture content, which is the total amount of water trapped in the spaces between soil particles. It is of crucial significance because of its connectivity to many hydrological, meteorological, and biological processes (Robock et al., 2000). It is useful for both public and private sectors related to weather, climate, flood control, reservoir management, early warning of droughts, irrigation scheduling, crop yield forecasting, geotechnical engineering, water quality, etc. Most significantly, management of irrigation based on the data obtained from soil moisture monitoring has been found to be helpful in the enhancement of crop productivities and reduction of leaching of agrichemicals (Bell et al., 1980; Brocca et al., 2010). The most tedious task of measuring soil moisture is at the surface, which has maximum spatial and temporal variations (Crow et al., 2012). Further, a large sample size also presents an obstruction in getting adequate information on soil moisture content of a particular area. Various types of soil moisture-estimating sensors are available in the market, namely frequency domain reflectometry (FDR) sensor, time domain reflectometry (TDR) sensor, gypsum blocks, neutron moisture gauge, etc. They are chosen based on physical properties of the soil, sample size, and aim of the soil moisture measurements. In previous decades, the volumetric method, which used the gravimetric method, was the only choice. Although it was an easily adapted and cost-effective method, it suffered from several drawbacks, such as applicability to fine-textured soil only with high water-retention capacity (Wagner et al., 1999). Remote sensing has recently been used as an alternative, especially when there is a requirement of assessment of a very large area. It offers fast estimation of soil moisture content and is cost-effective. However, it requires expert handling, especially in data analysis and calibration. Here we have focused only on field-based sensors, discussed further next.

5.1 Time Domain Reflectometry Sensor

A time domain reflectometry (TDR) sensor (Fig. 15.3A) is used to determine moisture content in the soil, as well as porous media, both in the laboratory and in agricultural land. It is an electronic device that works on the principle of radar based on transmitting signals into the medium and collecting reflected signals. Analysis of reflected signals, particularly their magnitude, shape, and sign, provides a complete image of the transmitting medium. The reflections are measured, generally plotted as a function of time or sometimes as a function of cable length. TDR determines dielectric constant and consequently permitivity and water content (direct related) of the medium, which is soil, via wave propagation transmitted by two parallel embedded metal probes with the utmost accuracy. The probes have a length of 10–30 cm, which is connected to the TDR via a coaxial cable. However, spatial and temporal variability of water as well as solute fluxes in the field often raise several difficulties in obtaining quantitative understanding of the dynamics of the water and salt regimes. It has been found that soil in the root zone has maximum variability due to active transpiration. Thus, it is almost impossible to get accurate estimates of soil water pressure and osmotic potentials. Proponents of the in situ neutron scattering method have claimed that field soil water can be measured accurately in any section of the soil zone, but the method has not achieved much publicity, as it requires a very large amount of sample, can only perform measurements at the soil surface (most crucial zone), requires intensive calibration, and is a radiation hazard. A porous ceramic salinity sensor can be used for measuring soil salinity. It has four probes made up of platinum, measures in situ electrical conductivity of the soil solution, and subsequently gives its salinity measurements. However, the

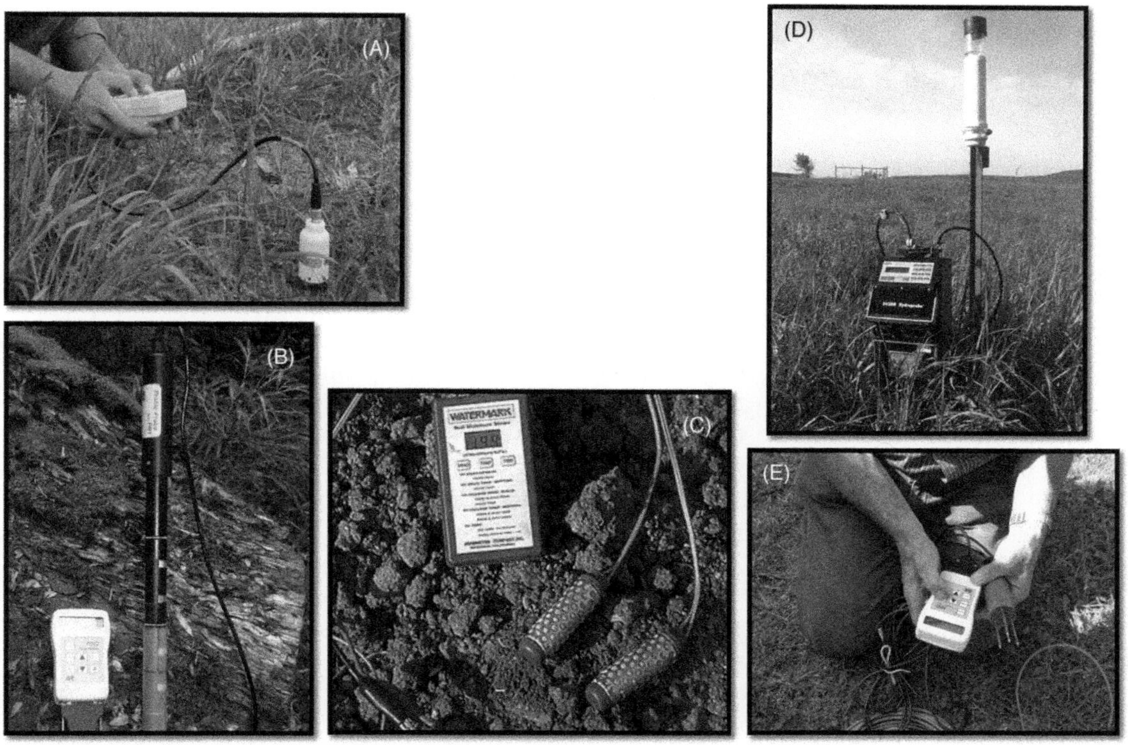

Figure 15.3. Sensors for soil moisture content. (A) Time domain reflectometry (TDR) sensor, (B) frequency domain reflectometry (FDR) sensor, (C) gypsum blocks, (D) neutron probes, and (E) amplitude domain reflectometry (ADR) sensor. Image obtained from http://www.google.co.in/soilsensors/images

direct measurement of soil water electrical conductivity is possible only when ceramic ions surrounding the probes are in equilibrium. Further, this method is limited to a relatively narrow range of soil water pressures. Here, very small amount of soil samples is required and the method can be used even for aggregated soils. The most common problems associated with measuring soil water content and salinity using different devices are sampling errors and lack of correlation. Thus, TDR is the best-suited technology for the simultaneous measuring of water content and soil salinity. Further, the method can be used for measuring volumetric water content of unsaturated soils with minimal sampling (Huisman et al., 2001; Robinson et al., 2002).

TDR is used in various other sectors these five examples (Noborio, 2001):

1. Maintenance of telecommunication lines: TDR sensors are used for in-place testing of several-kilometer-long telecommunication cables running very deep within the ground. TDRs

detect resistance on joints and connectors, level of corrosion, insulating leakage, shortcircuiting, and determination of wire taps in the cable lines, as they have capability of detecting moisture. Thus, they are helpful for various catastrophic failures. In TDR technology, the impulse velocity passing through the medium is primarily affected by the moisture content and temperature of the medium. Therefore, obtained results are highly affected by the boiling point and liquid level of the medium.

2. Anchor cables in dams: The Dam Safety Interest Group of CEA Technologies, Inc. (CEATI, a consortium of electrical power organizations) has used TDR technology to identify potential faults in concrete dams to anchor cables.
3. Geotechnical usage: TDR has been used in monitoring slope movement in geotechnical settings like highway cuts, rail beds, and open pit mines. They have the ability to determine soil moisture content, and are used to calculate the time required for a drop of water to reach a certain depth; thus the speed of water infiltration and effective measures for best management practices in reducing storm water surface runoff can be determined.
4. Semiconductor device analysis: TDR is used for locating defects in semiconductor devices by providing an electrical signature of individual conductive traces in the particular device.
5. Aviation wiring maintenance: TDRs are used on aviation wiring for both preventive maintenance and fault location.

5.2 Frequency Domain Reflectometry Sensors

Frequency domain reflectometry (FDR) sensors (Fig. 15.3B) are used for measuring soil moisture content, and contain an oscillating circuit and the sensing part of the sensor (embedded in the soil). There are two types of sensors.

1. Fringe capacitance sensor: Uses capacitance to measure the dielectric permittivity of the soil water. There is a sensing probe fixed at a suitable depth inside the soil, containing an oscillator circuit, an annular electrode, and a fringe-effect capacitor. The measurements are based on the change in the dielectric permittivity of water (which is 80 for pure water) with additional components.
2. Electrical impedance sensor: Uses electrical impedance measurement to calculate soil water content. It is based on the standing wave principle consisting of a sinusoidal oscillator (100 MHz), fixed impedance coaxial transmission line, and

probe wires (buried in the soil). The oscillator signal is transmitted along the coaxial line into the soil probe, and variations in the reflected-back signals are used in calculating the probe's impedance, which is then used to obtain the water content present in the soil.

FDRs are very cheap, with higher response times compared to TDRs. However, they require extensive calibration due to the complexity of generated electrical field around the probe with different soil types (Geng et al., 2005). Improvisation is in progress, particularly in optimizing usage of the frequency range. The FDR sensors working in the frequency range >150 MHz are being used, but efforts are being made to increase it to 500 MHz, which will be helpful for saline soils frequently found in a majority of agricultural fields due to higher usage of chemical fertilizers. FDRs are quite reliable in heavy and saline soils and has no component that has any toxicity. They present nondestructive and in situ measurements of soil water content and salinity with wide applicability in agricultural applications, such as hydrology, precision agriculture, and irrigation scheduling. FDRs are least affected by various soil disturbances as they are based on the dielectric properties of soil and the propagation characteristics of electromagnetic waves in the soil, which only change with water content and salinity, not with other parameters. It has been found that the relationship between the real part of the permitivity and soil volumetric water content is strongest in the case of quartz-dominated soils, while clay-dominated soils have maximum dispersion. Clayey soil has a good water-retentive ability, and thus is given the least priority for being chosen for water content measurements (Gabai et al., 2015; Zhou et al., 2015).

5.3 Gypsum Blocks

Gypsum blocks (Fig. 15.3C) are used for measuring soil moisture by estimating resistance between two electrodes present inside the blocks. Gypsum blocks can be of various sizes and shapes (cylindrical and rectangular) with either concentric or parallel electrodes connected by wires measuring resistance between the electrodes. The resistance between the two electrodes depends on the water content present in the gypsum block which is directly related to the soil water tension. Resistance increases with decreasing water content in the soil, that is, during soil drying caused due to low groundwater levels or poor irrigation. Data obtained by the gypsum blocks can be stored and used for the development of good irrigation facilities and their efficacies in the field. Commercially available gypsum blocks come with a calibration kit and multimeter current reading, and can be easily used by nonprofessionals. Reliable measurements can be done only if there is an optimal contact between sensor and soil. Once the site of gypsum blocks is located, they are fixed permanently in the soil at the desired depth. They have life of about 3–5 years, depending on the soil types. They are made of sturdy synthetic material, nonresistant to frost and salt, with a measuring range from 30 to 1500 kPa. They are best suited for drier soil than wetter soil. Gypsum blocks are located at several depths (upper fibrous root zone or lower part of the root zone) in the soil, giving information regarding the turning on and off of irrigation facilities depending on the soil conditions and preventing excess wastage of water. The most tedious task with gypsum blocks is their accurate location in the soil, which is based on the type of watering being used in the field. The gypsum block fixed closest to the soil surface is located in the middle of the wetting front, where it becomes wet with every stage of watering, whereas for trickle, microirrigation, and sprinklers the blocks are placed with thorough investigation of various soil levels. Root depth is another determining factor in locating gypsum blocks; for example, if roots extend >800 mm, then three gypsum blocks are installed at 300 and 600 mm and at the bottom of the root zone; roots with <800 mm extension require only two gypsum blocks installed in the middle of the fibrous root zone, usually at 200 or 300 mm depth. Gypsum blocks are the cheapest soil moisture measuring system and suction indicator, and they can be used not only for fields but for smaller areas, such as schools, colleges, etc. They have a large measuring range, are useful for dry cultures, and give a spontaneous response on wetting and drying of the soil. Tensiometers are another device used for soil moisture measurements, but they have a smaller range compared to gypsum blocks. Further, they cannot be used for dry soils. However, they are sensitive to temperature, salinity, and high levels of nitrogen fertilizers. Gypsum blocks have a unique ability of measuring soil moisture content even when the salinity of the irrigation water exceeds 2000 ppm or the soil salinity of a saturated soil solution is >6.0 dS/m (Stenitzer, 1993; Abraham et al., 2000).

5.4 Neutron Probes

Neutron probes (Fig. 15.3D) are used to measure the quantity of water present in soil, containing a pellet of americium-241 and beryllium. The alpha particles emitted by the decay of these pellets produce very fast-moving neutrons, which collide with the hydrogen nuclei present in the soil being used for measurements and lose their energy. During this process, the neutron velocity decreases by several thousand times and then returns back to the probe. It measures the amount of hydrogen present in the soil and hence is used for soil moisture measurements. Even though it has a very sophisticated design, it can be used by nonprofessionals such as farmers in their fields. The most frequent problem with neutron probes is their usage for soil water content measurements close to the soil surface, which has maximum spatial variability. Therefore, they have not achieved much further use. However, there is no manual labor required during their installation in the field, they are cost-effective, and they can be used in any soil type. A lot of research in this regard is being carried out around the world for their improvement. Despite of their lower usage, they have opened the scope of development in the sensor field on soil surface–based probes for easier assessment and minimal requirement of expertise with respect to soil layers, as well as extensive studies on plant rooting (Zreda et al., 2008).

5.5 Amplitude Domain Reflectometry Sensors

Amplitude domain reflectometry (ADR) sensors (Fig. 15.3E) measure soil moisture content based on the principle of electrical impedance. Electromagnetic waves traveling along a transmission line enter the soil medium, leading to a reduction of impedance (which has two components: electrical conductivity and dielectric constant), which is measured after its reflection onto the transmitter. The effect of conductivity is minimized using an appropriate selection of frequency. The incident and reflected wave interact and produce a voltage standing wave along the length of the transmission line. These sensors consist of an array of metallic parallel rods generating sinusoidal signals with frequency of 100 MHz, with an external shield extending deep into the soil. The arrangement of outer layers adds an additional impedance with values ranging based on the distance between the rods. The advantages of ADRs are minimal calibration, measurements in saline soils up to 20 dS/m, cost-effectiveness, least disturbance in the soil during installation, stability at higher temperatures, easier data analysis, in situ estimation of soil, and ability to be used by nonprofessionals. However, calibration is required depending on different soil types; measurements are affected by air gaps, stones, and channeling water; and ADRs are useful for a small sample size only (Wijaya et al., 2003).

5.6 Ground-Monitoring Soil Moisture Networks

Ground-monitoring soil moisture networks are being used to collect information related to various processes responsible for transfer of heat, mass, and energy between the terrestrial ecosystems and the atmosphere. Thus, they provide massive information on the parameters being used in the characterization of surface–atmosphere exchange. There are a number of sophisticated remote-sensing radiometers that have been developed for collecting information derived from surface heat fluxes and surface soil moisture content data. The data so obtained are analyzed based on various Earth Observation algorithms. Thorough studies are being conducted for the development and distribution of operational products that are not restricted to any particular country, with technology that can be transferred across the whole world (Dorigo et al., 2011; Stockli et al., 2008). Fig. 15.4 shows soil moisture content present in different countries of the world via remote sensing. The International Soil Moisture Network (ISMN) is one of the ground-monitoring networks being used globally with an effort of international cooperation by the Global Energy and Water Exchanges (GEWEX) project and European Space Agency (ESA). It is used in collecting data of in situ soil moisture content over very large areas, with the data portal being maintained on the technology provided by Vienna University. There are a number of scientists around the world that are involved for the collection,

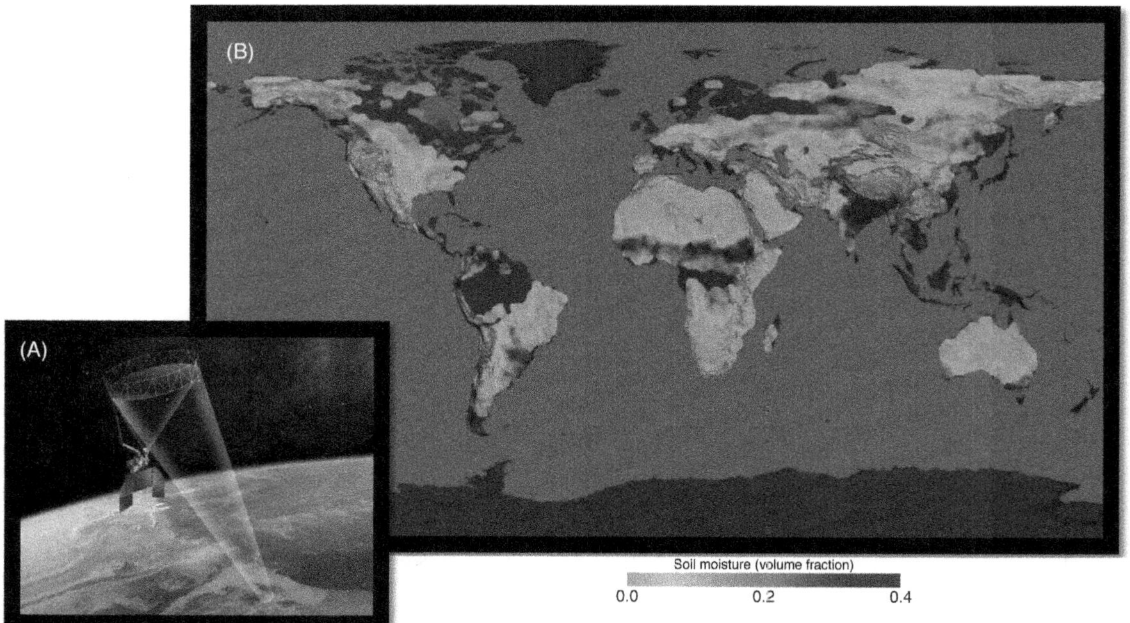

Figure 15.4. (A) Remote sensing has been used for obtaining soil moisture content present in (B) various countries across the world. Image obtained from http://www.nasa.gov/

maintenance, and analysis of harmonized data collected in the database. The data provided by ISMN are shared by the different network operating organizations on a voluntary basis and are free of cost. The data are available at http://ismn.geo.tuwien.ac.at/networks, including historical observations as well as near real-time measurements. The users are able to access harmonized data sets through this web portal having an additional ability of filtering the data sets (to eliminate spurious observations), conveniently. A web interface of the ISMN with a map showing the spatial distribution of the stations was set up in October 2012. Further, there are several other operational networks like Global Soil Moisture Data Bank, which shares its data with ISMN. Hence, ISMN has a complete package of information to be used for further studies. FLUXNET is another global network being used for measuring a number of parameters based on the physical properties of soil, such as soil moisture content in different ecosystems, characterization of land surface interaction processes, etc., in addition to soil moisture. Soil moisture content is the core parameter being measured at least at two depths (surface and root zone) with intervals of half an hour between each site, which is then passed to regional networks and subsequently to FLUXNET. Various countries have included networking by FLUXNET: Australia (OZNET, 64 stations), France (SMOSMANIA, 21 stations), Italy (UMBRIA, 7 stations), Spain (REMEDHUS, 18 stations), the United States (US Climate Reference Network, 114; SCAN, 182 stations; SNOTEL, 381 stations).

6 Future Prospects

Studies on various aspects of soil will continue to grow in the coming years with advancements in the technology and their accurate measurements of different parameters. Soil moisture content is the key factor in a mature understanding of topographic, climatological/meteorological, hydrological, biotic, abiotic, and anthropogenic factors. There is an urgent requirement of thorough studies on the different sites to be used for measurement methods. Various sensors available in the market come with advantages and disadvantages. Therefore, basic information should always be given to the user before their active usage in the ground to yield fruitful results. Soil monitoring via operational networks (FLUXNET and ISMN being the densest monitoring networks) provides simultaneous in situ measurements of soil moisture, in addition to other ancillary parameters across the large land surface. They provide an easy and rapid access to harmonized and quality-checked long-term data. However, it has not been adopted across the whole world, and is restricted to few countries such as the United States, France, Italy, Australia, and Spain. Clearly, there is a need for more studies on operational networks by the scientific and user communities for accurate measurements of soil moisture content spatially over different ecosystem conditions. Further, a better understanding of other ancillary parameters characterizing land surface interactions of the Earth system is required. Various other novel techniques are also being developed for measuring soil moisture based on cosmic ray hydrometeorology, distributed temperature sensing, etc. (Montzka et al., 2011; Rosolem et al., 2013). The former is based on the inverse relationship between density of low-energy cosmic ray neutrons in the atmosphere, while the latter is based on thermal conductivity and its correlation with soil moisture content. They have claimed to have given estimates of soil moisture over areas of several hundred square meters. Recently, the United States has set up a large monitoring network of cosmic ray probes with claims of accuracy of ±99.98%, covering a very large land surface. The probes can be used with minimal power requirements with a good remote sensing ability. However, there is a requirement of intensive studies during installation with respect to adequate depths and locations. It is expected that these emerging technologies for soil assessment would help various countries across the world with their economies based on agriculture, such as India, and enhance crop productivity by several fold.

References

Abraham, N., Hema, P.S., Saritha, E.K., Subramannian, S., 2000. Irrigation automation based on soil electrical conductivity and leaf temperature. Agric. Water Manag. 45, 145–157.

Abuarab, M., Mostafa, E., Ibrahim, M., 2013. Effect of air injection under subsurface drip irrigation on yield and water use efficiency of corn in a sandy clay loam soil. J. Adv. Res. 4, 493–499.

Albiach, R., Canet, R., Pomares, F., Ingelmo, F., 2000. Microbial biomass content and enzymatic activities after the application of organic amendments to a horticultural soil. Bioresour. Technol. 75, 43–48.

Alt, C., Stuètzel, H., Kage, H., 2000. Optimal nitrogen content and photosynthesis in cauliflower (*Brassica oleracea* L. botrytis). Scaling up from a leaf to the whole plant. Ann. Bot. 85, 779–787.

Ayres, E., Dromph, K.M., Bardgett, R.D., 2006. Do plant species encourage soil biota that specialise in the rapid decomposition of their litter? Soil Biol. Biochem. 38, 183–186.

Baier, W., 1965. The interrelationship of meteorological factors, soil moisture and plant growth. Int. J. Biometeorol. 9, 5–20.

Barron-Gafford, G.A., Scott, R.L., Jenerette, G.D., Huxman, T.E., 2011. The relative controls of temperature, soil moisture, and plant functional group on soil CO_2 efflux at diel, seasonal, and annual scales. J. Geophys. Res. 116, 1–16.

Bell, K.R., Blanchard, B.J., Schmugge, T.J., Witzak, M.W., 1980. Analysis of surface soil moisture variations within large field sites. Water Resour. Res. 16, 796–810.
Brocca, L., Melone, F., Moramarco, T., Morbidelli, R., 2010. Spatial-temporal variability of soil moisture and its estimation across scales. Water Resour. Res. 46, W02516.
Bronick, C.J., Lal, R., 2005. Soil structure and management: a review. Geoderma 124, 3–22.
Burkholder, W.H., 1920. The effect of two soil temperatures on the yield and water relations of healthy and diseased bean plants. Ecology 1, 113–123.
Campbell, A.S., Schwertmann, U., Campbell, P.A., 1997. Formation of cubic phases on heating ferrihydrite. Clay Miner. 32, 615–622.
Chantigny, M.H., 2003. Dissolved and water-extractable organic matter in soils: a review on the influence of land use and management practices. Geoderma 113, 357–380.
Choi, H.I., Kumar, P., Liang, X.-Z., 2007. Three-dimensional volume-averaged soil moisture transport model with a scalable parameterization of subgrid topographic variability. Water Resour. Res. 43, 1–15.
Crow, W.T., Berg, A.A., Cosh, M.H., Loew, A., Mohanty, B.P., Panciera, R., de Rosnay, P., Ryu, D., Walker, J.P., 2012. Upscaling sparse ground-based soil moisture observations for the validation of coarse-resolution satellite soil moisture products. Rev. Geophys. 50, RG2002.
DeBano, L.F., Savage, S.M., Hamilton, D.A., 1976. The transfer of heat and hydrophobic substances during burning. Soil Sci. Soc. Am. J. 40, 779–782.
Dif, A.E., Bluemel, W.F., 1991. Expansive soils under cyclic drying and wetting. Geotech. Test. J. 14, 96–102.
Doran, J.W., Zeiss, M.R., 2000. Soil health and sustainability: managing the biotic component of soil quality. Appl. Soil Ecol. 15, 3–11.
Dorigo, W.A., Wagner, W., Hohensinn, R., Hahn, S., Paulik, C., Xaver, A., Gruber, A., Drusch, M., Mecklenburg, S., van Oevelen, P., Robock, A., Jackson, T., 2011. The international soil moisture network: a data hosting facility for global in-situ soil moisture measurements. Hydrol. Earth Syst. Sci. 15, 1675–1698.
Farrell, M., Prendergast-Miller, M., Jones, D.L., Hill, P.W., Condron, L.M., 2014. Soil microbial organic nitrogen uptake is regulated by carbon availability. Soil Biol. Biochem. 77, 261–267.
Filip, Z., 2002. International approach to assessing soil quality by ecologically-related biological parameters. Agric. Ecosyst. Environ. 88, 169–174.
Fontaine, S., Mariotti, A., Abbadie, L., 2003. The priming effect of organic matter: a question of microbial competition? Soil Biol. Biochem. 35, 837–843.
Fowells, H.A., Stephenson, R.E., 1934. Effects of burning on forest soils. Soil Sci. 38, 175–181.
Franzluebbers, A.J., 2002. Soil organic matter stratification ratio as an indicator of soil quality. Soil Till. Res. 66, 95–106.
Frey, S.D., Lee, J., Melillo, J.M., Six, J., 2013. The temperature response of soil microbial efficiency and its feedback to climate. Nat. Clim. Change 3, 395–398.
Gabai, H., Botsev, Y., Hahami, M., Eyal, A., 2015. Optical frequency domain reflectometry at maximum update rate using I/Q detection. Opt. Lett. 15, 1725–1728.
Gao, X., Wu, P., Zhao, X., Wang, J., Shi, Y., 2014. Effects of land use on soil moisture variations in a semi-arid catchment: implications for land and agricultural water management. Land Degrad. Dev. 25, 163–172.
Geng, J., Spiegelberg, C., Jiang, S., 2005. Narrow line width fiber laser for 100-km optical frequency domain reflectometry. Photon. Technol. Lett. 17, 1827–1829.
Gonzalez-Perez, J.A., Gonzalez-Vila, F.J., Almendros, G., Knicker, H., 2004. The effect of fire on soil organic matter—a review. Environ. Int. 30, 855–870.

Harper, R.J., Beck, A.C., Ritson, P., Hill, M.J., Mitchell, C.D., Barrett, D.J., Smettem, K.R.J., Mann, S.S., 2007. The potential of greenhouse sinks to underwrite improved land management. Ecol. Eng. 29, 329–341.
Harrison, M.J., Buuren, V., 1995. A phosphate transporter from the mycorrhizal fungus *Glomus versiforme*. Nature 378, 626–629.
Haynes, R.J., Naidu, R., 1998. Influence of lime, fertilizer and manure applications on soil organic matter content and soil physical conditions: a review. Nutr. Cycl. Agroecosyst. 51, 123–137.
Heiskanen, J., 1995. Irrigation regime affects water and aeration conditions in peat growth medium and the growth of containerized Scots pine seedings. New Forest. 9, 181–195.
Herrick, J.E., 2000. Soil quality: an indicator of sustainable land management? Appl. Soil Ecol. 15, 75–83.
Hosking, J.S., 1938. The ignition at low temperatures of the organic matter in soils. J. Agric. Sci. 28, 393–400.
Huisman, J.A., Sperl, C., Bouten, W., Verstraten, J.M., 2001. Soil water content measurements at different scales: accuracy of time domain reflectometry and ground-penetrating radar. J. Hydrol. 245, 48–58.
Johnson, P.C., Stanley, C.C., Kemblowski, M.W., Byers, D.L., Colthart, J.D., 1990. A practical approach to the design, operation, and monitoring of in-situ soil-venting systems. Ground Water Monit. Remediat. 10, 159–178.
Karlen, D.L., Mausbach, M.J., Doran, J.W., Cline, R.G., Harris, R.F., Schuman, G.E., 1995. Soil quality: a concept, definition, and framework for evaluation. Soil Sci. Soc. Am. J. 61, 4–10.
Kuzyakov, Y., 2006. Sources of CO_2 efflux from soil and review of partitioning methods. Soil Biol. Biochem. 38, 425–448.
Li, Z., Shuman, L.M., 1996. Heavy metal movement in metal-contaminated soil profiles. Soil Sci. 161, 656–666.
Loneragan, J.F., Webb, M.J., 1993. Interactions between zinc and other nutrients affecting the growth of plants. Dev. Plant Soil Sci. 55, 119–134.
Maire, V., Martre, P., Kattge, J., Gastal, F., Esser, G., Fontaine, S., Soussana, J.F., 2012. The coordination of leaf photosynthesis links C and N fluxes in C_3 plant species. PLoS One 7, e38345.
Marios, S., 2002. Interactions between groundwater and surface water: the state of the science. Hydrogeol. J. 10, 52–67.
Marschener, H., Dell, B., 1994. Nutrient uptake in mycorrhizal symbiosis. Plant Soil 159, 89–102.
McBride, M.B., 1989. Reactions controlling heavy metal solubility in soils. Adv. Soil Sci. 10, 1–56.
Megías, A.G., Müller, C., 2010. Root herbivores and detritivores shape above-ground multitrophic assemblage through plant-mediated effects. J. Anim. Ecol. 79, 923–931.
Montzka, C., Moradkhani, H., Weihermüller, L., Franssen, H.H., Canty, M., Vereecken, H., 2011. Hydraulic parameter estimation by remotely-sensed top soil moisture observations with the particle filter. J. Hydrol. 399, 410–421.
Nduwumuremyi, A., Ruganzu, V., Mugwe, J.N., Rusanganwa, A.C., 2013. Effects of unburned lime on soil pH and base cations in acidic soil ISRN. Soil Sci. 1, 1–7.
Nielsen, D.R., Hopmans, J.W., Kutílek, M., Wendroth, O., 1997. A brief review of soil water, solute transport and regionalized variable analysis. Sci. Agric. 54, 89–115.
Noborio, K., 2001. Measurement of soil water content and electrical conductivity by time domain reflectometry: a review. Comput. Electron. Agric. 31, 213–237.

Paré, D., Boutin, R., Larocque, G.R., Raulier, F., 2006. Effect of temperature on soil organic matter decomposition in three forest biomes of eastern Canada. Can. J. Soil Sci. 86, 247–256.
Rajan, S.S.S., 1987. Phosphate rock and phosphate rock/sulphur granules as phosphate fertilizers and their dissolution in soil. Fert. Res. 11, 43–60.
Robinson, D.A., Jones, S.B., Wraith, J.M., Or, D., Friedman, S.P., 2002. A review of advances in dielectric and electrical conductivity measurement in soils using time domain reflectometry. Vadose Zone J. 2, 444–475.
Robock, A., Vinnikov, K.Y., Srinivasan, G., Entin, J.K., Hollinger, S.E., Nina, A., Speranskaya, N.A., Liu, S., Namkhai, A., 2000. The global soil moisture Data Bank. Bull. Am. Meteorol. Soc. 81, 1281–1299.
Rosolem, R., Shuttleworth, W.J., Zreda, M., Franz, T.E., Zeng, X., Kurc, S.A., 2013. The effect of atmospheric water vapor on neutron count in the cosmic-ray soil moisture observing system. J. Hydrometeorol. 14, 1659–1671.
Roy, B.B., Barde, N.K., 1962. Some characteristics of the black soils of India. Soil Sci. 93, 142–147.
Saxton, K.E., Rawls, W.J., 2005. Soil water characteristic estimates by texture and organic matter for hydrologic solutions. Soil Sci. Soc. Am. J. 70, 1569–1578.
Schipper, L.A., Hobbs, J.K., Rutledge, S., Arcus, V.L., 2014. Thermodynamic theory explains the temperature optima of soil microbial processes and high Q_{10} values at low temperatures. Glob. Change Biol. 20, 3578–3586.
Schmidt, M.W., Torn, M.S., Abiven, S., Dittmar, T., Guggenberger, G., Janssens, I.A., Kleber, M., Kögel-Knabner, I., Lehmann, J., Manning, D.A., Nannipieri, P., Rasse, D.P., Weiner, S., Trumbore, S.E., 2011. Persistence of soil organic matter as an ecosystem property. Nature 478, 49–56.
Stenitzer, E., 1993. Monitoring soil moisture regimes of field crops with gypsum blocks. Theor. Appl. Climatol. 48, 159–165.
Stockli, R., Lawrence, D.M., Niu, G.Y., Oleson, K.W., Thornton, P.E., Yang, Z.L., Bonan, G.B., Denning, A.S., Running, S.W., 2008. Use of FLUXNET in the Community Land Model development. J. Geophysi. Res. 113, 1–19.
Swartjes, F.A., 1999. Risk-based assessment of soil and groundwater quality in the Netherlands: standards and remediation urgency. Risk Anal. 19, 1235–1249.
Tilman, D., Cassman, K.G., Matson, P.A., Naylor, R., Polasky, S., 2002. Agricultural sustainability and intensive production practices. Nature 418, 671–677.
Wagner, W., Lemoine, G., Rott, H., 1999. A method for estimating soil moisture from ERS scatterometer and soil data. Remote Sens. Environ. 70, 191–207.
West, T.O., Post, W.M., 2002. Soil organic carbon sequestration rates by tillage and crop rotation. Soil Sci. Soc. Am. J. 66, 1930–1946.
White, J.G., Zasoski, R.J., 1999. Mapping soil micronutrients. Field Crop. Res. 60, 11–26.
Wijaya, K., Nishimura, T., Kato, M., 2003. Estimation of dry bulk density of soil using amplitude domain reflectometry probe. J. Jap. Soc. Soil Phys. 5, 63–73.
Ye, C., Li, S., Yang, Y., Shu, X., Zhang, J., Zhang, Q., 2015. Advancing analysis of spatio-temporal variations of soil nutrients in the water level fluctuation zone of China's three gorges reservoir using self-organizing map. PLoS One 10, e0121210.
Yuste, J.C., Baldocchi, D.D., Gershenson, A., Goldstein, A., Misson, L., Wong, S., 2007. Microbial soil respiration and its dependency on carbon inputs, soil temperature and moisture. Glob. Change Biol. 13, 1–18.
Zandonadi, D.B., Santos, M.P., Busato, J.G., Peres, L.E.P., Façanha, A.R., 2013. Plant physiology as affected by humified organic matter. Theor. Exp. Plant Physiol. 25, 12–25.

Zhao, Y., Peth, S., Hallett, P., Wang, X., Giese, M., Gao, Y., Horn, R., 2011. Factors controlling the spatial patterns of soil moisture in a grazed semi-arid steppe investigated by multivariate geostatistics. Ecohydrology 4, 36–48.

Zhou, H., Sun, Y., Tyree, M.T., Sheng, W., Cheng, Q., Xue, X., Schumann, H., Schulze Lammers, P., 2015. An improved sensor for precision detection of in situ stem water content using a frequency domain fringing capacitor. New Phytol. 206, 471–481.

Zreda, M., Desilets, D., Ferré, T.P.A., Scott, R.L., 2008. Measuring soil moisture content non-invasively at intermediate spatial scale using cosmic-ray neutrons. Geophys. Res. Lett. 35, 1–5.

16

NANOSENSORS FOR DETECTION OF PESTICIDES IN WATER

Clarice Steffens*, Juliana Steffens*, Adriana Marcia Graboski*, Alexandra Manzoli*, Fabio Lima Leite**

**Department of Food Engineering, URI, Erechim, Erechim, Brazil; **Department of Physics Mathematics and Chemistry (DFMQ), Nanoneurobiophysics Research Group, Federal University of São Carlos (UFSCar), Sorocaba, Brazil*

1 Water in the World

Water is the most abundant compound on Earth equivalent to about three-quarters of its surface. According to Shiklomanov and Rodda (2003), 97.5% of all water on Earth is salt water, leaving only 2.5% as freshwater. Only 0.4% of that, 2.5% is accessible as surface water or water being actively conveyed in the atmosphere. The remainder is found in glaciers (68.7%), groundwater (30.1%), and permafrost (0.8%). Out of that very scarce 0.4%; 67.4% is contained in lakes, 12.2% in soil, 9.5% in the atmosphere, 8.5% in humid areas, 8% in plants and animals and only 1.6% in rivers and surface currents (Fig. 16.1). The distribution of water on the Earth's surface is extremely uneven, which can cause great risks of shortages, if their planning and management are not efficient.

The total water estimated in the world was around 1,386,000,000 km^3, only 1,030,000 km^3 are of sweet water, who distribute unevenly in different regions of the world (USGS, 2014). The distribution of freshwater resources in the world at continental level are 45% America, followed by 28% Asia, 15.5% Europe and 9% Africa (FAO, 2003). The freshwater demand is associated with the population size. Last century, world population has tripled and growing at a rate of 80 million per year, and is expected to reach above 9.4 billion in 2050 (USCB, 2013). However, in the last century, water usage levels have increased at over twice the rate of population. Water scarcity could affect around 1.8 billion people that living in water stressed countries or regions in 2025, and over 66% of the world's population could end up living under water-restricted conditions (UN-Water, 2007).

New Pesticides and Soil Sensors. http://dx.doi.org/10.1016/B978-0-12-804299-1.00017-5

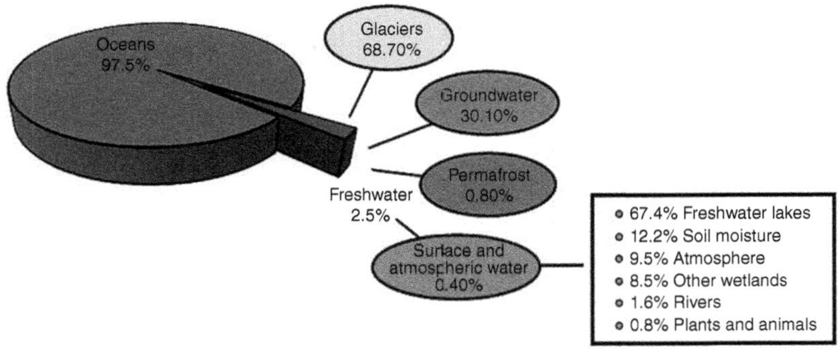

Figure 16.1. Distribution of water on Earth.

Economic activities developed by the population, which use water can be divided between agriculture and industry, which apply larger amount and also the domestic consumption (Alcamo et al., 2003). According to a Food and Agriculture Organization of the United Nations (FAO) (2015), agriculture is responsible for about 71% of global water withdrawals, 19% industrial and 11% for domestic use.

Industrialization and urbanization together with the intensification of agricultural activities, increasing water demand while growing the release of contaminant levels in water bodies (Holt, 2000). This carries many problems to the environment and population. It can be seen that the receiving bodies are becoming more contaminated with domestic sewage, industrial wastes, pesticides, hormones, chemical fertilizers, and waste (Pal et al., 2014).

1.1 Contaminants in Water

Nutrients, heavy metals, bacteria, and priority pollutants (compounds, such as industrial chemicals, pesticides, petroleum hydrocarbons with known health effects) had been the focus on water pollution in the past (Pal et al., 2014). But, actually research revealed new sources as pharmaceutical ingredients, pesticides and metabolites, disinfection-by-products, algal toxins, and taste-and-odor compounds (Jung et al., 2015; Oliveira et al., 2015; Somashekar et al., 2015; Khraisheh et al., 2014; Matić et al., 2014; Onesios et al., 2009; Lin et al., 2013a; Tang et al., 2013; Hasan et al., 2012).

Recently, scientific studies of water contaminant refer to a group called emerging contaminants. Among the definitions about these contaminants the United States Geological Survey (USGS) (2014), describe "emerging contaminants" as any synthetic or naturally occurring chemical or any microorganism that is not commonly monitored in the environment but has the potential to enter the environment and cause known or suspected adverse ecological and(or) human health effects, synthesis of new chemicals or changes in use and disposal of existing chemicals can create new sources of "emerging contaminants."

These contaminants are a large group of compounds, including pharmaceuticals, drugs of abuse, personal care products, plasticizers, surfactants, pesticides, steroids, hormones, perfluorinated compounds, flame retarders, industrial additives, gasoline additives, as well as their processing products, among others. The occurrence of these contaminants in freshwater is a major problem with understood consequences. Some examples can be visualized in Table 16.1 (González et al., 2012; Lapworth et al., 2012; Matamoros et al., 2012; Pal et al., 2010; Rosal et al., 2010; la Farré et al., 2008).

Such compounds are found in low concentrations (microgram per liter and nanogram per liter), but with harmful potential effect on human health and the environment (Murray et al., 2010; Stanford et al., 2010). Approximately 1.8 million of children under 5 years die every year from water-related disease (Corcoran et al., 2010).

Other effects with potential risks to human health, terrestrial, and marine creatures are observed. These effects comprise from headaches, nausea, anemia, skin irritation and lungs, serious reductions in neurological, liver functions, effects on the endocrine system of humans, animals, birds and have also shown estrogenic and reproductive effects on marine organisms. It has also been mentioned cases of genotoxic health effects, such as congenital defects, reproductive abnormalities, increased incidence of gastrointestinal and bladder carcinomas, reproductive tumoanomalias, effects on thyroid and respiratory system, and even death of people (Pal et al., 2014; Sauvé and Desrosiers, 2014; Flint et al., 2012; Lindstrom et al., 2011; Bolong et al., 2009; Richardson, 2003).

Emerging contaminants, as well as other contaminants, classify the sources of pollution in point and nonpoint (Birkett and Lester, 2003; Holt, 2000). Point sources enter into the environment through the watercourses. Examples are industrial and domestic effluents, accidental spills, mining, floods. Nonpoint sources has no specific entry point, may involve a way that results in partial deposition before reaching the watercourse, as an example we can mention atmospheric deposition and surface water flows, particularly from agricultural practices (Birkett and Lester, 2003; Holt, 2000).

Table 16.1 Classes of emerging compounds according to the study of la Farré et al. (2008) and Unep (2012)

Compounds	Examples
Drugs of abuse	Amphetamine
	Tetrahydrocannabinol
	Cocaine
Flame retardants	Chloroalkanes
	Hexabromocyclcdodecane
	Polybrominateddiphenyl ethers
	Tetrabromobisphenol A
	Tris (2-chloroethyl)phosphate
Gasoline additives	Dialkyl ethers
	Methyl-t-butyl ether
Industrial additives and agents	Chelating agents (EDTA)
	Aromatic sulfonates
Personal-care products, Fragrances, insect repellants, soaps, antimicrobials, sun-screen agents	Benzophenone
	N,N-diethyltoluamide
	Methylbenzylidene
	Nitro
	Polycyclic musks
	Macrocyclicmusks
	Triclosan
Pharmaceuticals, Analgesics and antiinflammatory drugs, human and veterinary antimicrobials, antiepileptics, blood-lipid regulators and psychiatric drugs, antitumoral drugs, cardiovascular drugs (β-blockers) and β2-symphatomimetics, X-ray contrast agents	Acetaminophen
	Acetylsalicylicacid
	Diclofenac
	Diazepam
	Carbamazepine
	Benzafibrate
	Iopromide
	Iopamidol
Steroids and hormones	Diethylstilbestrol
	Estradiol
	Estriol
	Estrone

Table 16.1 Classes of emerging compounds according to the study of la Farré et al. (2008) and Unep (2012) (*cont.*)

Compounds	Examples
Surfactants and surfactante metabolites	Alkylphenolethoxylates
	Alkylphenols (nonylphenolandoctylphenol)
	Alkylphenol carboxylates
Pesticides	Atrazine
	Di-ethylatrazine
	Metolachlor
	Cyanazine
	Alachlor
	Diazinon
	Alachlor
	Cyanazine
	Diazinon
	Dichloro-diphenyl-trichloroethane (DDT)
	Dieldrin
	Chlordane
	Endosulfan sulfate
New classes	Nanomaterials
	1,4-dioxane
	Swimming-pool-disinfection by-products

Source: Reprinted with permission from Elsevier.

The concentration, transportation, final processing, and disposal of a contaminant introduced into the water depend mainly on the environmental properties and contaminant characteristics (Rand et al., 1995).

These emerging compounds reach the environment and are transported and distributed by various ways. In urban areas, the soil particles are transported preferentially to surface water because there is little soil exposure to the environment and the erosion process occurs less often. Contamination can also occur by the accumulation of waste, during transit and radioactive emissions. In rural area the pollutants are discharged through leaching into the water bodies, which hinders their removal (Birkett and Lester, 2003).

Both industrial and agricultural sector, produce water in the process which can carry toxic wastes, such as heavy metals, hormones, pesticides, and a variety of other substances which may be harmful to the environment and population (Somashekar et al., 2015; Matić et al., 2014; Matamoros et al., 2012; Liu et al., 2011; Järup, 2003). Heavy metals (lead, cadmium, mercury, and nickel) are toxic and carcinogenic, even in low concentrations, as they are not biodegradable and can accumulate in organisms (Gammoudi et al., 2014; Badruddoza et al., 2013; Ozay et al., 2009; Liu et al., 2008). The hormones (natural and synthetic) comes from domestic effluents (Erickson, 2002), may cause some effects in humans, such as the reduction of sperm, increased incidence of breast, testicular and prostate cancer, as well as endometriosis (Moraes et al., 2015; Wen et al., 2014; Lin et al., 2013b). The pesticides used for controlling living organisms considered undesirable in the environment are mainly applied in agriculture and can be considered as one of the main factors involved in environmental pollution in the world (Mostafalou and Abdollahi, 2013). They have high toxicity making them carcinogenic, mutagenic and teratogenic, causing various types of chronic disease and may accumulate in the environment (Unal et al., 2011; Rosa et al., 2010; Pimentel, 2005; Abdollahi et al., 2004; Eskenazi et al., 1999; Biziuk et al., 1996).

2 Pesticides as Water Pollutants

Pesticides are defined as a large group of natural or synthetic chemical compounds used to eliminate biological threats and other pests, which attack agricultural crops (Fenik et al., 2011; LeDoux, 2011). FAO (2007) define as any substance or mixture of substances intended for preventing, destroying, or controlling any pest, including vectors of human or animal disease, unwanted species of plants or animals, causing harm during or otherwise interfering with the production, processing, storage, transport, or marketing of food, agricultural commodities, wood and wood products or animal feedstuffs, or substances that may be administered to animals for the control of insects, arachnids, or other pests in or on their bodies. The term includes substances intended for use as a plant growth regulator, defoliant, desiccant, and agent for thinning fruit or preventing the premature fall of fruit. Also used as substances applied to crops either before or after harvest to protect the commodity from deterioration during storage and transport.

Pesticides can be classified in different ways, according to Gevao et al. (2000):

- Organisms group who control: insecticides (fighting insects, larvae, and ants); fungicides (to fight fungi), herbicides (weed fighting), etc.
- Toxicity: which should have on the labels an indicative colored band of their toxicity class: red band (extremely toxic), yellow band (highly toxic), blue band (moderately toxic), and green band (low toxicity).
- Chemical group: ionic (cationic, basic, acidic, and miscellaneous) and nonionic (chlorinated, organophosphorus, dinitroanilides, carbanilates, benzonitriles, esters, acetamides, carbothioates, thiocarbamates, anilides, ureas, and methylcarbamates).

Pesticides regardless of the type are added intentionally in the environment with the objective of destroying or controlling undesired life forms, also become a problem for the public health. The main undesirable consequences of the pesticides use are the residual in soil, water, air, vegetables, animals, food, and also the destruction of microorganisms in the soil, mortality of beneficial insects, among others.

Pesticides enter into the aquatic environment in several ways: through the use in agricultural, industrial, and municipal sewage when applied to the control of aquatic herbs and insects, by accidents in warehouses, during transport or even by the improper disposal of packaging (Harnpicharnchai et al., 2013; Kosikowska and Biziuk, 2010; Bedos et al., 2002).

When released into the environment these pesticides can cause undesirable and harmful effects on humans and other populations (animals, insects, and plants). They are toxic, carcinogenic, cause neurodegenerative diseases, such as Parkinson's, Alzheimer's, and amyotrophic lateral sclerosis, also act on the respiratory system, causing diseases, such as asthma and chronic obstructive pulmonary disorder, as well as reproductive inhibition. Cases of diabetes, cardiovascular disease, immune system suppression, and teratogenic effects are also reported in the literature [Hernández et al., 2013; Mostafalou and Abdollahi, 2013; Mostafalou, 2012; Agrawal, 2010; Food and Agriculture Organization of the United Nations (FAO), 1996].

Due pesticides are poorly soluble in water, the concentration of most of the pesticides in water is low (Helbling, 2015). Pesticides are bioconcentrated and persistent in the environment due mainly to its chemical stability, low solubility in water, and high lipophilicity (Ghiselli and Jardim, 2007). The maximum allowable concentration of any individual pesticide in drinking water in the European Union is 0.1 μg/L and all of pesticides combined are 0.5 μg/L. The US Environmental Protection Agency (EPA) and Health Canada (Health Canada, 1995, 2014) has established maximum contaminant levels (MCLs). The analytical methodologies used to detect these compounds do not reach detection limits of this magnitude; another fact that generates controversy is the fact that it does not consider the toxicity of each product. Resolution (CONAMA) No. 20 of 1986, provides a classification of fresh, brackish and marine waters, establishing maximum limits of contaminants for each class corresponds a certain quality to be maintained in the body of water depending on your destination (Brasil, 1986).

The reason for concern is that pesticides are resistant to conventional water treatment. The total biodegradation of these substances in each ecosystem is not guaranteed, with its coadjuvants also generate transformation products which in turn interact with the organic matter under specific conditions. They may also become increasingly toxic and pollute natural resources. Therefore, the water, even treated, could contain residual contaminants that when reach their limits of concentration, become toxic (Sinclair et al., 2006).

In this sense become important techniques for detection, identification and qualification of these pollutants in water.

3 Analytical Techniques for Water Pollutant Detection

The monitoring of pesticides residues on samples of environmental nature is of great importance. In many cases, the application of analytical methods that use simple, efficient and sensitive extraction techniques is necessary. The pesticides extraction techniques from the environment are quite important for the quality of the analytical method since such techniques must select a representative fraction of the sample (Tankiewicz et al., 2011; Jönsson and Mathiasson, 1999).

Extraction techniques are sample preparation procedures in which the relevant analytes are isolated and concentrated at adequate levels, to be then, determined using the analytical equipments (Sibiya et al., 2013). This takes place normally because matrices in brute form present interference and incompatibility with analytical equipment. The sample preparation is made in order to be compatible with the analytical techniques that provide chemical data. It is an important step, oftentimes limiting the analytical method, since it has direct impact on accuracy, precision, and quantification limits (Tankiewicz et al., 2011).

Currently, there is a tendency for extraction methods that use lesser amounts of samples, which provide a selective and specific extraction, as well as methods that increase the possibility for automation. Consequently, reduce the operation manual, is less aggressive to the environment with the use of lower amounts of organic solvents. Among the main techniques of microextraction it is possible to mention solid phase (SPME) and in liquid phase (LPME), that are compatible with many analytical methods. These are constantly used to determine organic composts on water samples. SPME integrates sampling, extraction, concentration, and sample introduction into a single solvent-free step. Analytes in the sample are directly extracted and concentrated to the extraction fiber. The method saves preparation time and disposal costs and can improve detection limits. SPME technique was introduced by Arthur and Pawlyszin (1990) in the final of 20th century. Since then, due to the diversity of fibers coating, this technique became versatile in several types of analysis (Neves Dias et al., 2015). This equipment consists of a length (100 μm of diameter) of fused silica fiber coated with a polymer material, in some cases mixed with a solid adsorbent (extracting phase). The fiber is attached to a stainless steel plunger sheathed by a protective needle.

SPME technique is normally applied for extraction of analytes of low and medium polarity. Extraction occurs through passive diffusion, and can be either direct or indirect. Direct extraction is used either for nonvolatile analytes or for volatile analytes on noncomplex samples, where the fiber absorbs the analytes directly from the sample solution. Indirect extraction is used for volatile analytes, where the fiber absorbs the headspace analytes over the volatile sample, which needs to be heated. The extraction efficiency is essentially determined by the fiber's sample partition coefficient.

The fiber coating material is the most important factor on the SPME extraction technique (Zhao et al., 2013; Doong et al., 2000). It is responsible for the extraction and preconcentration of analytes, that after to be adequately desorbed directly of the fibers are analyzed by chromatographic techniques (Arthur and Pawlyszin, 1990). The analytes adsorbed in the extractor layer can be desorbed in two ways, thermally in a hot injection port of GC, for subsequent analysis, or by elution with an organic solvent, which is subsequently injected into the HPLC. There are a limited number of commercially available fibers that are relatively expensive and easily breakable (Kumar et al., 2008).

In the last years, an effort can be seen in terms of using various materials as coating for fibers in order to decrease costs and increase the robustness and efficiency of the analytes extraction using SPME technique. An array of coating materials has been tested for the SPME fibers, from polymers (Mohammadi et al., 2009; Theodoridis et al., 2000; Djozan and Ebrahimi, 2008) to carbon materials, among them stand out: carbon nanotubes (Chen et al., 2009), grafite (Kuo and Shiea, 1999), and graphene (Wu et al., 2012; Zhang and Lee, 2011). This diversity of materials is responsible for successful use of the SPME technique on the extraction of many toxic substances from water samples, to be then properly determined through the analytical techniques.

The coatings extraction with graphene has been intensively investigated due to interesting properties presented by this carbon material (Novoselov et al., 2004). SPME samples preparation technique developed with graphene-coated fibers present an excellent sensitivity level on extraction of different herbicides (atrazine, prometon, ametryn, and prometryn) in water samples, prior to the determination by High-Performance Liquid Chromatography with Diode-Array Detection (HPLC-DAD). The use of this new fiber was very positive, since there is a great effort in search analytical techniques that can offer good efficiency in herbicides separation and concentration (Wu et al., 2012). The study conducted by (Li et al., 2015) using a C18 composite SPME fiber, showed an excellent performance on the extraction of six organochlorine pesticides (OCPs) (hexachlorobezene, *trans*-chlordane, *cis*-chlordane,1,1,1-trichloro-2-(2-chlorophenyl)-2-(4-chlorophenyl)ethane (*o,p*-DDT), 1,1,1-Trichloro-2,2-bis(4-chlorophenyl) ethane (p,p-DDT), and mirex) in water samples. The six OCPs have been appropriately determined with gas chromatography–mass spectrometry (GC–MS) after the extraction phase, obtaining wide linearity (2–500 ng L^{-1}) and good sensitivity. A stainless steel wire was used as the substrate, and a mixture of the C18 particle and 184 silicone were used as coating materials. C18 is a type of surface modified with amorphous silica that has good separation characteristics, constantly used in solid phase extraction (SPE) (Rissato et al., 2005). The Fig. 16.2 shows the C18 composite SPME fibers preparation process, in which a section of capillary column was used to fix the C18 particle (3.5 mm) and the 184 silicone mixture onto the stainless steel wire and to ensure a constant coating thickness; the SPME procedure, which exhibited excellent OCPs extraction performance; OCPs separation and analysis using gas chromatography–mass spectrometry (GC–MS).

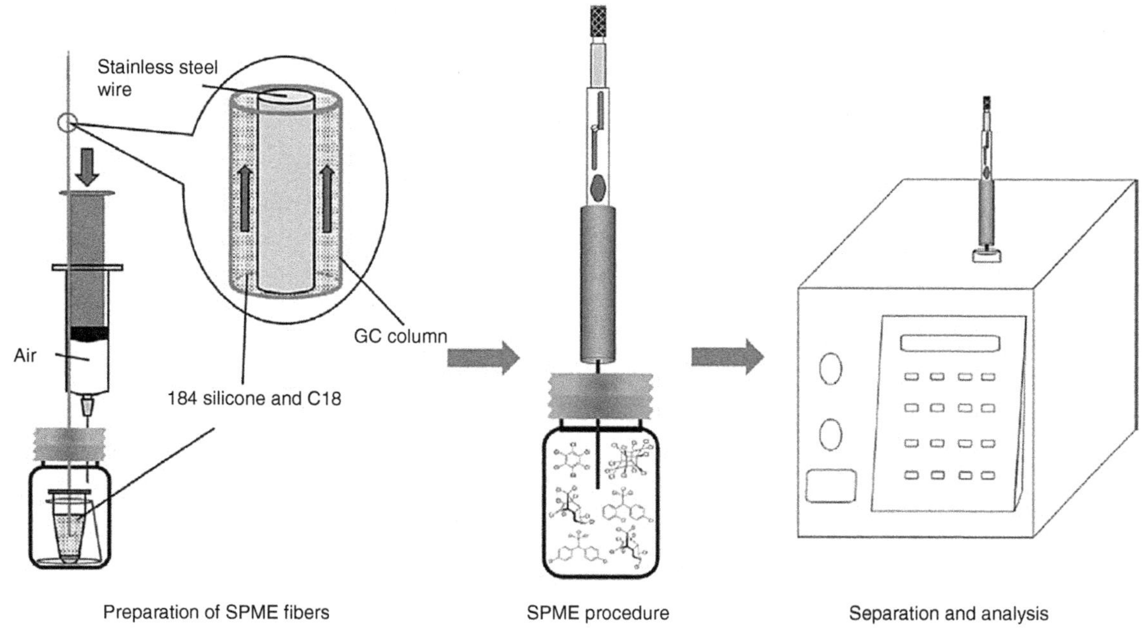

Figure 16.2. SPME fibers preparation process, SPME procedure, and separation and analysis (Li et al., 2015). Reprinted with permission from Elsevier.

In this diversity of coatings for SPME fibers, an attempt to use natural biodegradable materials from renewable sources, also known as green or environmentally friendly coatings can be noted. Among the examples of green coating used on SPME fibers, the potential for the use of cork has been noticed. Cork being itself an excellent biosorbent material in extraction of organochlorine pesticides at ultratrace levels in water samples, where detection was made using a chromatography technique with electron capture detection (Neves Dias et al., 2015).

Another interesting approach to sample preparation is the liquid phase microextraction (LPME), which aims to miniaturize liquid-liquid extractions, reduces longtime and organic solvent volume. The development of LPME followed the one of SPME. The first scientific publications using the LPME technique appeared in 1996 (Liu and Dasgupta, 1996; Jeannot and Cantwell, 1996). In the beginning, the LPME systems used a tiny drop of organic solvent suspended on the tip of a GC syringe as the extracting phase, which was immersed in an aqueous solution for the passive diffusion based extraction. After the extraction phase, the organic drop suspended on the syringe's tip was injected in the GC. These LPME systems are simple and reduce the consumption of organic solvents. However, they present low stability, as the drop suspended on the syringe's tip can be easily lost during extraction.

In 1999, Pedersen-Bjergaard and Rasmussen introduced a new methodology for liquid phase microextraction, which was named "hollow fiber liquid-phase microextraction" (HF-LPME) (Pedersen-Bjergaard and Rasmussen, 1999). This new technology solved the problem caused by the suspended drop low stability, as the extracting phase (or acceptor solution) is placed inside a hollow porous fiber of a lumen. Such fiber needs to be hydrophobic and compatible with the organic solvent that will be used for the liquid membrane formation. Normally, polypropylene capillary membranes (inner diameter of 600 nm) are compatible with the extracting solution volume (μL). Also, nominal and maximum pore sizes of 0.2 and 0.64 μm, respectively, providing an efficient micro filtration and only allows the penetration of small molecules (target analytes) through the hollow fiber pores. 200 nm fiber wall thickness provides excellent mechanical stability (Psillakis and Kalogerakis, 2003).

The liquid membrane is formed when dipping the hollow fiber into an organic solvent of low polarity for a few seconds. The high porosity of the fiber is responsible for immobilize the organic solvent as a thin film. The extracting phase is mechanically protected inside the hollow fiber, being separated from the sample through the liquid membrane (organic solvent), thus preventing its dissolution in the sample.

The HF-LPME technique can be performed in either two or three phases, according to the characteristics of the analyte in use, since these two systems differ on the type of acceptor solution (Halvorsen et al., 2001; Grønhaug Halvorsen et al., 2001; Rasmussen et al., 2000). Fig. 16.3 shows the basic set-up for HF-LPME. In the two-phase extraction system the same organic solvent is used on the acceptor solution and on the liquid membrane. In order to obtain favourable results using this extraction method the analyte must be mildly or highly hydrophobic, containing acidic or basic groups or neutral compounds of similar

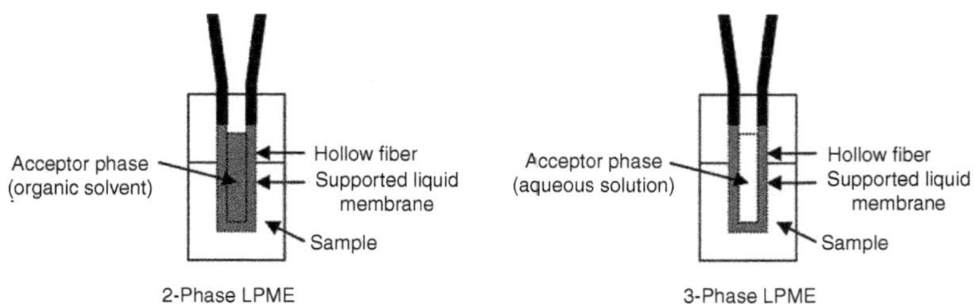

Figure 16.3. Schematic illustration of 2- and 3-phase LPME (Pedersen-Bjergaard and Rasmussen, 2008). Reprinted with permission from Elsevier.

hydrophobicity (Ho et al., 2002b). In the three-phase system, acidic or basic aqueous solutions are used as extracting solutions.

The HF-LPME extraction technique is very versatile, allowing the use of the same extraction device for both two-phase and three-phase systems, providing compatibility with various techniques, such as GC, HPLC, and capillary electrophoresis. The two-phase system is suitable for the extraction of neutral substances and both the acidic and basic compounds can be extracted using both systems (Pedersen-Bjergaard and Rasmussen, 2008).

Advantages presented by this extraction technique are the high analyte enrichments that were obtained without solvent evaporation or its reconstitution (Ho et al., 2007), clean extraction, especially on three-phase systems (Psillakis and Kalogerakis, 2003), as well as low consumption of organic solvents (Pedersen-Bjergaard and Rasmussen, 2008). It allows the use of a dynamic system through stirring, both in the two-phase and three-phase modes, which improves the extraction efficiency and increases reproducibility when compared to the static mode. The HF-LPME extraction technique also enables the use of higher stirring speeds, since the acceptor phase is located inside the hollow fiber (Li et al., 2008). The stirring accelerates the extraction kinetics facilitating the analytes diffusion from the donor phase to the acceptor phase, therefore diminishing the time span to attain thermodynamic equilibrium especially for the higher molecular mass analytes (Lambropoulou and Albanis, 2005; Zhao and Lee, 2002; Shen and Hian, 2002). The use of ultrasonic bath is recommended for the sample stirring. The stirring induced by a magnetic bar can cause cross-contamination on the samples and the appearance of air bubbles, which tend to adhere to the hollow fiber's surface. It accelerates the solvent evaporation process presenting inaccurate measurements (Lambropoulou and Albanis, 2005; Shen and Hian, 2002; Pedersen-Bjergaard and Rasmussen, 2000).

Hou et al. (2003) developed a hollow fiber-protected dynamic LPME controlled by a programable syringe pump for extracting pesticides from water prior to the GC–MS analysis. Thus, present a higher enrichment and better reproducibility when compared to the static system (hollow fiber-protected static LPME). It demonstrated to be a clean-up technique with outstanding potential for pesticides extraction from unclean matrices, such as slurry. As disadvantages cited the relatively long extraction times, normally between 20 and 60 min (Pai-Shan and Shang-Da, 2006; Ho et al., 2002a).

Choosing the appropriate solvent for the HF-LPME technique is very important, since there is a reduced number of solvents that are immiscible and compatible with the polypropylene membrane (Psillakis and Kalogerakis, 2003; Pedersen-Bjergaard and

Rasmussen, 1999). The organic solvents need present low solubility in water and low volatility in order to be used in the HF-LPME system. The use of a mix of solvents has been done efficiently (Psillakis and Kalogerakis, 2003; Ugland et al., 2000).

Basheer et al. (2007) developed a methodology capable to determine mildly polar pesticides, which showed higher analytes enrichment mainly in complex matrices. A binary solvent-based two-phase hollow fiber-protected membrane liquid-phase microextraction technique, coupled with GC–MS has been used to determine organophosphorus pesticides in domestic wastewater samples. They were extracted from 10 mL of wastewater using an extracting phase composed of binary-solvent (toluene:hexane, 1:1) mixture.

Thus, the chromatographic techniques, such as GC–MS and high performance liquid chromatography-mass spectrometry (HPLC-MS) have been employed efficiently on the sensitive measurement of pesticides residues. However, chromatographic techniques employ a pretreatment for the analyte's isolation and enrichment. This pretreatment has a direct impact on analytes accuracy, precision, and quantification. In this context, interesting microextraction techniques have been developed to reduce amounts of organic solvents, as well as the phases involved in the sample preparation processes.

Sensing devices, such as nanossensors have emerged as an interesting tool showing high sensitivity and selectivity on the detection of many analytes, as well as the potential for miniaturization and skipping the samples pretreatment step. They are devices that incorporate a sensing element associated to a transduction system that allows the signal processing produced by the interaction between the sensing element and analyte. The technology for development of these devices is verified as cutting edge on the research for analytical instrumentation. This highly sensitive detection is due to the inclusion of nanostructured materials that raise the number of sites available for the molecular interactions originated from the nanomaterials high area/surface ratios (Wang, 2005). There are many interesting sensing devices that have been developed in order to determine pesticides (Haddaoui and Raouafi, 2015; Deda et al., 2013; Durán and Marcato, 2013; Ricciardi et al., 2013; Da Silva et al., 2013), of which will be described on the following part in more detail.

4 Nanobiosensors

The development of sensing devices has attracted great interest due to its highly sensitive, detection ability for specific molecules in a wide range of applications, including environmental monitoring in terms of determining emerging pollutants without the need for sample preparation procedures. The use of these devices is quite interesting, since normally the isolation and concentration procedures of pollutants at suitable levels for detection are not needed.

Sensors are defined as devices that measure both directly and indirectly the interaction with the sensing layer. Such reaction occurs over a transducer that converts any type of energy into a measurable output signal. The concept of the sensor can be extending depending on the sensing layer type. The biosensors present sensing layer that is comprised of either by biological molecules (biological elements, organisms, tissues, cells, organelles, membranes, enzymes, enzyme components, receptors, antibodies, nucleic acids, organic molecules) or biochemical materials, which in some cases can result in an increase on the biosensor uniqueness. The following descriptive definition for biosensors states: "a biosensor is a device capable of providing specific, quantitative or semi-quantitative analytical information using an element of biological recognition that is in direct contact with the transducing element" (Thévenot et al., 1996). Generally, are very reliable means of measuring specific analytes faster and at lower cost than traditional methods (IUPAC, 1997). Transducers forms can be by potentiometric, amperometric, conductimetric, impedimetric, optical, calorimetric, acoustic, mechanical, and molecular electronic. The Fig. 16.4 shows a schematic representation of the biosensor parts.

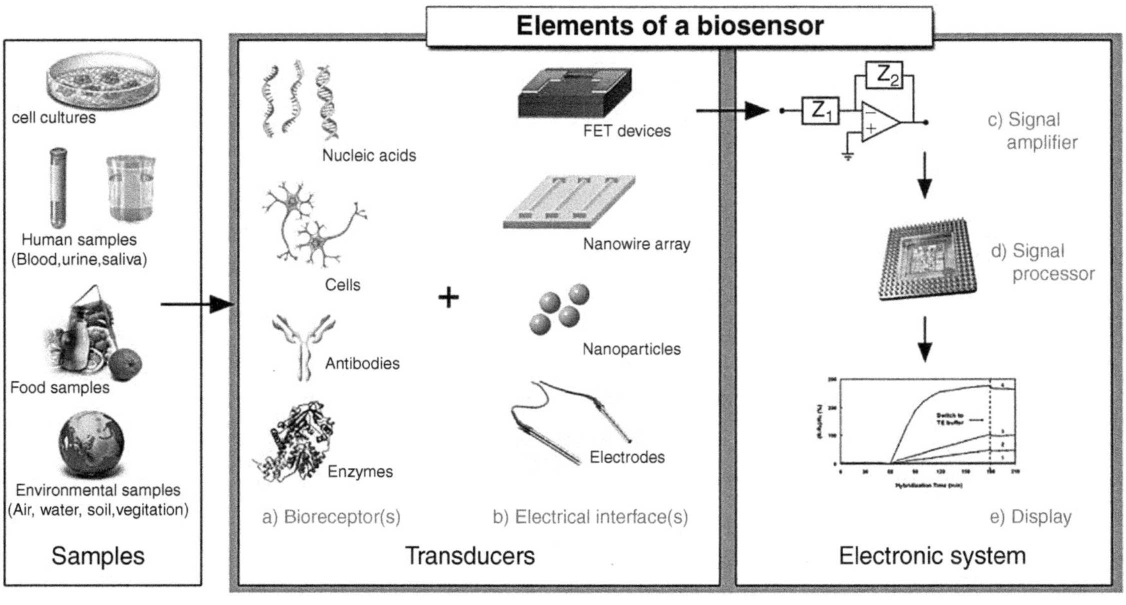

Figure 16.4. Schematic diagram of a biosensor device (Grieshaber et al., 2008). Reprinted with permission from Elsevier.

When biosensors are investigated using nanoscale, such devices are then call nanobiosensors. The sensitivity and performance of nanobiosensors can be increased by the miniaturization of such devices and/or the use of nanomaterials as sensing layers. The nanomaterials reduced size with dimensions defined by the nanotechnology between 1 and 100 nm, makes them materials with quite interesting properties and different from the same materials in a larger scale. The size reduction increases these materials with specific surface area, since many of the nanomaterials atoms are located on/or near the surface.

Currently, with the nanotechnology development has increasing studies with nanobiosensors and nanomaterials. The interest and relevance of nanomaterials in the fabrication of nanobiosensors lie in their extraordinary properties that make them ideally suited and very promising for sensing applications. Nanomaterials, such as nanotubes, nanobels, nanoprobes, nanowires, nanorods, nanograins, nanoparticles, submicrosized and nanometers thickness film and nanofibers, (Malik et al., 2013) and quantum dots have been intensively investigated for their use in nanobiosensors. Nanomaterials, such as nanotubes, nanowires, nanorods, nanoparticles, and quantum dots have been intensively investigated for their use in nanobiosensors (Zhang et al., 2009). Among them, nanoparticles, due to their diversity in structure and dimension, have been prominent as a sensing layer for the specific recognition of several molecules by amplifying their recognition signal strength. Thereby, creating highly sensitive nanobiosensors (Malik et al., 2013).

Nanobiosensors works on the nanoscale size and can sense analytes in traces with fast, precise and accurate biological identification (Bueno et al., 2015; Steffens et al., 2014a).

The classification for nanobiosensors includes the following criteria (Rumayour et al., 2005):

- method used to detect desired interactions
- type of interaction established between the sensor element and analyte
- transduction system
- nature of the compound recognition (biological or nonbiological)

Among the several types of biosensors, the nanomechanical sensors based on microcantilevers, which are used on atomic force microscopy (AFM) have been presenting very interesting results on the detection of many specific substances. These nanomechanical sensors have excellent performances, such as real time response, low detection limits, and high sensitivity. They can provide compact and portable devices for the specific identification of many substances (Devreese, 2007). Since these nanobiosensors are devices that enable the immobilization of specific molecules, they also provide a focused and specific recognition, avoiding nonspecific cross-connections. They also present the advantage to detect multiple analytes and can be reused and mimic organic environments depending on the nanobiosensor's design (Bogue, 2009).

The possibility of AFM use on either topographic or nontopographic sample surface analyses makes it a quite versatile technique. Topographic analysis refers to a structural and dynamic characterization of the samples surface through its imaging. Nontopographic analysis relates to the use of AFM as a nanoscale sensor, called nanomechanical systems, which allow the processes analyses at an intermolecular level of interaction. Both the AFM tip and the cantilever (needless of its tip) can be chemically modified. It originates the AFM tip nanobiosensors on the first case and the cantilever-based nanobiosensors on the latter case.

4.1 Nanobiosensors of Cantilevers

Recent advances in the design and development of cantilevers make them capable of detecting small mechanical deflections (around 10^{-4} N/m). Cantileveres are typically prepared from silicon material and/or silicon nitride materials or polymeric, with dimensions from 100 to 500 μm in length and thickness of 0.5–5 μm, and may form a "V" (triangle) or "T" (rectangular) (Lang et al., 2002).

The AFM can be used to measure forces between the cantilever (spring constant) and the sample. The beam deflection technique is the most common method used to measure cantilever deformation (Ziegler, 2004). The deformations measure in the cantilever follows Hooke's law $F = k \cdot x$, where F is the restoring force, x is the displacement from the equilibrium position, and k is the cantilever spring constant. The deflection of a cantilever can be measured with an optical sensor when it is a small deflection; the vertical displacement of the tip (Z) is directly proportional to the force on it (F) and is thus a direct measurement of the strength of interaction between the tip and a surface (Fig. 16.5) (Steffens et al., 2012). The cantilever is move by piezocrystal elements with nanometer resolution. At the end of the cantilever is a probe. The principle of operation of a cantilever sensor is based on the adsorption of analytes at the surface of the cantilever (coated with a sensing layer), which usually leads to an induced surface stress and an increase of the apparent mass of the cantilever (Dong et al., 2010; Hansen et al., 2001). The change in mass leads to deflection of the cantilever in the Z direction.

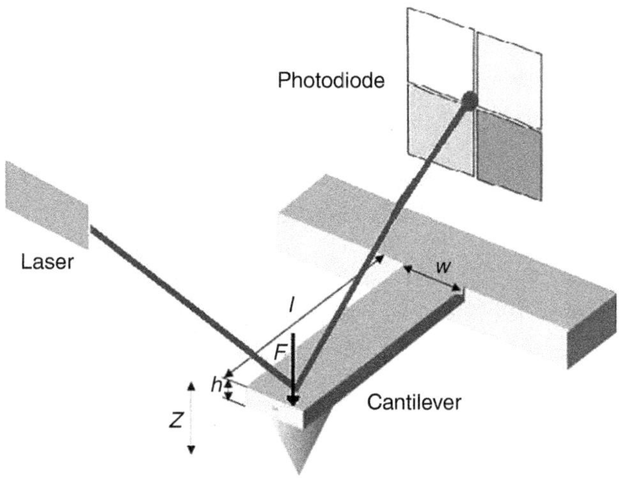

Figure 16.5. Illustration of the displacement of the cantilever (*h*, *w*, and *l* are thickness, width, and length of the cantilever, respectively) (Steffens et al., 2012).

Other technique as piezoresistive method, also can be used for measuring the cantilever deflection, were the beam deflection is indicated by the change in the resistance. To measure this deflection with integrated piezoresistors, an amplifier circuit with high amplification factor is needed (Sierakowski et al., 2014).

Based on AFM principle of work is possible to measure forces between the cantilever tip and sample surface (contact mode) or resonance frequency of a vibrating cantilever (dynamic mode). Based in this principle the cantilever sensors operate in same mode, where interaction with analyte changes the bending (static mode) or resonance frequency (resonant mode). In this way, the modes of operation of cantilevers sensors can be classified based on their principles in translating the recognition event into micro or nanomechanical motion (Gopinath et al., 2014). The Fig. 16.6 demonstrates the sensor operating modes based on the cantilever.

Second Lang et al. (2007) the static deflection upon the formation of surface stress during adsorption of a molecular layer or external influences and chemical/physical reactions in cantilevers surfaces is termed static mode (Fig. 16.6A). In the dynamic mode, the mass of the oscillating cantilever (resonance frequency) changes owing to additional mass deposited or mass removed changes (Fig. 16.6B). In the heat mode, the temperature change causes a thermal expansion in the cantilever material (Fig. 16.6C). Diffusion of molecules into a polymer layer leads to swelling of the polymer and bending the cantilever (Fig. 16.6D). In the thermogravimetric

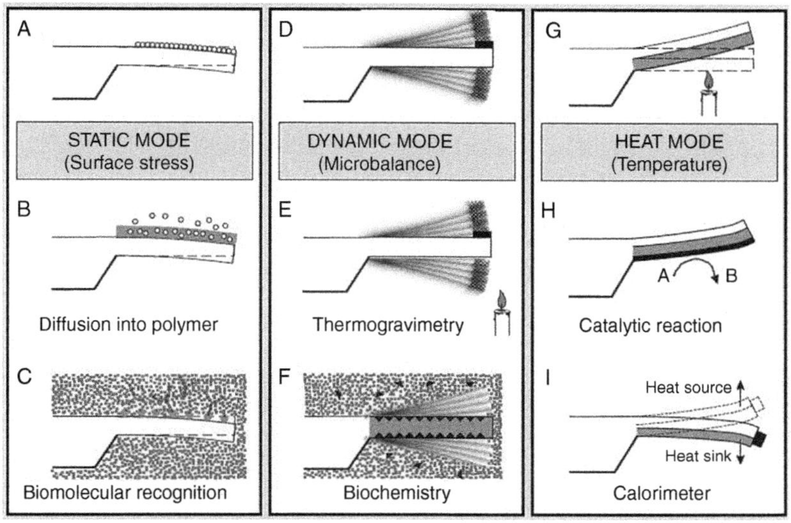

Figure 16.6. Basic operations modes of cantilever sensors. Reprinted from Lang et al. (2007) with permission.

mode, a change in the temperature while a sample is attached to the apex of the cantilever allows information to be gathered on decomposition or oxidation process (Fig. 16.6E). Catalytic active surface on a bimetallic cantilever bends due to heat production during a reaction (Fig. 16.6F). Biomolecular recognition mode, the biomolecules with sensitive coating of the cantilever causing a bending (Fig. 16.6G). Biochemistry mode, measurements in liquids yield details on mass changes during biochemical processes (Fig. 16.6H). Calorimeter mode, a tiny sample attached to the apex of the cantilever is investigated, taking advantage of the bimetallic effect. Tracking the deflection as a function of temperature allows the observation of phase transitions in the sample in a calorimeter mode (Fig. 16.6I) (Lang et al., 2007).

The AFM nanobiosensors present as main advantage the larger detection limits at molecular level. This system can detect interactions to the piconewtons order (pN) (Gruber et al., 2011). The molecular interactions (adsorption or binding) induced change in surface tension of the cantilever. These interactions results in electrostatic repulsion or attraction, steric effects and intermolecular (Tang et al., 2004), interactions between molecules on the cantilever surfaces that alter the surface stresses on the cantilever.

Also, nanomechanical sensors have advantages of performance as instantaneous response (in real time) and portability (in some cases). In these devices are immobilized specific molecules, in this way offer particular recognition, avoiding nonspecific binding. They are considered intelligent, therefore can be used as independent detection systems or integrated to data networks (Bogue, 2009). On the other hand, they have disadvantage in relation to the sensing systems, used for operation. It should be studied in detail to choose the best geometry, adequate functionalization method, and suitable molecules to act as a sensitive element.

4.1.1 Functionalization of the AFM Cantilever or Nanomechanical Systems

The appropriate functionalization of the AFM cantilever surface makes the devices capable to transduce a chemical signal into a mechanical motion, creating highly sensitive nanobiosensors. The functionalization of these mechanical transducers is considered one of the most important stages, as it directly affects these devices' sensitivity, detection limit, reproducibility, and selectivity on detecting the forces, motion, mechanical properties, and mass that emerge in both biomolecular interactions, as well as fundamental biological processes. The appropriate surface functionalization coupled with the extremely reduced size of these mechanical systems provides an outstanding mass resolution reaching single atom levels. In addition, nanomechanical systems can exhibit extremely low mechanical compliances translating biomolecular recognition events into measurements displacements (Carrascosa et al., 2006; Tamayo et al., 2013). The Fig. 16.7 showed a demonstration of the work principle of the coated and uncoated cantilever sensor.

According to Carrascosa et al. (2006), an appropriate surface functionalization occurs when placed the receptor molecule layer (sensing layer) with the follow conditions:

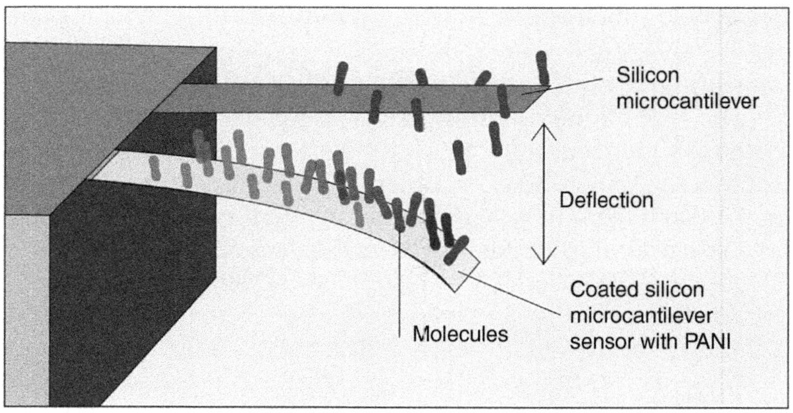

Figure 16.7. Schematic representation of the working principle of uncoated and coated microcantilevers sensors (Steffens et al., 2014b).

- Thin, avoiding change in the cantilever mechanical properties.
- Uniform, in order to generate a surface stress as large as possible.
- Compact, avoiding interactions with the solid substrate underneath it. The receptor molecule layer should have enough degree of freedom to allow the target molecules free access on the environment. The functionalization should allow the receptor activity to be maintained on the long run, making the sensor to be reused a number of times.

According to Tamayo et al. (2013) an appropriate functionalization is comprised of the following stages:

- Chemical modification of the surface in order to obtain reactive functional groups that strongly bind to the bio recognition element.
- Immobilization of the bio recognition element.
- Bare areas must be blocked with antifouling molecules to minimize nonspecific adsorption should they remain on the cantilever surface.

There are many common aspects between the functionalization of nanomechanical systems with the functionalization of biosensors. Are necessary some requirements for tonanomechanical systems works correctly (Tamayo et al., 2013):

- The cleaning of this material must be made with accuracy and care because they are fragile.
- It is necessary to preserve the biological activity on the cantilever surface during and after functionalization.
- Very ultra low volumes of samples and reagents are necessary to perform measures with these nanomechanical systems.

The functionalization can be performed on materials, such as silicon dioxide, silicon nitride, gold, etc. Over this material can be deposited alkaline chain molecules with thiol groups (-SH) on gold substrates (Dubois and Nuzzo, 1992) or silanos (-SIOX) on silicon substrates (Weetall and Detar, 1975) (Raiteri et al., 2001). It is a very versatile methodology; it enables the connection of various types of receptor molecules to the substrate as it forms monolayers of different lengths and final groups with specific chemical properties. The cantilever surface functionalization with gold is very common in nanomechanical sensors that operate on static mode. In this operation method the bending is the result of a change on the surface tension between the opposite sides of the cantilever. Such variation is reached through the deposition of a 20–30 nm thin layer of gold on only one cantilever sides, which can be placed using various techniques, such as thermal, e-beam or sputtering deposition methods. Normally a 2–5 nm thin layer of either chromium or titanium is used as an intermediate layer in order to improve the adhesion between the gold and surface. The use of thiol with different functional groups make the development of surfaces possible with different properties and functions, enabling almost specific interactions between the sensing surface and the biological material, with a high degree of control over its molecular structure (Awsiuk et al., 2012). The perfect pairing between the alkanethiols (normally with a 20–30 degree inclination in relation to the surface's usual one) and the gold reticle resulting in a highly ordered structure have made this system subject to a great number of studies using spectroscopic, microscopic, and electrochemical means. The forming of monolayers organized through the silanization process is more commonly used for the functionalization of cantilever that operate on a dynamic module, in other words, both sides of the cantilever are coated (Tamayo et al., 2013). Silicon oxide existent on the surface of the materials that form the cantilevers, such as silicon and silicon nitride absorbs water molecules forming silane groups (Si-OH) of high density (Rye et al., 1997). They react with organosilicon molecules form a silicon-oxygen-silicon carbon linkage. Organosilicon molecules are composed by organic, reactive, and a terminal group that can be replaced by different groups providing suitable properties for the surface modification (Pesek and Matyska, 1997).

For sensitive element it is possible to immobilize a great variety of enzymes, such as acetylcholinesterase, cholinesterase, acid phosphatase, ascorbate oxidase, acetolactate synthase, urease, and aldehyde dehydrogenase. Where, pesticide detection is based on measurements of enzyme inhibition or direct measurements of compounds involved in the enzymatic reaction (Sassolas, 2012). Microorganisms, such as *Moraxella sp.* and *P. putida* were immobilized by chemical (covalent binding and cross-linking) and physical (adsorption and entrapment) methods (Lei et al., 2006). Antibodies or antigens, nucleic acid sequences that bind non-nucleic acid targets with high affinity and specificity also are biorecognition element for pesticides detection.

4.2 Applications of Cantilevers Nanobiosensors in Pesticide Detection

Nanomechanical sensors of cantilevers have enabled a wide range of applications for detection of water pollutants with high sensitivity. Karnati et al. (2007) studied the detection of organophosphorus compounds using microcantilever coated with organophosphorus hydrolase. They functionalized both sides of the cantilever surface using the layer-by-layer technique, which is alternately dipped into a polycation (polyethyleneimine) and

Table 16.2 Detection Limit of Nanobiosensors to the Pesticide Paraoxon

Nanobiosensor	Sensitive Material	Detection Limit	References
Cantilever sensor	Polyethyleneimine	10^{-7} M	Karnati et al. (2007)
Fluorescence	Liposomes	6.7×10^{-10} M	Vamvakaki and Chaniotakis (2007)
Fluorescence	*n*(CdSe)ZnS core–shell Quantun dots	10^{-8} M	Ji et al. (2005)
Fiber-optic	Gold nanoparticles covalently coupled with acetylcholinesterase	0.234 ppb	Lin et al. (2006)
Eletrochemical	Carbon nanotube/organo-phosphorus hydrolase	0.15 μmol/L	Deo et al. (2005)

polyanion solution [poly(sodium styrene sulfonate)], and the process is repeated several times for multilayer formation. The organophosphorus hydrolase enzyme was depositing by immersion onto the layers. The authors observed that the microcantilever biosensor presented a detection limit of 10^{-7} M for paraoxon, with a bilayer thickness around 25 nm. This detection limit was very interesting compared with other nanobiosensors (Table 16.2).

Xu et al. (2014) evaluated the detection of organophorous vapors (harmful at very low concentration of ppm or even ppb level) with resonant microcantilever coated with ordered mesopores and studied the capacity of detoxification to pesticides. They observed that long time of reaction with vapors would cause excessive consumption of the Si-OH groups on the silica surface and lead to significant decrease in detoxification performance (Fig. 16.8). The experiment conducted at 298 K using 80 ppb dimethyl methylphosphonate showed response time shorter than 6 min. However, the sensing signals always cannot recover completely after the vapor exposition.

Dichlorodiphenyltrichloroethane is a chlorinated compound with insecticidal properties that has been used worldwide for controlling insect pests. In this way, Alvarez et al. (2003) used a microcantilever coated with a gold layer (25 nm of thickness) to covalently immobilized dichlorodiphenyltrichloroethane conjugated with bovine serum albumin using thiol self-assembled

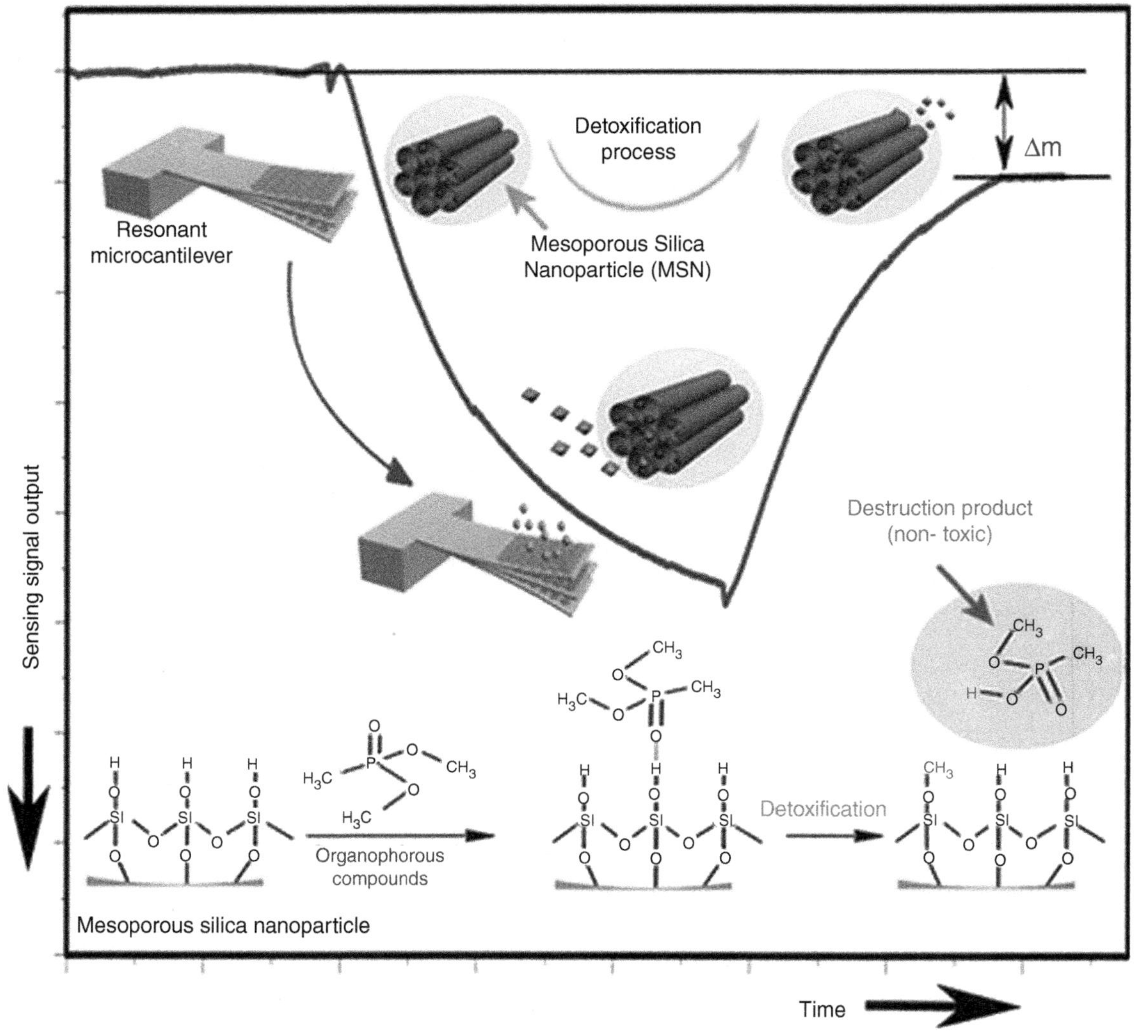

Figure 16.8. Response of the microcantilever to dimethyl methylphosphonate vapors (Xu et al., 2014). Reprinted with permission from Elsevier.

monolayers. The detection was monitoring by exposure to a solution of a monoclonal antibody and the device present response at concentration of 25 nM (Fig. 16.9), thus indicates sensitivity at nanomolar range.

Antibody to an antigen-coated cantilever was investigated as a transducer for a pesticide bioassay by Bache et al. (2011). The cantilever was functionalized using microspotting and passive adsorption to the gold layer and observed that the differential signal (deflection) was not repeatable.

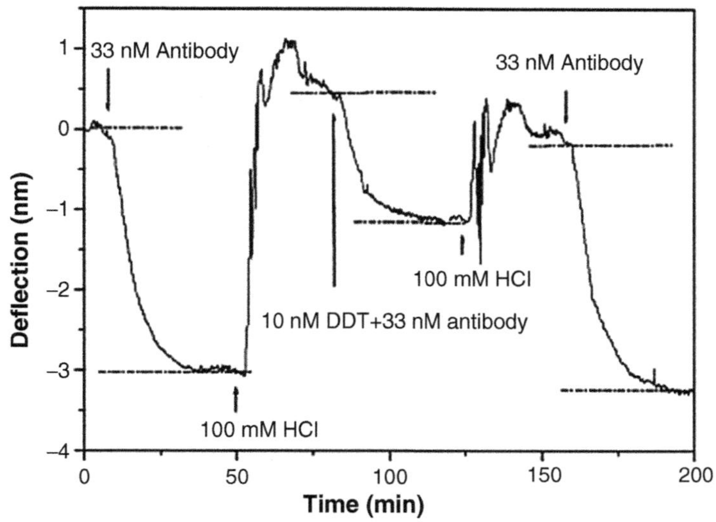

Figure 16.9. Dichlorodiphenyltrichloroethane pesticide detection using a single microcantilever sensor by real-time competitive immunoassay (Carrascosa et al., 2006). Reprinted with permission from Elsevier.

2,4-dichlorophenoxyacetic acid (2,4-D) is a herbicide widely used to control the growth of broadleaf and woody plants and present moderately toxic. The detection by an immunosensor was investigated by Raiteri et al. (1999). For this purpose on one side of the cantilever was cover with a gold layer (<30 nm) and then deposited a monolayer of cysteamine. The detection was evaluated using a buffer solution and monoclonal antibody against the herbicide. The nanobiosensor bends 40 nm when exposed to 25 μg/mL of antibody, which corresponds to a 20 mN/m of compressive stress, and exposed to phosphate buffer solution does not influence the deflection.

Atrazine is a herbicide used in agriculture to control broad leaf weeds in corn, sorghum, sugarcane, citrus, etc. Raman Suri et al. (2008) have used a polyclonal atrazine based antibody as a "ligand" covalently linked to the cantilever surface with 2 nm thick titanium layer and 20 nm thick gold layer. The experiments were performed inject into the fluid cell concentrations of atrazine solution (4.65 pM–46.5 μM) and evaluated the cross-reactivity. The cantilever deflected when atrazine antigen binding with this antibody showing a detection limit of 4.65 pM.

In the literature are few developments of different atrazine sensors. The Table 16.3 present different detection limits for the sensors and can be observed that the nanomechanical sensor based in cantilever is the most sensitive.

Table 16.3 Examples of Nanobiosensors Developed for Atrazine Determination With Detection Limit (Bhalla and Zazubovich, 2011)

Transduction System and Nanobiosensors	Recognition Biocomponent	Detection Limit	References
Electrochemical immunosensor	Biotinylated-Fab fragment K47 antibody	20 ng/mL	Hleli et al. (2006)
Piezoelectric immunosensor	Self-assembled layer of cysteamine	0.025 ng/mL	Přibyl et al. (2003)
Conductimetric immunosensor	Antibodies labelled with gold nanoparticles	0.1–1 μg/L	Valera et al. (2008)
Cantilever sensor	Antibody–antigen	pM	Raman Suri et al. (2008)
Electrochemiluminescence flow injection immunoassay	Antibodies	0.1 ppb–6 nM	Wilson et al. (1997)
Direct hapten-coated microtiter plates in Immunoassay	Antibodies	20 ng/L–0.09 nM	Kaur et al. (2008)
Photosynthetic II biosensor	Photosynthetic II reaction centers or membrane fragments	247 ng/L–1.15 nM	Bhalla and Zazubovich (2011)
Imprinted quartz crystal microbalance sensor	Self-assembling monolayer formation of allylmercaptane on gold	0.028 nM	Gupta et al. (2015)
Boron-doped diamond electrode, electrochemical sensor	Boron-doped diamond electrode	10 nM	Švorc et al. (2013)
Piezoelectric transducers	Natural antibodies	20 ppb	Yaqub et al. (2011)

4.3 AFM Tip Nanosensors Based on the Atomic Force Spectroscopy

The measurement of the necessary force to physical separate the interaction between two molecules, one immobilized on a substrate and the other on the AFM cantilever tip is the principle of the Atomic Force Spectroscopy (AFS) technique, which is an AFM technique module. The interactions between the AFM cantilever tip and a molecule immobilized on a substrate result in a force curve, which provide information about the properties of materials, such as elasticity, hardness, Hamaker constant, adhesion, and surface charge density (Deda et al., 2013).

The AFM tip sensors are based on the AFS, which detects specific intermolecular interactions, allowing the mapping of functional groups on a substrate at both micro and nanometre scales. Thus, the AFS based AFM tip nanosensors are highly sensitive and selective devices (Leite et al., 2007; Ditzler et al., 2011; Jauvert et al., 2012) since it allows the quantification of forces between the tip and the sample.

These sensors are quite promising for detecting and monitoring pesticides in concentrations low enough to be safe. Da Silva et al. (2013) using AFM-based nanobiosensor tip of silicon nitrite modified with the acetolactate synthase enzyme for detection of metsulfuron-methyl herbicide. The detection of metsulfuron-methyl herbicide by an acetolactate synthase inhibitor was performed with a specific interaction between the enzyme and the herbicide. This was obtained by the tip functionalization with acetolactate synthase and force curve measurements. The nanobiosensors high sensitivity with AFM tip is related to the functionalization efficiency, since it is responsible for the specific interactions between the tip and the substrate. For the metsulfuron-methyl detection it was deposited onto mica substrate. The modification on the AFM tips with acetolactate synthase enzyme was made through 3-aminopropyltriethoxysilane (APTES) and glutaraldehyde, according to Fig. 16.10.

Nanobiosensors based on chemically modified AFM tips were developed to detect atrazine by Deda et al. (2013). AFM tips were functionalized in two ways: with antiatrazine antibody for the detection of atrazine and with acetolactate synthase enzyme for the detection of imazaquin and metsulfuron-methyl herbicides. The analysis of adhesion force values showed an increase of approximately 175% to the AFM functionalized tip with the antibody specific to the atrazine and approximately 132 and 145% to the AFM tip modified with enzyme used to detect imazaquin and metsulfuron-methyl, respectively. These high adhesion values are due to specific interactions between the biomolecules functionalized on the AFM tips and the different herbicides. Thus, the modified tips became efficient nanobiosensors, selective and specific to detect pesticides.

AFM tip immunobiosensors based on AFS have been used to determine the two most used herbicides atrazine (MPAD) and 2,4-D (Kaur et al., 2004). AFS technique was used to measure the adhesion forces between the antibodies immobilized on Au-coated

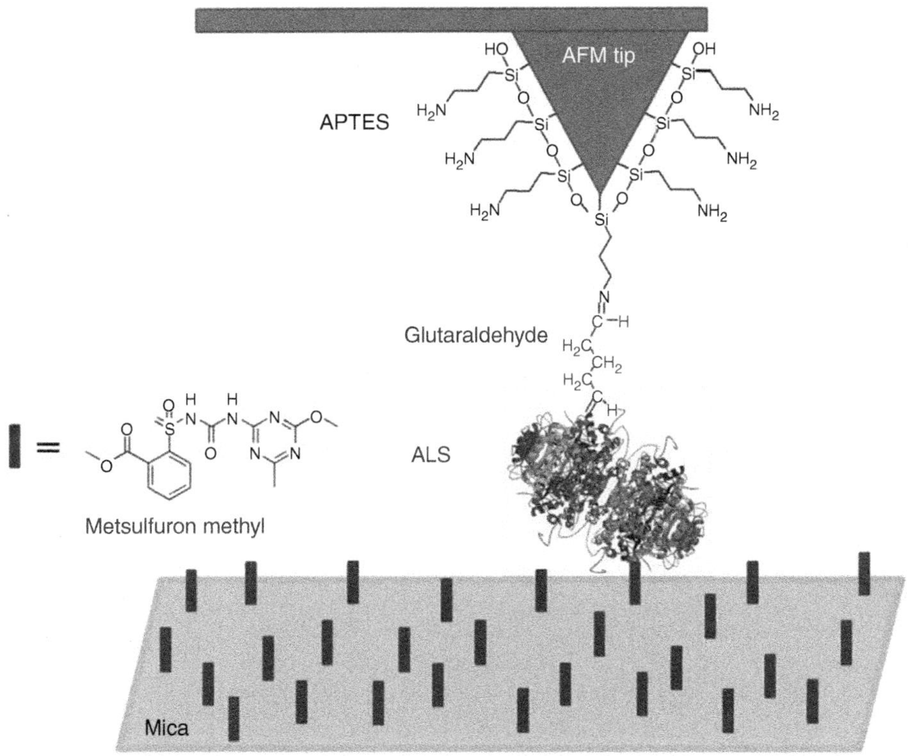

Figure 16.10. Functionalization scheme of AFM tip and the detection of metsulfuron-methyl herbicide on the mica surface (Da Silva et al., 2013).

glass via Protein A and their respective antigens that have been immobilized on the cantilever tip. AFM tips were then covalently functionalized with either bovine serum albumin-MPAD (BSA-MPAD) or BSA-2,4-D conjugates using aminopropyltriethoxysilane (APTES) and glutaraldehyde. In this study, purified hapten-specific antibodies have been used, which were covalently linked with BSA. The use of these small organic molecules (haptens) was due to antibodies being highly specific making it very unlikely to recognize more than one site on the pesticide molecule. This specific connection between antibodies and small pesticide haptens has contributed to the development of many important immunosensors for environmentally sensitive small toxic molecules (Lee et al., 2001). The results showed that the developed AFM tip immune biosensor was efficient in the analyses of the strength of antibody–hapten interactions and they showed that the anti-MPAD antibody had a higher functional affinity as compared to the anti-2,4-D antibody.

4.4 Nanobiosensors with Nanomaterials for Pesticides Detection

In the literature it was also found that other types of nanobiosensors for organophosphorus pesticides target acetylcholinesterase. This enzyme is used to catalyze the hydrolysis of the neurotransmitter acetylcholine into choline and acetic acid. It can be also used as a biological sensing since when in contact with organophosphates and carbamates, their toxicity inhibits the enzyme during synapsis (Vargas-Bernal et al., 2012). Vamvakaki and Chaniotakis (2007) developed liposome-based nanobiosensor for detection different pesticides (paraoxon and dichlorvos). The enzyme acetylcholinesterase was encapsulated in egg phosphatidylcholine liposomes and used as fluorescent biosensors. The nanobiosensor can detect concentrations down to 10^{-10} M of both pesticides.

Firdoz et al. (2010) immobilized acetylcholine esterase by layer by layer [Poly(diallyldimethylammonium chloride)–single walled carbon nanotubes] technique to construct an amperometric biosensor for detection of paraoxon. The biosensor showed good sensitivity and stability toward the monitoring of carbaryl pesticides in water with the detection limit of 10^{-12} g/L (0.2 ppb). Also the authors observed that the enzymatic activity was inhibited in the presence of paraoxon and retained 94% of its original activity after six cycles of inhibition with 500 ppb, showing activity after 2 months storage in dry state at 4°C.

Multienzyme biosensing systems provide versatility for detection of multianalytes. In this way Zhang et al. (2015) applied bilayers multiwalled carbon nanotube with organophosphate hydrolase and acetylcholine esterase by the layer by layer technique for discriminative detection of organophosphorus and nonorganophosphorus pesticides. The bienzymatic biosensor presented a linear response range 0.5–40 μM for paraoxon and 10–80 μM for carbaryl with 0.5 and 10 μM of detection limit, respectively.

Silica coated silver nanoparticles is a very sensitive material and has been studied to increase the fluorescence signal of organophosphorus hydrolase with a histidine tail–pyraninebioconjugate to detected organophosphorus pesticides by Thakur et al. (2013). These metallic nanostructures alter the fluorescence either by enhancing the excitation rate, so resulted in lowering detection limit 2 ppb for paraoxon and 10 ppb for methyl parathion.

Khaksarinejad et al. (2015) also investigated the organo phosphorous hydrolase for detection of paraoxon, immobilizing the enzyme on nanomangetic-silica core–shell using glutaraldehyde as cross-linker. Lower detection limits (5×10^{-6} μM) was achieved using spectrofluorometric organophosphorous hydrolase-based assay.

Immunochromatographic fluorescent test strip based on biosensor for direct detection of organophosphorus (trichloropyridinol) in human saliva was developed by Zhang et al. (2013). Gold nanoparticles were deposited on test strip and treated with phosphate-buffered saline containing polyethylene glycol, Tween-20, and casein. Then antibodies were conjugates with gold nanoparticles. Second the authors, the biosensor presents a linear range of 0.625–20 ng/mL, with a detection limit of 0.47 ng/mL in the best condition.

Another sensitive coating of polymer was used to obtain a dual-template imprinted dendrimer nanofiber on gold surface of quartz crystal microbalances. This sensor was used for determination of organo-chlorinated pesticides (dichlorodiphenyltrichloroethane and hexachorobenzene) showing detection limit lower than 0.75 ng/mL, reproductivity of six analysis and stability of 60 in air (Prasad and Jauhari, 2015).

Songa et al. (2009a) developed a electrochemical nanobiosensor depositing poly(2,5- dimethoxyaniline) (PDMA) doped with poly(4-styrenesulfonic acid) onto gold electrode surface followed by electrostatic attachment of horseradish peroxidase onto the nanocomposite film. This nanobiosensor was applied to detect glyphosate and the results showed a detection limit of 1.0 μg/L. Still Songa et al. (2009b) develop an amperometric nanobiosensors, immobilizing the enzyme horseradish peroxidase for determination of glyphosate and glufosinate. They observed detection limits of 0.1 μg/L (10^{-10} M) and good reproducibility of these nanobiosensors.

Tyrosinase is inhibited by different compounds, such as carbamate and atrazine pesticides. Haddaoui and Raouafi (2015) studied enzymatic biosensor for chlortoluron, based on herbicide-induced inhibition of tyrosinase activity during the oxidation of phenol to *o*-quinone. They observed that the biosensor presented reproducibility higher of 0.998, sensitivity of 0.099 ppb and limit of detection of 0.1 ppb.

5 Conclusions

Water is an unprecedented natural resource of most importance for the survival of all species, however it has been very contaminated. In recent years, the scientific community has been aiming at the development of reliable and faster methodologies for monitoring emerging contaminants in aquatic environments.

Among the emerging contaminants, pesticides are investigated due the indiscriminate use, stability in the environment, and toxicity. Pesticides threaten biodiversity and the balance of natural ecosystems. In this context the nanobiosensors are devices that can be applied for pesticide detection in water at very low concentrations. This detection can be reached through the efficient functionalization of the biological matter with nanomaterials and/or nanostructured materials.

Biosensors present many advantages over conventional detection methods, which are generally determined by chromatographic techniques, such as GC–MS and HPLC-MS. Among the different advantages the sample preparation stage is not necessary, shorter analysis time frame, on-line application and lower operational costs in relation to more conventional methods. Furthermore, the technology of development biosensors provides the miniaturization of this equipment, becoming portable enabling their use on field.

Nanomechanical sensors showed great capabilities on the recognition of biomolecular interactions through changes in their surface stress or mass. A very high selectivity, sensitivity, and excellent detection limits are achieved by their small size and type of surface functionalization. The functionalization with an appropriate sensing layer is a crucial stage for the use of nanomechanical devices on many applications.

Acknowledgments

The authors would like to thank URI Erechim, Embrapa Instrumentation, responsible for the National Nanotechnology Laboratory for Agribusiness (LNNA) for the infrastructure and facilities, UFSCar, FAPESP, CNPq, Capes, Fapergs, Finep for the financial support.

References

Abdollahi, M., Ranjbar, A., Shadnia, S., Nikfar, S., Rezaie, A., 2004. Pesticides and oxidative stress: a review. Med. Sci. Monit. 10 (6), A141–A147.

Agrawal, A., 2010. Water pollution with special reference to pesticide contamination in India. J. Water Resour. Prot. 02 (05), 432–448.

Alcamo, J., Döll, P., Henrichs, T., Kaspar, F., Lehner, B., Rösch, T., Siebert, S., 2003. Development and testing of the WaterGAP 2 global model of water use and availability. Hydrol. Sci. J. 48 (3), 317–337.

Alvarez, M., Calle, A., Tamayo, J., Lechuga, L.M., Abad, A., Montoya, A., 2003. Development of nanomechanical biosensors for detection of the pesticide DDT. Biosens. Bioelectron. 18 (5–6), 649–653.

Arthur, C., Pawlyszin, J., 1990. Solid phase microextraction with thermal desorption using fused silica optical fibers. Anal. Chem. 62 (19), 2145–2148.

Awsiuk, K., Bernasik, A., Kitsara, M., Budkowski, A., Petrou, P., Kakabakos, S., Prauzner-Bechcicki, S., Rysz, J., Raptis, I., 2012. Spectroscopic and microscopic characterization of biosensor surfaces with protein/amino-organosilane/silicon structure. Colloids Surf. B Biointerf. 90 (1), 159–168.

Bache, M., Taboryski, R., Schmid, S., Aamand, J., Jakobsen, M.H., 2011. Investigations on antibody binding to a micro-cantilever coated with a BAM pesticide residue. Nanoscale Res. Lett. 6 (1), 386.

Badruddoza, A.Z.M., Shawon, Z.B.Z., Tay, W.J.D., Hidajat, K., Uddin, M.S., 2013. Fe_3O_4/cyclodextrin polymer nanocomposites for selective heavy metals removal from industrial wastewater. Carbohydr. Polym. 91 (1), 322–332.

Basheer, C., Alnedhary, A.A., Rao, B.S.M., Lee, H.K., 2007. Determination of organophosphorous pesticides in wastewater samples using binary-solvent liquid-phase microextraction and solid-phase microextraction: a comparative study. Anal. Chim. Acta 605 (2), 147–152.

Bedos, C., Cellier, P., Calvet, R., Barriuso, E., Gabrielle, B., 2002. Mass transfer of pesticides into the atmosphere by volatilization from soils and plants: overview. Agronomie 22 (1), 21–33.

Bhalla, V., Zazubovich, V., 2011. Self-assembly and sensor response of photosynthetic reaction centers on screen-printed electrodes. Anal. Chim. Acta 707 (1–2), 184–190.

Birkett, J.W., Lester, J.N., 2003. Endocrine disruptors in wastewater and sludge treatment processes. Environ. Health Perspect. 111 (10), 13427.

Biziuk, M., Przyjazny, A., Czerwinski, J., Wiergowski, M., 1996. Occurrence and determination of pesticides in natural and treated waters. J. Chromatogr. A 754 (1-2), 103–123.

Bogue, R., 2009. Nanosensors: a review of recent research. Sens. Rev. 29 (4), 310–315.

Bolong, N., Ismail, A.F., Salim, M.R., Matsuura, T., 2009. A review of the effects of emerging contaminants in wastewater and options for their removal. Desalination 238 (1–3), 229–246.

Brasil, 1986. Resolution (CONAMA) No. 20 of 1986.

Bueno, C. De C., Garcia, P.S., Steffens, C., Deda, D.K., Leite, F. de L., 2015. Nanossensores. in:Róz, A.L., Leite, F.L., Ferreira, M., Oliveira, O.N. (Eds.). Grandes Áreas da Nanociência. Elsevier Editora Ltda, Rio de Janeiro, pp. 145–187.

Carrascosa, L.G., Moreno, M., Álvarez, M., Lechuga, L.M., 2006. Nanomechanical biosensors: a new sensing tool. Trends Anal. Chem. 25 (3), 196–206.

Chen, W., Zeng, J., Chen, J., Huang, X., Jiang, Y., Wang, Y., Chen, X., 2009. High extraction efficiency for polar aromatic compounds in natural water samples using multiwalled carbon nanotubes/Nafion solid-phase microextraction coating. J. Chromatogr. A 1216 (52), 9143–9148.

Corcoran, E., Nellemann, C., Baker, E., Bos, R., Osborn, D., Savellt, H., 2010. Sick Water? The Central Role of Wastewater Management in Sustainable Development. United Nations Environ. Program. UN-HABITAT, GRID GRID-Arendal.

Da Silva, A.C.N., Deda, D.K., Da Róz, A.L., Prado, R.A., Carvalho, C.C., Viviani, V., Leite, F.L., 2013. Nanobiosensors based on chemically modified AFM probes: a useful tool for metsulfuron-methyl detection. Sensors 13 (2), 1477–1489.

Deda, D.K., Pereira, B.B.S., Bueno, C.C., da Silva, A.N., Ribeiro, G.A., Amarante, A.M., Franca, E.F., Leite, F.L., 2013. The use of functionalized AFM tips as molecular sensors in the detection of pesticides. Mater. Res. 16 (3), 683–687.

Deo, R.P., Wang, J., Block, I., Mulchandani, A., Joshi, K.A., Trojanowicz, M., Scholz, F., Chen, W., Lin, Y., 2005. Determination of organophosphate pesticides at a carbon nanotube/organophosphorus hydrolase electrochemical biosensor. Anal. Chim. Acta 530 (2), 185–189.

Devreese, J.T., 2007. Importance of nanosensors: Feynman's vision and the birth of nanotechnology. MRS Bull. 32 (09), 718–725.
Ditzler, L.R., Sen, A., Gannon, M.J., Kohen, A., Tivanski, A.V., 2011. Self-assembled enzymatic monolayer directly bound to a gold surface: activity and molecular recognition force spectroscopy studies. J. Am. Chem. Soc. 133 (34), 13284–13287.
Djozan, D., Ebrahimi, B., 2008. Preparation of new solid phase micro extraction fiber on the basis of atrazine-molecular imprinted polymer: application for GC and GC/MS screening of triazine herbicides in water, rice and onion. Anal. Chim. Acta 616 (2), 152–159.
Dong, Y., Gao, W., Zhou, Q., Zheng, Y., You, Z., 2010. Characterization of the gas sensors based on polymer-coated resonant microcantilevers for the detection of volatile organic compounds. Anal. Chim. Acta 671 (1–2), 85–91.
Doong, R.a, Chang, S.M., Sun, Y.C., 2000. Solid-phase microextraction for determining the distribution of sixteen US Environmental Protection Agency polycyclic aromatic hydrocarbons in water samples. J. Chromatogr. A 879 (2), 177–188.
Dubois, L.H., Nuzzo, R.G., 1992. Synthesis, structure, and properties of model organic surfaces. Ann. Rev. Phys. Chem. 43, 437–463.
Durán, N., Marcato, P.D., 2013. Nanobiotechnology perspectives. Role of nanotechnology in the food industry: a review. Int. J. Food Sci. Technol. 48 (6), 1127–1134.
Erickson, B.E., 2002. Analyzing the ignored environmental contaminants. Environ. Sci. Technol. 36 (7), 140–145.
Eskenazi, B., Bradman, A., Castorina, R., 1999. Exposures of children to organophosphate pesticides and their potential adverse health effects. Environ. Health Perspect. 107 (Suppl February), 409–419.
Food and Agriculture Organization of the United Nations (FAO), 2003. Review of world water resources by country. 127.
FAO, 2007. Coping with Water Scarcity: Challenge of the Twenty-First Century. 1–29.
Fenik, J., Tankiewicz, M., Biziuk, M., 2011. Properties and determination of pesticides in fruits and vegetables. Trends Anal. Chem. 30 (6), 814–826.
Firdoz, S., Ma, F., Yue, X., Dai, Z., Kumar, A., Jiang, B., 2010. A novel amperometric biosensor based on single walled carbon nanotubes with acetylcholine esterase for the detection of carbaryl pesticide in water. Talanta 83 (1), 269–273.
Flint, S., Markle, T., Thompson, S., Wallace, E., 2012. Bisphenol A exposure, effects, and policy: a wildlife perspective. J. Environ. Manage. 104, 19–34.
Food and Agriculture Organization of the United Nations (FAO), 1996. Control of Water Pollution from Agriculture. 101.
Food and Agriculture Organization of the United Nations (FAO), 2015. Aquastat—Water withdrawal by sector, around 2007. Available from: http://www.fao.org/nr/water/aquastat/tables/WorldData-Withdrawal_eng.pdf
Gammoudi, I., Blanc, L., Moroté, F., Grauby-Heywang, C., Boissière, C., Kalfat, R., Rebière, D., Cohen-Bouhacina, T., Dejous, C., 2014. High sensitive mesoporous TiO_2-coated love wave device for heavy metal detection. Biosens. Bioelectron. 57, 162–170.
Gevao, B., Semple, K.T., Jones, K.C., 2000. Bound pesticide residues in soils: a review. Environ. Pollut. 108 (1), 3–14.
Ghiselli, G., Jardim, W.F., 2007. Interferentes endócrinos no ambiente. Quim. Nova 30 (3), 695–706.
González, S., López-Roldán, R., Cortina, J.L., 2012. Presence and biological effects of emerging contaminants in Llobregat River basin: a review. Environ. Pollut. 161, 83–92.

Gopinath, P.G., Mastani, S.A., Anitha, V.R., 2014. MEMS microcantilevers sensor modes of operation and transduction principles. Int. J. Comput. Eng. Sci. 4 (2), 1–11.

Grieshaber, D., MacKenzie, R., Vörös, J., Reimhult, E., 2008. Electrochemical biosensors—sensor principles and architectures. Sensors 8 (3), 1400–1458.

Grønhaug Halvorsen, T., Pedersen-Bjergaard, S., Rasmussen, K.E., 2001. Reduction of extraction times in liquid-phase microextraction. J. Chromatogr. B Biomed. Sci. Appl. 760 (2), 219–226.

Gruber, K., Horlacher, T., Castelli, R., Mader, A., Seeberger, P.H., Hermann, B.A., 2011. Cantilever array sensors detect specific carbohydrate-protein interactions with picomolar sensitivity. ACS Nano 5 (5), 3670–3678.

Gupta, V.K., Yola, M.L., Eren, T., Atar, N., 2015. Selective QCM sensor based on atrazine imprinted polymer: its application to wastewater sample. Sens. Act. B Chem. 218, 215–221.

Haddaoui, M., Raouafi, N., 2015. Chlortoluron-induced enzymatic activity inhibition in tyrosinase/ZnO NPs/SPCE biosensor for the detection of ppb levels of herbicide. Sens. Act. B Chem. 219, 171–178.

Halvorsen, T.G., Pedersen-Bjergaard, S., Rasmussen, K.E., 2001. Liquid-phase microextraction and capillary electrophoresis of citalopram, an antidepressant drug. J. Chromatogr. A 909 (1), 87–93.

Hansen, K.M., Ji, H.F., Wu, G., Datar, R., Cote, R., Majumdar, A., Thundat, T., 2001. Cantilever-based optical deflection assay for discrimination of DNA single-nucleotide mismatches. Anal. Chem. 73 (7), 1567–1571.

Harnpicharnchai, K., Chaiear, N., Charerntanyarak, L., 2013. Residues of organophosphate pesticides used in vegetable cultivation in ambient air, surface water and soil in Bueng Niam Subdistrict, Khon Kaen, Thailand. Southeast Asian J. Trop. Med. Public Health 44 (6), 1088–1097.

Hasan, Z., Jeon, J., Jhung, S.H., 2012. Adsorptive removal of naproxen and clofibric acid from water using metal-organic frameworks. J. Hazard. Mater. 209-210, 151–157.

Health Canada, 1995. Approach to the Derivation of Drinking Water Guidelines. Heal. Environ. Consum. Saf. Branch.

Health Canada, 2014. Guidelines for Canadian Drinking Water Quality—Summary Table. Water and Air Quality Bureau. Heal. Environ. Consum. Saf. Branch, 1–15.

Helbling, D.E., 2015. Bioremediation of pesticide-contaminated water resources: the challenge of low concentrations. Curr. Opin. Biotechnol. 33, 142–148.

Hernández, A.F., Parrón, T., Tsatsakis, A.M., Requena, M., Alarcón, R., López-Guarnido, O., 2013. Toxic effects of pesticide mixtures at a molecular level: their relevance to human health. Toxicology 307, 136–145.

Hleli, S., Martelet, C., Abdelghani, A., Burais, N., Jaffrezic-Renault, N., 2006. Atrazine analysis using an impedimetric immunosensor based on mixed biotinylated self-assembled monolayer. Sens. Act. B Chem. 113 (2), 711–717.

Ho, T.S., Pedersen-Bjergaard, S., Rasmussen, K.E., 2002a. Liquid-phase microextraction of protein-bound drugs under non-equilibrium conditions. Analyst 127 (5), 608–613.

Ho, T.S., Pedersen-Bjergaard, S., Rasmussen, K.E., 2002b. Recovery, enrichment and selectivity in liquid-phase microextraction: comparison with conventional liquid-liquid extraction. J. Chromatogr. A 963 (1–2), 3–17.

Ho, T.S., Vasskog, T., Anderssen, T., Jensen, E., Rasmussen, K.E., Pedersen-Bjergaard, S., 2007. 25,000-Fold pre-concentration in a single step with liquid-phase microextraction. Anal. Chim. Acta 592 (1), 1–8.

Holt, M.S., 2000. Sources of chemical contaminants and routes into the freshwater environment. Food Chem. Toxicol. 38 (1), 21–27.

Hou, L., Shen, G., Lee, H.K., 2003. Automated hollow fiber-protected dynamic liquid-phase microextraction of pesticides for gas chromatography-mass spectrometric analysis. J. Chromatogr. A 985 (1–2), 107–116.
IUPAC, 1997. biosensor. in:IUPAC Compendium of Chemical Terminology. Research Triagle Park, NC: IUPAC.
Järup, L., 2003. Hazards of heavy metal contamination. Br. Med. Bull. 68, 167–182.
Jauvert, E., Dague, E., Séverac, M., Ressier, L., Caminade, A.M., Majoral, J.P., Trévisiol, E., 2012. Probing single molecule interactions by AFM using bio-functionalized dendritips. Sens. Act. B Chem. 168, 436–441.
Jeannot, M.A., Cantwell, F.F., 1996. Solvent microextraction into a single drop. Anal. Chem. 68 (13), 2236–2240.
Ji, X., Zheng, J., Xu, J., Rastogi, V.K., Cheng, T., Defrank, J.J., Leblanc, R.M., 2005. (CdSe) ZnS quantum dots and organophosphorus hydrolase bioconjugate as biosensors for detection of paraoxon. J. Phys. Chem. 109, 3793–3799.
Jönsson, J.Å., Mathiasson, L., 1999. Liquid membrane extraction in analytical sample preparation. Trends Anal. Chem. 18 (5), 325–334.
Jung, C., Son, A., Her, N., Zoh, K.-D., Cho, J., Yoon, Y., 2015. Removal of endocrine disrupting compounds, pharmaceuticals, and personal care products in water using carbon nanotubes: a review. J. Ind. Eng. Chem. 27, 1–11.
Karnati, C., Du, H., Ji, H.F., Xu, X., Lvov, Y., Mulchandani, A., Mulchandani, P., Chen, W., 2007. Organophosphorus hydrolase multilayer modified microcantilevers for organophosphorus detection. Biosens. Bioelectron. 22 (11), 2636–2642.
Kaur, J., Singh, K.V., Schmid, A.H., Varshney, G.C., Suri, C.R., Raje, M., 2004. Atomic force spectroscopy-based study of antibody pesticide interactions for characterization of immunosensor surface. Biosens. Bioelectron. 20 (2), 284–293.
Kaur, J., Boro, R.C., Wangoo, N., Singh, K.R., Suri, C.R., 2008. Direct hapten coated immunoassay format for the detection of atrazine and 2,4-dichlorophenoxyacetic acid herbicides. Anal. Chim. Acta 607 (1), 92–99.
Khaksarinejad, R., Mohsenifar, A., Rahmani-Cherati, T., Karami, R., Tabatabaei, M., 2015. An organophosphorus hydrolase-based biosensor for direct detection of paraoxon using silica-coated magnetic nanoparticles. Appl. Biochem. Biotechnol. 176 (2), 359–371.
Khraisheh, M., Kim, J., Campos, L., Al-Muhtaseb, A.H., Al-Hawari, A., Al Ghouti, M., Walker, G.M., 2014. Removal of pharmaceutical and personal care products (PPCPs) pollutants from water by novel TiO2-Coconut Shell Powder (TCNSP) composite. J. Ind. Eng. Chem. 20 (3), 979–987.
Kosikowska, M., Biziuk, M., 2010. Review of the determination of pesticide residues in ambient air. Trends Anal. Chem. 29 (9), 1064–1072.
Kumar, A., Gaurav, Malik, A.K., Tewary, D.K., Singh, B., 2008. A review on development of solid phase microextraction fibers by sol–gel methods and their applications. Anal. Chim. Acta 610 (1), 1–14.
Kuo, C.P., Shiea, J., 1999. Application of direct electrospray probe to analyze biological compounds and to couple to solid-phase microextraction to detect trace surfactants in aqueous solution. Anal. Chem. 71 (19), 4413–4417.
la Farré, M., Pérez, S., Kantiani, L., Barceló, D., 2008. Fate and toxicity of emerging pollutants, their metabolites and transformation products in the aquatic environment. Trends Anal. Chem. 27 (11), 991–1007.
Lambropoulou, D.A., Albanis, T.A., 2005. Application of hollow fiber liquid phase microextraction for the determination of insecticides in water. J. Chromatogr. A 1072 (1), 55–61.
Lang, H.P., Hegner, M., Meyer, E., Gerber, C., 2002. Nanomechanics from atomic resolution to molecular recognition based on atomic force microscopy technology. Nanotechnology 13 (5), R29–R36.

Lang, H., Hegner, M., Gerber, C., 2007. Nanomechanical Cantilever Array Sensors. Springer Handbook of Nanotechnology. Springer Berlin Heidelberg, Berlin, Heidelberg, pp. 443–460.

Lapworth, D.J., Baran, N., Stuart, M.E., Ward, R.S., 2012. Emerging organic contaminants in groundwater: a review of sources, fate and occurrence. Environ. Pollut. 163, 287–303.

LeDoux, M., 2011. Analytical methods applied to the determination of pesticide residues in foods of animal origin. A review of the past two decades. J. Chromatogr. A 1218 (8), 1021–1036.

Lee, H.S., Kim, Y.A., Chung, D.H., Lee, Y.T., 2001. Determination of carbamate pesticides by a cholinesterase-based flow injection biosensor. Int. J. Food Sci. Technol. 36 (3), 263–269

Lei, Y., Chen, W., Mulchandani, A., 2006. Microbial biosensors. Anal. Chim. Acta 568 (1–2), 200–210.

Leite, F.L., Borato, C.E., Da Silva, W.T.L., Herrmann, P.S.P., Oliveira, O.N., Mattoso, L.H.C., 2007. Atomic force spectroscopy on poly(o-ethoxyaniline) nanostructured films: sensing nonspecific interactions. Microsc. Microanal. 13 (4), 304–312.

Li, G., Zhang, L., Zhang, Z., 2008. Determination of polychlorinated biphenyls in water using dynamic hollow fiber liquid-phase microextraction and gas chromatography-mass spectrometry. J. Chromatogr. A 1204 (1), 119–122.

Li, S., Lu, C., Zhu, F., Jiang, R., Ouyang, G., 2015. Preparation of C18 composite solid-phase microextraction fiber and its application to the determination of organochlorine pesticides in water samples. Anal. Chim. Acta 873, 57–62.

Lin, T.J., Huang, K.T., Liu, C.Y., 2006. Determination of organophosphorous pesticides by a novel biosensor based on localized surface plasmon resonance. Biosens. Bioelectron. 22, 513–518.

Lin, Y.C., Chien, G.P.C., Chiang, P.C., Chen, W.H., Lin, Y.C., 2013a. Multivariate analysis of heavy metal contaminations in seawater.pdf. Mar. Pollut. Bull. 76, 266–275.

Lin, Z., He, Q., Wang, L., Wang, X., Dong, Q., Huang, C., 2013b. Preparation of magnetic multi-functional molecularly imprinted polymer beads for determining environmental estrogens in water samples. J. Hazard. Mater. 252-253, 57–63.

Lindstrom, A.B., Strynar, M.J., Libelo, E.L., 2011. Polyfluorinated compounds: past, present, and future. Environ. Sci. Technol. 45, 7954–7961.

Liu, H., Dasgupta, P.K., 1996. Analytical chemistry in a drop. Solvent extraction in a microdrop. Anal. Chem. 68 (11), 1817–1821.

Liu, C., Bai, R., San Ly, Q., 2008. Selective removal of copper and lead ions by diethylenetriamine-functionalized adsorbent: behaviors and mechanisms. Water Res. 42 (6–7), 1511–1522.

Liu, J., Zhang, X.H., Tran, H., Wang, D.Q., Zhu, Y.N., 2011. Heavy metal contamination and risk assessment in water, paddy soil, and rice around an electroplating plant. Environ. Sci. Pollut. Res. 18 (9), 1623–1632.

Malik, P., Katyal, V., Malik, V., Asatkar, A., Inwati, G., Mukherjee, T.K., 2013. Nanobiosensors: Concepts and Variations. ISRN Nanomater. 2013, 9 p.

Matamoros, V., Arias, C.A., Nguyen, L.X., Salvadó, V., Brix, H., 2012. Occurrence and behavior of emerging contaminants in surface water and a restored wetland. Chemosphere 88 (9), 1083–1089.

Matić, I., Grujić, S., Jauković, Z., Laušević, M., 2014. Trace analysis of selected hormones and sterols in river sediments by liquid chromatography-atmospheric pressure chemical ionization–tandem mass spectrometry. J. Chromatogr. A 1364, 117–127.

Mohammadi, A., Ameli, A., Alizadeh, N., 2009. Headspace solid-phase microextraction using a dodecylsulfate-doped polypyrrole film coupled to ion mobility spectrometry for the simultaneous determination of atrazine and ametryn in soil and water samples. Talanta 78 (3), 1107–1114.

Moraes, F.C., Rossi, B., Donatoni, M.C., de Oliveira, K.T., Pereira, E.C., 2015. Sensitive determination of 17β-estradiol in river water using a graphene based electrochemical sensor. Anal. Chim. Acta 881, 37–43.

Mostafalou, S., 2012. Concerns of environmental persistence of pesticides and human chronic diseases. Clin. Exp. Pharmacol. 01 (S5), 10–11.

Mostafalou, S., Abdollahi, M., 2013. Pesticides and human chronic diseases: evidences, mechanisms, and perspectives. Toxicol. Appl. Pharmacol. 268 (2), 157–177.

Murray, K.E., Thomas, S.M., Bodour, A.A., 2010. Prioritizing research for trace pollutants and emerging contaminants in the freshwater environment. Environ. Pollut. 158 (12), 3462–3471.

Neves Dias, A., Simão, V., Merib, J., Carasek, E., 2015. Use of green coating (cork) in solid-phase microextraction for the determination of organochlorine pesticides in water by gas chromatography-electron capture detection. Talanta 134, 409–414.

Novoselov, K.S., Geim, A.K., Morozov, S.V., Jiang, D., Zhang, Y., Dubonos, S.V., Grigorieva, I.V., Firsov, A.A., 2004. Electric field effect in atomically thin carbon films. Science 306 (5696), 666–669.

Oliveira, T.S., Murphy, M., Mendola, N., Wong, V., Carlson, D., Waring, L., 2015. Characterization of Pharmaceuticals and Personal Care products in hospital effluent and waste water influent/effluent by direct-injection LC-MS-MS. Sci. Total Environ. 518-519, 459–478.

Onesios, K.M., Yu, J.T., Bouwer, E.J., 2009. Biodegradation and removal of pharmaceuticals and personal care products in treatment systems: a review. Biodegradation 20 (4), 441–466.

Ozay, O., Ekici, S., Baran, Y., Aktas, N., Sahiner, N., 2009. Removal of toxic metal ions with magnetic hydrogels. Water Res. 43 (17), 4403–4411.

Pai-Shan, C., Shang-Da, H., 2006. Determination of ethoprop, diazinon, disulfoton and fenthion using dynamic hollow fiber-protected liquid-phase microextraction coupled with gas chromatography–mass spectrometry. Talanta 69 (3), 669–675.

Pal, A., Gin, K.Y.H., Lin, A.Y.C., Reinhard, M., 2010. Impacts of emerging organic contaminants on freshwater resources: review of recent occurrences, sources, fate and effects. Sci. Total Environ. 408 (24), 6062–6069.

Pal, A., He, Y., Jekel, M., Reinhard, M., Gin, K.Y.H., 2014. Emerging contaminants of public health significance as water quality indicator compounds in the urban water cycle. Environ. Int. 71, 46–62.

Pedersen-Bjergaard, S., Rasmussen, K.E., 1999. Liquid–liquid–liquid microextraction for sample preparation of biological fluids prior to capillary electrophoresis. Anal. Chem. 71 (14), 2650–2656.

Pedersen-Bjergaard, S., Rasmussen, K.E., 2000. Liquid-phase microextraction and capillary electrophoresis of acidic drugs. Electrophoresis 21 (3), 579–585.

Pedersen-Bjergaard, S., Rasmussen, K.E., 2008. Liquid-phase microextraction with porous hollow fibers, a miniaturized and highly flexible format for liquid-liquid extraction. J. Chromatogr. A 1184 (1–2), 132–142.

Pesek, J.J., Matyska, M.T., 1997. Methods for the modification and characterization of oxide surfaces. Interface Sci. 5 (2/3), 103–117.

Pimentel, D., 2005. Environmental and economic costs of the application of pesticides primarily in the United States. Environ. Dev. Sustain. 7 (2), 229–252.

Prasad, B.B., Jauhari, D., 2015. A dual-template biomimetic molecularly imprinted dendrimer-based piezoelectric sensor for ultratrace analysis of organochlorine pesticides. Sens. Act. B Chem. 207, 542–551.

Pr˘ibyl, J., Hepel, M., Halámek, J., Skládal, P., 2003. Development of piezoelectric immunosensors for competitive and direct determination of atrazine. Sens. Act. B Chem. 91 (1–3), 333–341.

Psillakis, E., Kalogerakis, N., 2003. Developments in liquid-phase microextraction. Trends Anal. Chem. 22 (9), 565–574.

Raiteri, R., Nelles, G., Butt, H.-J., Knoll, W., Skadal, P., 1999. Sensing of biological substances based on the bending of microfabricated cantilevers. Sens. Act. B Chem. 61 (1–3), 213–217.

Raiteri, R., Grattarola, M., Butt, H.J., Skládal, P., 2001. Micromechanical cantilever-based biosensors. Sens. Act. B Chem. 79 (2–3), 115–126.

Raman Suri, C., Kaur, J., Gandhi, S., Shekhawat, G.S., 2008. Label-free ultra-sensitive detection of atrazine based on nanomechanics. Nanotechnology 19 (23), 235502.

Rand, G., Wells, P., McCarty, L., 1995. Introduction to aquatic toxicology. In: Rand, G.M. (Ed.), Fundamentals of aquatic toxicology: Effects, environmental fate, and risk assessment. Publishing Taylor & Francis, London, pp. 3–66.

Rasmussen, K.E., Pedersen-Bjergaard, S., Krogh, M., Ugland, H.G., Grønhaug, T., 2000. Development of a simple in-vial liquid-phase microextraction device for drug analysis compatible with capillary gas chromatography, capillary electrophoresis and high-performance liquid chromatography. J. Chromatogr. A 873 (1), 3–11.

Ricciardi, C., Castagna, R., Ferrante, I., Frascella, F., Luigi Marasso, S., Ricci, A., Canavese, G., Lorè, A., Prelle, A., Lodovica Gullino, M., Spadaro, D., 2013. Development of a microcantilever-based immunosensing method for mycotoxin detection. Biosens. Bioelectron. 40 (1), 233–239.

Richardson, S.D., 2003. Disinfection by-products and other emerging contaminants in drinking water. Trends Anal. Chem. 22 (10), 666–684.

Rissato, S.R., Galhiane, M.S., Apon, B.M., Arruda, M.S.P., 2005. Multiresidue analysis of pesticides in soil by supercritical fluid extraction/gas chromatography with electron-capture detection and confirmation by gas chromatography – mass spectrometry. J. Agric. Food Chem. 53 (1), 62–69.

Rosa, A., Quidute, P., Magalhães, R., Júnior, M., 2010. Contaminantes ambientais e os interferentes endócrinos. Arq. Bras. Endocrinol Metab. 54 (1), 6–16.

Rosal, R., Rodríguez, A., Perdigón-Melón, J.A., Petre, A., García-Calvo, E., Gómez, M.J., Agüera, A., Fernández-Alba, A.R., 2010. Occurrence of emerging pollutants in urban wastewater and their removal through biological treatment followed by ozonation. Water Res. 44 (2), 578–588.

Rumayour, V.G., Iglesias, E.G., Galán, O.R., 2005. Aplicaciones de Biosensores en la Industria Agroalimentaria. Elecé Indutria Grafica, Madrid.

Rye, R.R., Nelson, G.C., Dugger, M.T., 1997. Mechanistic aspects of alkylchlorosilane coupling reactions. Langmuir 13 (11), 2965–2972.

Sassolas, A., 2012. Biosensors for pesticide detection: new trends. Am. J. Anal. Chem. 3, 210–232.

Sauvé, S., Desrosiers, M., 2014. A review of what is an emerging contaminant. Chem. Cent. J. 8 (1), 8–15.

Shen, G., Hian, K.L., 2002. Hollow fiber-protected liquid-phase microextraction of triazine herbicides. Anal. Chem. 74 (3), 648–654.

Shiklomanov, I.A., Rodda, J.C., 2003. World Water Resources at the Beginning of the Twenty-First Century. Internatio. Hydrol. Series. Cambridge University Press, New York.

Sibiya, P., Cukrowska, E., Jönsson, J.Å., Chimuka, L., 2013. Hollow-fibre liquid-phase microextraction for the determination of polycyclic aromatic hydrocarbons in Johannesburg Jukskei River, South Africa. Chromatographia 76 (7–8), 427–436.

Sierakowski, A., Kopiec, D., Janus, P., Ekwińska, M., Płuska, M., Grabiec, P., Gotszalk, T., 2014. Piezoresistive cantilever working in a shear force mode for in situ characterization of exposed micro- and nanostructures. Meas. Sci. Technol. 25 (4), 044018.

Sinclair, C.J., Boxall, A.B.A., Parsons, S.A., Thomas, M.R., 2006. Prioritization of pesticide environmental transformation products in drinking water supplies. Environ. Sci. Technol. 40 (23), 7283–7289.

Somashekar, K.M., Mahima, M.R., Manjunath, K.C., 2015. Contamination of water sources in mysore city by pesticide residues and plasticizer—a cause of health concern. Aquat. Procedia 4, 1181–1188.

Songa, E.a., Somerset, V.S., Waryo, T., Baker, P.G.L., Iwuoha, E.I., 2009a. Amperometric nanobiosensor for quantitative determination of glyphosate and glufosinate residues in corn samples. Pure Appl. Chem. 81 (1), 123–139.

Songa, E.A., Waryo, T., Jahed, N., Baker, P.G.L., Kgarebe, B.V., Iwuoha, E.I., 2009b. Electrochemical nanobiosensor for glyphosate herbicide and its metabolite. Electroanalysis 21 (3–5), 671–674.

Stanford, B.D., Snyder, S.A., Trenholm, R.A., Holady, J.C., Vanderford, B.J., 2010. Estrogenic activity of US drinking waters: a relative exposure comparison. J. Am. Water Work. Assoc. 102 (11), 55–65.

Steffens, C., Leite, F.L., Bueno, C.C., Manzoli, A., Herrmann, P.S.P., 2012. Atomic Force Microscopy as a tool applied to nano/biosensors. Sensors 12 (6), 8278–8300.

Steffens, C., Leite, F.L., Manzoli, A., Sandoval, R.D., Fatibello, O., Herrmann, P.S.P., 2014a. Microcantilever sensors coated with doped polyaniline for the detection of water vapor. Scanning 36 (3), 311–316.

Steffens, C., Manzoli, A., Oliveira, J.E., Leite, F.L., Correa, D.S., Herrmann, P.S.P., 2014b. Bio-inspired sensor for insect pheromone analysis based on polyaniline functionalized AFM cantilever sensor. Sens. Act. B Chem. 191, 643–649.

Švorc, Ľ., Rievaj, M., Bustin, D., 2013. Green electrochemical sensor for environmental monitoring of pesticides: Determination of atrazine in river waters using a boron-doped diamond electrode. Sens. Act. B Chem. 181, 294–300.

Tamayo, J., Kosaka, P.M., Ruz, J.J., San Paulo, Á., Calleja, M., 2013. Biosensors based on nanomechanical systems. Chem. Soc. Rev. 42 (3), 1287–1311.

Tang, Y., Fang, J., Xu, X., Ji, H.F., Brown, G.M., Thundat, T., 2004. Detection of femtomolar concentrations of HF using an SiO_2 microcantilever. Anal. Chem. 76 (9), 2478–2481.

Tang, W., Zhao, Y., Wang, C., Shan, B., Cui, J., 2013. Heavy metal contamination of overlying waters and bed sediments of Haihe Basin in China. Ecotoxicol. Environ. Saf. 98, 317–323.

Tankiewicz, M., Fenik, J., Biziuk, M., 2011. Solventless and solvent-minimized sample preparation techniques for determining currently used pesticides in water samples: a review. Talanta 86 (1), 8–22.

Thakur, S., Kumar, P., Reddy, M.V., Siddavattam, D., Paul, A.K., 2013. Enhancement in sensitivity of fluorescence based assay for organophosphates detection by silica coated silver nanoparticles using organophosphate hydrolase. Sens. Act. B Chem. 178, 458–464.

Theodoridis, G., Koster, E.H., Jong, G.J., 2000. Solid-phase microextraction for the analysis of biological samples. J. Chromatogr. B. Biomed. Sci. Appl. 745 (1), 49–82.

Thévenot, D.R., Toth, K., Durst, R.A., Wilson, G.S., 1996. International union of pure and applied chemistry physical chemistry division, steering committee on biophysical chemistry analytical chemistry division, commission V.5 (electroanalytical chemistry) Electrochemical biosensors: proposed definitions and classification Synopsis of the report. Sens. Act. B Chem. 30 (1), 81.

Ugland, H.G., Krogh, M., Rasmussen, K.E., 2000. Liquid-phase microextraction as a sample preparation technique prior to capillary gas chromatographic-determination of benzodiazepines in biological matrices. J. Chromatogr. B Biomed. Sci. Appl. 749 (1), 85–92.

Unal, F., Yüzbaşıoğlu, D., Yılmaz, S., Akıncı, N., Aksoy, H., 2011. Genotoxic effects of chlorophenoxy herbicide diclofop-methyl in mice in vivo and in human lymphocytes in vitro. Drug Chem. Toxicol. 34 (4), 390–395.

Unep, 2012. Environment for the future we want. Progress Press LTD, Valletta.

United States Geological Survey (USGS), 2014. The Water Cycle. Available from: http://water.usgs.gov/edu/watercycleportuguese.html

UN-Water, 2007. Coping with Water Scarcity: Challenge of the Twenty-First Century, Rome, Italy. Available from: http://www.fao.org/nr/water/docs/escarcity.pdf

United States Census Bureau (USCB), 2013. International Data Base Population Estimates and Projections Methodology. Available at: Unep, 2012. Environment for the future we want. Available from: http://www.census.gov/population/international/data/worldpop/table_population.php

Valera, E., Ramón-Azcón, J., Sanchez, F.J., Marco, M.P., Rodríguez, Á., 2008. Conductimetric immunosensor for atrazine detection based on antibodies labelled with gold nanoparticles. Sens. Act. B Chem. 134 (1), 95–103.

Vamvakaki, V., Chaniotakis, N.A., 2007. Pesticide detection with a liposome-based nano-biosensor. Biosens. Bioelectron. 22 (12), 2848–2853.

Vargas-Bernal, R., Rodríguez-Miranda, E., Herrera-Pérez, G., 2012. Evolution and expectations of enzymatic biosensors for pesticides. In: Soundararajan, R.P. (Ed.), Pestices—Advances in Chemical and Botanical Pesticides. Intech, pp. 329–356.

Wang, J., 2005. Nanomaterial-based amplified transduction of biomolecular interactions. Small1 (11), 1036–1043.

Weetall, H.H., Detar, C.C., 1975. Covalent attachment of proteins to inorganic supports directly by activation with cyanogen bromide. Biotechnol. Bioeng. 17, 295–297.

Wen, Y., Niu, Z., Ma, Y., Ma, J., Chen, L., 2014. Graphene oxide-based microspheres for the dispersive solid-phase extraction of non-steroidal estrogens from water samples. J. Chromatogr. A 1368, 18–25.

Wilson, R., Barker, M.H., Schiffrin, D.J., Abuknesha, R., 1997. Electrochemiluminescence flow injection immunoassay for atrazine. Biosens. Bioelectron. 12 (4), 277–286.

Wu, Q., Feng, C., Zhao, G., Wang, C., Wang, Z., 2012. Graphene-coated fiber for solid-phase microextraction of triazine herbicides in water samples. J. Sep. Sci. 35 (2), 193–199.

Xu, Y., Li, Z., Duan, W., 2014. Thermal and Thermoelectric Properties of Graphene. Small 10 (11), 2182–2199.

Yaqub, S., Latif, U., Dickert, F.L., 2011. Plastic antibodies as chemical sensor material for atrazine detection. Sens. Act. B Chem. 160 (1), 227–233.

Zhang, H., Lee, H.K., 2011. Plunger-in-needle solid-phase microextraction with graphene-based sol-gel coating as sorbent for determination of polybrominated diphenyl ethers. J. Chromatogr. A 1218 (28), 4509–4516.

Zhang, X., Guo, Q., Cui, D., 2009. Recent advances in nanotechnology applied to biosensors. Sensors 9 (2), 1033–1053.

Zhang, W., Tang, Y., Du, D., Smith, J., Timchalk, C., Liu, D., Lin, Y., 2013. Direct analysis of trichloropyridinol in human saliva using an Au nanoparticles-based immunochromatographic test strip for biomonitoring of exposure to chlorpyrifos. Talanta 114, 261–267.

Zhang, Y., Arugula, M.a., Wales, M., Wild, J., Simonian, A.L., 2015. A novel layer-by-layer assembled multi-enzyme/CNT biosensor for discriminative detection between organophosphorus and non-organophosphrus pesticides. Biosens. Bioelectron. 67, 287–295.

Zhao, L., Lee, H.K., 2002. Liquid-phase microextraction combined with hollow fiber as a sample preparation technique prior to gas chromatography/mass spectrometry. Anal. Chem. 74 (11), 2486–2492.

Zhao, R.S., Liu, Y.L., Chen, X.F., Yuan, J.P., Bai, A.Y., Zhou, J.B., 2013. Preconcentration and determination of polybrominated diphenyl ethers in environmental water samples by solid-phase microextraction with Fe_3O_4-coated bamboo charcoal fibers prior to gas chromatography-mass spectrometry. Anal. Chim. Acta 769, 65–71.

Ziegler, C., 2004. Cantilever-based biosensors. Anal. Bioanal. Chem. 379 (7–8), 946–959.

17

CHEMICAL SENSORS FOR SOIL ANALYSIS: PRINCIPLES AND APPLICATIONS

Larisa Lvova*, Marina Nadporozhskaya**

**University "Tor Vergata," Department of Chemical Science and Technologies, Rome, Italy; **St. Petersburg State University, Faculty of Biology, St. Petersburg, Russia*

1 Introduction

1.1 Soil Definition, Brief Description of Soil Functions, Sustainable Management of Soils

The soil is a complicated object to study and evaluate. One of the soil definitions accepted in classical Russian soil science begins with the words "soil is the especial natural body ....". The peculiarity of soil is in its spatial and temporal heterogeneity and multiplicity of forming factors, which often can influence different directions and lead to different results. The spatial heterogeneity caused by varying the parent geological rocks, vegetation, relief changes, animals, and human activity. Temporal heterogeneity can demonstrate itself in short intervals during long periods, noted by scientific and poetic figurative terms (Targulian and Goryachkin, 2008). Soil has properties that change rapidly within a few hours or days. In figurative terms, this is called the "soil-moment." On the other hand, soil may keep some properties for a long time—years and centuries—holding traces of past influences. This is called the "soil memory." There is no doubt that for environmental monitoring of a particular object, such as soil, for its economic management, for planning measures for the soil protection, reclamation, and rehabilitation, the new methods—fast, relatively inexpensive, and suitable for mass analysis—are required. To measure properly the soil physical characteristics and chemical properties, and to plan the field and laboratory works and data processing, it is necessary to find the most corresponding definition to such a complex object.

New Pesticides and Soil Sensors. http://dx.doi.org/10.1016/B978-0-12-804299-1.00018-7

What is soil? Many definitions of soil were formulated over more than one century of soil science. Some definitions emphasized the description of soil as a natural object carrying fertility. Others take into account the possibility of mathematical simulation and determine the soil as a function of soil-forming factors. Still others emphasize systematic and hierarchical structure of the soil. On the basis of these multiple and diverse determinations we have compiled the determination of the soil, in our opinion, the most satisfying goals of environmental research to nature conservation, as follows: "Soil is the complex three-phase multifunctional open system formed during the time in the surface crust of weathering rocks due to an interaction of the parent mineral materials with organisms under impact of climate and anthropogenic activity and modifying by the landform."

The advantage of this definition is in the proclamation of the soil as the system, that is, a set of functionally corelated elements. This allows the analysis of soil, based on the theory of the benefits system unity, with an understanding of the complexity and hierarchy of the device in soil systems. It is significant that the soil system is the dynamics and developing system. Natural soils are changed by human activities and can be transformed totally and can keep the new properties (not always helpful to maintain the stability of life) for a long time. At this point, the soils are nonrenewable natural resources at the human time scale.

The European Soil Charter of 1972, adopted by the Council of Europe, for the first time had accepted that any biological, physical, or chemical degradation of the soil should be recognized as the primary ecological hazard (www.eusoils.jrc.ec.europa.eu; Soil Atlas of Europe, 2005). In this case, measures to restore and protect the soil must be taken immediately. Pedosphere in contrast to the atmosphere and hydrosphere is the more conservative form. Soil can accumulate and store all types of pollutants for a long time, and later, after exceeding the critical loads, irremediably collapse. Contaminants reside in soil much longer than in air and water, so the effects of the mobilization can be hidden for a long time. Private ownership of the soil is also an important factor, which makes it difficult to monitor and protect the object.

It is important to remember that soil is not the only particularly complex system, but it is a fundamental part of any terrestrial ecosystem and it performs important functions. The term "functions of soil " generally means the general capabilities of soil or its main roles played in terrestrial ecosystems, which are important for various areas of human activities (agriculture, forestry and municipal economy, mining), as well as for implementing environmental protection measures and rehabilitation of a disturbed landscape (Blum, 1990). Six basic soil functions are:

1. biomass production
2. biogeochemical barrier
3. buffer medium and the medium to transform chemical compounds
4. living environment of organisms and gene reservoir
5. the foundation techno-industrial and socio-cultural parts of human life
6. source of raw materials and historical environment

The last two functions are important in terms of technical, commercial, socio-economic, and cultural aspects of human activity. The first four are important for environmental features. Soils are nonrenewable resources and should be managed taking into account the need to maintain their ecological functions and specific characteristics peculiar to different soil types.

Ecological soil functions persisted for many centuries. In the early 20th century, accelerating socio-economic development of society stated to impact significantly on larger and larger territories. The development of industry, urbanization, and the increase in areas occupied by dumps and mining operations, the growth of agricultural lands were reasons for really large changes in natural ecosystems. Positive changes may be found in some cases. For example, the organization of city and suburban parks increases the local biological diversity. Terracing of slope territories leads to the creation of steadier natural-anthropogenic soil and vegetable complexes. But such cases are quite rare. More often, human activity leads to violation of soil functions and deterioration of soil properties. Violation of soil functions reduces the soil quality as bases of stability of ecosystems, their efficiency, and the ability to maintain quality of life. The first logical step to harmonize soils requires an assessment of soil suitability for certain systems of land use and parametrization of influences for the preservation of soil functions.

Modern global processes, such as population growth, urbanization, and climate variability, complicate the management of soil resources. Soils are increasingly being violated because of erosion, compaction, pollution, salinization, and sealing, the result of which may be a dehumification and loss of biodiversity, as well as the loss of or improper performance of some ecological functions.

The first logical step to harmonize soil use consists in an assessment of soil suitability for certain systems of land use and parameterization of the extent of influences for preservation of functions of soils.

A large spatial and temporal variability of soils complicates their research and protection. The soil diversity is formed due to differences in soil-forming factors: climate and geological origin, living organisms influence, time, and land-use history. Different soil types require different approaches when planning their economic use and protection. The also require different managements and protection measures.

For elemental environmental control and an assessment of the vulnerability degree of soils, the following minimum set of its properties was chosen: pH, portion of the grain size fraction less than 0.01 mm, mineralogical structure of clay fraction, soil texture, and total content and quality of soil organic matter (SOM). By this data, for example, a rough estimation of the area of soil vulnerable to the action of the main damaging factors was carried out in the first approximation (Fraters, 1994).

In short, there is an urgent need for better soil protection to secure irreplaceable soil-based services (Eswaran et al., 1993). According to the insurance hypothesis, declines in ecosystem functioning due to reduced biodiversity are more likely to occur under fluctuating, extreme, or rapidly changing environmental conditions. The depletion of biological diversity often leads to a decrease in the organic matter content in the soil. Other negative changes of soil properties can also cause dehumidification. Soil organic carbon (OC), the major component of SOM, is extremely important in all soil processes. Organic material in the soil is essentially derived from residual plant and animal material, synthesized by microbes, and decomposed under the influence of temperature, moisture, and ambient soil conditions. The annual rate of organic matter loss can vary greatly, depending on cultivation practices, the type of plant/crop cover, drainage status of the soil, and weather conditions. There are two groups of factors that influence inherent organic matter content: natural factors (climate, soil parent material, land cover and/or vegetation, and topography), and human-induced factors (land use, management, and degradation). Decline in SOM is one of the major threats defined within the Soil Thematic Strategy (www.esdac-catalog.jrc.ec.europa.eu/esdac_subthemes.jsp?DI=3). Other major threats to soils are: salinization, soil erosion, landslide, compaction, and contamination (www.ec.europa.eu/environment/soil/three_en.htm).

The European Commission wants to define a policy for the sustainable management of soils by adopting a legally binding Soil Framework Directive, such as exists for air and water. Scientific and technological knowledge on soil biodiversity and functioning in relation with the earlier-mentioned ecosystem services is required to reach this goal (www.eusoils.jrc.ec.europa.eu). The sustainable use of soil functions is not a scientific but a political issue. Scientists can only explain the detail of the causes and possible impacts of human activities on soil functions. Scientists can prepare the scenarios for the spatial and temporal harmonization in the cited six soil uses of the functions, excluding or minimizing some negative effects, for example, sealing, acidification, contamination or pollution, salinization, and others (Blum, 2005).

According to damaging impacts, soil quality monitoring is strongly required. The main components to monitor in soils are: SOM amount and composition, humic substances fractioning, main nutrients (C, N, P, K, Ca) and microelements (transition metals and other minor elements) content, physical–chemical parameters (pH, Ox–Red potential, porosity, humidity, etc.).

The standard methods of soil analysis include first, classical wet chemistry methods, and various instrumental methods, such as molecular emission spectrometry, atomic absorption spectrometry (AAS), nuclear magnetic resonance spectroscopy, high performance liquid chromatography (HPLC), and gas chromatography (GC) combined with mass spectrometry (MS). These methods are often complex due to the extraction and pretreatment processes involved; they are time- and effort-consuming, and require sophisticated and often expensive equipment and qualified personnel involvement.

Due to the historically extreme increase of damaged soil areas, and the natural soils heterogeneity and variability, the new techniques and methods for soil assessment are of critical interest. One of the ways of the modern environmental monitoring of soil may be the use of sensors: physical, biological (including bioassays), and chemical. Therefore, inexpensive chemical sensors, simple in fabrication and handling, provide notable sensitivity and rapid response time, and can be effective tools in soil analysis, because they may be employed for in-field analysis with no or minimum sample pretreatment, simultaneously measure several analytes, and provide the real-time results at reasonable costs. The control of soil components and conditions with sensors can permit an optimization of irrigation and fertilization management systems, effective soil utilization, mapping, and preservation. The description of different sensors types and the methods of their application for the soil analysis are discussed in this chapter. The works on sensory soil analysis performed in the past 15 years are reviewed and the critical analysis of the sensory approach is provided.

1.2 Sensors Involved in Soil Analysis

The general definition of sensor has undergone several changes. The Instrument Society of America defines a sensor as a device that provides a usable output in response to a specified measurand. The output is defined as an "electrical quantity" and measurand as a "physical quantity, property, or condition, which is measured" (ISA, 1975). This definition can be generalized by extending "electrical quantity" to any type of signal, such as mechanical and optical and extending "physical quantity, property, or condition which is measured" to those of nature—chemical and biochemical and so on (NMAB, 1995; Patranabis, 2004). According to the IUPAC recommendations of 1991, chemical sensor is "a device that transforms chemical information, ranging from the concentration of a specific sample component to total composition analysis, into an analytically useful signal" (Hulanichi et al., 1991). The chemical information mentioned earlier, may originate from a chemical reaction of the analyte or from a physical property of the system investigated. Lately, the so-called Cambridge definition of a chemical sensor was suggested. According to it, chemical sensors are miniaturized devices that can deliver real-time and online information on the presence of specific compounds or ions even in complex samples (Cammann et al., 1996). Sensors can be classified into physical, chemical, and biosensors. In soil analysis last two types are the most often employed.

Chemical sensors can be classified into electrochemical, gravimetric, and optical (Göpel et al., 1989). Two main classes of electrochemical sensors are potentiometric (static measurement of voltage at zero current) and voltammetric (dynamic measurement of current upon applied voltage) (Liu, 2000). Often, conductimetric sensors are also involved in soil analysis. These devices measure analyte conductivity and are based on Kohlrausch law, relating the conductance to the electrolyte concentration (Liu, 2000).

Gravimetric, or mass-sensitive sensors "transform the mass change at a specially modified surface into a change of a property of the support material" (Hulanichi et al., 1991). Mass sensors are often based on acoustic wave devices that vibrate at a certain frequency. The accumulation of the analyte on a piezoelectric substrate modified with chemically absorbent film causes the mass change on the surface that is directly proportional to the transducer resonant frequency variation. This relationship is given by Sauerbrey law (Sauerbrey, 1959). The two major types of mass sensors are bulk acoustic wave and surface acoustic wave called thus due to the type of propagation in crystal acoustic wave (NMAB, 1995). Quartz crystal microbalances sensors are the most often used construction of bulk acoustic wave.

Optical sensors rely on changes in the various light properties (photon radiation intensity) to detect the analyte of interest. The light intensity can be modulated by absorption, or the direction of wave propagation, or wavelength can be modulated by scattering, refraction, or reflection. The detected photons could be emitted by fluorescence, phosphorescence, or chemi-/bioluminescence. Each of these photon sources has a known relationship to a given chemical reaction, facilitating chemical sensing with high selectivity. Most often, optical chemical sensors are found in a fiber-optic arrangement. In this construction light is generated by a light-emitting diode or laser and is sent through the fiber, on the tip of which the sensing film is deposited. The reflected light can then be measured by a photodetector. The injection near the sensor, the reagent that reacts either chemically or biologically with the analyte can also be performed. The reaction products are detected to give an estimate of the initial analyte concentration. Lately the involvement of familiar optical devices (digital- and web-cameras) and image interpretation (often based on color differences) has been intensely utilized for different monitoring purposes, and soil analysis in particular (Motellier et al., 1995; Hung et al., 2010; Viscarra Rossel et al., 2008; Yokota et al., 2007).

In biosensors a biologically induced recognition event is converted into a usable (bio)chemical signal. Bioassays are biological tools for the determination of the effect (positive or adverse) of an analyzed substance or a mixture by quantifying that effect on living organisms (Farré et al., 2005). Biosensors and bioassays have been widely applied for soil bioassessment analysis (Magrisso et al., 2008).

In the following sections the sensory applications on the analysis of main soil nutrients, microelements, and pollutants, as far as different physico-chemical parameters are summarized. The last section is devoted to the multisensory approach employed to soil characterization. The main attention is gained to the analysis performed with chemical sensors of different types, and also other popular techniques, including bioassays and image processing discussed.

2 Sensory Analysis of Main Soil Nutrients

Besides carbon, the main constituent of SOM, the three most essential soil macronutrients that play a fundamental role in the balanced soil system formation are nitrogen, phosphorus, and potassium (N, P, K). These macronutrients are essential for soil stability and fertility, and play an important role in healthy plant growth. Nitrogen is fundamental in the chlorophyll synthesis and is an essential element of enzymatic proteins that catalyze and regulate the plant growth processes. It is present in SOM and in inorganic forms, such as nitrite (NO_2^-), nitrate (NO_3^-), and ammonia

(NH_4^+). Among them nitrate is the most stable and plant-available form. Phosphorous plays a significant role in root growth stimulation. It is present in soil mainly in the form of orthophosphate in pH range of 6.0–7.0, and this form is the most easily plant-available. The requirement of potassium for plant growth may be in quantities equivalent to and sometimes greater than nitrogen. Potassium regulates the water uptake, CO_2 exchange, is important in sugars production and transport, and also in enzymatic processes that enable photosynthesis.

The monitoring of these nutrient levels in soils provides useful information on actual soil conditions, permits to make a conclusion on the necessity of the fertilizers incorporation for agricultural crop production, and helps to avoid an uncontrolled addition of these substances leading to runoff of nutrients excess into surface and groundwater and causing an undesirable environmental damages. Moreover, information obtained in real time can permit design-intelligent soil mapping, irrigation, and fertilization management systems.

As earlier mentioned, the standard laboratory methods are powerful tools in soil analysis, but their use is not always possible due to pretreatment requirements, costly equipment, and the qualified technical support required. Moreover, these methods often provide results with a significant delay.

Sensory soil assessment would be an effective, low-cost, and convenient substitution to the standard laboratory techniques and wet chemistry methods. Despite the evident benefits, there are few reports on the systems to measure soil main nutrients, and even fewer works report the direct in-field or on-the-go soil analysis. Sinfield et al. (2010) have published a comprehensive overview on sensing technologies for nitrogen (N), phosphorous (P), and potassium (K) analysis in cultivated soils. In this review the macronutrient assessment technologies were categorized according to the target compound and the employed sensing approach (chemical, electrical, or optical). Lobsey et al. (2010) published a review of 34 publications on the application of 2 types of electrochemical sensors, ion-selective electrodes (ISEs), and ion-sensitive field effect transistors (ISFETs), for rapid in situ soil analysis. The limitations of this technology, especially for on-the-go proximal soil sensing are also discussed. Here we briefly summarize the previous works on soil sensory analysis and review the new research.

An in-depth study of the past 15-year publications shows that the chemical sensors in the soil analysis are mainly used for the determination of the individual components of the soil, mainly in the ionic form, and then were related to the total content of the analyte (e.g., total nitrogen, carbon, phosphorus, potassium, and so forth). Thus, total carbon (Plata et al., 2008), nitrate and total N (Artigas et al., 2003; Yagodina et al., 2000; Adamchuk et al., 2005; Birrell and Hummel, 2001; Price et al., 2003; Sethuramasamyraja et al., 2008), potassium (Ciesla et al., 2007; Lemos et al., 2004; Kim et al., 2007), phosphates and phosphorous (Zou et al., 2007; Lemos et al., 2009), calcium (Artigas et al., 2001a,b; Lemos et al., 2007), several metals (McGraw et al., 2008; Nedeltcheva et al., 2005; Wilson et al., 2010; Md Noh and Tothill, 2006; Singh et al., 2014; Md Noh et al., 2005; Kopylovich et al., 2011), and pH (Staggenborg et al., 2007; Silva and Molin, 2013) sensors for analysis in soil were reported. Indirect determination of soil components, such as inorganic phosphates (Engblom, 1999), and various forms of alumina (Garotti et al., 1992) using cobalt- and fluoride-selective electrodes, respectively, also have been suggested previously.

2.1 Total Carbon

The method for determining total carbonate in soil samples by means of a ZnO-based microcantilever device was reported by Plata et al. (2008). The method was based on the selective generation of CO_2 (g) from samples and the measure of the pressure effect on the microcantilever sensor located in a closed system. The carbonate analysis can be performed in the 3–75 mg range, with a precision of 1.7%, expressed as relative standard deviation (RSD). It was applied to the analysis of different soil samples, obtaining results in agreement with those of calcium carbonate content measured by the Bernard's calcimeter official method. The low detection limit (LOD), defined as the mass of $CaCO_3$ was 0.91 mg, whereas the quantification limit (LOQ) calculated as 10 times the standard deviation of the blank was 3.0 mg.

2.2 Nitrates and Total Nitrogen

Artigas et al. (2003) have developed a device incorporating three thick-film nitrate-selective sensors each at a different depth and featuring a copper plate as the reference electrode and the possibility to transmit sensor signal via radio. This probe was calibrated in field and tested up the fertilizers addition. Then the developed thick-film sensors were employed for the analysis of nitrate content in soil extracts, and the results were compared to the standard Kjeldahl method. The similar trends obtained by both methods confirm the sensors capability to measure in situ and in automated manner the chemical parameters of soil.

Yagodina et al. (2000) developed air-gap sensors on the base of pH electrode and nitrate–ISE for determining nitrogen oxides and nitrite in complex environmental samples, including water extracts of soils with nitrates. The nitrite amount determined with developed sensors was a good correlation to the results obtained by standard Griess method.

Adamchuk et al. (2005) have performed nitrate–nitrogen content detection using nitrate-selective electrode simulating in-field soil analysis in laboratory conditions (Sethuramasamyraja et al., 2008). Birrell and Hummel (2001) have demonstrated that ISFETs in combination with flow-injection analysis represent a valid alternative for nitrate concentration evaluation in manually extracted solutions ($R^2 > 0.9$) in 14 Illinois surface soils. Price et al. (2003) have developed a nitrate extraction system that in combination with ISFET technology was used to map soil nitrate on-the-go.

Another application of ISFETs and ISEs for precise dosage of liquid fertilizing agents in horticulture greenhouse was reported by Gieling et al. (2005). In this paper, a fertigation strategy aimed to keep the concentration of the individual ions in the drainage water of a set of plants constant at a level that is nonlimiting to ion-transport, and nutrient uptake was elaborated. Chemical sensors were employed to measure nitrate, potassium, ammonia, and calcium in nutrient supply and drain in a greenhouse with a real crop. The variation in nutrient concentration in supply and drain provided information on the uptake of ions by the plants and provide a feedback on the nutrient demand of the plants to be satisfied. The system was able to provide reliable information for a 1-week period; the main problems faced during the testing were the life expectation of the sensors and the stability and robustness of the system mechanics. In other research the total nitrogen amount was determined by means of multisensory approach; these works are described in detail in a later section.

2.3 Potassium

The feasibility of use of the valinomycin-based ISE for determination of assimilated potassium in Egner-Riehm soil extracts was demonstrated by Ciesla et al. (2007). Flame photometry was used as a reference method. Results obtained from potentiometric and photometric methods in soil extracts correlated linearly ($R^2 = 0.84$).

Lemos et al. (2004) have reported potentiometric in-soil potassium sensor system based on ion-selective PVC membranes deposited over graphite-epoxy solid inner contact. The sensors were incorporated in PVC tubes at three depths: 5, 20, and 50 cm, thus allowing the monitoring of the potassium profile in different soil horizons. The good linear relationship was obtained for in-field potassium content evaluated with developed sensor system and by a current flame photometry ($R^2 = 0.992$ and $R^2 = 0.995$, for 5- and 20-cm depths correspondingly).

Kim et al. (2007) have tested the ISEs for simultaneous detection of K and N in soil samples coming from Missouri and Illinois. Unfortunately the potassium concentrations evaluated with ISE were 50% below the concentration determined by standard methods. Authors have proposed the use of a calibration factor to obtain actual nutrient concentrations.

2.4 Phosphates and Total Phosphorus

A disposable on-chip microsensor with planar cobalt (Co) microelectrodes and Ag/AgCl reference for phosphate detection in soil extracts was reported by Zou et al. (2007) (Fig. 17.1). The sensor had a response range of 10^{-5}–10^{-2} M (0.31–310 ppm phosphate-P), and permitted the analysis of inorganic and organic phosphate compounds [KH_2PO_4, adenosine 5'-triphosphate (ATP), and adenosine 5'-diphosphates (ADP), respectively] in soils. Unfortunately the device lifetime was quite short, approximately 30 min.

Lemos et al. (2009) have developed a selective PVC-based chemical sensor of phosphorus coming from orthophosphate

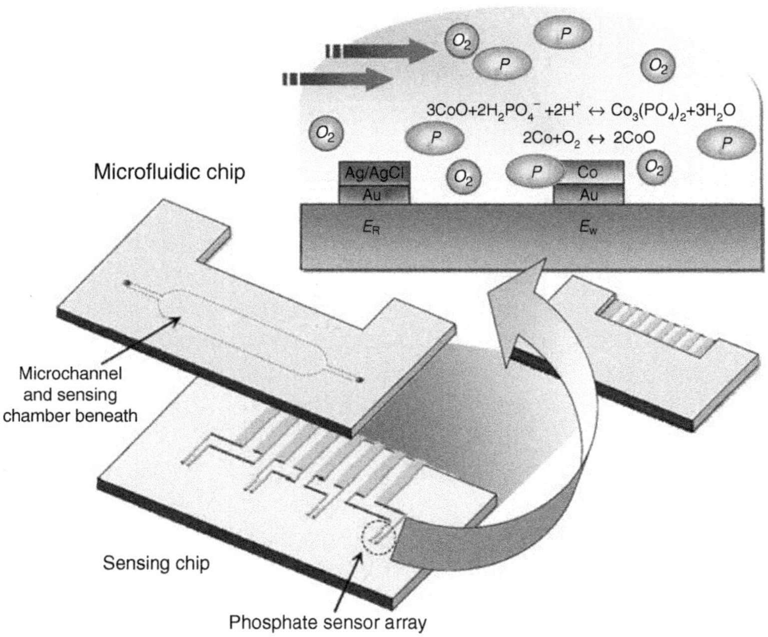

Figure 17.1. On-chip phosphate sensor with planar Co electrodes on polymer substrate. Reprinted from Zou et al. (2007) with permission from Elsevier.

(PO_4^{3-}). The phosphorus amounts determined by standard spectrophotometry method were compared with the potentials registered by the sensor. The results indicate good response and the potential applicability of these probes to assist in the monitoring of soil nutrients, helping to establish rational processes in the use of fertilizers in crops.

Bogrekci and Lee (2005) have tested a total of 345 soil samples collected from the drainage basin of the Lake Okeechobee with a phosphorous concentration in the range from 1 to 2709 mg/kg by means of UV, VIS, and NIR spectroscopy. Phosphorus concentrations of the samples were correlated with the absorbance of the same soil sample. Chemometric approach for obtained data treatment was employed. In particular, partial least squares regression analysis was used. Two-thirds of the experimental spectroscopic data was used for calibration while one-third of the data was for validation. The obtained correlation coefficient of determination (R^2) were 0.87 and 0.93 for original and constituent (from original soil signatures were subtracted spectra of the leached soils samples with removed nutrients) spectra, respectively. The root mean square errors (RMSEs) were 222 and 172 mg/kg, demonstrating efficiency of P detection from combined spectroscopic data and employment of unleached/leached spectra subtraction method.

2.5 Calcium, pH, and Other Macroelements

Ion-sensitive electrochemical sensors with photocurable sensing membranes based on aliphatic diacrylated polyurethane for evaluation of calcium activity in water samples extracted from agricultural soils were fabricated by Artigas et al. (2001a, 2001b). ISEs, with a solid internal reference and ISFETs, were used to evaluate the membrane; the sensors have shown a functional period over more than 8 months with quasi-Nernstian (26–27 mV/dec) sensitivities and working range from 5×10^{-6} to 8×10^{-2} mol/L. The results of calcium sensory analysis in agricultural soils extracts were compared with those yielded by standard methods, finding a good correlation between the two analytical procedures.

A sensory system comprising temperature, moisture, and all solid-state ISEs for pH and calcium ions analysis in soil in real conditions was developed by Lemos et al. (2007) with a scope to complement the precision agriculture needs. The system demonstrated a good correlation with the standard methodologies for pH (soil extraction with 0.05 mol/L calcium chloride solution and further pH measurement of extract with a combined glass electrode) and calcium (an extraction with a mixed ion exchange resin and analysis by flame atomic absorption spectrometer, FAAS). It also showed the possibility to notice the soil buffer capacity at different soil depths and to correct determination of Ca^{2+} amounts in different soil depths with varied relative moisture by employment of a calibration model based on multiple linear regressions. The developed sensorial system proved thus to be useful for agrochemical analysis of a complex and heterogeneous matrix, such as soil.

3 Microelements and Pollutants Analysis in Soils

The analysis of soil microelements content as far as pollutant detection and monitoring are another two great areas of chemical sensors implementation.

3.1 Heavy Metals Detection

The need for the determination of heavy metals in soils increased during the past few years due to the importance of these elements in balanced soil systems, and because of growing environmental problems. Chemical sensors are simple and effective tools to detect and measure toxic contaminants in-field, and research on sensory assessment of heavy metals and other pollutants has been performed previously. Thus, Md Noh and Tothill (2006) have reported a screen-printed gold sensor for analysis of lead(II) by square-wave stripping voltammetry. The working electrode was fabricated with gold ink deposited by use of thick-film technology, the LOD of the sensor were 2 and 5.8 μg/L for two linear concentration ranges of sensor (10–50 and 25–300 μg/L, respectively). The sensor was tested in a variety of wastewater and soil sample extracts from polluted sites and showed the relatively high correlation coefficient with standard ICP–MS method ($r^2 = 0.9681$, $n = 9$) over a wide range of Pb concentrations. Unfortunately, the undesirable effect of cadmium, if present at high concentrations in the samples, on sensor response toward Pb(II) was registered. The same authors proposed a screen-printed carbon electrode modified with in situ codeposition of mercury and cysteine (Md Noh et al., 2005). These devices were prepared in a three-electrode configuration (graphite carbon, WE, carbon counter and Ag/AgCl reference), tested with stripping chronopotentiometric technique and exhibited good sensitivity toward Cd(II) in the concentration range of 0.4–800 μg/L and detection limit of 0.4 μg/L. The detection of Cd(II) in wastewater and soil samples collected from a contaminated site and extracted with acetic acid was performed.

A semiquantitative method for in-field screening of contaminated sites by heavy metals based on single-use screen-printed sensors coupled with differential pulse anodic stripping voltammetry (DPASV), have been reported by Cooper et al. (2007). The simultaneous determination of Cd and Pb in soil and water samples was possible in the microgram per liter per kilogram range with recoveries of 64% and 52%, respectively, and RSD of <8% for both analytes ($n = 10$). In order to allow field-based device usage, a simplified soil extraction procedure, using 1 mol/L aqua regia and a 3-min ultrasonic sample agitation, was developed. A good correlation was obtained between developed combined extraction–DPASV procedure and standard ICP–AES tested in 82 analysis soil samples; the correlation coefficients of 0.978 and 0.973 for Cd and Pb, respectively, was obtained. An attempt to perform simultaneously the analysis of copper (Cu) was not satisfactory due to significant peak distortions reducing the confidence of the method for this metal.

On the contrary, the possibility of simultaneous detection of Pb(II), Cd(II), and Cu(II) with detection limits of 0.3, 1, and 0.5 μg/L on the miniaturized graphite working electrode modified with a cellulose-derivative mercury coating and coupled with square wave anodic stripping voltammetry (SWASV) analysis, was demonstrated by Palchetti et al. (2005). Examples of on-site environmental applications of device were also illustrated.

Previously, Silva et al. (2001) reported a 6 μm-diameter iridium microdisc sensor onto which Hg microdrops were electroplated for simultaneous analysis of Cd, Pb, and Cu metal trace concentrations. These sensors employed SWASV and were used to analyze extracts from soils collected in the Rouyn-Noranda region (Que., Canada) at different depth (from the surface down to 1 m). The satisfactory agreement was found between the metal amounts measured with developed method and graphite furnace AAS; the possibility to measure reliably the metal concentration as low as 50 ppt in soil extracts was declared.

A development of a novel 1-phenyl-2-(2-hydroxyphenylhydrazo)butane-1,3-dione (H_2L) ionophore-based Cu-selective poly(vinyl) chloride (PVC) membrane electrode, which has permitted authors to perform a precise potentiometric analysis of Cu in soils polluted by oil (Kopylovich et al., 2011).

Recently, Singh et al. (2014) exploited benzothiazol-based chelating ionophores, such as 1,3-bis[2-(1,3-benzothiazol-2-yl)-phenoxy]propane (L1) and 1,2′-bis[2-(1,3-benzothiazol-2-yl)-phenoxy]2-ethoxyethane(L2) as neutral ionophores in the fabrication of Cu^{2+} ISEs. The optimization of membrane composition, working conditions, and transducer material (classical inner liquid contact sensors vs. coated graphite electrodes, CGE, and coated pyrolytic graphite electrodes, CPGE) has been performed. The sensor with the best potentiometric characteristics, CPGE coated with L2:PVC:1-CN:NaTPB = 6:39:53:2 (w/w; mg) membrane, had a LOD of 6.3 nM/L and theoretical Nernstian slope of 29.5 mV/decade of activity between pH 2.0 and 8.5. The sensor has been employed for the estimation of Cu^{2+} ion in real samples, and among them in three soil samples extracted with a mixture of nitric acid, perchloric acid, and concentrated hydrofluoric acid. A good agreement of sensor response with AAS results was found.

McGraw et al. (2008) have developed both liquid- and solid-contact ISEs for Pb detection in soil samples from abandoned mining sites. Three different techniques for the extraction of an analyte from soil were tested to find out the techniques and solvents compatible with portable devices. Soil Pb^{2+} levels between 30 and 29,100 mg/kg were measured with developed sensors and these results were in good agreement with reference AAS measurements.

Another sensor for Pb analysis in soils was reported by Wilson et al. (2010). In this work two PVC membrane ISEs for Pb(II) ion based on two bis-thioureas: 1,3-bis(*N*'-benzoylthioureido)benzene and 1,3-bis(*N*'-furoylthioureido)benzene as ionophores were tested. These sensors exhibited a Nernstian response to Pb(II) over a wide concentration range (4×10^{-6} to 10^{-2} M), revealed acceptable selectivities for Pb(II) over a wide variety of other metal ions and could be used in a pH range of 2.2–6.0. Both electrodes were assayed in direct potentiometric determination of Pb in soils (10–30 mg/kg range) with very good performance (0.99935 correlation coefficient in the comparison against ICP–MS method).

Nedeltcheva et al. (2005) have used a combination of anodic and cathodic stripping voltammetry on hanging mercury drop electrode to measure the amount of mobile forms of Zn, Pb, Cd, and Cu in soil samples extracted with ammonium nitrate. The standard deviation of the results was not higher than 10% depending on the metal content in the sample. Voltammetric results were in good agreement with the AAS analysis.

A Pt wire coated with phenyl hydrazone derivative–carbon composite in a PVC membrane was proposed for monitoring Pb arising in environment from the contaminated soils and Pb-containing rocks that undergo weathering (Abbaspour et al., 2010).

Liu et al. (2009) reported a DNA-based sensor that allowed detection of Pb^{2+} ions in Montana Soil samples and spiked Hg^{2+} ions in pond water samples. This sensor employed a thrombin-binding aptamer (TBA) probe labeled with the donor carboxyfluorescein (FAM) and 4-([4-(dimethylamino)phenyl]azo)benzoic acid (DABCYL) quencher at its 5′ and 3′ termini, respectively. Upon binding of Pb^{2+} and Hg^{2+} ions the TBA changed from a random

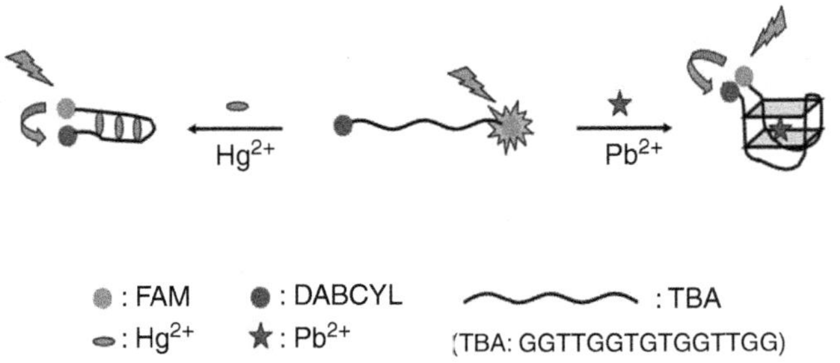

Figure 17.2. Sensing mechanism of the TBA probe for the detection of Hg^{2+} and Pb^{2+} ions. Reprinted from Liu et al. (2009) with permission from ACS.

coil structure into a G-quartet structure and a hairpin-like structure. In this sensor the changes in structure of TBA labeled with the donor FAM unit at one termini and DABCYL quencher on the other side upon the exposure to metal ion was employed. The TBA aptamer changed from a random coil structure into a G-quartet upon binding of Pb^{2+} ions, while Hg^{2+} ions resulted in hairpin-like structure formation (Fig. 17.2). As a result a decrease in fluorescence intensity allowed the selective detection of the quencher ions at low concentrations of 300 pM and 5.0 nM using this TBA probe in the presence of phytic acid and a random DNA/NaCN mixture, respectively.

3.2 Hydrocarbons Pollution Analysis

Soil pollution with anthropogenic petroleum hydrocarbon spills has become a serious environmental problem; the contamination may occur due to the leakage from storage tanks and pipelines or even accidental discharge during transportation. The assessment of hydrocarbons soil pollution is important also to evaluate the contaminated soil bioavailability. An elegant method to detect the level of the hydrocarbon contamination present in the soil was suggested by Kaur et al. (2015). The soil microbial activity in a hydrocarbon-contaminated soils and the amount of CO_2 emitted as a result of biota respiration was used as an indicator of contamination. An inexpensive nondispersive infrared CO_2 sensor was successfully deployed to differentiate the control and diesel-contaminated soils in terms of CO_2 emission after glucose addition (Fig. 17.3).

3.3 Herbicides Detection With (bio)chemical Sensors

There is growing concern about the fate and toxicity of herbicides and their possible entering the food chain. The availability of

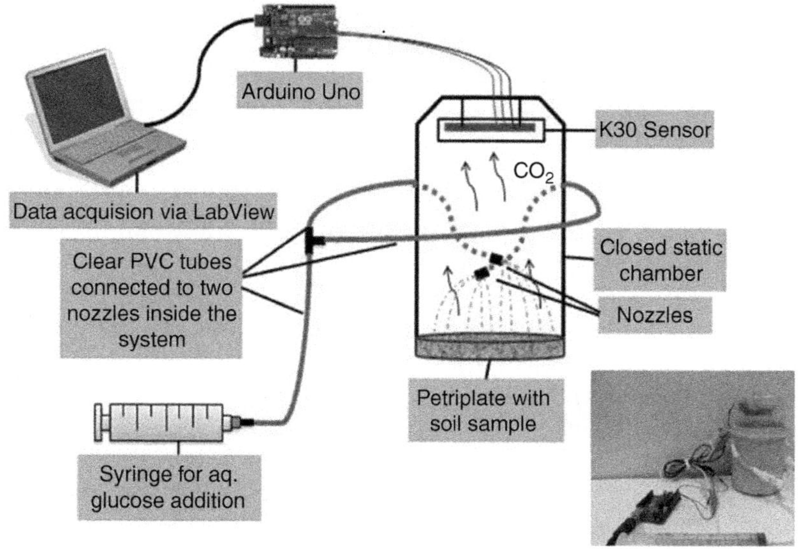

Figure 17.3. Glucose-induced CO_2 emission sensing system for soils integrated with NDIR-based K_3O CO_2 sensor. Reprinted from Kaur et al. (2015).

herbicides in soil depends on several factors, including the composition of both the organic and inorganic materials, the rates of adsorption and mobility, and the rate of herbicide degradation. Else, one should take into account synergistic or antagonistic interactions that may occur between herbicides, their metabolites, and other additives. Therefore, to measure the analytes sensitively is important. The traditional methods of herbicides estimation in soils allow quantification of sorption rates using physicochemical parameters for particular soil types in the laboratory, they do not accurately relate to the natural soil conditions in the field. In this regard, the sensory approach to herbicides analysis in soils seems to be attractive.

Tang et al. (2008) has reported a disposable electrochemical immunosensor based on conductive chitosan/gold nanoparticles (Au NPs) composite membrane for the sensitive detection of herbicide in agricultural samples. In this device a self-synthesized picloram antibody was encapsulated in the immunomembrane to form an immunoconjugate by a competitive immunoreaction in sample solution, followed by the immobilization of horseradish peroxidase (HRP)-labeled secondary antibody. Under optimal conditions, picloram could be detected in the range from 0.005 to 10 μg/mL with the correlation coefficient of 0.9937, and the detection limit is 5 ng/mL.

The analysis of phosphorus-containing amino acid type herbicides, glyphosate, and glufosinate on double-template molecularly imprinted polymer nanofilm-modified pencil graphite electrode and DPASV in aqueous, soil, and serum samples were reported in Prasad et al. (2014). The simultaneous imprinting of herbicide targets has permitted a reliable sensitive and selective analytes detection without matrix complications. The developed sensor linear ranges toward glyphosate and glufosinate, respectively, were 3.98–176.23 and 0.54–3.96 ng/L for simultaneous analysis with detection limits as low as 0.35 and 0.19 ng/L.

A membrane-based immunosensor for isoproturon, a common herbicide, was reported by Baskeyfield et al. (2011). The authors have used the heterogeneous competitive enzyme-linked immunosorbent assay (ELISA) principle and a screen-printed carbon working electrode with carbon counter and silver–silver chloride pseudoreference electrode system for sensor development. On the working electrode the membrane containing an immobilized isoproturon–ovalbumin conjugate was fixed and HRP-labeled polyclonal antibody was then applied for the competitive assay. Sensor was tested in a flow injection mode, and the limit of isoproturon detection was (LLD_{90}) 0.84 ng/mL. The sensor was validated in spiked extracted soil samples and in isoproturon-contaminated samples.

Gianetto et al. (2014) have developed the voltammetric competitive immunosensor selective for atrazine. It was based on the immobilization of a conjugate atrazine–bovine serum albumin on a nanostructured gold substrate previously functionalized with poliamidoaminic dendrimers (Gianetto et al., 2014). The response of the developed immunosensor for atrazine was explored over the 102–103 ng/mL range. Good sensitivity was proved, as limit of detection and limit of quantitation of 1.2 and 5 ng/mL, respectively, were estimated for atrazine. Response of the sensor was reliable, highly selective, and suitable for the detection and quantification of atrazine at trace levels in complex matrices, such as territorial waters, corn-cultivated soils, corn-containing poultry, and bovine feeds and corn flakes for human use.

Sacks et al. (2000) have reported an amperometric enzyme biosensor for the direct measurement of parathion. Parathion (O,O-diethyl O-4-nitrophenyl phosphorothioate) has a wide range of applications against numerous insect species on several crops. Like all organophosphate insecticides, parathion irreversibly inhibits the enzyme acetylcholinesterase, which is essential for central nervous system function in humans and insects. Parathion is highly toxic by all routes of exposure and is readily absorbed through the skin. Human fatalities have been caused by ingestion, dermal adsorption, and inhalation of parathion. The developed biosensor was based on parathion hydrolase from *Pseudomonas* sp. isolated from contaminated soil. The enzyme was immobilized on a carbon electrode, where the hydrolysis of parathion to *p*-nitrophenol was performed. The latter amount was detected by measuring anodic oxidation current and related to the parathion concentration. The achieved LOD of parathion was > 1 ng/mL.

A methyl parathion (MP) sensor based on multiwalled carbon nanotubes–CeO_2–Au nanocomposite (MWCNTs–CeO_2–Au) was developed by Dong et al. (2013). The electrochemical stripping voltammetric detection of MP with developed sensor in water and soil samples was reported. The sensor has demonstrated an ultralow detection limit of 3.02×10^{-11} M for MP.

The detection of other microelements and pollutants in soils, and among them rare metals, such as dysprosium (Gupta et al., 2009), palladium dysprosium (Bojdi et al., 2014), trinitrotoluene (TNT) explosives dysprosium (Alizadeh et al., 2010) by means of chemical sensors have been also reported previously.

3.4 Sensors for Soil Moisture

Soil moisture is the key hydroecological compartment, responding dynamically to sequences of the complex processes in the soil. Field moisture is one of the most important general characteristics of the soil. Growth and development of the biota, the rate of soil processes, accumulation and removal of organic and inorganic compounds is largely dependent on the soil moisture. Field soil moisture has an extremely variable value over the time. It depends on the receipt of rainfall, irrigation, and groundwater in the soil and the water consumption from the soil by evaporation, transpiration, and runoff. Balance in soil moisture is determined by climate, soil position in the landscape, the type of vegetation, human activities, and the seasons. In addition, soil moisture depends on the properties of the soil: water capacity, water permeability, and wettability. Soil moisture determines the efficiency of plants, and regulates species diversity phyto-, zoo-, and microbial-complexes. Features of soil water regime are determined removal or accumulation of substances in the soil profile. The processes of transformation of substances in the soil (dissolution, crystallization, oxidation, reduction, etc.) are associated with soil moisture dynamics. Soil moisture is rapidly changing quantity characterizing the properties of soil-moment. When measuring the moisture content the following should take into account special dynamism of its values, the relationship with the temperature of air and soil, amount of rainfall, uneven distribution over the surface of the soil, and in the soil profile. To obtain accurate data need not only the traditional methods, but also new, based on the measurement of undisturbed samples in the field. The data obtained by different methods may differ measurement; results may differ not only by methods and mistakes but also due to high spatial variability of water distribution in natural soils.

The most useful definition of soil moisture is the volumetric water content W:W (%) = $100(V_w/V_s)$, where V_w is the total volume of water in the soil and V_s is the total volume of all soil components. Typical values of W range up to 60% because of the porosity of most soils, that is, the volume of liquid and gaseous fractions related to the total volume, is between 40% and 60%. To measure the water content in the soil either direct (thermogravimetric) or indirect methods should be used. The thermogravimetric method is the most common and reliable. It used for the standard calibration. The disadvantage is that the thermogravimetric method requires the removal of soil samples, it is time consuming and is not repeatable. Indirect methods are based on the measurement of electrical conductivity, thermal conductivity, or absorption of radiation. The time domain reflectometry (TDR) and electromagnetic methods, such as impedance measurements are the most important from indirect methods for soil water measurement.

Because of the limited applicability for field measurements of thermogravimetry and capacitive sensors operated with laboratory instruments, and the possible problems associated with TDR when applied to highly conductive and very wet soil, a new sensor for field measurements of the water content of natural soils has been developed by Eller and Denoth (1996). In this research the measurement was the complex permittivity at a frequency of 32MHz. The impedance was measured by a twin T-bridge optimized to a large range of permittivities of natural soils. An analysis of measured soil permittivities showed a dominant influence of liquid water content on dielectric permittivity, whereas soil-specific parameters, such as grain-size distribution, chemical composition, and bulk density have only a negligible influence at this comparable high measurement frequency. The loss factor, however, strongly depended on both the type of soil and the water content. In addition, comparative studies with commonly used measurement methods, such as the thermogravimetric method and TDR showed satisfactory agreement.

Another example of indirect measured moisture sensor was demonstrated in the study of de Matos Oliveira et al. (2014). They tested the capability of porous ceramics sensor devices, developed in the National Institute for Space Research to monitor the soil water dynamics. They found that the ceramics devices are promising concerning their potential in the environmental parameters monitoring.

The soil profile moisture sensor was first designed based on a high-frequency capacitor by Wang et al. (2012). The experiment results showed that the sensor output voltage linearly increased with soil temperature changes ranged from 5°C to 45°C, and it decreased with electrical conductivity increasing more than 2 mS/cm. The sensor output voltage decreased with bulk density increasing. The largest error of measurement was 4.7%, correlation coefficient R^2 was 0.967 between sensor and traditional gravimetric method.

Few new sensors to measure soil moisture have been developed in recent years. Some of the research devoted to the problems of handling large amounts of field data obtained with sensors, improving the accuracy of the calibration of sensors, and eliminating the random errors in the field measurements. For example, the study conducted by Rivera et al. (2012) has applied $\Delta\theta$ time series and wavelet filtering in order to identify the representative sample points and depths through an analysis of hourly soil moisture. The $\Delta\theta$ time series was allowed to assess the spatio-temporal influence of the monitoring points location, while the wavelet periodograms allowed to get insight about the response of the monitoring points at different time scales. Analysis of their case study permits to reallocate 16 sensors (out of 28) without a significant loss of information.

3.5 Soil Salinity and pH Sensors

Soil salinity is an important indicator in arid regions especially, where salinity of the soil may increase significantly and pose a danger to plants. The soil salinity is defined by measuring the electrical conductivity of soil water extract or saturated soil water extract. The factors that produce measurement errors are temperature, moisture, and texture of the soil. The development of more precise methods for evaluating soil salinity is important. The salinity of soil is a dynamic parameter, which characterizes the "soil-moment," so, the soil salinity measuring should be conducted taking into account all influencing factors. This may be achieved by using various sensors on one measuring device and via a selective analysis of sensor readings.

Wilczek et al. (2012) have defined the salinity on the basis of electrical conductivity with respect to the real part of the soil complex dielectric permittivity. The frequency-domain reflectometry (FDR) sensor designed for soil salinity assessment of sandy soils in a wide range of soil moisture and bulk electrical conductivity.

The complex dielectric permittivity spectra in the frequency range 10–500 MHz have been determined in soil. The status of soil salinity was calculated as the salinity index, a partial derivative of the soil bulk electrical conductivity with respect to the real part of the complex dielectric permittivity of soil. Five sandy soils have been tested, the relationship between bulk electrical conductivity and dielectric permittivity was linear. It was demonstrated that the salinity index may be applied for FDR measurements and may be adapted to field use after loam and clayey soils testing.

Visconti et al. (2014) have defined salinity of soil on the basis of electrical conductivity of soil solution or bulk soil with respect to the real part of the soil complex dielectric permittivity. Commercial dielectric sensors of the FDR and capacitance–conductance types have estimated the dielectric permittivity and electrical conductivity in the pot experiment.

The analysis of soil pH is important to assess the chemical status of soil and to prevent extremely high and low soil pH values. Unfortunately, the standard methods of soil pH analysis require the procedures of sampling and extraction; moreover, the final laboratory procedure (even if this measure is often performed with a standard pH glass electrode) is limited by personnel and lab analysis costs. Automation of pH measurement may help to solve this question. In order to lower the cost of the work and create a field map of pH distribution, Staggenborg et al. (2007) have measured Kansas soil pH directly in the field using a mobile platform on which the pH sensor was incorporated.

The study of Silva and Molin (2013) has compared manual and automatic methods of an ion-selective sensor in determining soil pH. The manual operation showed better performance. In both of the operations, pH determination in soils with low clay content showed highest correlation with known true values.

4 Colorimetric and Optical Sensors for Soil Analysis

A review on proximal active optical sensors application for agricultural sensing was published by Holland et al. (2012). In this review, 26 researches related to the application of optical sensors for crop production and soil conditions evaluations were discussed. Some significant examples of optical sensors employed for soil parameters analysis were mentioned here.

A fiber-optic pH sensor for investigation of soil and its interstitial water was reported by Motellier et al. (1995). The sensor was constructed of stainless steel guidelines on the end of which the sensing tip (optode) with immobilized resin semibeads coated with phenol red pH indicator was introduced. Sensor had special characteristics for measurements at high pressure (up to 17 bar) and was employed to analyze groundwater pH at Mol, Belgium. Sensor characteristics, such as the influence of pressure on the measured signal, in situ applicability, possible limitations, and further developments were described.

Hung et al. (2010) have developed a selective colorimetric method for the detection of aqueous mercuric, silver, and Pb ions by using label-free Au NPs and selected alkanethiols induced the degree of Au NPs aggregation in the presence of target cation. This aggregation resulted in a declining ratio of the extinction coefficients at 650–520 nm (Ex650/520, a measure of the molar ratio of the aggregated to the dispersed Au NPs) and visible color changes, thus permitting the selective detection of Ag^+, Hg^{2+}, and Pb^{2+} ions, at concentrations down to the nanomolar range in river water and Montana soil.

An interesting study on nondestructive measurements of soil color and predictions of soil OC and iron (Fe) contents with digital cameras was performed by Viscarra Rossel et al. (2008). The indirect measurements of soil OC and Fe were performed using soil color as the proxy. The RGB signal was transformed to variables from other color space models and a redness index (RI) and these were used to derive pedotransfer functions for soil OC and Fe. The best results for soil OC content prediction was obtained with the VIP-PLSR technique; the model parameters were quite good, providing R^2 and RMSE values of 0.91 and 0.46%. The iron prediction with different regression methods was less successful with the best results for full factorial regression (FFR) with R^2 of 0.71 and an RMSE of 0.068%.

Yokota et al. (2007) have reported an optical sensor based on photometric detection of six soil nutrients: ammonia nitrogen (NH_4–N), nitrate nitrogen (NO_3–N), available phosphorus (P_2O_5), available iron (Fe), exchangeable manganese (Mn), and exchangeable calcium (CaO). The light emitting diodes light source of the wavelength that fits the absorption band of chemical reagents whose color develops by reaction with soil nutrients. The results are compared with those calculated using absorbance of solutions measured by spectrophotometer, and agreement is observed.

5 Bacterial Sensors (Bioassays) for Soil Analysis

Environmental hazard of heavy metals in soils depends to a large extent on their bioavailability, that is, to detect a bioavailable fraction of total contaminant concentration. Different microorganisms, and also genetically engineered ones, can provide a quantifiable signal to the presence of the target chemical(s), and hence, may serve as powerful tools for bioavailability assessment. Numerous bacterial metal-sensor strains have been developed in the past, displaying high detection sensitivities for a broad spectrum of environmentally significant metal targets. A comprehensive review on bacterial bioassays employment was published by Magrisso et al. (2008). Here we report some examples of soils bioavailability assessment and pollutants analysis with bioassays performed in the past 15 years.

5.1 Bioavailable Heavy Metals Determination

The determination of bioavailable metals, namely Cd and Pb was performed in 50 agricultural soils sampled near zinc and Pb smelters in Northern France by means of recombinant bacterial sensors, *Bacillus subtilis* BR151-(pTOO24) and *Staphylococcus aureus* RN4220 (pTOO24), in which the luminescence is induced in the presence of metals (Ivask et al., 2004). Comparison of the data on total metal concentrations in the soils determined with AAS and the bacterial sensors, results indicate that the bioassays can serve as a complement method rather than replace the chemical analysis of environmental samples. The same group has conducted the combined chemical and ecotoxicological hazard evaluation study, which was conducted on 60 smelter-influenced soils containing different amounts (from 1 to 1000 mg/kg) of Cd, Pb, and Zn (Kahru et al., 2005). Various species were tested for bioassays, among them algae *Selenastrum capricornutum*, *B. subtilis* (pTOO24) for Cd, *S. aureus* (pT0024) as Pb–Cd sensor. The bioavailability of metals was evaluated, and the possibility of bioassays to signal hazards already at subtoxic level was indicated.

Liu et al. (2012) have tested a modified bacteria *Pseudomonas putida* as a Zn-specific biosensor. The specific strain *P. putida* X4 (pczcR3GFP) was constricted by fusing a promoterless-enhanced green fluorescent protein (egfp) gene with the czcR3 promoter in the chromosome of *P. putida* X4. In water extracts of four different soils amended with Zn, the reporter strain detected about 90% of the Zn content.

The new sensors for the specific detection of mercury and arsenic (As) were prepared by engineering soil bacteria *Pseudomonas fluorescens* with reporter gene systems by Petänen et al. (2001). These reporter plasmids express metal presence by luminescence phenotype; they were transferred into *Escherichia coli* DH5α and *P. fluorescens* OS8. It was shown that the good ability of the strain OS8 to quantitatively detect specific heavy metals in spiked soil and soil extracts in real-time in comparison to a traditional chemical analysis that requires sampling, sample pretreatment, is time-consuming and demands qualified personnel efforts. Being also a good humus soil colonizer, *P. fluorescens* is a good candidate for measuring soil heavy metal bioavailability. One year later the same researchers have tested two different strains of *P. fluorescens* OS8, pTPT11, and pTPT31, respectively for mercury and As detection in three different soil types (humus, mineral, and clay) (Petänen and Romantschuk, 2002). The lowest mercury concentration measured using pTPT31 strain (0.003 μg/kg) was considerably lower than by chemical method (0.05 μg/kg), and had a useful detection range similar to that of chemical methods. The obtained results suggest that the bacteria can be used as an alternative traditional method for different types of samples.

Hou et al. (2014) have constructed an *E. coli*-based biosensor to measure the bioavailability of As in soil. *E. coli* biosensors were employed to assess the impact of different long-term fertilization regimes containing N, NP, NPK, M (manure), and NPK + M treatments on the bioavailability of As. In conclusion, NKP fertilization was recommended as a more suitable regime in As-polluted soil especially with high As concentration, and this *E. coli* arsRp::luc-based biosensor was a more realistic approach in assessing the bioavailability of As in soil since it would not overrate the risk of As to the environment.

The mutant *E. coli* strain whole-cell biosensor utilizing a modified ArsR repressor that is highly selective toward trivalent methyl and aromatic arsenicals that are actively employed as herbicides, and as growth promoters, respectively was reported by Chen et al. (2014). The biosensor was adapted for in vitro detection of organoarsenicals by fluorescence anisotropy of ArsR–DNA interactions. Its detection limits were 10^{-7} M and linearity to 10^{-6} M for phenylarsenite and 510^{-6} M for methylarsenite.

Wei et al. (2010) have fused the mercury-inducible promoter, P_{merT}, and the regulatory gene, *merR*, with a promoterless reporter gene EGFP in order to construct a luminescent whole cell reporter (BMB-ME) on the base of *P. putida* chromosome for mercury analysis in the red soil of China. Several parameters, including both the specific transport of toxic metals inside and outside of the host microorganism cell, as far as the influence of such abiotic factors as soil pH, the amount of clay, and dissolved OC, from roots that were tested. The new sensor strain had a detection range similar to the reversed-phase HPLC with the lowest detectable concentration of Hg^{2+} of 200 nM. Any influence of nanomolar levels of Cu^2, Fe^{2+}, Mn^{2+}, Sn^{2+}, Zn^{2+}, Co^{2+}, Ag^+, Ba^{2+}, Mg^{2+}, and Pb^{2+} ions was detected.

The other group of *Pseudomonas*, *P. fluorescens*, was used for monitoring of bioavailable Cu, total dissolved Cu, and free Cu ions activity in aqueous extracts of amended with various amounts of manure (Brandt et al., 2008). Total Cu concentrations in soil are poor predictors of toxicity to soil biota, and consequently bioavailability-based risk assessment should be considered the ultimate goal for proper environmental protection of soil resources. The developed *P. fluorescens* biosensor was permitted to assess the bioavailable Cu species; the measurements performed with biosensor were backed by analysis of manure and Cu amounts.

During the past two decades a number of recombinant bacterial sensors, which allow the specific detection and quantification of the bioavailability of heavy metals has been developed. Thus, Peltola et al. (2005) have presented a comparison of the operational speciation of Cu and Pb determined with sequential extraction and their bioavailability determined with bioluminescent Cu- and Pb-specific bacterial (*E. coli, S. aureus*) and bioluminescent Cu fungal (*Saccahromyces cerevisiae*) sensors. The fungal method was a relatively new. The use of both prokaryotic (bacterial) and eukaryotic (yeast) sensor cells had allowed to compare the bioavailability of Cu to different organisms in 20 samples of urban soils, with the concentrations of 14–5323 mg/kg of Pb and 8–12,987 mg/kg of Cu, respectively. One of the unsolved questions of that study is in what the limiting factor was the detection capability of the bacterial sensors, because the bioavailability of Pb and Cu from natural soils was at present out of reach. When studying the bioavailability of chemical elements in soils, it would also be good to know the natural soil concentrations. Thus, when further developing these methods it has to be considered as a direct challenge to lower the detection limits.

Another example of applied research in this field was the microbial biosensors to assess changes in the water-soluble biotoxicity of metals as a consequence of ameliorant (activated carbon, bonemeal, bentonite, and calcium polysulfide) dosing (Maletić et al., 2015). The ameliorants were compared to assess their effectiveness in immobilizing metals in soils. At the ameliorant concentrations used to effectively immobilize the metals, the biosensor performance was not impaired. Microbial biosensors offered a rapid and relevant screening tool to validate the reduced toxicity associated with the ameliorant dosing and could be calibrated to complement chemical analysis.

In research of Coelho et al. (2015), the different bacteria may have different responses to the concentration ranges of the analyzing metals and their compounds. Thus, the responses of two bacterial bioreporters, pCHRGFP1 *E. coli* and pCHRGFP2

Ochrobactrum tritici, were within the range of 0.5–2 μM and 2–10 μM chromate, respectively.

5.2 Bioassays and Bioluminescent Determination of Herbicides

Not all bacterial biosensors are sufficiently sensitive for routine analysis, except on highly contaminated sites. The biosensors combining cell and antibody are able to diagnose the factors that determine the bioavailable fraction of the herbicides. Strachan et al. (2002) investigated the responses of cellular and immunological biosensors to four commonly used herbicides (atrazine, diuron, mecoprop, and paraquat). Immunosensors were based on stabilized recombinant single chain antibodies (stAbs) specific for the four above-mentioned groups of herbicides, namely antiatrazine, mecoprop, diuron, and paraquat stAbs. These receptors, used in combination, can be employed for soil toxicity assessment and quantification of herbicides present in aqueous and methanol extracts from soil. The soil toxicity was evaluated with *lux*-marked bacterial biosensor *E. coli* HB101. The HPLC analysis was employed as reference method, and satisfactory correlation of standard analysis results and herbicides amounts recovered from immunoassay analysis was obtained.

The biosensor developed by Chen et al. (2014) detects reduced forms of MSMA and roxarsone and offers a practical, low-cost method for detecting activated forms and breakdown products of organoarsenical herbicides and growth promoters. The biosensor requires optimization, such as elimination of the two-plasmid system by integration of the repressor-reporter genes into the chromosome before it could be used in the field, and further development is in progress.

The glyphosate [(*N*-phosphonomethyl)] is the most frequently used nonselective postemergence herbicide all around the world. Due to the continued accumulation in water and crop glyphosate has been considered as a "toxicologically harmless." The analytical methodology is nearly exclusive for this analyte and this chemical cannot be determined by a multiresidue method. Gonzalez-Martınez et al. (2005) have developed a fully automated immunosensor for the herbicide glyphosate based on the immunocomplex capture assay protocol. The sensor carried out an online analyte derivatization prior to the assay and used a selective antiglyphosate serum, a glyphosate peroxidase enzyme tracer, and fluorescent detection. Under optimal conditions, the detection limit achieved is 0.021 μg/L with an analysis rate of 25 min/assay, autonomy of more than 48 h, and sensor reusability >500 analytical cycles. The immunosensor was able to discriminate structurally related molecules, such as aminomethylphosphonic acid, the main metabolite of glyphosate, and other related herbicides, such as glufosinate and glyphosine. Interferences from naturally occurring species (anions, cations, and humic substances) and their elimination were also studied. The immunosensor was successfully applied to water and soil sample analysis, with good recoveries at levels lower than 1 μg/L. Results obtained with the immunosensor correlate well with data from a magnetic particle ELISA and LC/LC/MS chromatographic method.

6 Multisensory Soil Analysis

Nowadays more and more interest has been generated for the use of chemometric approach and application of chemical sensors arrays for environmental monitoring, including soil analysis (Lvova et al., 2014). Chemometric methods are used to treat simultaneously several soil parameters, such as main nutrients, various forms of humates, the oxidation potential of the medium, pH, color, moisture, clay and/or sand content, concentrations of certain microelements (Ca, Mg, Mn, Na, Fe, Al, etc.), in order to obtain final soil characterization output. Depending on the purpose, the analysis may be carried out as a qualitative (soil types ranking and classification) and quantitative (determination of certain components content).

The mathematical methods employed in chemometric approach deal with a vast volume of data obtained either from standard instrumental and laboratory methods of soil analysis or from the chemical sensors or multisensory systems.

The most-often applied chemometric techniques are artificial neural networks (ANNs), principal component analysis (PCA), cluster and hierarchical cluster analysis (CA, HCA), support vector machine (SVM), various regression methods: partial least squares (PLS), multiple linear regression (MLR), principal component regression (PCR), and so on. The detailed description of these chemometric methods can be found elsewhere (Esbensen, 2004).

6.1 Chemometric Approach for Soils Classification

Probably one of the first works were the chemometric approach, which was applied in soil analysis and was reported by Cal (1995) almost 20 years ago. In this research the authors have employed the back propagation ANN method in order to give a quantitative soil classification based on three main soil parameters: plastic index, liquid limit water capacity, and clay content. First the ANN was calibrated with 6 kinds of clay (heavy clay, light clay, heavy subclay, medium subclay, light subclay, and subsandy soil) as learning samples, then 20 unknown soils were used as test samples. It was concluded, so that more satisfying results can be obtained, the neural network model was expected to be referred to as an effective technique for soil classification.

After this pioneering work several attempts on soils classification by means of multisensory systems and chemometrics were done. Thus, Kovačević et al. (2010) have reported application of SVMs in the estimate of values of soil properties and soil-type classification based on known values of particular chemical and physical properties in sampled profiles. The following soil parameters were used to classify 151 soil samples collected in the Negotin municipality in eastern Serbia: SOM, pH, total N, available soil potassium, available soil phosphorus, exchangeable bases, cation-exchange capacity, sand and soil particles of different size content. It was demonstrated that soil-type classifications based on samples with known values of particular chemical and physical soil properties, exhibit a high degree of linearity. Classification models such as logistic regression or linear SVMs could be used to automate this task with satisfactory accuracy.

Bansod and Pandey (2013) have used several parameters such as site-specific spatial variability of apparent electrical conductivity, crop yield, pH, moisture, temperature, and dielectric constant to construct spatial distribution maps for precision agriculture purposes. The necessity of such an analysis was explained by a well-known phenomenon of within-field variability in soil chemical properties and crop productivity. PCA and fuzzy c-means (FCM) clustering algorithm were then performed to delineate management zones. The georeferenced sensor data were analyzed for within-field classification. It was found that apparent electrical conductivity was correlated to the crop yield variability pattern. The obtained result enables reduction in number of soil analysis needed to create application maps for certain cultivation operations. Bhattacharya and Solomatine (2006) have conducted experiments to classify soil types based on cone penetration testing (CPT) data. In CPT, a metallic cone is pushed into the soil and an indication of the in situ soil strength is obtained by measuring the force needed to let it advance at a constant rate. Decision trees, ANN, and SVMs chemometric techniques were employed for soil classification purposes. The satisfactory results (from 60% to 80% of correctly classified soils) were obtained.

6.2 Soil Assessment by Sensor Arrays

Despite the obvious advantages of such systems, only few examples of an array of sensors for soil analysis have been published previously. Thus, about two decades ago an automated work-station for soil analysis (AWSSA) has been developed by McGrath and Skotnikov (1996). This system automatically unpacked, prepared, processed, and analyzed in sequential order soil samples and then determine therein parameters, such as pH, particle size, overall humus, alkali-soluble humus fraction, sesquioxides, carbonates, as well as the content of NO_3^-, NH_4^+, K, P, Ca, and Mg macrocomponents. The concentration of macronutrients are determined by means of ISEs, while automated photocolorimeter was used for the determination of sesquioxides, alkali-soluble fraction of humus, overall humus, and P. Authors stress that a developed system was economical and fast and it does one sample per minute after initial process setup time. Development of such a system was a significant step toward automation of soil analysis, however, this approach requires laboratory conditions and the use of a large number of reagents.

Artigas et al. (2001a,b) have proposed an application of ISFETs to measure Ca^{2+}, K^+, NO_3^- nutrients, and pH levels in soils. The robust, small size, and low output impedance ISFETs had photocurable polymeric selective membranes deposited on transducer fabricated with microelectronic technology. ISFETs response was tested in horticulture soils and compared with standard methods; the results confirmed the feasibility of ISFET sensors for in-soil monitoring (Fig. 17.4).

An attempt to perform a direct soil measurement (DSM) with commercial implementation for on-the-go mapping of soil pH using ISEs has been tested by Adamchuk et al. (2005). The simultaneous soil mapping for pH, available potassium, nitrate–nitrogen, and sodium contents was performed in six sets of soil samples simulating in-field measurements in laboratory conditions. Response, calibration, precision, and accuracy of the DSM were analyzed based on the results of a laboratory test. It was found that a satisfactory correlation among average DSMs and corresponding reference measurements with a regression correlation coefficient (R^2) equal to 0.93–0.96 for soil pH, while the potential applicability of other ISEs declined in the order: potassium > nitrate > sodium. Authors explain such a founding by few probes selected and stress the importance of further test to investigate suitable application approaches. Later the same research group conducted agitated soil measurements (ASM) on potassium-containing soil samples and proved it enhanced effectiveness over DSM (Sethuramasamyraja et al., 2008). Authors have performed in-field ASM measurements of soil pH, potassium and nitrate contents, and achieved R^2 values versus standard methods equal to 0.95.

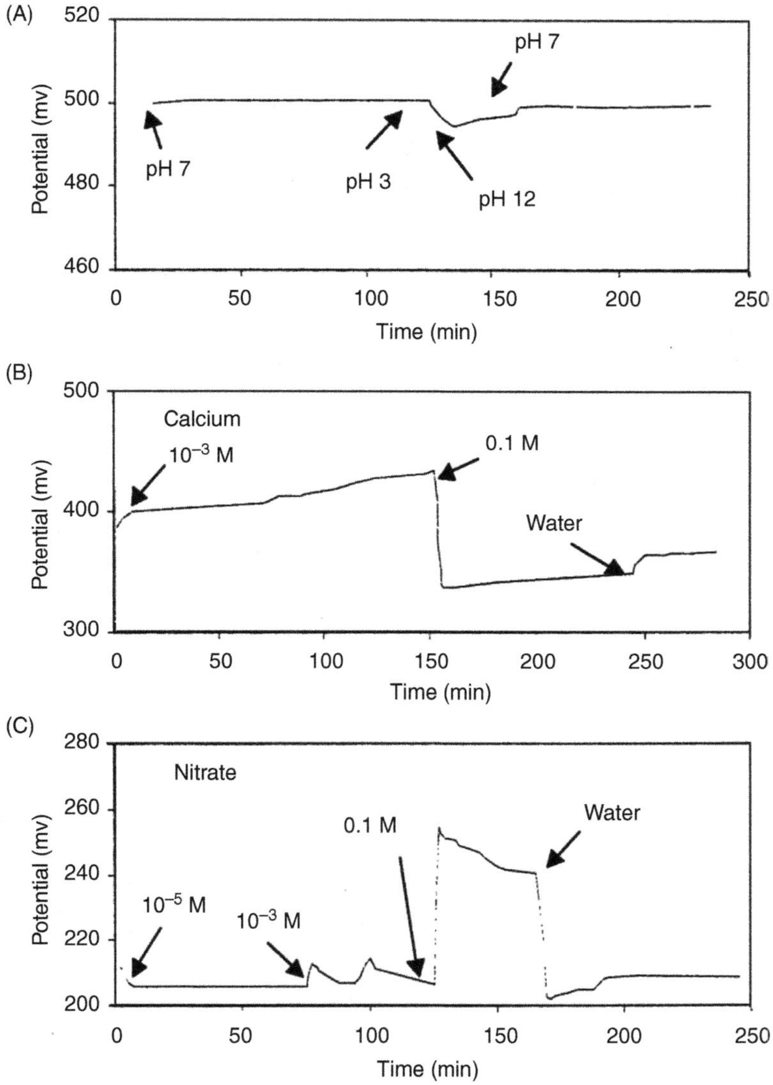

Figure 17.4. Response of pH, calcium- and nitrate-ISFETs in soil along the addition of fertilizer solutions. (A) With different pH, (B) with different calcium concentrations, and (C) with different nitrate concentrations. Reprinted from Artigas et al. (2001a,b) with permission from Elsevier.

Chikae et al. (2007) have reported a maturity sensor system for composts analysis. Three parameters, namely pH, the concentration of ammonia ions, and phosphatase activity, were simultaneously evaluated in composts in order to conclude on their maturity. The pH and NH_4^+ concentrations of the fresh extracts from compost were measured by an ion-meter and a pH-meter, respectively, and the apparent phosphatase activity in crude test solutions was determined using screen-printed carbon strips (SPCSs) coated with α-naphthyl phosphate (α-NP) in Nafion film and differential pulse voltammetry (DPV). In total, 24 compost samples were collected in various composting days and tested both with developed sensor system, and by the conventional germination tests. The germination index (GI) of composts was expressed by using multiple regression analysis for correlation between maturity sensor system response and conventional germination tests. GI often used to evaluate the compost maturity when GI value is 50%, the compost can be characterized as phytotoxin free. Authors showed that the composts' GIs evaluated by developed sensor system correlated well with the GIs measured by standard germination tests ($r = 0.873$) (Fig. 17.5). This founding permitted authors to propose the portable maturity sensor system for rapid evaluation of compost stability directly at the composting site.

Gutierrez et al. (2007) tested an array of eight potentiometric sensors based on polymeric (PVC) membranes (electronic tongue) for the supervision of the nutrient solution composition produced by a fertigation system. Multilayer ANN model was employed to treat sensor array data and predicted the concentration values of ammonium, potassium, and nitrate, and the undesired saline sodium and chloride compounds in nutrient solution, drainage solution, and tap water. Despite difficulties to predict chloride content, the proposed approach appeared to be a feasible method for the in-line assessment of nutrients and undesired compounds

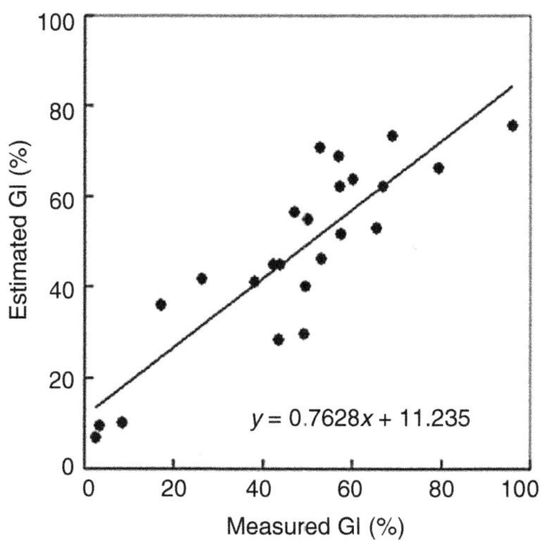

Figure 17.5. Correlation between the measured and the estimated GI values.
Reprinted from Chikae et al. (2007) with permission from Elsevier.

in fertigation solutions. One year later the same researches have reported an extended research in which some changes were introduced in the sensor array to improve its response toward chloride ions and to incorporate phosphate in the model (Gutierrez et al., 2008). Two measurement sessions with electronic tongue were performed in different seasons: winter and summer. The differences obtained in the calculated concentrations of the ions considered were explained using crop physiological arguments. It was found that the sensor based on Ag/AgCl is a good alternative to the PVC sensor based on tridodecylmethylammonium chloride (TDMAC) exchanger sensor for chloride; unfortunately the metallic cobalt wire sensor to phosphate permitted only semiquantitative analysis. Determination of Pb^{2+}, Cd^{2+}, Cu^{2+}, and Zn^{2+} in soils by PVC potentiometric sensor array at the mg/kg level was performed by the same research group (Wilson et al., 2012). The mixed response system was modeled employing ANN method; results were compared and validated against AAS reference methodology, with correlations $R^2 > 0.948$ for the four heavy metals considered.

Previously in our laboratory the studies on the use of portable analytical system based on an array of metallic potentiometric sensors for the SOM analysis, and the detection of mobile forms of soil humic substances in particular, have been conducted (Lvova et al., 2014). An evaluation of total amount of OC in soils and organic fertilizers is important in agricultural chemistry, because this value represents a potential fertility of soils and may serve as a measure of fertilizers' effectiveness. The ability of soil humic substances to form stable complexes with several transition metal cations is well known. The binding strength of humic substances with metal ions varies in the range from 200 to 600 μmol/L. On the basis of this property we employ an array of Cu, tin, Fe, aluminum, brass, and stainless steel wires for classification of aqueous extracts of organic fertilizers and several soils differing in the C/N ratio and the content of labile pools and stable organic substances. Five types of commercially available organic fertilizers (Humate 80, Nobel, Green Belt, Agrocore, and Humate + 7), Flucka humic acid preparation and aqueous extracts from: (1) two plug-in garden soils from Russian boreal zone (Arhangelsk) and middle Europe (Oldenburg); (2) typical chernozem (WRB, Haplic Chernozems, HC); and (3) soddy-podzolic (WRB, Albic Luvisol, AL) were analyzed with potentiometric metallic multisensor system. The effectiveness of the system for monitoring of labile soil fertility and soil types classification was shown. As it can be seen from Fig. 17.6, all soil extracts are separated from the group of organic fertilizers along the PC1 axis, which may be attributed to the lower content of humus. HC and AL soils are well distinguished also

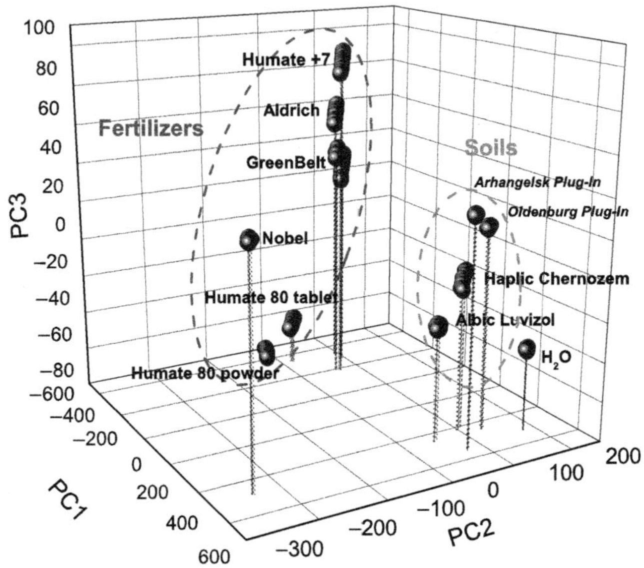

Figure 17.6. PCA scores plot of identification among the aqueous extracts of several organic fertilizers and real soils by means of potentiometric metallic multisensor system. Reprinted from Lvova et al. (2014) with permission from the authors.

along the PC2, which may be correlated to the pH of the samples as far as to the HS lability, since HC contains less amount of labial fulvic acids. The lower amount of humates in organic fertilizers can be noted along PC3 axis.

A very interesting study on the interaction between humic substances and poly(*o*-ethoxyaniline) (POEA) conducting polymer, was conducted by Venancio et al. (2005). The interactions between POEA and fulvic and humic acids were confirmed by atomic force microscopy, UV-Vis, and Raman spectroscopies. The sensor formed by an array of different sensing units and PCA was able to detect and distinguish humic substances in aqueous solution.

Mimendia et al. (2011) used an array of potentiometric chemical sensors with cross-sensitivity to cations and anions for the recognition of different soil types and definitions of some parameters of soil fertility in these soils. Very recently the same group have reported a multichannel sensor measurements of array composed of 20 ISEs plus an ANN used as a pattern recognition method for soil analysis (Mimendia et al., 2014). The qualitative discrimination between six distinct soil types extracted with different extracting agents ($BaCl_2$ saline solution and an acetic acid) based on their extractable components was attempted. The acetic acid extraction method gave a correct classification rate and sensitivity both of 94% and a specificity of 100%. A possibility of quantitative determination of several physicochemical properties of agricultural interest, such as OC content, K^+, Mg^{2+}, NO_3^-, and Cl^- ions was also demonstrated, showing satisfactory agreement with the reference methods.

Kim et al. (2007) simultaneously measured potassium and total N content in Missouri and Illinois soils. Lately this soil macronutrient sensing system was employed for the analysis of 36 soil samples from a single site, the Northern Illinois Agronomy Research Center (NIARC) and have demonstrated the ability to estimate variations in soil NO_3–N, P, and K within a single test site (Kim et al., 2013). The array of ISEs fabricated with new membranes and cobalt rod, in conjunction with the previously developed normalization methods and calibration models, accurately estimated NO_3–N, P, and K in solution without need to recalibrate the ISE system through standard laboratory analysis of soil samples from the new test site. This study showed that it was possible to transfer existing calibration equations to new membranes and electrodes through application of the baseline correction and two-point normalization methods and an adjustment for differences in extraction efficiency. This finding enhances the applicability of the ISE-based soil macronutrient sensing system and methodology for rapid soil analysis.

Beni et al. (2005) has developed and tested a portable prototype of electrochemical trace metal analyzer, that implements anodic stripping voltammetry at suitable sensor electrodes and permits the detection of Cu in acetic acid soil extracts, both in the laboratory and in the field.

6.3 Multisensory Soil Analysis With Gas Sensors

Yang et al. (2001, 2004) have tested SnO_2 Figaro-type ceramic gas sensor system for the monitoring of aromatic volatile organic contaminants (VOCs), such as benzene, toluene, ethyl benzene, and xylene and their mixtures in the exhaust gas from a soil vapor extraction process. Reasonably good correlation factors > 0.98 were obtained between the GC analyses and the sensor responses for each component thus indicating a utility of developed approach to detect contaminated soil sites.

In the same period Gurbuz et al. (2004) have fabricated and tested diamond-based chemical sensor for benzene and toluene VOCs analysis and for possible environmental hazard and petroleum indications in soil. For both analytes the sensor detection mechanisms were developed, and the calculated small values of activation energies for two gases confirmed the sensor fast response and high sensitivity.

De Cesare et al. (2008) have tested a combination of solid phase microextraction (SPME) and electronic nose (EN) techniques to analyze clay loam forest soil artificially contaminated with phenanthrene. In particular, the degradation of phenanthrene by soil microorganisms was analyzed. EN was based on an array of Quartz Crystal Microbalance sensors modified with six different metalloporphyrins, hydrophilic polyethylenimine, and hydrophobic polymethylphenylsiloxane films. Results obtained by e-nose were compared to those collected by SPME–GC/MS analysis. PCA and PSA–DA chemometric methods were applied to EN and SPME–GC/MS data, respectively. Results suggest that the two techniques can be considered as complementary rather than represent mutually exclusive alternatives to each other.

7 Conclusions

The wide range-applications of sensors, chemical and biosensors in particular, for soil analysis performed over the past two decades have been reported in this chapter. Sensors represent a low-cost, fast, and nondestructive way for the evaluation of main soil nutrients concentrations, measuring moisture, salinity, pH, and other soil parameters, assessment of fertility and evaluation of anthropogenic impact on soil conditions. Recently sensors have been widely used for on-the-go and on-field soil assessment, for precision agriculture, horticulture, soil mapping, and proper soil recourses management purposes, thus attesting to be an effective and promising substitutive technique to standard analysis methods employed in soil analysis. Moreover, the possibility to simultaneously measure several soil parameters by multisensory approach in combination to chemometric techniques opens new perspectives in sensors application for soil types ranking and classification and quantitative analysis.

Acknowledgments

This work was partly supported by the RFBR project No.15-04-08707.

References

Abbaspour, A., Mirahmadi, E., Khalafi-nejad, A., Babamohammadi, S., 2010. A highly selective and sensitive disposable carbon composite PVC-based membrane for determination of lead ion in environmental samples. J. Hazard. Mater. 174, 656–661.

Adamchuk, V.I., Lund, E.D., Sethuramasamyraja, B., Morgan, M.T., Dobermann, A., Marx, D.B., 2005. Direct measurement of soil chemical properties on-the-go using ion-selective electrodes. Comput. Electron. Agric. 48, 272–294.

Alizadeh, T., Zare, M., Ganjali, M.R., Norouzi, P., Tavana, B., 2010. A new molecularly imprinted polymer (MIP)-based electrochemical sensor for monitoring 2,4,6-trinitrotoluene (TNT) in natural waters and soil samples. Biosens. Bioelectron. 25, 1166–1172.

Artigas, J., Beltran, A., Jiménez, C., Bartroli, J., Alonso, J., 2001a. Development of a photopolymerisable membrane for calcium ion sensors. Application to soil drainage waters. Anal. Chim. Acta 426, 3–10.

Artigas, J., Beltran, A., Jimenez, C., Baldi, A., Mas, R., Domınguez, C., Alonso, J., 2001b. Application of ion sensitive field effect transistor based sensors to soil analysis. Comput. Electron. Agric. 31, 281–293.

Artigas, J., Jimenez, C., Lemos, S.G., Nogueira, A.R.A., Torre-Neto, A., Alonso, J., 2003. Development of a screen-printed thick-film nitrate sensor based on a graphite-epoxy composite for agricultural applications. Sens. Actuat. 88, 337–344.

Bansod, B.S., Pandey, O.P., 2013. An application of PCA and fuzzy C-means to delineate management zones and variability analysis of soil. Eurasian Soil Sci. 46, 556–564.

Baskeyfield, D.E.H., Davis, F., Magan, N., Tothill, I.E., 2011. A membrane-based immunosensor for the analysis of the herbicide isoproturon. Anal. Chim. Acta 699, 223–231.

Beni, V., Ogurtsov, V.I., Bakunin, N.V., Arrigan, D.W.M., Hill, M., 2005. Development of a portable electroanalytical system for the stripping voltammetry of metals: determination of copper in acetic acid soil extracts. Anal. Chim. Acta 552, 190–200.

Bhattacharya, B., Solomatine, D.P., 2006. Machine learning in soil classification. Neural Netw. 19, 186–195.

Birrell, S.J., Hummel, J.W., 2001. Real-time multi-ISFET/FIA soil analysis system with automatic sample extraction. Comput. Electron. Agric. 32 (1), 45–67.

Blum, W.E.H., 1990. The challenge of soil protection in Europe. Environ. Conserv. 17, 72–74.

Blum, W.E.H., 2005. Functions of soil for society and the environment. Rev. Environ. Sci. Biotechnol. 4, 75–79.

Bogrekci, I., Lee, W.S., 2005. Spectral soil signatures and sensing phosphorus. Biosyst. Eng. 92 (4), 527–533.

Bojdi, M.K., Behbahani, M., Sahragard, A., Amin, B.G., Fakhari, A., Bagheri, A., 2014. A palladium imprinted polymer for highly selective and sensitive electrochemical determination of ultra-trace of palladium ions. Electrochim. Acta 149, 108–116.

Brandt, K.K., Holm, P.E., Nybroe, O., 2008. Evidence for bioavailable copper-dissolved organic matter complexes and transiently increased copper bioavailability in manure-amended soils as determined by bioluminescent bacterial biosensors. Environ. Sci. Technol. 42, 3102–3108.

Cal, Y., 1995. Soil classification by neural network. Adv. Eng. Softw. 22, 95–97.

Cammann, G.G., Guilbault, E.A., Hal, H., Kellner, R., Wolfbeis, O.S., 1996. The Cambridge Definition of Chemical Sensors, Cambridge Workshop on Chemical Sensors and Biosensors. Cambridge University Press, New York.

Chen, J., Sun, S., Li, C.-Z., Zhu, Y.-G., Rosen, B.P., 2014. Biosensor for organoarsenical herbicides and growth promoters. Environ. Sci. Technol. 48, 1141–1147.

Chikae, M., Kerman, K., Nagatani, N., Takamura, Y., Tamiya, E., 2007. An electrochemical on-field sensor system for the detection of compost maturity. Anal. Chim. Acta 581, 364–369.

Ciesla, J., Ryzak, M., Bieganowski, A., Tkaczyk, P., Walczak, R.T., 2007. Use of ion-selective electrodes for determination of content of potassium in Egner-Riehm soil extracts. Res. Agric. Eng. 53, 29–33.

Coelho, C., Branco, R., Natal-da-Luz, T., Sousa, J.P., Morais, P.V., 2015. Evaluation of bacterial biosensors to determine chromate bioavailability and to assess ecotoxicity of soils. Chemosphere 128, 62–69.

Cooper, J., Bolbot, J.A., Saini, S., Setford, S.J., 2007. Electrochemical method for the rapid on site screening of cadmium and lead in soil and water samples. Water Air Soil Pollut. 179, 183–195.

De Cesare, F., Pantalei, S., Zampetti, E., Macagnano, A., 2008. Electronic nose and SPME techniques to monitor phenanthrene biodegradation in soil. Sens. Actuat. B 131, 63–70.

de Matos Oliveira, R., de Andrade, M.C.N., de Souza Oliveira, G., 2014. A capacitive-type humidity sensor using porous ceramics for environmental monitoring. Advanced Materials Research. 6th International Conference on Electroceramics, ICE 2013, Joao Pessoa, Brazil; Code 106904. 975, pp. 194–198.

Dong, J., Wang, X., Qiao, F., Liu, P., Ai, S., 2013. Highly sensitive electrochemical stripping analysis of methyl parathion at MWCNTs–CeO_2–Au nanocomposite modified electrode. Sens. Actuat. B 186, 774–780.

Eller, H., Denoth, A., 1996. A capacitive soil moisture sensor. J. Hydrol. 185, 137–146.

Engblom, S.O., 1999. Determination of inorganic phosphate in a soil extract using a cobalt electrode. Plant Soil 206, 173–179.

Esbensen, K., 2004. Multivariate Data Analysis in Practice, fifth ed Camo Press, AS, Trondheim, 590 p.

Eswaran, H., Berg, E., Van Den, Reich, P., 1993. Organic carbon in soils of the world. Soil Sci. Soc. Am. J. 57 (N 1), 192–194.

Farré, M., Brix, R., Barcelo, D., 2005. Screening water for pollutants using biological techniques under European Union funding during the last 10 years. Trends Anal. Chem. 24, 532–545.

Fraters, D., 1994. Generalized soil map of Europe: Aggregation of the FAO-Unesco soil units based on the characteristics determining the vulnerability to soil degradation processes, RIVM, Report 71240300. RIVM, Biltoven, The Netherlands.

Garotti, F.V., Massaro, S., Serrano, S.H.P., 1992. Determination of aluminum in soils with fluoride-ion selective electrode. Analysis 20, 287–290.

Gianetto, M., Umiltà, E., Careri, M., 2014. New competitive dendrimer-based and highly selective immunosensor for determination of atrazine in environmental, feed and food samples: the importance of antibody selectivity for discrimination among related triazinic metabolites. Anal. Chim. Acta 806, 197–203.

Gieling, Th.H., van Straten, G., Janssen, H.J.J., Wouters, H., 2005. ISE and Chemfet sensors in greenhouse cultivation. Sens. Actuat. B 105, 74–80.

Gonzalez-Martınez, M.A., Brun, E.M., Puchades, R., Maquieira, Ä., Ramsey, K., Rubio, F., 2005. Glyphosate immunosensor. Application for water and soil analysis. Anal. Chem. 77, 4219–4227.

Göpel, W., Hesse, J., Zemel, J.N., 1989. Sensors: A Comprehensive SurveyVCH, New York.

Gupta, V.K., Pal, M.K., Singh, A.K., 2009. Comparative evaluation of Dy(III) selective poly(vinyl) chloride based membrane electrodes of macrocyclic tetraimine Schiff's bases. Talanta 79, 528–533.

Gurbuz, Y., Kang, W.P., Davidson, J.L., Kerns, D.V., 2004. Diamond microelectronic gas sensor for detection of benzene and toluene. Sens. Actuat. B 99, 207–215.

Gutierrez, M., Alegret, S., Caceres, R., Casadesus, J., Marfa, O., del Valle, M., 2007. Application of a potentiometric electronic tongue to fertigation strategy in greenhouse cultivation. Comput. Electron. Agric. 57, 12–22.

Gutierrez, M., Alegret, S., Caceres, R., Casadesus, J., Marfa, O., del Valle, M., 2008. Nutrient solution monitoring in greenhouse cultivation employing a potentiometric electronic tongue. J. Agric. Food Chem. 56, 1810–1817.

Holland, K.H., Lamb, D.W., Schepers, J.S., 2012. Radiometry of proximal active optical sensors (AOS) for agricultural sensing. IEEE J. Select. Top. Appl. Earth Observ. Remote Sens. 8, 1793–1802.

Hou, Q.-H., Ma, A.-Z., Lv, D., Bai, Z.-H., Zhuang, X.-L., Zhuang, G.-Q., 2014. The impacts of different long-term fertilization regimes on the bioavailability of arsenic in soil: integrating chemical approach with *Escherichia coli* arsRp::luc-based biosensor. Appl. Microbiol. Biotechnol. 98, 6137–6146.

Hulanichi, A., Geab, S., Ingman, F., 1991. Chemical sensors definitions and classification pure. Appl. Chem. 63, 1247.

Hung, Y.-L., Hsiung, T.-M., Chen, Y.-Y., Huang, Y.-F., Huang, C.-C., 2010. Colorimetric detection of heavy metal ions using label-free gold nanoparticles and alkanethiols. J. Phys. Chem. C 114, 16329–16334.

ISA, 1975. Instrument Society of America. Electrical Transducer Nomenclature and Terminology ANSI Standard MC6.1. Research Triangle Park, North Carolina. Available from: www.isa.org

Ivask, A., Francois, M., Kahru, A., Dubourguier, H.-C., Virta, M., Douay, F., 2004. Recombinant luminescent bacterial sensors for the measurement of bioavailability of cadmium and lead in soils polluted by metal smelters. Chemosphere 55, 147–156.

Kahru, A., Ivask, A., Kasemets, K., Pollumaa, L., Kurvet, I., Francois, M., Dubourguier, H.-C., 2005. Biotests and biosensors in ecotoxicological risk assessment of field soils polluted with zinc, lead, and cadmium. Environ. Toxicol. Chem. 24, 2973–2982.

Kaur, J., Adamchuk, V.I., Whalen, J.K., Ismail, A.A., 2015. Development of an NDIR CO_2 sensor-based system for assessing soil toxicity using substrate-induced respiration. Sensors 15, 4734–4748.

Kim, H.J., Hummel, J.W., Sudduth, K.A., Motavalli, P.P., 2007. Simultaneous analysis of soil macronutrients using ion-selective electrodes. Soil Sci. Soc. Am. J. 71, 1867–1877.

Kim, H.J., Sudduth, K.A., Hummel, J.W., Drummond, S.T., 2013. Validation testing of a soil macronutrient sensing system. Trans. ASABE 56, 23–31.

Kopylovich, M.N., Mahmudov, K.T., Pombeiro, A.J.L., 2011. Poly(vinyl) chloride membrane copper-selective electrode based on 1-phenyl-2-(2-hydroxyphenylhydrazo)butane-1,3-dione. J. Hazard. Mater. 186, 1154–1162.

Kovačević, M., Bajat, B., Gajić, B., 2010. Soil type classification and estimation of soil properties using support vector machines. Geoderma 154, 340–347.

Lemos, S.G., Nogueira, A.R., Torre-Neto, A., Parra, A., Artigas, J., Alonso, J., 2004. In-soil potassium sensor system. J. Agric. Food Chem. 52, 5810–5815.

Lemos, S.G., Nogueira, A.R.A., Torre-Neto, A., Parra, A., Alonso, J., 2007. Soil calcium and pH monitoring sensor system. J. Agric. Food Chem. 55, 4658–4663.

Lemos, S.G., Menezes, E.A., Chaves, F.S., Nogueira, A.R.A., Torre-Neto, A., Parra, A., Alonso, J., 2009. In situ soil phosphorus monitoring probe compared with conventional extraction procedures. Comm. Soil Sci. Plant Anal. 40, 1282–1294.

Liu, C.C., 2000. Electrochemical Sensors. In: Bronzino, J.D. (Ed.), The Biomedical Engineering Handbook: second ed CRC Press LLC, Boca Raton.

Liu, C.-W., Huang, C.-C., Chang, H.-T., 2009. Highly selective DNA-based sensor for lead(II) and mercury(II) ions. Anal. Chem. 81, 2383–2387.

Liu, P., Huang, Q., Chen, W., 2012. Construction and application of a zinc-specific biosensor for assessing the immobilization and bioavailability of zinc in different soils. Environ. Pollut. 164, 66–72.

Lobsey, C.R., Viscarra Rossel, R.A., McBratney, A.B., 2010. Proximal soil nutrient sensing using electrochemical sensors. In: Viscarra Rossel, R.A., McBratney, A.B., Minasny, B. (Eds.), Proximal soil sensing. Springer, pp. 77–88.

Lvova, L., Kirsanov, D., Legin, A., Di Natale, C. (Eds.), 2014. Multisensor Systems for Chemical Analysis—Materials and Sensors. Pan Stanford Publishing, Singapore, 430 p.

Magrisso, S., Erel, Y., Belkin, S., 2008. Microbial reporters of metal bioavailability. Microb. Biotechnol. 1 (4), 320–330.

Maletić, S.P., Watson, M.A., Dehlawi, S., Diplock, E.E., Mardlin, D., Paton, G.I., 2015. Deployment of microbial biosensors to assess the performance of ameliorants in metal-contaminated soils. Water Air Soil Pollut. 226, 85–98.

McGrath, D., Skotnikov, A., 1996. Automated work-station for soil analysis. Commun. Soil Sci. Plant Anal. 27, 1795–1812.

McGraw, C.M., Radu, T., Radu, A., Diamond, D., 2008. Evaluation of liquid- and solid-contact, Pb^{2+}-selective polymer-membrane electrodes for soil analysis. Electroanalysis 20 (3), 340–346.

Md Noh, M.F., Tothill, I.E., 2006. Development and characterisation of disposable gold electrodes, and their use for lead(II) analysis. Anal. Bioanal. Chem. 386, 2095–2106.

Md Noh, M.F., Kadara, R.O., Tothill, I.E., 2005. Development of cysteine-modified screen-printed electrode for the chronopotentiometric stripping analysis of cadmium(II) in wastewater and soil extracts. Anal. Bioanal. Chem. 382, 1175–1186.

Mimendia, A., Gutierrez, J.M., Alcaniz, J.P., del Valle, M., 2011. Discrimination of soils and assessment of some soil fertility parameters using an electronic tongue. AIP Conf. Proc. 1362, 191–192.

Mimendia, A., Gutierrez, J.M., Alcaniz, J.P., del Valle, M., 2014. Discrimination of soils and assessment of soil fertility using information from an ion selective electrodes array and artificial neural networks. Clean Soil Air Water 42, 1808–1815.

Motellier, S., Noir, M.H., Pitsch, H., Durdault, B., 1995. pH determination of clay interstitial water using a fiber-optic sensor. Sens. Actuat. B 29, 345–352.

Nedeltcheva, T., Atanassova, M., Dimitrov, J., Stanislavova, L., 2005. Determination of mobile form contents of Zn, Cd, Pb and Cu in soil extracts by combined stripping voltammetry. Anal. Chim. Acta 528, 143–146.

NMAB, 1995. Expanding the vision of sensor materials, 1995. National Materials Advisory Board, National Academy Press, Washington, DC, 134 p. Available from: www.nap.edu

Palchetti, I., Laschi, S., Mascini, M., 2005. Miniaturised stripping-based carbon modified sensor for in field analysis of heavy metals. Anal. Chim. Acta 530, 61–67.

Patranabis, D., 2004. Sensors and Transducers. PHI Learning, Delhi, India, 344 p.

Peltola, P., Ivask, A., Aström, M., Virta, M., 2005. Lead and Cu in contaminated urban soils: extraction with chemical reagents and bioluminescent bacteria and yeast. Sci. Total Environ. 350, 194–203.

Petänen, T., Romantschuk, M., 2002. Use of bioluminescent bacterial sensors as an alternative method for measuring heavy metals in soil extracts. Anal. Chim. Acta 456, 55–61.

Petänen, T., Virta, M., Karp, M., Romamtschuk, M., 2001. Construction and use of broad host range mercury and arsenite sensor plasmids in the soil bacterium *Pseudomonas fluorescens* OS8. Microb. Ecol. 41, 360–368.

Plata, M.R., Hernando, J., Zougagh, M., Contento, A.M., Villasenor, M.J., Sanchez-Rojas, J.L., Rıos, A., 2008. Characterization and analytical validation of a microcantilever-based sensor for the determination of total carbonate in soil samples. Sens. Actuat. B 134, 245–251.

Prasad, B.B., Jauhari, D., Tiwari, M.P., 2014. Doubly imprinted polymer nanofilm-modified electrochemical sensor for ultra-trace simultaneous analysis of glyphosate and glufosinate. Biosens. Bioelectron. 59, 81–88.

Price, R.R., Hummel, J.W., Birrell, S.J., Ahmad, I.S., 2003. Rapid nitrate analysis of soil cores using ISFETs. Trans. ASAE 46 (3), 601–610.

Rivera, D., Granda, S., Arumí, J.L., Sandoval, M., Billib, M., 2012. A methodology to identify representative configurations of sensors for monitoring soil moisture. Environ. Monitor. Assess. 184 (11), 6563–6574.

Sacks, V., Eshkenazi, I., Neufeld, N., Dosoretz, K., Rishpon, J., 2000. Immobilized parathion hydrolase: an amperometric sensor for parathion. Anal. Chem. 72, 2055–2058.

Sauerbrey, G., 1959. Verwendung von Schwingquarzen zur Wägung dünner Schichten und zur Mikrowägung. Z. Phys. 155, 206–222.

Sethuramasamyraja, B., Adamchuk, V.I., Dobermann, A., Marx, D.B., Jones, D.D., Meyer, G.E., 2008. Agitated soil measurement method for integrated on-the-go mapping of soil pH, potassium and nitrate contents. Comput. Electron. Agric. 60, 212–225.

Silva, F.C.S., Molin, J.P., 2013. Real time soil sensing for determination of tropical soils pH. In: Proc. of 9th European Conference on Precision Agriculture, Lleida, Spain, July 7–11, 2013, Precision Agriculture, vol. 13, pp. 41–48.

Silva, P.R.M., El Khakani, M.A., Chaker, M., Dufresne, A., Courchesne, F., 2001. Simultaneous determination of Cd, Pb and Cu metal trace concentrations in water certified samples and soil extracts by means of Hg-electroplated–Ir microelectrode array based sensors. Sens. Actuat. B. 76, 250–257.

Sinfield, J.V., Fagerman, D., Colic, O., 2010. Evaluation of sensing technologies for on-the-go detection of macro-nutrients in cultivated soils. Comput. Electron. Agric. 70, 1–18.

Singh, A.K., Sahani, M.K., Bandi, K.R, Jain, A.K., 2014. Electroanalytical studies on Cu (II) ion-selective sensor of coated pyrolytic graphite electrodes based on $N_2S_2O_2$ and $N_2S_2O_3$ heterocyclic benzothiazol ligands. Mater. Sci. Eng. C 41, 206–216.

Soil Atlas of Europe, 2005. European Soil Bureau Network European Commission, 2005, 128 pp. Office for Official Publications of the European Communities, L-2995 Luxembourg ©European Communities, 2005/Catalogue Number LB-37-01-744-EN-C ISBN 92-894-8120-XEUR 21676E. Available from: www.eusoils.jrc.ec.europa.eu/projects/soil_atlas/download/2.pdf

Staggenborg, S.A., Carignano, M., Haag, L., 2007. Predicting soil pH and buffer pH in situ with a real-time sensor. Agron. J. 99 (3), 854–861.

Strachan, G., Capel, S., Maciel, H., Porter, A.J.R., Paton, G.I., 2002. Application of cellular and immunological biosensor techniques to assess herbicide toxicity in soils. Eur. J. Soil Sci. 53, 37–44.

Tang, L., Zeng, G.M., Shen, G.L., Li, Y.P., Hang, Y.Z., Huang, D.L., 2008. Rapid detection of picloram in agricultural field samples using a disposable immunomembrane-based electrochemical sensor. Environ. Sci. Technol. 43, 1207–1212.

Targulian, V.O., Goryachkin, S.V. (Eds.), 2008. Soil Memory: Soil as a Memory of Biosphere-Geosphere-Anthroposphere Interaction. Publishing house GEOS, Moscow (In Russian).

Venancio, E.C., Consolin Filho, N., Constantino, C.J.L., Martin-Neto, L., Mattoso, L.H.C., 2005. Studies on the interaction between humic substances and conducting polymers for sensor application. J. Braz. Chem. Soci. 16, 24–30.

Viscarra Rossel, R.A., Fouad, Y., Walter, C., 2008. Using a digital camera to measure soil organic carbon and iron contents. Biosyst. Eng. 100, 149–159.

Visconti, F., Martínez, D., Molina, M.J., Ingelmo, F., de Paz, J.M., 2014. A combined equation to estimate the soil pore-water electrical conductivity: calibration with the WET and 5TE sensors. Soil Res. 52, 419–430.

Wang, X., Liu, F., Han, X., 2012. Influence of soil physical and chemical properties on performance of soil profile moisture sensor. Nongye Jixie Xuebao/Trans. Chin. Soc. Agric. Machine. 43 (11), 97–101.

Wei, H., Cheng, H., Mao, T., Zhong, W.-H., Lin, X.-G., 2010. A chromosomally based luminescent bioassay for mercury detection in red soil of China. Appl. Microbiol. Biotechnol. 87, 981–989.

Wilczek, A., Szypłowska, A., Skierucha, W., Cies´la, J., Pichler, V., Janik, G., 2012. Determination of soil pore water salinity using an FDR sensor working at various frequencies up to 500 MHz. Sensors 12, 10890–10905.

Wilson, D., de los Ángeles Arada, M., Alegret, S., del Valle, M., 2010. Lead(II) ion selective electrodes with PVC membranes based on two bis-thioureas as ionophores: 1,3-bis(*N'*-benzoylthioureido)benzene and 1,3-bis(*N'*-furoylthioureido)benzene. J. Hazard. Mater. 181, 140–146.

Wilson, D., Gutierrez, J.M., Alegret, S., del Valle, M., 2012. Simultaneous determination of Zn(II), Cu(II), Cd(II) and Pb(II) in Soil samples employing an array of potentiometric sensors and an artificial neural network model. Electroanalysis 24, 2249–2256.

Yagodina, O.V., Nikolskaya, E.B., Shor, N.B., 2000. Gas-gap sensors for the determination of nitrogen oxides and nitrites. Anal. Chim Acta 409, 143–147.

Yang, J.-W., Cho, H.-J., Choi, G.-Yo., Lee, S.-H., 2001. Cost-effective monitoring for a soil vapor extraction (SVE) system. A simplified modeling and gas sensor test. Environ. Monitor. Assess. 70, 201–210.

Yang, J.-W., Cho, H.-J., Lee, S.-H., Lee, J.-Yo., 2004. Characterization of SnO_2 ceramic gas sensor for exhaust gas monitoring of SVE process. Environ. Monitor. Assess. 92, 153–161.

Yokota, M., Okada, T., Yamaguchi, I., 2007. An optical sensor for analysis of soil nutrients by using LED light sources. Measure. Sci. Technol. 18, 2197–2201.

Zou, Z., Han, J., Jang, A., Bishop, P.L., Ahn, C.H., 2007. A disposable on-chip phosphate sensor with planar cobalt microelectrodes on polymer substrate. Biosens. Bioelectron. 22, 1902–1907.

18

SURFACE PLASMON RESONANCE BASED NANOSENSORS FOR DETECTION OF TRIAZINIC PESTICIDES IN AGRICULTURAL FOODS

Fatma Yılmaz*, Yeşeren Saylan, Semra Akgönüllü**, Duygu Çimen**, Ali Derazshamshir**, Nilay Bereli**, Adil Denizli****

**Abant İzzet Baysal University, Department of Chemistry Technology, Bolu, Turkey; **Hacettepe University, Department of Chemistry, Ankara, Turkey*

1 Introduction

Pesticides are chemicals that control insects, weeds, fungi, and other pests that destroy crops and include a large number of compounds like fungicides, nematicides, insecticides, molluscicides, rodenticides, herbicides, and plant growth hormones. Pesticides are spread in the environment with the aim of controlling undesired living species. The use of these compounds may pose risks to human health and the environment because their toxicity is not always specific to the target organisms. The most common pesticides like organochlorines (OC) which are used to overcome many diseases like malaria and typhus, have been banned or at least reduced during the last 50 years due to their recalcitrant nature. Increased productivity was obtained by the application of various organophosphorus (OP) compounds during the 1960s, carbamates during the 1970s, and pyrethroids during the 1980s, along with the synthesis of other pesticides (1970s–1980s), which have reduced the pest hazards (Aktar et al., 2009). Pesticides are essential tools for the control of vector-borne diseases and noxious insects so without the use of pesticides, up to 50% of the agricultural products would be lost and also pesticides have several other uses, including protection of plants and products from biological degradation.

New Pesticides and Soil Sensors. http://dx.doi.org/10.1016/B978-0-12-804299-1.00019-9

The first molecules extracted from plants or mined (arsenic, mercury, oil derivatives, etc.) were used as pesticides and the first pesticide to be synthesized was 1,1,1-trichloro-2,2-bis[4-chlorophenyl]ethane (DDT) in 1874. Muller and coworkers discovered its insecticidal properties in 1978 (International Programme on Chemical Safety, 1978). The bioaccumulation potential of DDT, together with the risk of effects on human and animal health and also environment, led to the restriction of its use in many countries since the beginning of the 1960s. At the beginning of the 1970s, OP compounds largely replaced DDT accompanied by low level of accumulation in biological organisms and in the environment, and these compounds showed very good insecticidal activity. Introduction of these highly toxic compounds into the market caused a rapid growth of acute poisoning cases and fatalities. Consequently, acetylcholinesterase inhibitors, such as the carbamate insecticides were developed with lower toxic potential for humans and nontarget species and were introduced in the market. Meanwhile, OP compounds that were easily degradable by biological enzymes such as carboxylesterase were developed. Since carboxylesterase is found in mammalian tissues, OP compounds show good insecticidal activity and low toxicity to mammals but are poorly represented in insects; however, their toxicity remains unchanged for untargeted nonmammalian species, such as bees. In 1978, a compound similar to natural pyrethrum, fenvalerate was introduced in the market. Later, other pyrethroids were developed; there are currently roughly 40 available in the market. Insecticide development history similar to the history of the development of other pesticides, such as fungicides and herbicides, clearly shows that research has always been oriented at two major complementary objectives: pest control efficacy and risk reduction to human and environment. Therefore, pest management strategies rely on risk assessment of pesticide use as a fundamental component. At present, pesticides are classified according to their acute mammalian toxicity as suggested by WHO (2006) (Table 18.1). Pesticides can also be classified according to the target pest, as reported in Table 18.2 (Vasilescu and Medvedovici, 2005).

Herbicides are the class of pesticides that are used to kill weeds and other undesirable life forms in agricultural crops, including insects, while fungicides are employed to restrict the growth of molds and mildew. A herbicide, is intended to prevent, control, destroy, repel, or mitigate the growth of weeds within a crop, consists of any individual substance or mixture. The use of insecticides is seen to be gradually declining and herbicides will gain popularity in the future (Zhang et al., 2011). There are many criteria involved

Table 18.1 Classification of Pesticides According to Hazard

	Rat LD_{50} (mg kg^{-1} body weight)			
	Oral Administration		Dermal Administration	
Class of Pesticides	Solid Form	Liquid Form	Solid Form	Liquid Form
Extremely hazardous	≤5	≤20	≤10	≤40
Highly hazardous	5–50	20–200	10–100	40–400
Moderately hazardous	50–500	200–2000	100–1000	400–4000
Slightly hazardous	>500	>2000	>1000	>4000

Physical state of products and formulations are shown as solid and liquid form.

Table 18.2 Pesticide Classification According to the Target Pest

Larvicides	Acaricides
Miticides	Attractants
Molluscicides	Defoliants
Nematicides	Desiccants
Plant growth regulators	Fungicides
Repellents	Herbicides
Rodenticides	Insecticides

in the classification of herbicides, including classifications according to the way of action and chemical structure (Vasilescu and Medvedovici, 2005).

Due to the excessive use of these chemicals in agriculture, humans may be exposed to low concentrations of these biocidal residues through the food chain. The health effects of these residues are currently being investigated. Surveys have revealed that more prevalent cases of insomnia, dizziness, headaches, hand tremors, fatigue, and other neurological symptoms in children among the farming community are due to the use of agricultural insecticides and pesticides. Hepel et al. (2012) established that reactive oxygen species (ROS) generation which are potent enough to cause damage to DNA (Nurzhanova et al., 2013) may be induced by catechol-containing compounds.

Nowadays, a large amount of various harmful organic chemicals including herbicides, insecticides and fungicides are used in agriculture. Their prolonged use involves the hazards of retention in soils because of persistency in the environment. So, they could pass probability into surface and ground waters due to washing and leaching processes. For these reasons, their monitoring of them is one of the most important tasks of modern analytical chemistry (Barek et al., 2007; Martini et al., 2015; Zhang et al., 2014). So enhanced attention is given to health risks associated with exposure of a human population to harmful substances occurring in the environment.

Atrazine (ATZ), simazine (SMZ), and cyanazine (SNZ) are the most known triazinic herbicides that have been used in the annual control of some grasses and broadleaf weeds with toxic effects on organisms. They are stable and persistent in the environment for a longer period (half-life varying among 20 and 100 days) due to their low reactivity, water solubility, and slow degradation (Xinga et al., 2012). Even in small quantities, it may act as a carcinogen and an endocrine disruptor (Lin and Chu, 2011). There is a still growing need to develop sensitive and selective analytical methods for environmental monitoring of residual pesticides.

In recent years, various analytical methods for the determination of triazinic herbicides were reported in research literature. These particularly involve spectrophotometric (Zhang and Pan, 2011) and chromatographic methods, such as high-performance liquid chromatography (HPLC) (Wulfeck-Kleier et al., 2010; Mou et al., 2011; Zhao et al., 2011) and gas chromatography (GC) (Real et al.,2012), which have become the most widely used analytical methods for the determination of trace amounts of triazinic herbicides because of their absolute best sensitivity and selectivity. However in these techniques, complicated sample preparations including preconcentration steps are required prior to the analysis. Expensive, time consuming, and solvent waste-producing methods and also the demands for highly skilled personnel often restrict their use in routine analytical practice.

Molecular imprinting has attracted growing attempts to prepare molecular complementary parts of the interested molecules into the highly cross-linked polymeric structure. The method mainly depends on the molecular recognition by which polymerization occurs around the interested target molecules called templates (Wulff et al., 1997). Specific cavities are created inside the polymeric matrices after removal of template molecules (Ozcan et al., 2006), which have memories that are capable of selectively rebinding the template molecules (Ersöz et al., 2008). By using this approach, recognition sites for many molecules including small molecules, such as metal ions (Asir et al., 2005), organic molecules (Cao et al., 2010), and large molecules like proteins (Whitcombe et al., 2011; Zhou et al., 2011; Uzun et al., 2009a) in a synthetic polymer can be created.

Although this technique has several advantages it also has some drawbacks. First, rebinding capacity of highly cross-linked rigid structures of the MIPs, with irregular shape, is reduced. Second, imprinted template molecules inside the polymer cannot be removed easily from their cavities. Therefore, some decrease in the analyte adsorption and desorption rates to the imprinted polymer was observed. Molecularly imprinted nanosized materials were preferred to overcome these problems, because, these materials have a high surface to volume ratio and more critically most of the imprinted sites are located at the surface (Sener et al., 2010; Guan et al., 2008; Lu et al., 2007; Chen et al., 2011; Xu et al., 2011).

Surface plasmon resonance (SPR), an optical phenomenon occurs when a p-polarized light goes through a prism and hits a metal layer covering the prism surface at a particular angle (Englebienne et al., 2003). SPR was introduced as the underlying technology for biomolecular interaction analysis in affinity biosensors, a new concept for the analysis of the functional properties of biomolecules in the early 1990s (Malmqvist and Biacore, 1999). SPR biosensors with unique properties, such as real-time measurement, high specificity, sensitivity, and no need for labeling, have become more popular for investigation of several analyte molecules (Banerjia et al., 2010; Shina et al., 2010; Hooper et al., 2009; Kim et al., 2009). Additionally, MIPs are used for creation of biorecognitive surfaces on the SPR biosensors (Uzun et al., 2009a,b; Riskin et al., 2010). Saylan et al. (2017) have focused their attention on producing SPR nanosensors for detection of ATZ, SMZ, and SNZ herbicides, which are chosen as model pesticides by molecular imprinting method.

2 Surface Plasmon Resonance

SPR has seen extensive growth since its initial observation by Wood (1902) with utilization of the optical phenomenon. It was initially exploited for a variety of spectroscopic and physical characterizations including enhanced holography (Cowan, 1972), surface enhanced Raman scattering (SERS) or coherent anti-Stokes Raman scattering (CARS) (Kiefer and Long, 1982), and surface plasmon microscopy (SPM) for high contrast imaging of thin dielectric films (Rothenbausler and Knoll, 1988; Hickel and Knoll, 1989). Refractive index (η) changes that occur in the vicinity of a thin metal film surface are probed with simple and direct-sensing SPR technique (Otto, 1968). This technique utilizes a thin film of metal, typically gold or silver, between two transparent media of different refractive index (i.e., glass prism and sample solution) to function as an optical sensor surface. A plane-polarized light beam entering the higher refractive index medium (glass prism) can undergo total internal refraction when critical angle is exceeded. Penetration of the evanescent wave, which is an electromagnetic field component of the light, into the gold film occurs under these conditions. At a specific angle of incidence, excitation of surface plasmon take place by interaction of this wave with free oscillating electrons at the gold film surface, resulting subsequently in a decrease in the reflected light intensity. SPR phenomena occurs only at a specific angle which is modified by the addition of the analyte onto the gold film surface, thereby allowing the monitoring of binding events. From a practical standpoint, the most frequently employed geometry in SPR is the Kretschmann prism arrangement. As illustrated in Fig. 18.1, this configuration uses an evanescent wave created by total internal reflection at a waveguide interface that excites charge density oscillation at the surface of the film. These electron oscillations are more commonly referred to as surface plasmons. The penetration depth of the evanescent field will depend on the wavelength of the light, the

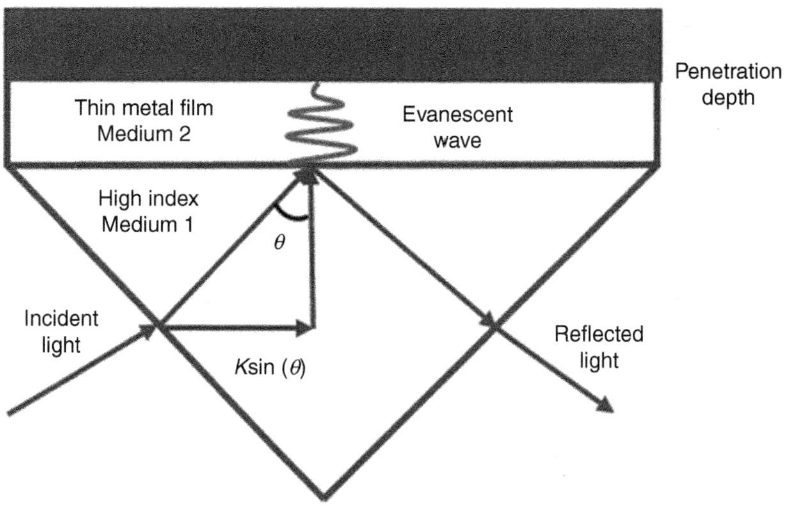

Figure 18.1. Total internal reflection at a dielectric boundary.

refractive index ratio of the waveguide to the surroundings, and the photon intensity in the mode.

The field energy will decay exponentially with distance from the surface, and thus penetration depth falls off rapidly as shown schematically in Fig. 18.1. An estimation of the penetration depth is given by the following expressions (Buck et al., 1990):

$$d_{\mathrm{p}} = \frac{\lambda}{4\pi\sqrt{\eta_1^2 \sin^2\theta - \eta_2^2}} \tag{18.1}$$

where η_1 and η_2 are the refractive index of medium 1 and medium 2, respectively. Typically, this will be approximately equal to one-fourth of the incident light wavelength.

Light that is p-polarized with respect to the metal surface is launched into the prism for coupling to the metal film, only p-polarized light can be utilized for plasmon generation because this particular polarization has the electric field vector oscillations normal to the metal film. This is referred to as the transverse magnetic (TM) wave of the electron plasma along the flat metal surface (Szentirmay, 1992; Welford, 1991). In contrast, the s-polarized transverse electric (TE) polarization cannot generate surface plasmons since its electric field vector is orientated parallel to the metal film. The wave vector of the oscillations, K_{sp}, is given by the expression:

$$K_{\mathrm{sp}} = \frac{\omega}{c}\sqrt{\frac{\varepsilon_{\mathrm{m}}\varepsilon_{\mathrm{s}}}{\varepsilon_{\mathrm{m}} + \varepsilon_{\mathrm{s}}}} \tag{18.2}$$

where ω is the frequency of the oscillations, c is the speed of light, ε_{s}, the dielectric function of the sample medium adjacent to the metal surface, and ε_{m} is the dielectric function of the metal. The wave vector for a component of incident light can be described by the equation:

$$K_x = \frac{\omega}{c}\eta_{\mathrm{p}}\sin\theta \tag{18.3}$$

where θ is the angle of incidence of the light onto the metal film and η, the refractive index of the prism. Surface plasmons, which oscillate and propagate along the upper surface of the metal film, absorb some of the p-polarized light energy from the evanescent field to change the total-internal-reflection light intensity I_{r}. Therefore, a plot of I_{r} versus incidence (or reflection) angle (θ_{r}) produces an angular intensity profile that exhibits a sharp dip at the resonance angle.

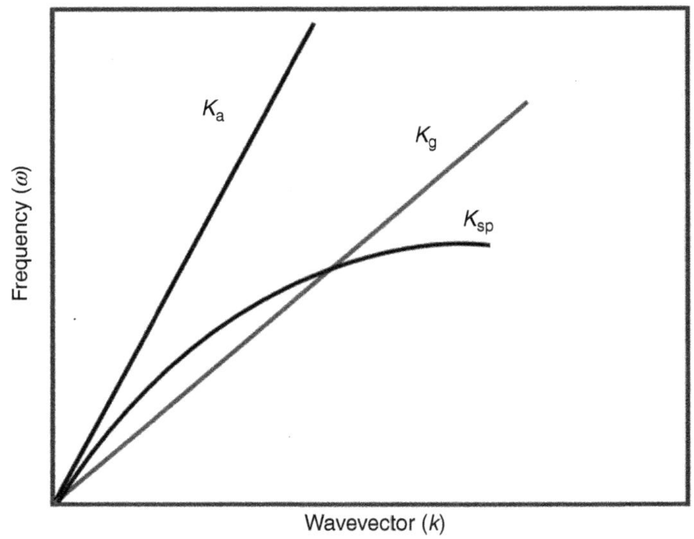

Figure 18.2. Dispersion curves for air, glass, and surface plasmon.

The presence of the prism (and its high refractive index value) is essential since it is not possible to generate surface plasmons directly with incident light radiation in the air. The wave vector for both the incident light and the surface plasmon field must be equal during SPR. However, as shown in Fig. 18.2, the dispersion curve of light in air ($K_a = \omega/c$) and that of plasmons in the metal do not intersect. Hence, there is no possibility of matching simultaneously both the wave vector and the frequency. In contrast, the intersection of the dispersion curves K_{sp} and K_g, also shown in Fig. 18.2, indicates the ability of glass to increase the light vector enabling the necessary matching for plasmon generation.

The surface plasmon wave vector can be related to the refractive index of the medium on the near vicinity of the metal film by simplification of the equation. Disregarding the imaginary portion of ε, K_{sp} can be rewritten as:

$$K_{sp} = \frac{\omega}{c}\sqrt{\frac{\eta_m^2 \eta_s^2}{\eta_m^2 + \eta_s^2}} \tag{18.4}$$

where η_m, is the refractive index of the metal and η_s is the refractive index of the sample. The imaginary component of the complex refractive index term can be related to absorbance.

The SPR profile is affected by the choice of metal due to its inherent optical properties, such as dielectric permittivity. Fig. 18.3 compares the SPR curve, a plot of reflected light intensity versus

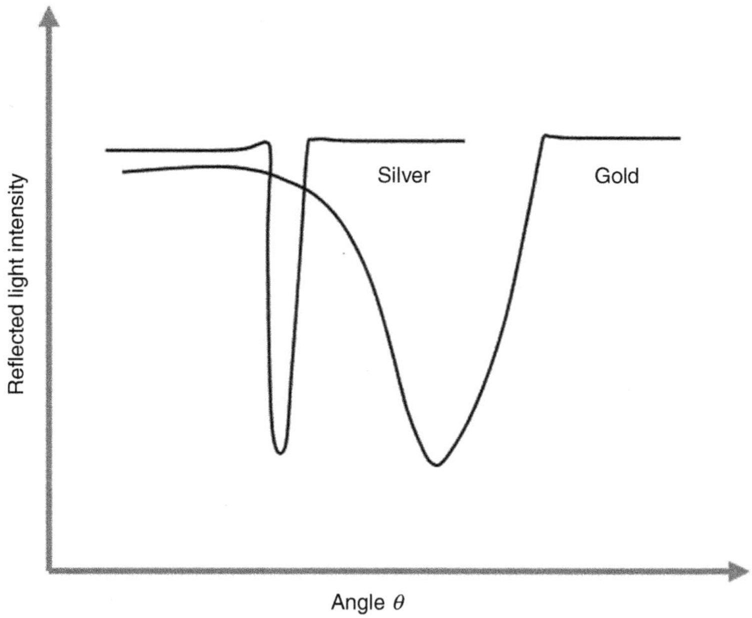

Figure 18.3. SPR curves for silver and gold (Earp and Dessy, 1996).

the incident angle for gold and silver films in air. The sharper resonance peak of silver is obvious and can be attributed to the intrinsic dampening of the surface plasmon oscillations on the metal film. All surface plasmon metals will tend to dampen these oscillations due to scattering of the electric field of the excitation light. A variety of metals, which have conduction band electrons capable of resonating with the light of the appropriate angle can produce SPR. To perform SPR assays, chemical compatibility with the chemistries is also needed. Gold is the preferred metal as other metals are not as practical. For example, some are too expensive (indium), violently reactive (sodium), too broad in their SPR response (copper, aluminum), or too susceptible to oxidation (silver) (Earp and Dessy, 1996).

The characteristic of this phenomenon, which makes SPR an analytical tool is that any change in the chemical composition of the environment within the range of the plasmon field causes a change in the angle of light that resonances with the plasmons. That is, a chemical composition change results in a shift in the angle of incidence at which light is absorbed and the magnitude of the shift is quantitatively related to the magnitude of the chemical change. In an immunoassay, a thin film of metal is applied to a prism that has been deposited onto a substrate (typically glass or plastic). Then antibodies specific to a particular analyte (e.g., hormone, drug, tumor marker, and so on) are nonspecifically adsorbed to the metal film. When the sensor is exposed to a sample containing that analyte, the binding of the antibody and the analyte causes a chemical composition change at the metal surface, within the plasmon field and the shift in the resonant angle of the incident light is measured. The size of the shift is proportional to the quantity of the analyte in the sample. Any pair of molecules that exhibit specific binding can be adapted to SPR measurement. These may be an antigen and antibody, a DNA probe and complementary DNA strand, an enzyme and its substrate, or a chelating agent and metal ion.

3 Molecular Imprinting

Molecular imprinting method, first reported by Wulff and Sarhan (1972), is regarded as one of the most facile methods to introduce molecular recognition sites into polymeric membranes (Wulff, 1995; Mosbach and Ramström, 1996; Sellergren, 1997; Piletsky et al., 1999). In order to introduce molecular recognition sites into polymeric materials, the first step involves the complexation of a target molecule (a print molecule or a template) with polymerizable monomers having functional moieties, which form covalent or noncovalent bonds with the print molecule in solution. During this step, functional monomers are assembled around the print molecule and as a result, predetermined orientation of the functional moieties is achieved. In the following step, cross-linkers are added to the complex solution with the mixture being polymerized to form highly cross-linked polymers such that the molecular shape of the print molecule and alignment of the functional moieties may be retained in the molecularly imprinted polymeric materials thus prepared. Removal of the print molecule from the imprinted polymers leads to completion of the complementary molecular recognition sites.

The interactions between analytes and/or template molecules and also the monomers can be described by single or multiple interactions of functional groups of both compounds. They can be different types of interaction such as hydrogen bonds, ionic and hydrophobic interaction. This implies that polymers generated from these monomers will always interact with the analyte or template molecule as well as with compounds that contain functional groups similar to those of the template.

The affinity increases with the number of interacting groups, however, each individual interaction can be strongly dependent on the properties of the solvent, for example, protic or aprotic, polarity, dielectric constants, presence of complex forming agents, and so on. These effects can occur through interaction with the polymer, the analyte, or both. Affinities between interacting groups can vary from zero to nanomolar equilibrium dissociation constants. Therefore, application of molecular imprints appears to have a potential for a range of analytical applications.

The number of functional molecules interact with a template molecule in solution (or in a gas). These functional molecules are arranged in an orderly manner with respect to each other so that their functional groups are complementary to the template. The interactions are hydrogen bonding, electrostatic, apolar, and any other noncovalent interactions. All the functional molecules would soon start moving randomly, and their ordering would disappear if suddenly the template molecule is removed from this system. As a result, the memory for the template is immediately gone. However, this randomization is minimized by connecting these functional molecules together by means of a polymer backbone by the molecular imprinting method. Nowadays, molecular imprinting may be classified into two types, namely, "covalent molecular imprinting" and "noncovalent molecular imprinting" depending on the nature of adducts between functional monomer and template. It is easy to obtain imprinted polymers with high specificity, due to stable complexes (covalent binding moieties) between the print molecule and target molecule being retained during polymerization. The covalent bond adopted for molecular imprinting should be reversible. Furthermore, formation and cleavage of the covalent bond should be fast for applications requiring membrane separation.

The first covalent imprinting shown in Fig. 18.4 was reported by Wulff et al. (1997). They synthesized covalent conjugate of p-vinylbenzeneboronic acid with 4-nitrophenyl-α-D-mannopyranoside (the template), and after copolymerization of this conjugate with methyl methacrylate ethylene dimethacrylate (a cross-linking monomer), the boronic acid ester in the polymer was cleaved, and the 4-nitrophenyl-α-D-mannopyranoside was removed.

The resultant polymer strongly and selectively bound this sugar exactly as desired. Two boronic acid groups having mutual conformation in the covalent conjugate were frozen in the polymer, and the structure of the template was memorized. Functional monomer and template are bound to each other covalently prior to polymerization (step 1). Then, this covalent conjugate is polymerized under the conditions where the covalent linkage is intact (step 2). After the cleavage of covalent linkage, template is removed from the polymer backbone.

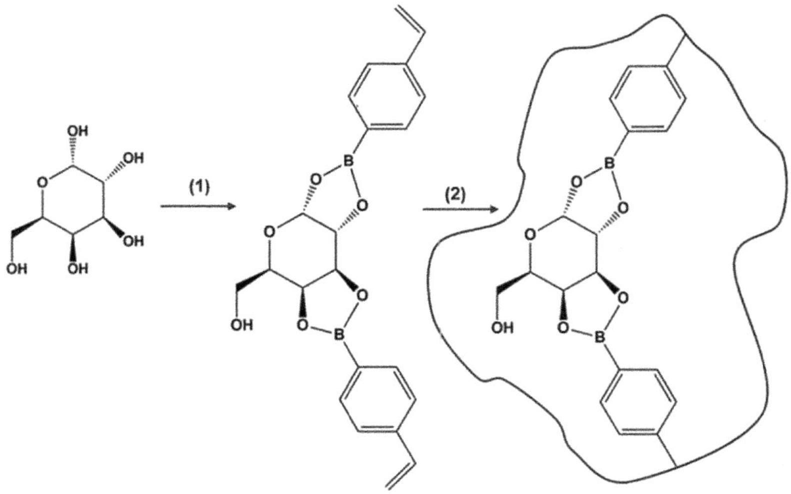

Figure 18.4. Concept of covalent imprinting (Wulff et al., 1997).

Performing the molecular imprinting method in a tailor-made fashion is quite simple and easy. Neither complicated organic synthesis nor complex molecular design is necessary. You can simply polymerize appropriate monomer(s) in the presence of the guest compound (or its analog) as the template, if you want to have a artificial receptor toward a certain guest compound used as template. Another combination of functional monomer and template can be used for another guest molecule. The corresponding receptor can be at hand almost automatically.

Molecular imprinting has been extensively reviewed in both the periodic press (Byrne et al., 2002; Mosbach et al., 2001; Ansell and Mosbach, 1996) and in a series of books (Sellergren, 2001; Komiyama et al., 2002; Yan and Ramström, 2005; Piletsky and Turner, 2006) and the number of original articles and patents have continued to increase (Piletsky et al., 2001; Bereli et al., 2011). Commonly, small (MW $\leq$ 1000) multifunctional template molecules have potential to give rise to MIPs having high affinity and specificity (Bowman et al., 1998), however, an increase in molecule size and functionality on the template leads to increased binding site heterogeneity in respective polymers (Takeuchi and Matsui, 1996). To establish polymer-template reciprocal functionality on which MIP function relies, polar noncovalent interactions are utilized commonly. Examples of this type of strategy includes amino acids (Kempe, 1996), drugs, such as theophylline and diazepam (Vlatakis et al., 1993), nucleotides (Spivak and Shea, 2001), and pesticides (Siemann et al., 1996). An alternative approach to establish reciprocal functionality relies initially on covalent interactions while subsequent rebinding has been demonstrated through either the reestablishment of covalent linkages or via a noncovalent mechanism (Wulff et al., 2005). Examples of the template types using this approach are sugars (Wulff and Schauhoff, 1991), monoalcohols (Alexander et al., 1999), and steroids (Cheong et al., 1997).

Noncovalent molecular imprinting was proposed by Mosbach (Arshady and Mosbach, 1981). The following interactions are enumerated as typical noncovalent interactions: hydrogen bonding, electrostatic interactions, hydrophobic interactions, metal coordinations, charge transfers, etc. Those noncovalent interactions should be, as a matter of course, reversible. By exploitation of these binding forces, as it has turned out, noncovalent interactions are prevalent in the biological world and the most efficient and preferred method for generating robust, biomimetic binding materials (Mosbach et al., 2001). It is assumed that selectivity change can only occur for molecularly imprinted polymers in comparison to nonimprinted polymers when the analyte and/or matrix components of the sample have an increased number of interaction points. So, single and part of the dual point interactions taking place between the analyte and the polymer will affect the selectivity. Analyte and matrix component interaction with nonimprinted parts of a polymer may overshadow the interactions of the analyte with the true imprint so that the selectivity is not as good as required for the application, resulting in irrespective imprinting efficacy. The number of binding sites play important role in the selective interaction of the analyte with the cavity present in the polymer backbone is typically less than 1% but can mount to 35% of the theoretical maximum amount of binding sites.

Noncovalent adducts were spontaneously formed by mixing those in a reaction mixture and satisfactory imprinting effects were obtained. In the imprinting process of monomer with template through hydrogen bonding and electrostatic interaction, a noncovalent monomer–template adduct was formed (Fig. 18.5).

Noncovalent interactions, for example, hydrogen bonding, electrostatic interaction, and coordination-bond formation are used in order to connect a functional monomer with a template. Thus, the adducts can be obtained in-situ simply by adding the components to reaction mixtures (step 1). The template is removed after the polymerization (step 2), by extracting with appropriate solvents (step 3). The guest binding by the polymer occurs through the corresponding noncovalent interactions (step 4). Table 18.3 shows advantages and disadvantages of covalent and noncovalent imprinting.

The advantages of covalent and noncovalent imprinting (fast guest binding) were combined. One of the shortcomings of covalent imprinting (slow guest binding and guest release) has been

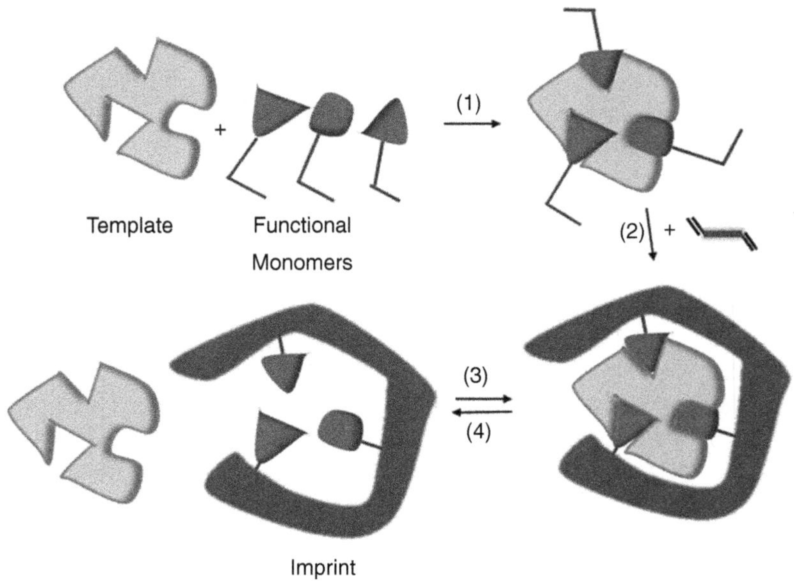

Figure 18.5. Concept of noncovalent imprinting.

Table 18.3 Advantages and Disadvantages of Covalent and Noncovalent Imprinting

	Covalent	Noncovalent
Synthesis of monomer-template conjugate	Necessary	Unnecessary
Polymerization condition	Rather free	Restricted
Removal of template after polymerization	Difficult	Easy
Guest-binding and guest-release	Slow	Fast
Structure of guest-binding site	Clearer	Less clear

solved by employing noncovalent interactions for guest binding and polymer was prepared as in covalent imprinting by this approach. The purpose is not restricted to the preparation of artificial receptors and is much wider in scope. There are no alternative methods which can freeze molecular movements in solutions (or in gases) and immobilize them according to design. The use of biomolecules as templates is also promising in molecular biology and pharmacology (Malmqvist and Biacore, 1999; Banerjia et al., 2010; Shina et al., 2010).

Monitoring pesticide residues in water is very important for human health protection as well as for environmental control. GC–ECD, GC–MS, or LC–MS analytical sytems are used to determine pesticides preceded by sample clean-up using liquid–liquid extraction, solid-phase extraction, solid-phase microextraction, or single-drop microextraction methods (Lopez-Blanco et al., 2003). Molecular imprinting is one of the promising options to incorporate selectivity and to enhance sensitivity of extraction methods. Molecularly imprinted polymers (MIPs) with molecular recognition brilliance are attractive materials designed to be used in many different fields, such as sensors, enantiomeric separations, biomedical and analytical applications, etc. Regarding analytical applications, thus far, MIPs have been applied successfully on solid-phase microextraction (SPME), but nowadays the main interest has focused more specifically on the up-and-coming technique of molecularly imprinted solid-phase microextraction (MISPME) (Spietelun et al., 2010).

Controlling polymeric film thickness in the molecularly imprinted SPME methods has severe difficulties as the desired graft polymerization was always accompanied by polymerization in solution when azo-initiators were used (Martin-Esteban, 2013). A number of procedures are explored by researchers in order to overcome the drawbacks of molecularly imprinted SPME methods. MIP-coated silica fibers produced by using surface reversible addition-fragmentation chain transfer polymerization (RAFT) offered a better control of the thickness of MIP coating. But all methods offer advantages with some restrictions, such as fragility, lack of porosity, and thereby poor accessibility of target analytes to binding sites, etc. due to the practical limitations of immobilization of tailor-made preparation onto fiber. Thus, stability and capacity of such fibers need improvement to produce molecularly imprinted SPME fibers that are robust, cost effective, most selective and sensitive, reproducible, thermally stable, easily synthesized and having better kinetics, capacity, and compatibility with environmental matrix.

Mazzotta et al. (2012) used the electropolymerization of conducting polymers to prepare MIP-coated fibers. Shaikh et al. (2014) reported successful employment of core–shell imprinted particles for enhanced and efficient preconcentration of endosulfan I and II pesticides through solid-phase microextraction technique prior to GC–μECD detection. They used a simple and cheap laboratory-made solid-phase microextraction device. The synthesized core–shell particles were characterized thoroughly and examined for its adsorption capacity and selectivity. The method was optimized using Plackett–Burman design and further verified with Central

Composite Surface design. The developed method was validated and found robust and highly sensitive to low limits of detection for endosulfan I and II. They solved the problems of low capacity, slow kinetics, poor accessibility of template molecules to binding sites, nonadherence of MIP on fiber surface, uncontrolled polymer thickness on the fiber surface, and fragility of molecularly imprinted fiber.

4 Applications of Surface Plasmon Resonance by Molecularly Imprinted Systems

Herbicides belong to an interesting class of pesticides frequently probed by sensor measurements owing to their increasing presence as a contaminant in water or in agricultural products. Among pesticides, triazinic compounds were intensively studied (Berg et al., 1995; Luo et al., 2001; Piletsky et al., 1995; Matsui et al., 1995). However, these studies were based on the use of conventional transducers: Shoji et al. (2003) studied the reduction behavior of ATZ using classical nonconducting polymeric sensing layer by electrochemistry. No work has yet been reported in the literature, concerning the use of MIPs for the quantitative detection of herbicides by optic-based nanosensors.

Molecular imprinting method, mainly depends on the molecular recognition, is a type of polymerization that occurs around the interested molecules called as template, has attracted growing attempts to prepare molecular complementary parts of the interested molecules into highly cross-linked polymeric structure (Wulff et al., 1997; Toorisaka et al., 1999). Specific cavities are created inside solid polymeric matrices after removal of template molecules, which have memories capable of selectively rebinding to the template molecules (Ozcan et al., 2006; Ersöz et al., 2008). By using this approach, recognition sites can be formed for many molecules including small molecules, such as metal ions, organic molecules, and large molecules like proteins.

Although this technique has several advantages, it also has some drawbacks. First, rebinding capacity of polymeric matrix is reduced due to the highly cross-linked rigid structures of the MIPs with irregular shape. Second, imprinted template molecule removal from the cavities formed inside the polymer is not easy. Therefore, some decrease in the analyte adsorption and desorption rates to the imprinted polymer was observed. To overcome these problems, molecularly imprinted nanosized materials were preferred, because, these materials have a high surface to volume ratio and more critically most of the imprinted sites are located at the surface. Hereby, the template molecules can be removed easily and higher adsorption rates can be obtained (Sener et al., 2010; Guan et al., 2008; Lu et al., 2007; Chen et al., 2011; Xu et al., 2011).

Optic phenomenon SPR occurs when a p-polarized light hits a metal layer covering the prism surface at a particular angle after passing through a prism (Englebienne et al., 2003). SPR was introduced in the early 1990s as the underlying new concept technology in affinity biosensors for the analysis of the functional properties of biomolecules using biomolecular interactions (Malmqvist and Biacore, 1999). The applications of SPR sensors having unique properties, such as real-time measurement, no need for labeling, high specificity, and sensitivity have been earning more popularity for investigation of several analyte molecules (Banerjia et al., 2010).

Relatively quick and real-time measurements can be taken with SPR (Sípová and Homola, 2013; Şener et al., 2011), however, using unstable receptor molecules, such as antibodies and cost limitation of coated chips which are used in SPR sensors have generated the need to investigate potential artificial recognition sites. Molecularly imprinted polymers (MIPs) as artificial synthetic receptors have been used in numerous applications ranging from liquid chromatography to sensor technology and have proven their potential for creation of biorecognitive surfaces on the SPR sensors (Uzun et al., 2009b; Riskin et al., 2010).

The physicochemical response change, such as mass, resistance, capacitance, and refractive index change, resulting from binding a target analyte are translated into a sensor signal often leads to MIP sensors showing relatively low sensitivity and specificity. This deficiency problem can be solved by using enzyme-labeled templates to amplify signal and increasing the number of cavities in the molecular imprinted film (Sharma et al., 2013).

Diffusion limitations occur with the increase of the membrane thickness although the amount of the imprinted sites increases because thick membranes lead to slow diffusion of the analytes to the recognition sites and to inefficient communication between the binding sites and transducers (Riskin et al., 2008). Yao et al. (2013) proposed an approach for the synthesis of magnetic MIPs with high density and accessible recognition sites for sensitive SPR detection of chlorpyrifos (CPF). Magnetic MIPs were synthesized by self-polymerization of dopamine on the surface of Fe_3O_4 nanoparticles (NPs) in the presence of template CPF molecule in the solution. This method enables the template-imprinting sites accessible to the target to situate at the surface or in the proximity of material's surfaces, and as a result fast association/dissociation kinetics can be expected. By applying external magnetic field to the imprinted Fe_3O_4@ polydopamine nanoparticles (Fe_3O_4@PDA NPs), enrichment and separation of target CPF molecules were carried out. Signal amplification due to the integration of Fe_3O_4@PDA NPs to SPR chip through the specific interactions between the CPF recognition cavities in the PDA matrix and the AChE immobilized on sensor chip was achieved successfully, and with this attempt molecularly imprinted nanoparticles having magnetic properties were combined with SPR for CPF detection.

Profenofos were detected in tap water by SPR sensor as a sensing material that uses molecularly imprinted ultrathin polymer which was anchored on a gold chip by surface-initiated radical polymerization developed by Dong et al. (2012). Surface-initiated radical polymerization method used to prepare an ultrathin MIP film on an SPR sensor is easier than photoinitiated polymerization.

MIP film anchored on a gold surface of SPR sensor chip was prepared by using surface-bound photoradical initiator to fabricate sensitive SPR sensor for organophosphorus pesticide (OPP) acephate by Wei et al. (2011). MIPs display both comparable molecular selectivity, and also chemical inertness, long-term stability, insolubility in water and most organic solvents compared to its biological counterparts, enzymes and antibodies. Triazinic herbicides are used to prevent pre- and postemergence of broadleaf weeds in crops and has become the most widely used herbicide (Rodríguez-González et al., 2014). Its wide spread use has led to the release of herbicides into waste water, sediments, and many water sources. The presence of herbicides in waste waters may affect the ecosystem and human health (Rivoira et al., 2015). Therefore, it is critical to develop sufficiently sensitive methods for the detection and determination of triazinic herbicides in waste water. Recently, a number of analytical methods have been developed to detect herbicides using gas micellar electrokinetic chromatography (Li et al., 2014), voltammetric competitive immunosensor (Giannetto et al., 2014), multivariate electronic spectroscopy (Amaral et al., 2014), gas chromatography–mass spectrometry (Bruzzoniti et al., 2006), thin-layer chromatography (Rezic et al., 2005), and high-performance liquid chromatography (Pinto and Jardim, 2000). But these methods have significant disadvantages in large material consumption, complexity, and expensiveness. A rapid and sensitive method to detect herbicides is important to ensure human and environmental safety. Molecularly imprinted quartz crystal microbalance (QCM) sensors using the molecules complexed with functional monomers have attracted great interests in recent years because of their simplicity and high sensitivity (Gupta et al., 2014).

Zhao et al. (2012) detected ametryn by preparing feasible, uniform, and controllable SPR sensing films with surface-initiated atom transfer radical polymerization (ATRP) method coupled to molecular imprinting to improve sensitivity and selectivity of SPR chip. Imprinted sensing film prepared on the gold chips revealed good imprinting effect and impressive selectivity for ametryn compared to the nonimprinted film with linear response in the range of 0.1–10 μM ($R^2 = 0.9985$). The selectivity efficiencies of ametryn and other structurally related analogs were 1.0 and 0.10–0.56, respectively.

Saylan et al. (2017) have focused their attention on combining of molecular imprinting into nanofilms and SPR nanosensor approaches and producing SPR nanosensors for herbicides, chosen as template molecules. Thus, the aim of their work is the design and development of an MIP based SPR nanosensor system for the selective detection of herbicides named SNZ, SMZ, and ATZ from aqueous solution by MIP method. They prepared herbicide [(SNZ), (SMZ), and (ATZ)] imprinted [PMAPAVIM] nanofilms which are attached on the surface of SPR nanosensor. Phenylalanine based monomer was chosen as functional monomer owing to its ability to establish hydrogen bonds with triazinic herbicides, forming a precursor complex. Herbicide imprinted SPR nanosensors were characterized by contact angle measurements, atomic force microscopy, and ellipsometry. The nanosensor has an ability to detect herbicide molecules from aqueous solution, even if it has herbicide concentration as low as 0.1 nM for SNZ, SMZ, and ATZ, respectively. Association kinetics analysis, Scatchard, Langmuir, Freundlich, Langmuir–Freundlich isotherms were applied to data. The calculated association constants were 0.148, 0.250, and 2.88 nM for SNZ, SMZ, and ATZ, respectively. The nonimprinted nanosensor was also prepared by them as a control to evaluate the selectivity of the imprinted nanosensor. Finally, the nanosensors were used for four adsorption–desorption–regeneration cycles and a reproducible response was observed.

By focusing on herbicides they expanded the coverage to discuss recent developments in sensor technology based on advanced functional materials. In the first section they synthesized *N*-methacryloyl-L-phenylalanine methyl ester (MAPA) comonomer from L-phenylalanine methyl ester and methacryloyl chloride (Türkmen et al., 2008). Preparation of herbicide imprinted SPR nanosensor was performed to produce SNZ, SMZ, and ATZ imprinted poly(*N*-methacryloyl-L-phenylalanine methyl ester-1-vinyl imidazole) (PMAPAVIM] nanofilm on the gold surface of SPR sensor. Procedure steps are: (1) surface modification of the SPR chip with allyl mercaptan (CH_2CHCH_2SH); (2) coordination of herbicides (templates) with MAPA comonomer to form SNZ-MAPA, SMZ-MAPA, ATZ-MAPA precomplexes; (3) mixing of precomplexes with hydrophobic VIM monomer to get mixture to be prepared as polymer nanofilm; (4) pouring monomer mixture onto the modified gold surface of the SPR sensor to contact with the allyl mercaptan; (5) irradiation with UV to initiate polymerization and fixing the imprinted orientation of monomers; and (6) removal of template molecule.

SPR chip surface modification was performed with allyl mercaptan according to the recipe prepared by Uzun et al. (2009b). Herbicides named SNZ (2,4-bis(ethylamino)-6-methoxy-s-triazine), SMZ (2,4-bis(ethylamino)-6-chloro-1,3,5-triazine), and ATZ (2-chloro-4-ethylamino-6-isopropylamino-1,3,5-triazine) were used for the preparation of herbicide imprinted nanofilm on allyl mercaptan modified SPR sensor and the following steps were used for the preparation.

Firstly, MAPA monomer was precomplexed with herbicides to preorganize and then precomplex monomer was mixed with vinyl-imidazole (VIM) and cross-linker, EGDMA monomer at room temperature for 2 h. The prepared mixture was put under the UV light (100 W, 365 nm) and polymerization was initiated at room temperature and continued for 4 h under nitrogen atmosphere. SPR sensor was dried in a vacuum oven after washing with 0.1 M HCl/methanol (1:1, v/v) and methanol, respectively, to remove unreacted monomers. Fig. 18.6 shows nanosensor chip making the system.

Template removal of the SPR nanosensor was performed via batch system setup using $CaCl_2$ solution as a desorption agent. Herbicide imprinted SPR nanosensors were immersed into the desorption solution and shaken at room temperature for 1 h. The SPR nanosensors were washed with deionized water and dried with N_2 under vacuum (200 mmHg, 25°C) after removal of herbicide molecules.

Surface characterization of SPR chip surfaces was performed with contact angle (CA) measurements with sessile drop method, atomic force microscopy (AFM) studies using tapping mode, and ellipsometry using an autonulling imaging ellipsometer at a wavelength of 658 nm with an angle of incidence of 60°. For imprinting of SNZ, SMZ, and ATZ herbicides onto the SPR chip, SPR chip surfaces were modified. Chip surfaces were characterized by CA, AFM, and ellipsometry measurements after modification steps. Fig. 18.7 shows CA measurements for SNZ, SMZ, and ATZ imprinted nanofilm attached sensors. According to the results,

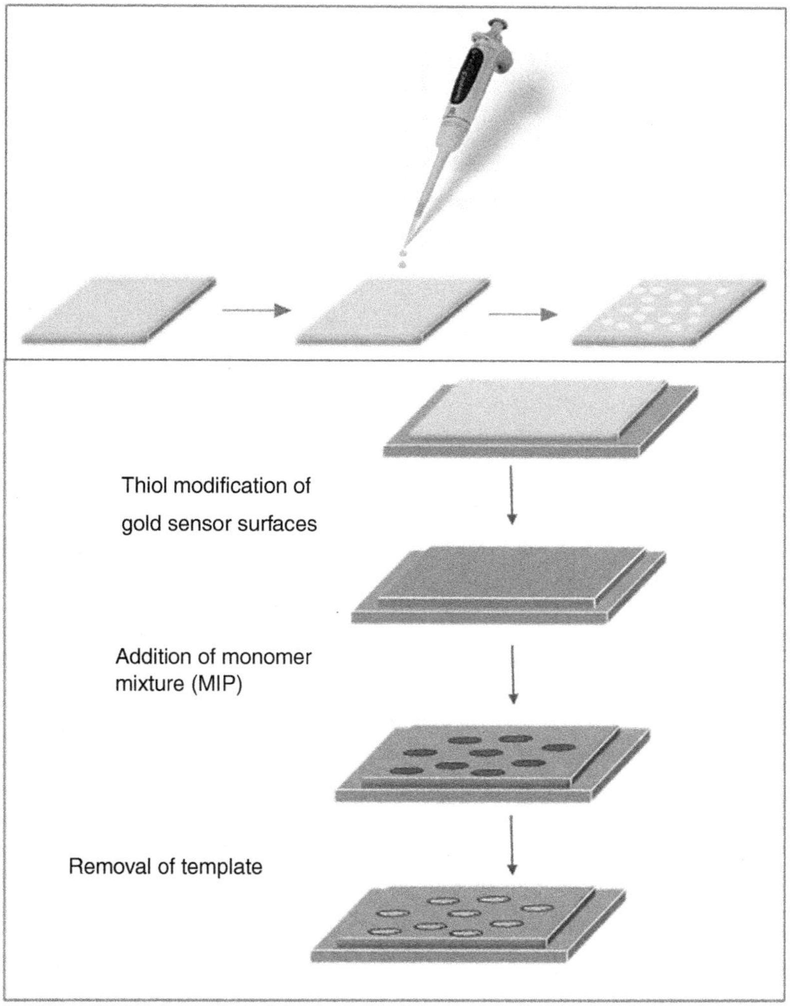

Figure 18.6. Schematic representation of the preparation of molecular imprinted SPR chip.

herbicide imprinting onto the SPR nanosensors were successfully performed. CA measurements for different sensors were summarized in Fig. 18.7. Due to the molecular imprinting of triazinic herbicides, the contact angle value of the chip surface decreased from 71.3° to 52.6°, 59.8°, 70.4° for nonimprinting, SNZ, SMZ, and ATZ imprinted nanosensors, respectively. Hydrophilicity and/or polarity of the surface increased due to the introduction of the herbicides having triazinic groups which cause significant decrease in contact angle value. After the production of nonimprinted

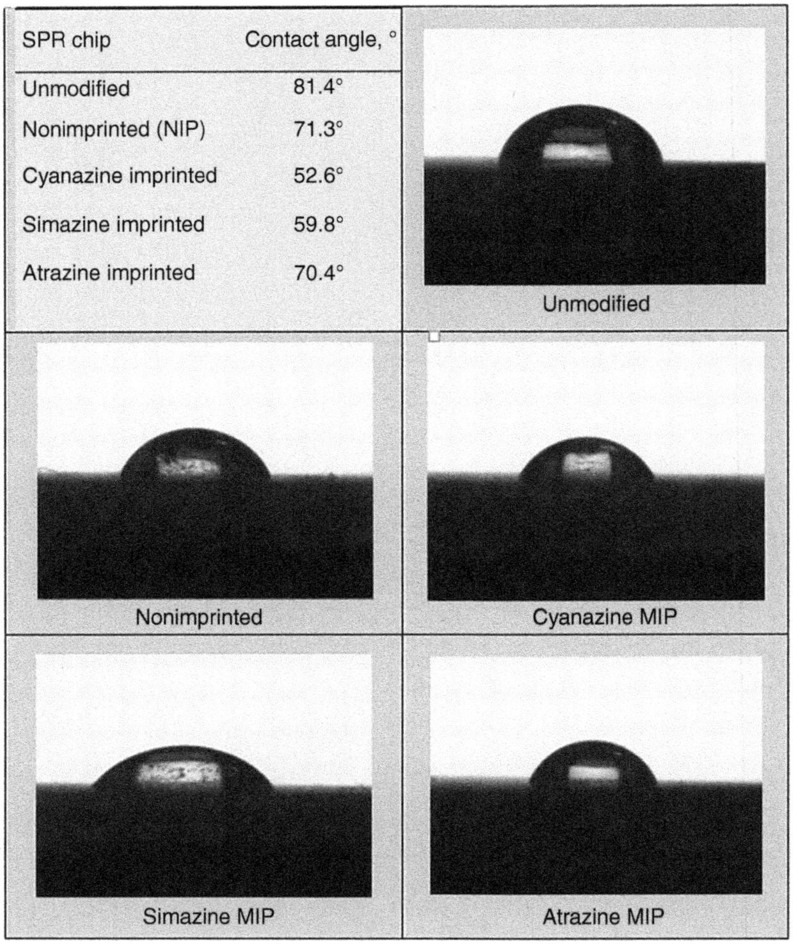

SPR chip	Contact angle, °
Unmodified	81.4°
Nonimprinted (NIP)	71.3°
Cyanazine imprinted	52.6°
Simazine imprinted	59.8°
Atrazine imprinted	70.4°

Figure 18.7. Contact angle measurements for unmodified, nonimprinted, SNZ, SMZ, and ATZ imprinted SPR chips.

polymeric nanofilm on chip surface, the contact angle value decreased from 81.4° to 71.3°. This implies that polymeric nanofilm formed on SPR nanosensor has hydrophilic character which stemmed from the hydrophilic monomers like vinylimidazole. AFM observations were carried out by using ambient AFM in dynamic mode. SPR chips used during this study were attached on a sample holder by silver paste. A rough polymeric surface was formed on the SPR chip surfaces due to the polymerization process. From the AFM image measurements, it was understood that the film formation is homogeneous and the surface deepness of the SPR chip surfaces was 112.72, 97.76, and 88.48 nm for SNZ, SMZ, and ATZ, respectively. These results show similarity with the ellipsometry measurements.

Ellipsometry measurements during the molecular imprinting process have been done to obtain surface thickness. Polymeric thin films are one of the most desirable forms of recognition elements in SPR sensors. The effect of thin films on sensor sensitivity is due to two main reasons. Since SPR sensitivity related to the surface plasmons is only effective in limited thickness (up to 200 nm), preparing thin films on sensor surface is one of the first things to do to prepare a good sensor system. Generally a good film thickness is accepted as values smaller than 50 nm. The thickness measurement of chip surfaces was carried out with single wavelength nulling type imaging ellipsometer in PCSA configuration. According to the data obtained the thickness of nonimprinted, SNZ, SMZ, and ATZ imprinted SPR nanosensors was estimated to be 115.687 ± 1.2, 125.600 ± 0.8, 121.760 ± 0.4, and 118.482 ± 0.9 nm, respectively.

Kinetic, isotherm, and selectivity studies with SPR nanosensors have been done for both herbicide imprinted (SNZ imprinted; SMZ imprinted; ATZ imprinted MIP) and nonimprinted (NIP) [PMAPAVIM] nanofilms. The $\Delta R\%$ values were monitored instantly and reached a plateau value in approximately 15 min. Concentration dependency of the herbicide-imprinted SPR nanosensor was evaluated by application of varied herbicide concentrations to the SPR system.

In order to determine the kinetic and equilibrium isotherm parameters, they examined SPR nanosensor data using a pseudo-first-order kinetic analysis and four different equilibrium isotherm models, Scatchard, Langmuir, Freundlich, and Langmuir–Freundlich, were applied to herbicide imprinted SPR sensor data (Li and Husson, 2006). The linear form of the applied model can be given as:

$$\text{Equilibrium kinetic analysis } \mathrm{d}\Delta R/\mathrm{d}t = k_\mathrm{a} C \Delta R_\mathrm{max} - (k_\mathrm{a} C + k_\mathrm{d})\Delta R \tag{18.5}$$

$$\text{Scatchard } \Delta R_\mathrm{ex}/C = K_\mathrm{A}(\Delta R_\mathrm{max} - \Delta R_\mathrm{eq}) \tag{18.6}$$

$$\text{Langmuir } \Delta R = \{\Delta R_\mathrm{max}[C]/K_\mathrm{D} + [C]\} \tag{18.7}$$

$$\text{Freundlich } \Delta R = \Delta R_\mathrm{max}[C]^{1/n} \tag{18.8}$$

$$\text{Langmuir} - \text{Freundlich } \Delta R = \{\Delta R_\mathrm{max}[C]^{1/n}/K_\mathrm{D} + [C]^{1/n}\} \tag{18.9}$$

ΔR is the response measured with binding; C is herbicide concentration (nM); $1/n$ is Freundlich exponent; k_a ($nM^{-1}.s^{-1}$) and k_d (s^{-1}) are forward and reverse kinetic rate constants; K_A (nM^{-1}) and K_D (nM) are forward and reverse equilibrium constants; subscripts ex, max, and eq indicate experimental, maximum, and equilibrium, respectively. When applying the equilibrium kinetic analysis, slopes of curves were calculated and plotting concentrations versus slopes of curves enabled the determination of k_a and k_d, respectively (Sener et al., 2010).

Real-time response of herbicide imprinted SPR nanosensor for aqueous solution of SNZ, SMZ, and ATZ herbicides was monitored. As clearly understood the sensors had a quick response when the herbicide solution was contacted to the sensor surface. The increase in herbicide concentration also caused an increase in SPR nanosensor response. After 15 min (900 s) a plateau was reached and desorption agent was injected on to the SPR nanosensor for flushing off bound molecules. After these steps, the system was washed with deionized water for 5 min. All of the steps, including equilibration–adsorption–desorption–regeneration, were completed in 50 min. As seen in Fig. 18.8, increase in concentrations for SNZ caused an increase in SPR responses. The SPR signal change was obtained as the Pixel Intensity Unit (PIU) in this SPR imager and these data were converted to the real change in reflectivity, $\Delta R\%$ because it is the absolute physical unit of measurement. To convert PIU to $\Delta R\%$ the following equation was used.

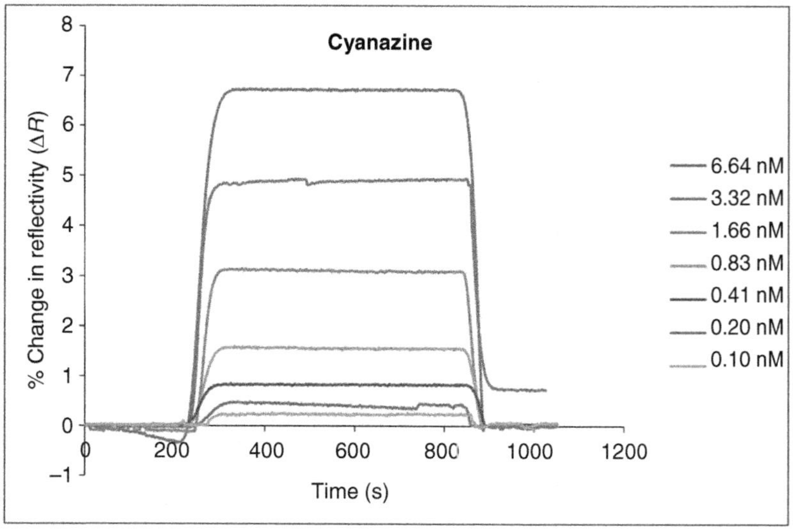

Figure 18.8. The real-time SNZ imprinted SPR nanosensor detection at different concentrations.

$$\text{Absolute } \Delta R\% = 100 \times \frac{\text{SPR sample pixel difference} \times 0.85}{s - \text{pol pixel intensity}/(1-d)} \quad (18.10)$$

Here d is the density of the filter used. In this study filter transmits only 25% of the light then $d = 0.75$.

The changes in percentage reflectivity value, taken from SPR nanosensors, serve the important information for analyzing the data. But, the data can be analyzed more precisely by using ΔR values, which show the difference between instant percentage reflectivity and initial reflectivity values (Meyer et al., 2006) (Fig. 18.8). With an increase in concentration from 0.1 to 6.64 nM, the resonance frequency change increases proportionally to the ratio of increment. So, a decrease in the concentration also decreased the driving force, that is, concentration gradient between herbicides and SPR chip surface. Cherif et al. prepared SPR sensor based novel peptide chips. They reported that with the increase in dilution ratio, from 1/100 to 1/1000, the resonance frequency signal decreased fourfold (Cherif et al., 2006). As can be seen in Fig. 18.8 there is a direct relationship between concentration and reflectivity change for SNZ imprinted nanosensor. At these concentration range it could not be reached to plateau for all herbicide types. This may be due to the fact that there are still binding sites for herbicides.

According to the results obtained by Saylan et al., SNZ imprinted SPR nanosensor responses show good linearity when compared to the others. For a linear calibration curve, instrument response y is assumed linearly related to the standard concentration x for a limited range of concentration (Federal Register Notices, 2000). It can be expressed in an equation model as $y = a + bx$. LOD values are computed by using this model. Therefore, the LOD can be expressed as LOD = $3S/b$, where S is the standard deviation of the response and can be estimated by the standard deviation of either y-residuals, or y-intercepts, of regression lines. According to the linear part of calibration curve with the $3S/b$ formula, the limit of detection (LOD) was determined as 0.095, 0.031, and 0.091 for SNZ, SMZ, and ATZ herbicides.

Kinetic and isotherm analysis of herbicide imprinted SPR nanosensors were used to determine host–guest interactions by Saylan and coworkers. If the total amount of binding side $[BS]_0$ is explicited in terms of the maximum analyte-binding capacity of the SPR sensor surface, such as the total amount of SNZ, SMZ, ATZ, all concentration terms can then be expressed as an SPR response signal ΔR, eliminating the need to convert from mass to molar concentration.

Under pseudo-first-order conditions where the free analyte concentration is held constant in the flow cell, the binding can be described by the following equation;

$$\mathrm{d}\Delta R/\mathrm{d}t = k_a C(\Delta R_{max} - \Delta R) - k_d \Delta R \tag{18.11}$$

where $\mathrm{d}\Delta R/\mathrm{d}t$ is the rate of change of the SPR response signal, ΔR and ΔR_{max} refers to the measured and maximum response signal after binding of analyte, C is the concentration of the analyte (nM), k_a and k_d values stand for association rate constant ($nM^{-1}{\cdot}s^{-1}$) and dissociation rate (s^{-1}) constants, respectively. Association constant K_A, can be calculated as $K_A = k_a/k_d$ (nM^{-1}) by using rate constants k_a and k_d. At equilibrium, $\mathrm{d}\Delta R/\mathrm{d}t = 0$ and the equation can be rewritten as:

$$\Delta R_{eq}/C = K_A \Delta R_{max} - K_A \Delta R_{eq} \tag{18.12}$$

Therefore, plotting of $\Delta R_{eq}/C$ versus ΔR_{eq} enables the association constant K_A and dissociation constant K_D can be calculated as $1/K_A$. Eq. (18.12) may be rearranged to give:

$$\mathrm{d}\Delta R/\mathrm{d}t = k_a C \Delta R_{max} - (k_a C + k_d)\Delta R \tag{18.13}$$

Thus, plotting of $d\Delta R/\mathrm{d}t$ against ΔR will be a straight line with slope $-(k_a C + k_d)$ for interaction-controlled kinetics. Concentration measurements can be obtained by using the relationship between the initial binding rate (at $\Delta R = 0$) which is directly proportional to the analyte concentration. Although it is difficult to determine ΔR_{max} experimentally since a high analyte concentration is required to fully saturate the surface, if ΔR_{max} is known, both k_a and k_d can be determined from a single association sensorgram. Measurement of the association sensorgram at several different analyte concentrations is a preferable approach to consider. Forward and back rates related to the S value can be calculated as the slope by plotting the change in the total detector response ($\mathrm{d}\Delta R/\mathrm{d}t$) versus ΔR as follows:

$$S = k_a C + k_d \tag{18.14}$$

A plot of S against C will be a straight line with slope k_a and intercept on the ordinate ($C = 0$) gives k_d: in practice, however, this cannot be used as a reliable measure of the dissociation rate constant if $k_a C > k_d$. This value can be obtained more accurately by direct measurement of the dissociation from saturated binding sites into a buffer solution flow that contains no analyte. The dissociation is quantified by:

$$\ln(\Delta R_0/\Delta R_t) = k_d(t - t_0) \quad (18.15)$$

where ΔR_0 is the initial response level at t_0 and ΔR at t times represents values obtained along the dissociation curve (Şener et al., 2011).

Association kinetics analysis is an approach based on the pseudo-first-order adsorption kinetics (Krishnamoorthy et al., 2010).

$$\Delta R_{ex}/C = K_A \Delta R_{max} - K_A \Delta R_{eq} \quad (18.16)$$

Calculation of the number of binding sites and analysis of the data for freely reversible host/guest binding interactions is generally performed by Scatchard (Sener et al., 2010). Figs. 18.9 and 18.10 show calculation of kinetic rate constants by association kinetics analysis approach and equilibrium analysis approach (Scatchard), respectively.

The adsorption models can be used to define recognition ability, interaction selectivity, and surface homogeneity of the molecular imprinting based nanosensors. Examination of Langmuir, Freundlich, and Langmuir–Freundlich isotherm models was carried out to test the experimental data. The Langmuir model, which is a homogeneous binding site model, is used commonly to fit MIP binding isotherms (Li and Husson, 2006). However, increasingly, studies show that most MIPs have heterogeneous binding sites. The Freundlich model is a heterogeneous model. It demonstrates excellent fit to MIP adsorption isotherm data in the low concentration region (nM–mM) (Umpleby et al., 2001) but is incapable of modeling saturation behavior and deviates from experimental isotherms in high concentration regions. The Langmuir–Freundlich (LF) model provides heterogeneity information and is able to model adsorption behavior over the entire concentration region up to saturation; it is probably the best choice for fitting the binding isotherm of adsorption. Freundlich model is used to show multilayer binding of analyte molecules. Langmuir–Freundlich can be applied to a system that provides heterogeneity information about adsorption behavior over wide concentration regions. Among the applied models, Langmuir is the best-fitted isotherm model with a high regression coefficient ($R^2 = 0.9999$) and well fitted $\Delta R_{max} = 8.330$ for ATZ, for SMZ ($R^2 = 0.9927$, $\Delta R_{max} = 8.904$), and also for SNZ ($R^2 = 0.9963$, $\Delta R_{max} = 7.178$). Monolayer binding of herbicide molecules onto MIP SPR sensor was shown with these results (Xu et al., 2011). The ΔR_{max} value obtained from the Langmuir model was very close to the experimental ones. In fact all isotherms, except Scatchard isotherms for all three herbicides, had high correlation coefficients. The linear fit with the Langmuir equation was comparably the best, which

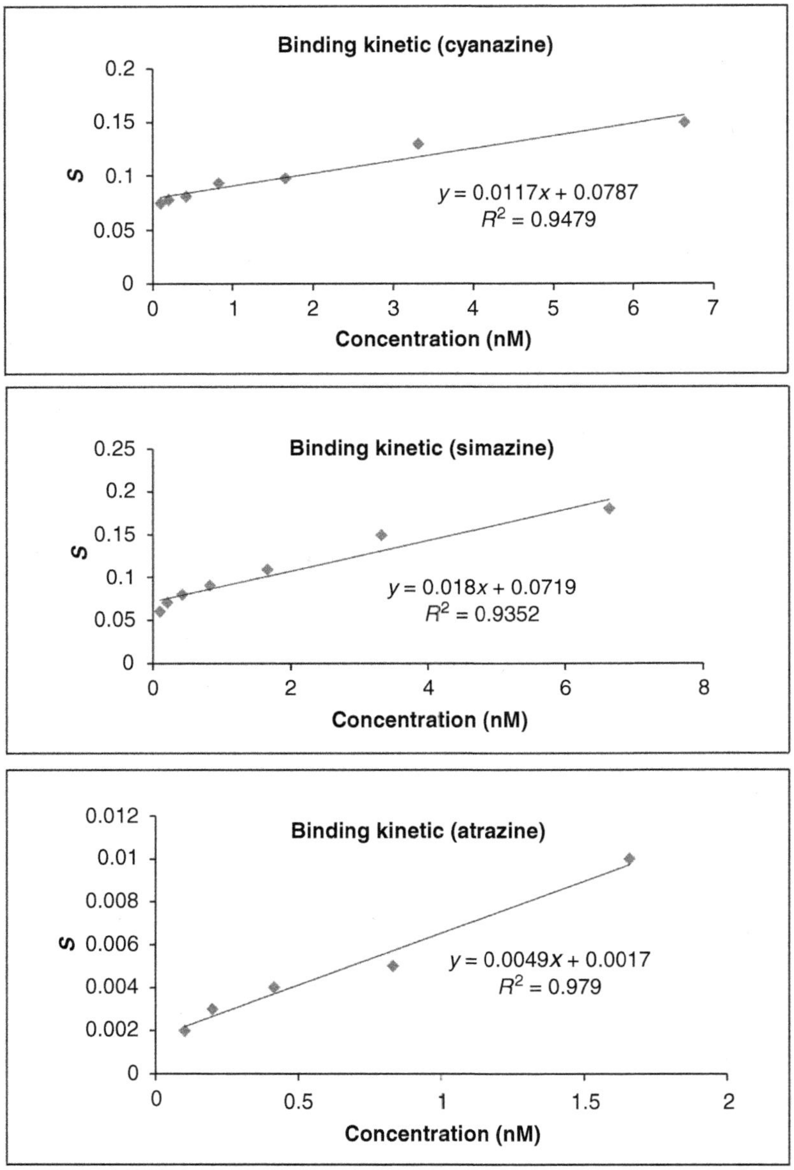

Figure 18.9. Determination of kinetic rate constants: Association kinetics analysis approach.

means that the binding of herbicide imprinted SPR nanosensors is monolayer, although Scatchard curve shows some surface heterogeneity. Surface heterogeneity shown by Scatchard curve can be explained by the imprinted SPR chip surfaces having different binding sites which have similar binding affinity to herbicide

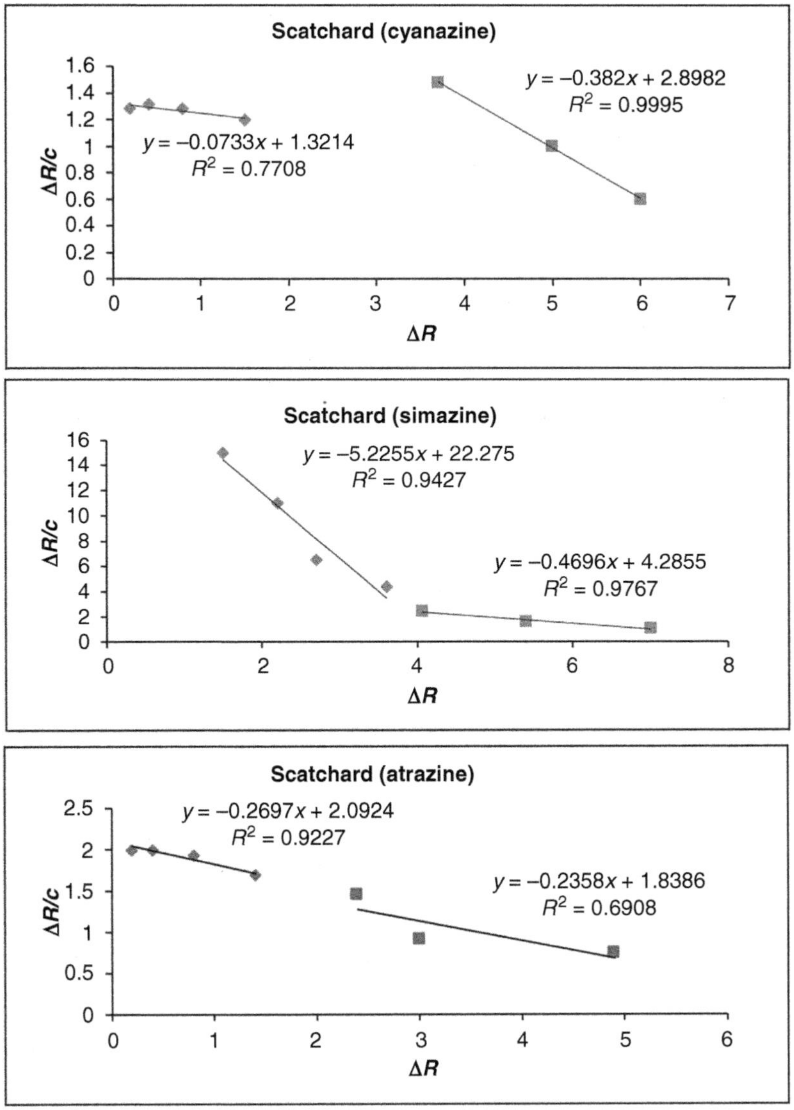

Figure 18.10. Determination of kinetic rate constants for SNZ, SMZ, and ATZ: Equilibrium analysis approach (Scatchard).

molecules. The K_A values were calculated as 0.283 nM^{-1} for SNZ, 0.498 nM^{-1} for SMZ, and 0.25 nM^{-1} for ATZ. Tables 18.4–18.6 show the calculated parameters for all models.

SNZ, SMZ, and ATZ herbicides were used for each other, respectively, to investigate the selectivity of herbicide SPR nanosensors. Competitor herbicide solution was applied to both herbicide imprinted and nonimprinted SPR nanosensors. The responses of

Table 18.4 Equilibrium and Association Kinetics Constants (Cyanazine)

Equilibrium Analysis (Scathard)		Association Kinetics	
ΔR_{max}	7.586	k_a (nM^{-1}.s^{-1})	0.0117
K_A (nM^{-1})	0.382	k_d (s^{-1})	0.0787
K_D (nM)	2.617	K_A (nM^{-1})	0.148
R^2	0.9995	K_D (nM)	6.726
		R^2	0.9479

Table 18.5 Equilibrium and Association Kinetics Constants (Simazine)

Equilibrium Analysis (Scathard)		Association Kinetics	
ΔR_{max}	9.137	k_a (nM^{-1}.s^{-1})	0.018
K_A (nM^{-1})	0.469	k_d (s^{-1})	0.071
K_D (nM)	2.132	K_A (nM^{-1})	0.250
R^2	0.9767	K_D (nM)	3.990
		R^2	0.9352

Table 18.6 Equilibrium and Association Kinetics Constants (Atrazine)

Equilibrium Analysis (Scathard)		Association Kinetics	
ΔR_{max}	8.03	k_a (nM^{-1}.s^{-1})	0.0049
K_A (nM^{-1})	0.26	k_d (s^{-1})	0.0017
K_D (nM)	3.84	K_A (nM^{-1})	2.88
R^2	0.9227	K_D (nM)	0.34
		R^2	0.979

the MIP and the nonimprinted SPR nanosensor were determined as the percentage of change in reflectivity ($\Delta R\%$). The distribution coefficient is utilized to evaluate the binding specificity of imprinted polymer:

$$K_d = \left[(C_i - C_f)/C_f\right] \times V/m \quad (18.17)$$

where, K_d (mL/g) is the distribution coefficient, C_i (μg/mL) is the concentration of herbicides in solution, and C_f (μg/mL) is the concentration of herbicides in solution after binding; V (mL) is the volume of protein solution; and m (g) is the mass of polymer. In SPR sensor applications, the concentration and mass parameters are modified because there is no significant difference between the initial and final concentration of herbicide solutions (Lin et al., 2005). The mass of the polymer, is not accurately detectable (Ertürk et al., 2011) in this system. Therefore, the selectivity coefficient k is described by the following equation.

$$k = \Delta R_{\text{template}} / \Delta R_{\text{competitor}} \quad (18.18)$$

The equation for relative selectivity coefficient, k' can be written as:

$$k' = k_{\text{MIP}} / k_{\text{NIP}} \quad (18.19)$$

In order to show the selectivity of the herbicide imprinted SPR nanosensors, structurally related triazine molecules SNZ, SMZ, and ATZ were used as competitor agents for each other. They were preferred for similar molecular weight and pK_a values with each other. The selectivity coefficients for herbicide imprinted and nonimprinted SPR nanosensors and the relative selectivity coefficients were given in Tables 18.7–18.9. As seen in tables, recognition sites for herbicides have been created during the imprinting process. Although nonimprinted SPR nanosensor may contain enough functional groups, no defined cavities exist to provide selective binding. The selectivity ratio for SNZ between SNZ/ATZ and SNZ/SMZ were determined to be 7.79 and 13.04; for SMZ between SMZ/ATZ and SMZ/SNZ were determined to be 1.75 and 2.0; and for ATZ between ATZ/SMZ and ATZ/SNZ were determined to be 7.14 and 7.58, respectively. The relative selectivity coefficients of herbicide-imprinted SPR nanosensors to nonimprinted nanosensors for ATZ between ATZ/SMZ and ATZ/SNZ were determined to be 7.90 and 7.95; for SMZ between SMZ/ATZ and SMZ/SNZ were determined to be 1.67 and 2.11; and for SNZ between SNZ/ATZ and SNZ/SMZ were determined to be 7.04 and 12.38, respectively. The relative selectivity coefficients

Table 18.7 Selectivity Coefficients of the MIP (SNZ Imprinted) and NIP (SNZ Nonimprinted) SPR Nanosensors

Molecular Imprinted			Nonimprinted		
Herbicide	**ΔR**	**k**	**ΔR**	**k**	**k'**
Cyanazine	6.00	—	1.77	—	—
Atrazine	0.77	7.79	1.60	1.11	7.04
Simazine	0.46	13.04	1.68	1.05	12.38

Table 18.8 Selectivity Coefficients of the MIP (SMZ Imprinted) and NIP (SMZ Nonimprinted) SPR Nanosensors

Molecular Imprinted			Nonimprinted		
Herbicide	**ΔR**	**k**	**ΔR**	**k**	**k'**
Simazine	7.00	—	1.68	—	—
Atrazine	4.00	1.75	1.60	1.05	1.67
Cyanazine	3.50	2.00	1.77	0.95	2.11

Table 18.9 Selectivity Coefficients of the MIP (ATZ Imprinted) and NIP (ATZ Nonimprinted) SPR Nanosensors

Molecular Imprinted			Nonimprinted		
Herbicide	**ΔR**	**k**	**ΔR**	**k**	**k'**
Atrazine	5.00	—	1.60	—	—
Cyanazine	0.70	7.14	1.77	0.90	7.90
Simazine	0.66	7.58	1.68	0.95	7.95

obtained for ATZ, SMZ, and SNZ molecules show that the cavities created in the imprinted nanofilm recognize imprinted molecules preferentially and have structural memory for template molecules. The molecular imprinting approach for herbicide molecules effectively presented monolayer recognition sites to the substrate in which the imprint will be formed. Molecular imprinting of herbicide molecules resulting in a material that is potentially homogenous and selective.

Reusability of the herbicide imprinted SPR nanosensors was performed with aqueous herbicide solutions by four repeated adsorption–desorption–regeneration cycles. For this purpose, herbicide solutions were interacted with the herbicide imprinted SPR nanosensors consecutively. The $\Delta R\%$ values obtained for the four cycles. The herbicide imprinted SPR nanosensors, can be reused successfully with reproducible results for consecutive herbicide solutions.

5 Conclusions

The presence of herbicides in waste waters may affect the ecosystem and human health. Therefore, it is critical to develop sufficiently sensitive methods for the detection and determination of triazinic herbicides in waste water. Due to the unique properties of SPR nanosensors, such as real-time measurement, high specificity and sensitivity, no need for labeling, their applications have been more popular for the investigation of several analyte molecules.

The aim of this chapter is to summarize the most relevant contributions in the development of herbicide detection sensor systems. Since the first application for the detecton of herbicides involving sensor systems, an increasing number of publications have been reported. Although there are many conventional methods for the detection of herbicides, optic-based SPR nanosensors enable high sensitivity, label-free detection, real-time monitoring, low volume sample consumption, quantitative evaluation, and determination of kinetic rate constants. To describe the challenges and opportunities, the discussion is extended further by Saylan et al. by exploring the sensing properties of herbicide imprinted [PMAPAVIM] nanofilms on the SPR sensor chip for detection of SNZ, SMZ, and ATZ herbicides from aqueous solutions. The isotherm models, performed by fitting the data to a variety of isotherm models, Scatchard, Langmuir, Freundlich, and Langmuir–Freundlich, were used to determine the kinetic and binding constants. Although Scatchard curve shows that herbicide imprinted SPR nanosensors have some surface heterogeneity, SPR nanosensors were well-fitted to the Langmuir adsorption model for all herbicide types. The selectivity studies show that the imprinted cavities recognize herbicides selectively. The prepared herbicide imprinted SPR nanosensors enable (1) high sensitivity, (2) label-free detection, (3) real-time monitoring, (4) low volume sample consumption, (5) quantitative evaluation, and (6) determination of kinetic rate constants. SPR based herbicide imprinted nanosensors are easy to perform and can be a cost-effective solution due to the reusability of the prepared sensor. In the light of obtained data, the herbicide imprinted SPR nanosensors can be used as a potential alternative for herbicides SNZ, SMZ, and ATZ sensing to protect environmental and human health.

References

Aktar, M.W., Sengupta, D., Chowdhury, A., 2009. Impact of pesticides use in agriculture: their benefits and hazards. Interdiscip. Toxicol. 2, 1–12.

Alexander, C., Smith, C.R., Whitcombe, M., Vulfson, E.N., 1999. Imprinted polymers as protecting groups for regioselective modification or polyfunctional substrates. J. Am. Chem. Soc. 121, 6640–6651.

Amaral, B.D., De Araujo, J.A., Peralta-Zamora, P.G., Nagata, N., 2014. Simultaneous determination of atrazine and metabolites (DIA and DEA) in natural water by multivariate electronic spectroscopy. Microchem. J. 117, 262–267.

Ansell, R.J., Mosbach, K., 1996. Towards artificial antibodies prepared by molecular imprinting. Pharm. News 3, 16–20.

Arshady, R., Mosbach, K., 1981. Synthesis of substrate-selective polymers by host-guest polymerization. Makromol. Chem. 182, 687–692.

Asir, S., Uzun, L., Turkmen, D., Say, R., Denizli, A., 2005. Ion-selective imprinted superporous monolith for cadmium removal from human plasma. Sep. Sci. Technol. 40, 3167–3185.

Banerjia, S., Penga, W., Kimb, Y.-C., Menegazzob, N., Bookshb, K.S., 2010. Evaluation of polymer coatings for ammonia vapor sensing with surface plasmon resonance spectroscopy. Sens. Actuat. B 147, 255–262.

Barek, J.F., Navratil, J.T., Peckova, K., Yosypchuk, B., Zima, J., 2007. Nontraditional electrode materials in environmental analysis of biologically active organic compounds. Electroanalysis 19, 2003–2014.

Bereli, N., Saylan, Y., Uzun, L., Say, R., Denizli, A., 2011. L-Histidine imprinted supermacroporous cryogels for protein recognition. Sep. Purif. Technol. 82, 28–35.

Berg, M., Mueller, S.R., Schwarzenbach, R.P., 1995. Simultaneous determination of triazines including atrazine and their major metabolites hydroxyatrazine, desethylatrazine, and deisopropylatrazine in natural waters. Anal. Chem. 67, 1860–1865.

Bowman, M.A.E., Allender, C.J., Brain, K.R., Heard, C.M., 1998. A high-throughput screening technique employing molecularly imprinted polymers as biomimetic selectors. Methodol. Surv. Bioanal. Drugs. Methodol. Surv. Bioanal. Drugs. 25, 37–43.

Bruzzoniti, M.C., Sarzanini, C., Costantino, G., Fungi, M., 2006. Determination of herbicides by solid phase extraction gas chromatography-mass spectrometry in drinking water. Anal. Chim. Acta 578, 241–249.

Buck, R.P., Hatfield, W.E., Umaana, M.L., 1990. Biosensor Technology. Marcel Dekker, New York.

Byrne, M.E., Oral, E., Hilt, J.Z., Peppas, N.A., 2002. Non-covalent molecular imprinting of glucose: recognition in aqueous media, in molecularly imprinted polymer science and technology. Polym. Adv. Technol. 13, 798–816.

Cao, F., Liao, J., Yang, K., Bai, P., Wei, Q., Zhao, C., 2010. Self-assembly molecularly imprinted nanofiber for 4-HA recognition. Anal. Lett. 43, 2790–2797.

Chen, L., Xu, S., Li, J., 2011. Recent advances in molecular imprinting technology: current status challenges and highlighted applications. Chem. Soc. Rev. 40, 2922–2942.

Cheong, S.H., McNiven, S., Rachkov, A., Levi, R., Yano, K., Karube, I., 1997. Testosterone receptor binding mimic constructed using molecular imprinting. Macromolecules 30, 1317–1322.

Cherif, B., Roget, A., Villiers, C.L., Calemczuk, R., Leroy, V., Marche, P.N., Livache, T., Villiers, M.B., 2006. Relationship between humoral response against hepatitis C virus and disease overcome. Clin. Chem. 52, 255–262.

Cowan, J.J., 1972. The surface plasmon resonance effect in holography. J. Opt. Commun. 5, 69–72.

Dong, J., Gao, N., Peng, Y., Guo, C., Lv, Z., Wang, Y., Zhou, C., Ning, B., Liu, M., Gao, Z., 2012. Surface plasmon resonance sensor for profenofos detection using molecularly imprinted thin film as recognition element. Food Control 25 (2), 543–549.

Earp, R.L., Dessy, R.E., 1996. Commercial biosensors: applications to clinical, bioprocess, and environmental samples. Surface Plasmon Resonance, 23, John Wiley and Sons, New York, pp. 1–27, (Chapter 4).

Englebienne, P., Van Hoonacker, A., Verhas, M., 2003. Surface plasmon resonance: principles methods and applications in biomedical sciences. Spectroscopy 17, 255–273.

Ersöz, A., Diltemiz, S.E., Özcan, A.A., Denizli, A., Say, R., 2008. Synergie between molecular imprinted polymer based on solid-phase extraction and quartz crystal microbalance technique for 8-OHdG sensing. Biosens. Bioelectron. 24, 742–747.

Ertürk, G., Uzun, L., Tümer, M.A., Say, R., Denizli, A., 2011. Fab fragments imprinted SPR biosensor for real-time human immunoglobulin G detection. Biosens. Bioelectron. 28 (1), 97–104.

Federal Register Notices 2000, 65, pp. 776–777.

Giannetto, M., Umiltà, E., Careri, M., 2014. New competitive dendrimer-based and highly selective immunosensor for determination of atrazine in environmental, feed and food samples: the importance of antibody selectivity for discrimination among related triazinic metabolites. Anal. Chim. Acta 806, 197–203.

Guan, G., Liu, B., Wang, Z., Zhang, Z., 2008. Imprinting of molecular recognition sites on nanostructures and its applications in chemosensors. Sensors 8, 8291–8320.

Gupta, V.K., Yola, M.L., Atar, N., 2014. A novel molecular imprinted nanosensor based quartz crystal microbalance for determination of kaempferol. Sens. Actuat. B 194, 79–85.

Hepel, M., Stobiecka, M., Peachey, J., Miller, J., 2012. Intervention of glutathione in press mutagenic catechol-mediated DNA damage in the presence of copper (II). Mutation Res. 2, 1–11.

Hickel, W., Knoll, W., 1989. Surface plasmon microscopic imaging of ultrathin metal coatings. Acta Metall. 37, 2141–2144.

Hooper, I.R., Rooth, M., Sambles, J.R., 2009. Dual-channel differential surface plasmon ellipsometry for bio-chemical sensing. Biosens. Bioelectron. 25, 411–417.

International Programme on Chemical Safety (IPCS), 1978. Environmental Health Criteria: No. 9. DDT and Derivatives. IPCS, Geneva, Switzerland.

Kempe, M., 1996. Antibody-mimicking polymers as chiral stationary phases in HPLC. Anal. Chem. 68, 1948–1953.

Kim, Y.H., Kim, J.P., Han, S.J., Sim, S.J., 2009. Aptamer biosensor for label-free detection of human immunoglobulin E based on surface plasmon resonance. Sens. Actuat. B 139, 471–475.

Kiefer, W., Long, D.A., 1982. Non-Linear Raman Spectroscopy and its Chemical Applications. D. Reidel Publishing Company, Dordrecht, Holland/Boston, USA/London, England, pp. 445–470.

Komiyama, M., Takeuchi, T., Asanuma, H., 2002. Molecular Imprinting: From Fundamentals to Applications. Wiley-VCH, Weinheim, pp. 75–118.

Krishnamoorthy, G., Carlen, E.T., Van Der Berg, A., Scasfoort, R.B.M., 2010. Surface plasmon resonance imaging based multiplex biosensor: integration of biomolecular screening, detection and kinetics estimation. Sens. Actuat. B 148, 511–521.

Li, X., Husson, S.M., 2006. Adsorption of dansylated amino acids on molecularly imprinted surfaces: a surface plasmon resonance study. Biosens. Bioelectron. 22, 336–348.

Li, Z., Zhang, S., Yin, X., Wang, C., Wang, Z., 2014. Micellar electrokinetic chromatographic determination of triazine herbicides in water samples. J. Chromatogr. Sci. 52, 926–931.

Lin, K.Y., Chu, W., 2011. Simulation and quantification of the natural decay of a typical endocrine disrupting chemical Atrazine in an aquatic system. J. Hazard. Mater. 192, 1260–1266.

Lin, L.P., Huang, L.S., Lin, C.W., Lee, C.K., Chen, J.L., Hsu, S.M., Lin, S., 2005. Determination of binding constant of DNA-binding drug to target DNA by surface plasmon resonance biosensor technology. Curr. Drug Target 5, 61–72.

Lopez-Blanco, M.C., Blanco-Cid, S., Cancho-Grande, B., Simal-Gandara, J., 2003. Application of single-drop microextraction and comparison with solid-phase microextraction and solid-phase extraction for the determination of a- and b-endosulfan in water samples by gas chromatography–electron-capture detection. J. Chromatogr. A 984, 245–252.

Lu, C., Zhou, W., Han, B., Yang, H., Chen, X., Wang, X., 2007. Surface-imprinted core–shell nanoparticles for sorbent assays. Anal. Chem. 79, 5457–5461.

Luo, C., Liu, M., Mo, Y., Qu, J., Feng, Y., 2001. Thickness-shear mode acoustic sensor for atrazine using molecularly imprinted polymer as recognition element. Anal. Chim. Acta 428, 143–146.

Malmqvist, M., Biacore, 1999. An affinity biosensor system for characterization of biomolecular interactions. Biochem. Soc. Trans. 27, 335–340.

Martin-Esteban, A., 2013. Molecularly-imprinted polymers as a versatile, highly selective tool in sample preparation. Trends Anal. Chem. 45, 169–181.

Martini, E., Merola, G., Tomassetti, M., Campanella, L., 2015. Agent orange herbicides, organophosphate and triazinic pesticides analysis in olive oil and industrial oil mill waste effluents using new organic phase immunosensors. Food Chem. 169, 358–365.

Matsui, J., Miyoshi, Y., Doblhoff-Dier, O., Takeuchi, T., 1995. A molecularly imprinted synthetic polymer receptor selective for atrazine. Anal. Chem. 67, 4404–4408.

Mazzotta, E., Malitesta, C., Díaz-Álvarez, M., Martin-Esteban, A., 2012. Electrosynthesis of molecularly imprinted polypyrrole for the antibiotic levofloxacin. Thin Solid Films 520, 1938–1943.

Meyer, M.H.F., Hartmann, M., Keusgen, M., 2006. SPR-based immunosensor for the CRP detection—a new method to detect a well known protein. Biosens. Bioelectron. 21, 1987–1990.

Mosbach, K., Ramström, O., 1996. The emerging technique of molecular imprinting and its future impact on biotechnology. Nat. Biotechnol. 14, 163–170.

Mosbach, K., Ye, L., Cormack, P., 2001. Molecular imprinting on microgel spheres. Anal. Chim. Acta 435, 187–196.

Mou, R.-X., Chen, M.-X., Cao, Z.-Y., Zhu, Z.-W., 2011. Simultaneous determination of triazine herbicides in rice by high-performance liquid chromatography coupled with high resolution and high mass accuracy hybrid linear ion trap-orbitrap mass spectrometry. Anal. Chim. Acta 706, 149–156.

Nurzhanova, A., Kalugin, S., Zhambakin, K., 2013. Obsolete pesticides and application of colonizing plant species for remediation of contaminated soil in Kazakhstan. Environ. Sci. Pollut. Res. 20, 2054–2063.

Otto, A., 1968. Excitation of nonradiative surface plasma waves in silver by the method of frustrated total reflection. Zeitschrift für Physik 16, 398–410.

Ozcan, A.A., Say, R., Denizli, A., Ersoz, A., 2006. L-Histidine imprinted synthetic receptor for biochromatography applications. Anal. Chem. 78, 7253–7258.

Piletsky, S., Turner, A.P.F., 2006. Molecular Imprinting of Polymers. Landes Bioscience, Austin, TX, USA, pp. 122–139, (Chapter 9).

Piletsky, S.A., Alcock, S., Turner, A.P., 2001. Molecular imprinting: at the edge of the third millennium. Trends Biotechnol. 19, 9–12.

Piletsky, S.A., Panasyuk, T.L., Piletskaya, E.V., Nicholls, I.A., Ulbricht, M., 1999. Receptor and transport properties of imprinted polymer membranes: a review. J. Membr. Sci. 157, 263–278.

Piletsky, S.A., Piletskaya, E.V., Elgersma, A.V., Yano, K., Karube, I., Parhometz, Y.P., Elskaya, A.V., 1995. Atrazine sensing by molecularly imprinted membranes. Biosens. Bioelectron. 10, 959–964.

Pinto, G.M.F., Jardim, I.C.S.F., 2000. Mobile phase optimization for the seperation of same herbicide sample using HPLC. J. Liq. Chromatogr. Relat. Technol. 23, 1353–1363.

Real, B.D., Ortiz, M.C., Sarabia, L.A., 2012. Develop of a multiway chemometric-based analytical method fulfilling regulatory identification criteria: application to GC–MS pesticide residue analysis. J. Chromatogr. B 910, 122–137.

Rezic, I., Horvat, A.J.M., Babíc, S., Ka'stelan-Macan, M., 2005. Determination of pesticides in honey by ultrasonic solvent extraction and thin-layer chromatography. Ultrason. Sonochem. 12, 477–481.

Riskin, M., Tel-Vered, R., Bourenko, T., Granot, E., Willner, I., 2008. Imprinting of molecular recognition sites through electropolymerization of functionalized Au Nanoparticles: development of an electrochemical TNT sensor based on π-donor-acceptor interactions. J. Am. Chem. Soc. 130, 9726–9733.

Riskin, M., Tel-Vered, R., Frasconi, M., Yavo, N., Willner, I., 2010. Stereoselective chiroselective surface plasmon resonance (SPR) analysis of amino acids by molecularly imprinted Au-nanoparticle composites. Chem. Eur. J. 16, 7114–7120.

Rivoira, L., De Carlo, R.M., Cavalli, S., Bruzzoniti, M.C., 2015. Simple SPE–HPLC determination of some common drugs and herbicides of environmental concern by pulsed amperometry. Talanta 131, 205–212.

Rodríguez-González, N., González-Castro, M.J., Beceiro-González, E., Muniategui-Lorenzo, S., Prada-Rodríguez, D., 2014. Determination of triazine herbicides in sea weeds: development of a sample preparation method based on matrix solid phase dispersion and solid phase. Talanta 121, 194–198.

Rothenbausler, B., Knoll, W., 1988. Surface–plasmon microscopy. Nature 332, 615–617.

Saylan, Y., Akgönüllü, S., Çimen, D., Derazshamshir, A., Bereli, N., Yılmaz, F., Denizli, A., 2017. Development of surface plasmon resonance sensors based on molecularly imprinted nanofilms for sensitive and selective detection of pesticide. Sens. Actuat. B. *Accepted.*

Sellergren, B., 1997. Imprinted polymers-stable, reusable antibody—mimics for highly selective separations. Am. Lab. 29, 14.

Sellergren, B., 2001. Towards Artificial Antibodies Prepared by Molecular Imprinting. Elsevier, Amsterdam, Holland, pp. 113–183.

Sener, G., Ozgur, E., Yilmaz, E., Uzun, L., Say, R., Denizli, A., 2010. Quartz crystal microbalance based nanosensor for lysozyme detection with lysozyme imprinted nanoparticles. Biosens. Bioelectron. 26, 815–821.

Şener, G., Uzun, L., Say, R., Denizli, A., 2011. Use of molecular imprinted nanoparticles as biorecognition element on surface plasmon resonance sensor. Sens. Actuat. B 160, 791–799.

Shaikh, H., Memon, N., Bhanger, M.I., Nizamani, S.M., Denizli, A., 2014. Core–shell molecularly imprinted polymer-based solid-phase microextraction fiber for ultra trace analysis of endosulfan I and II inreal aqueous matrix through gas chromatography–micro electroncapture detector. J. Chromatogr. A 1337, 179–187.

Sharma, P.S., Dabrowski, M., D'Souza, F., Kutner, W., 2013. Surface development of molecularly imprinted polymer films to enhance sensing signals. Trends Anal. Chem. 51, 146–157.

Shina, Y.B., Kimb, H.M., Junga, Y., Chunga, B.H., 2010. A new palm-sized surface plasmon resonance (SPR) biosensor based on modulation of a light source by a rotating mirror. Sens. Actuat. B 150, 1–6.

Shoji, R., Takeuchi, T., Kubo, I., 2003. Atrazine sensor based on molecularly imprinted polymer-modified gold electrode. Anal. Chem. 75, 4882–4886.

Siemann, M., Andersson, L.I., Mosbach, K., 1996. Selective recognition of the herbicide atrazine by noncovalent imprinted polymers. J. Agric. Food Chem. 44, 141–145.

Sípová, H., Homola, J., 2013. Surface plasmon resonance sensing of nucleic acids: a review. J. Anal. Chim. Acta 773, 9–23.

Spietelun, A., Pilarczyk, M., Kloskowski, A., Namies¸nik, J., 2010. Current trends in solid-phase microextraction (SPME) fibre coatings. Chem. Soc. Rev. 39, 4524–4537.

Spivak, D.A., Shea, K.J., 2001. Investigation into the scope and limitations of molecular imprinting with DNA molecules. Anal. Chim. Acta 435, 65–74.

Szentirmay, Z., 1992. Surface plasmon spectroscopy of metal/dielectric structures. Spectrochim. Acta 48, 9–17.

Takeuchi, T., Matsui, J., 1996. Molecular imprinting: an approach to "tailor-made" synthetic polymers with biomimetic functions. Acta Polym. 47, 471–480.

Toorisaka, E., Yoshida, M., Uezu, K., Goto, M., 1999. Artificial biocatalyst prepared by the surface molecular imprinting technique. Chem. Lett. 5, 387–388.

Türkmen, D., Denizli, A., Oztürk, N., Akgöl, S., Elkak, A., 2008. Phenylalanine containing hydrophobic nanospheres for antibody purification. Biotechnol. Prog. 24, 1297–1303.

Umpleby, R.J., Baxter, S.C., Chen, Y., Shah, R.N., Shimizu, K.D., 2001. Characterization of the heterogeneous binding site affinity distributions in molecularly imprinted polymers. Anal. Chem. 73, 4584–4591.

Uzun, L., Say, R., Unal, S., Denizli, A., 2009a. Hepatitis B surface antibody purification with hepatitis B surface antibody imprinted poly(hydroxyethyl methacrylate-*N*-methacryloyl-l-tyrosine methyl ester) particles. J. Chromatogr. B 877, 181–188.

Uzun, L., Say, R., Unal, S., Denizli, 2009b. Production of surface plasmon resonance based assay kit for hepatitis diagnosis. Biosens. Bioelectron. 24, 2878–2884.

Vasilescu, M.N., Medvedovici, A.V., 2005. Herbicides. In: Alan, P.T., Colin, P. (Eds.), Encyclopedia of Analytical Science. Elsevier, Oxford, UK, pp. 243–260.

Vlatakis, G., Andersson, L.I., Muller, R., Mosbach, K., 1993. Drug assay using antibody mimics made by molecular imprinting. Nature 361, 645–647.

Wei, C., Zhoub, H., Zhoua, J., 2011. Ultrasensitively sensing acephate using molecular imprinting techniques on a surface plasmon resonance sensor. Talanta 83 (5), 1422–1427.

Welford, K., 1991. Surface plasmon-polaritons and their uses. Opt. Quantum Electron. 23, 1–27.

Whitcombe, M.J., Chianella, I., Larcombe, L., Piletsky, S.A., Noble, J., Porter, R., Horgan, A., 2011. The rational development of molecularly imprinted polymer-based sensors for protein detection. Chem. Soc. Rev. 40, 1547–1571.

World Health Organization (WHO), 2006. The WHO Classification of Pesticides by Hazard. http://www.who.int/ipcs/publications/pesticides_hazard_rev_3.pdf

Wood, R.W., 1902. On a remarkable case of uneven distribution of light in a diffraction grating spectrum. Philos. Mag. 4, 396–402.

Wulfeck-Kleier, K.A., Ybarra, M.D., Speth, T.F., Magnuson, M.L., 2010. Factors affecting atrazine concentration and quantitative determination in chlorinated water. J. Chromatogr. A 1217, 676–682.

Wulff, G., 1995. Molecular imprinting in cross-linked materials with the aid of molecular templates—a way towards artificial antibodies. Angew. Chem. Int. Ed. Engl. 34, 1812–1832.

Wulff, G., Gross, T., Schonfeld, R., 1997. Enzyme models based on molecularly imprinted polymers with strong esterase activity. Int. Ed. Engl. 36, 1962–1964.

Wulff, G., Sarhan, A., 1972. Use of polymers with enzyme analogous structures for the resolution of racemates. Angew. Chem. Int. Ed. Engl. 11, 341–342.

Wulff, G., Schauhoff, S., 1991. Enzyme-analog built polymers. Racemic resolution of free sugars with macroporous polymers prepared by molecular imprinting–selectivity dependence on the arrangement of functional groups versus requirements. J. Org. Chem. 56, 395–400.

Wulff, G., Yan, M., Ramström, O., 2005. The covalent and other stoichiometric approaches. In: Yan, M., Ramström, O. (Eds.), Molecularly Imprinted Materials: Science and Technology. Dekker, New York, pp. 59–92.

Xinga, H., Wang, X., Sun, G., Gao, X., Xua, S., Wang, X., 2012. Effects of atrazine and chlorpyrifos on activity and transcription of glutathione S-transferase in common carp (*Cyprinus carpio* L.). Environ. Toxicol. Pharmacol. 33, 233–244.

Xu, S.S., Li, J., Chen, L., 2011. Molecularly imprinted core–shell nanoparticles for determination of trace atrazine by reversible addition-fragmentation chain transfer surface imprinting. J. Mater. Chem. 21, 4346–4351.

Yan, M., Ramström, O. (Eds.), 2005. Molecularly Imprinted Materials: Science and Technology. Marcel Dekker, New York, USA, pp. 395–418.

Yao, G.H., Liang, R.P., Huang, C.F., Wang, Y., Qiu, J.D., 2013. Surface plasmon resonance sensor based on magnetic molecularly imprinted polymers amplification for pesticide recognition. Anal. Chem. 85, 11944–11951.

Zhang, G., Pan, J., 2011. Simultaneous spectrophotometric determination of atrazine and cyanazine by chemometric methods. J. Spectrochim. Acta 78, 238–242.

Zhang, W., Asiri, A.M., Liu, D., Du, D., Lin, Y., 2014. Nanomaterial-based biosensors for environmental and biological monitoring of organophosphorus pesticides and nerve agents. Trends Anal. Chem. 54, 1–10.

Zhang, W.J., Jiang, F.B., Ou, J.F., 2011. Global pesticide consumption and pollution: with China as a focus. Proc. Intl. Acad. Ecol. Environ. Sci. 1, 125–144.

Zhao, G., Song, S., Wang, C., Wu, Q., Wang, Z., 2011. Determination of triazine herbicides in environmental water samples by high-performance liquid chromatography using graphene-coated magnetic nanoparticles as adsorbent. Anal. Chim. Acta 708, 155–159.

Zhao, N., Chen, C., Zhou, J., 2012. Surface plasmon resonance detection of ametryn using a molecularly imprinted sensing film prepared by surface-initiated atom transfer radical polymerization. Sens. Actuat. B 166–167, 473–479.

Zhou, D., Guo, T., Yang, Y., Zhang, Z., 2011. Surface imprinted macroporous film for high performance protein recognition in combination with quartz crystal microbalance. Sens. Actuat. B 153, 96–102.

19

SCIENTOMETRIC OVERVIEW IN NANOPESTICIDES

Ozcan Konur
Yildirim Beyazit University, Faculty of Engineering and Natural Sciences, Department of Materials Engineering, Keçiören Ankara, Turkey

1 Overview

1.1 Issues

The field of pesticides has been one of the most dynamic research fields in recent years with a focus on the causal relationships between pesticide exposure and human and animal health, with over 68,000 papers as indexed by the Science Citation Index–Expanded (SCIE) as of February 2016 (Anastassiades et al. 2003; Betarbet et al. 2000; Chiou et al. 1986; Henry et al. 2012; Isman 2006; Lehotay et al. 2010; Mullin et al. 2010; Rezaee et al. 2006; Tanner et al. 2011; Whitehorn et al. 2012).

Similarly, the field of nanomaterials and nanoprocesses has been one of the most dynamic research fields with a focus on carbon nanotubes, graphene, fullerenes, MoS_2 transistors, plasmonics, and solar nanomaterials in recent years, with over 1,000,000 papers as indexed by the SCIE as of February 2016 (Atwater and Polman, 2010; Bae et al., 2010; Dreyer et al., 2010; Geim and Novoselov, 2007; Iijima, 1991; Kroto et al. 1985; Novoselov et al., 2004; Oregan and Gratzel, 1991; Radisavljevic et al., 2011; Yella et al. 2011).

At the intersection of these research fields, a new specialized research field on nanopesticides, focusing on the detection and extraction of pesticides through the use of nanomaterials and nanoprocesses, has emerged in recent years with just over 2000 papers (Aragay et al. 2012; Basheer et al. 2006; Chen et al. 2010; Joshi et al. 2005; Kiso et al. 2001; Lin and Lu, 2004; Liu and Lin, 2005, 2006; Liu et al. 2012; Wang et al. 2011; Wu et al. 2011; Xie et al. 2010).

There have been many scientometric studies relating to research in nanomaterials and nanoprocesses (Hullmann and Meyer, 2003; Porter et al. 2008; Rafols and Meyer, 2010; Schummer, 2004).

New Pesticides and Soil Sensors. http://dx.doi.org/10.1016/B978-0-12-804299-1.00020-5

However, there has been only one scientometric study on pesticides in general, despite the huge public importance of this field (Sinha, 2012).

Therefore, it is not surprising that there have been no scientometric studies on nanopesticides as indexed by the SCIE as of February 2016, as in the fields of nanomaterials and nanoprocesses, pesticides, and others (Baltussen and Kindler 2004a,b; Dubin et al. 1993; Gehanno et al. 2007; Konur 2011, 2012a–o, 2013, 2014, 2015a–m, 2016a–l; Paladugu et al. 2002; Wrigley and Matthews 1986).

As North's New Institutional Theory highlights, it is important to have up-to-date information about current public policy issues to develop a set of viable solutions to satisfy the needs of all key stakeholders relating to nanopesticides (North 1994; Konur, 2000, 2002a–c, 2006a–b, 2007a–b, 2012c–d).

Brief information on a selected set of 25 citation classics in the field of nanopesticides is presented following a brief scientometric overview of the research in pesticides in general, nanomaterials and nanoprocesses, and nanopesticides in particular to inform key stakeholders as the first-ever study of its kind.

1.2 Methodology

The search for relevant materials was carried out in two major steps using v.5.21 of the Web of Science in February 2016.

In the first step, a broad search was carried out for the underlying research fields of nanomaterials and nanoprocesses and pesticides.

The relevant search set for nanomaterials and nanoprocesses was "TS = (*nano* or *graphene* or "quantum* *dot*" or *fullerene* or *silicene* or pcbm or pc71bm or "pc(71)bm") NOT TS = (*nanog* or *nanokelvin* or *nanoamper* or *nanomolar* or *nanomole* or nanolit* or Nano3 or nanoplankton or nonanonym* or nonanomal*) Timespan: All years. Indexes: SCI-EXPANDED, SSCI", while the relevant search set for pesticides was "TS = (*pesticide*) Timespan: All years. Indexes: SCI-EXPANDED, SSCI".

Key bibliometric data was extracted from these search activities, focusing on reviews and articles as the final set of references.

In the second step, these search sets were intersected to find references for the field of nanopesticides.

The most highly cited 25 papers were arranged in order of decreasing number of citations. Summary information about the located citation classics is presented in order of decreasing number of citations for the arranged topical areas, respectively.

Information relating to document type, affiliation of the authors, number and gender of the authors, country of the authors, journal in which the paper was published, subject area of the journal in which the paper was indexed, concise topic of the paper, and total number of citations received for the paper for the Web of Science databases was given in a table for each paper.

1.3 Pesticide Research in General—Overview

Using keywords related to pesticides, 75,519 references were located; 68,532 of these references were articles and reviews. Meeting abstracts, editorial materials, news items, and letters, as well as other works, formed the remaining part of the sample. 4195 papers were also presented at the conferences.

The most prolific three authors, Barcelo D., Barr D.B., and Li J., produced 307, 185, and 183 papers, respectively. The list of the most prolific authors was dominated by European, Chinese, and US authors. In total, 44,158 authors contributed to pesticide research.

The most prolific country in terms of number of publications was the United States, with 17,778 papers forming 26.0% of the sample. China, Spain, India, Germany, and Canada followed the United States with 10.8, 7.0, 5.6, 5.2, and 5.1% of the sample, respectively. Europe dominated the most prolific country list.

English was the dominant language of scientific communication in this field, comprising 95.4% of the sample, while German, Japanese, and Portuguese were the other major languages.

The most prolific national or regional institutions were the University of California system, the United States Department of Agriculture, the University of California system, the Chinese Academy of Sciences, the United States Environmental Protection Agency, and the Centre National de la Recherche Scientifique, with 1919, 1851, 1424, 1202, and 1080 citations, respectively.

Similarly, the most prolific single institutions were the University of California–Davis, the University of North Carolina, the China Agricultural University, the Universidade de São Paulo, and the University of Florida, with 775, 589, 516, 509, and 501 citations, respectively. The US institutions dominated the most-prolific institution list. In total, 7758 institutions contributed to the research in this area.

Like nanomaterials research, research in the field of pesticides has boomed since 1990, comprising 95.8% of the sample. There was a general increasing trend in the number of papers over time, starting with 268 papers in 1980 and reaching a peak with 4811 papers in 2015. There was a significant rise in 1991, possibly due to the inclusion of abstracts in abstract pages of indices for the first time. The publication rates were 4.2, 20.0, 37.5, and 38.2% for the 1980s, 1990s, 2000s, and 2010s, respectively.

The most prolific journals in terms of the number of publications were *Chemosphere*, the *Journal of Chromatography A*, the *Journal of Agricultural and Food Chemistry*, *Environmental Science Technology*, and *Science of the Total Environment*, with 1974, 1880, 1340, 1213, and 1158 citations, respectively. It is notable that journals related to the environment dominated the top journal list. In total, 3043 journals published papers on pesticides.

The most prolific subject categories in terms of the number of publications were Environmental Sciences, Chemistry Analytical, Toxicology, Entomology, and Food Science Technology, with 20,966, 16,025, 15,733, 7,414, and 4,865 citations, respectively. In total, papers were indexed under 211 subject categories, showing the huge diversity in categories.

The most cited papers in this field were dominated by the detection and extraction of pesticides as well as the impact of exposure to pesticides on human health in a number of areas. For example, Betarbet et al. (2000) discuss the causal relationships between pesticide exposure and Parkinson's disease with 1834 citations. This top paper was followed by Anastassiades et al. (2003), Rezaee et al. (2006), Isman (2006), and Chiou et al. (1986) focusing on the determination of pesticide residues in produce; determination of organic compounds; botanical insecticides, deterrents, and repellents; and water solubility enhancement, respectively.

There was a similar trend for the hottest papers published in the 2010s, but the focus has been more on the impact of pesticide exposure on humans and honeybees. For example, the hottest paper, with 254 citations, was related to the analysis of pesticide residues in fruits and vegetables (Lehotay et al. 2010). Tanner et al. (2011), Henry et al. (2012), Mullin et al. (2010), and Whitehorn et al. (2012) followed the hottest paper, focusing on causal relationships between pesticide exposure and Parkinson's disease, causal relationships between pesticide exposure and productivity in honeybees, causal relationships between pesticide exposure and the health of honeybees, and causal relationships between pesticide exposure and productivity in honeybees, respectively.

1.4 Nanomaterials and Nanoprocesses Research in General—Overview

Using the keywords related to nanomaterials and nanoprocesses, 1,093,647 references were located; 1,031,976 of these references were articles and reviews. Meeting abstracts, news items, and corrections, as well as other works, formed the remaining part of the.

The most prolific three authors, Zhang Y., Wang Y., and Liu Y., produced 5560, 5558, and 5358 papers, respectively. The list of the most prolific authors was dominated by Chinese and US authors.

The most prolific country in terms of number of publications was China, with 256,734 papers forming 24.9% of the sample. The United States closely followed China with 217,755 papers forming 21.1% of the papers. Japan, Germany, South Korea, and India were the other most prolific countries with 8.0, 7.5, 6.0, and 5.5% of the papers, respectively. It is surprising that China surpassed the United States in this field.

English was the dominant language of scientific communication in this field, comprising 97.9% of the sample. Chinese was the other key language with 1.5% of the sample.

The most prolific national or regional institutions were the Chinese Academy of Sciences, the Centre National de la Recherche Scientifique, the United States Department of Energy, the Russian Academy of Sciences, and the University of California system, with 55,689, 34,951, 24,649, 23,347, and 22,698 citations, respectively.

On the other hand, the most prolific single institutions were Tsinghua University, the Indian Institute of Technology, Zhejiang University, Nanyang Technological University, and the National University of Singapore with 10,378, 9,696, 8,320, 8,238, and 8,110 citations, respectively.

Nanomaterial research has boomed since 1990, comprising 99.8% of the sample with the seminal paper on the nanomaterials by Iijima (1991). There was a general increasing trend in the number of papers over time, starting with 143 papers in 1980 and reaching a peak with 129,788 papers in 2015.

Research from the 1980s, 1990s, 2000s, and 2010s comprised 0.2, 3.9, 34.2, and 60.8% of the sample, respectively with a significant rise (more than threefold) in 1991, possibly due to the inclusion of abstracts in abstract pages of indices for the first time.

The most prolific journals in terms of the number of publications were *Applied Physics Letters*, *Physical Review B*, the *Journal of Applied Physics*, the *Journal of Physical Chemistry C*, and *RSC Advances* with 25,156, 23,365, 17,532, 16,409, and 14,379 citations, respectively. It is notable that the top journals in this field relate to physics, not nanoscience and nanotechnology.

The most prolific subject categories were Materials Science Multidisciplinary, Physics Applied, Chemistry Physical, Chemistry Multidisciplinary, and Nanoscience Nanotechnology, with 302,224, 215,007, 206,755, 165,474, and 152,240 citations, respectively.

Perhaps the most important finding from these data is that only 14.8% of the papers were indexed under the subject category of Nanoscience and Nanotechnology, providing justification for the development of the search strategy outside this subject category through the keyword search.

The most cited papers in nanomaterials were dominated by carbon nanotubes, graphene, fullerenes, and solar nanomaterials. For example, Iijima (1991) discusses carbon nanotubes in a seminal paper with 25,170 citations. This top paper was followed by Novoselov et al. (2004), Oregan and Gratzel (1991), Geim and Novoselov (2007), and Kroto et al. (1985) focusing on graphene, solar cells, graphene, and fullerenes, with 20,143, 15,494, 14,706, and 9,607 citations, respectively.

There was a similar trend for the hottest papers in nanomaterials published in the 2010s. For example, the hottest paper with 3123 citations was related to graphene oxide (Dreyer et al. 2010). Yella et al. (2011), Atwater and Polman (2010), Bae et al. (2010), and Radisavljevic et al. (2011) followed the hottest paper focusing on solar cells, plasmonics, graphene films, and MoS_2 transistors, with 3113, 3040, 2875, and 2504 citations, respectively.

1.5 Research on Nanopesticides in General—Overview

Using keywords related to nanopesticides, 2312 references were located; 2174 of these references were articles and reviews. This finding suggests that this field has been a specialized field of research with relatively a small sample size and with a specific set of shareholders such as authors, institutions, and countries etc.

The most prolific three authors, Du D., Lin Y.H., and Wang C., produced 49, 36, and 33 papers, respectively. The list of the most prolific authors was dominated by Chinese and the US authors. In total, 1799 authors produced two or more papers.

The most prolific country in terms of the number of publications was China, with 944 papers forming 40.8% of the sample. The United States, India, and Iran followed China with 13.3, 8.7, and 5.5% of the sample, respectively. It seems that China surpassed the United States significantly in terms of the number of publications in this field. However, Europe dominated the most prolific country list. In total, 83 countries produced two or more papers in this field.

English was the dominant language of scientific communication in this field with 97.8% of the sample. The other key language was Chinese with 1.6% of the sample.

The most prolific single institution was the Central China Normal University with 76 papers. China Agricultural University, the Universidade de São Paulo, the Indian Institute of Technology, Jilin University, and Hebei Agricultural University followed the top institution, with 52, 31, 30, 30, and 29 citations, respectively.

On the other hand, the Chinese Academy of Sciences, the Council of Scientific Industrial Research, the United States Department of Energy, the Pacific Northwest National Laboratory, and Consejo Superior de Investigaciones Cientificas were the most prolific national or regional institutions, with 121, 42, 38, 33, and 31 citations, respectively. In total, 722 institutions published two or more papers in this field.

Unlike general nanomaterials research booming after 1991, research in the field of nanopesticides has boomed only in the 2010s, comprising 79.0% of the sample. Additionally, 20.4% of the research papers were published in the 2000s with a further 0.5% published in the 1990s. These findings suggest that research in this field has been relatively recent and, more importantly, will continue to gain importance in the near future.

The most prolific journal in terms of the number of publications was *Biosensors Bioelectronics,* publishing 76 papers. *Talanta,* the *Journal of Chromatography A, Sensors and Actuators B Chemical, Analytica Chimica Acta,* and *Analytical Methods* followed the top journal with 75, 71, 69, 56, and 55 citations, respectively. It is notable that the top journal list was dominated by journals related to sensors and analytical chemistry. In total, 230 journals published two or more papers in this field.

The most prolific subject category in terms of the number of publications was Chemistry Analytical, with 852 papers forming 36.9% of the sample. Chemistry Multidisciplinary, Environmental Sciences, Electrochemistry, Engineering Chemical, and Nanoscience Nanotechnology followed the top subject category with 13.0, 12.5, 12.2, 9.6, and 8.7% of the sample, respectively. In total, papers were indexed under 66 subject categories, highlighting the interdisciplinarity of this research field.

The citation impact of the papers published in this field has been significant, with 17.4 citations per paper and an H-index of 82.

The most cited papers in this field were dominated by applications of nanomaterials and nanoprocesses in the detection and extraction of pesticides. For example, Liu and Lin (2006) discuss nanobiosensors based on self-assembling acetylcholinesterase (AChE) on carbon nanotubes in a paper with 260 citations. This top paper was followed by Liu and Lin (2005), Lin and Lu (2004), Basheer et al. (2006), Kiso et al. (2001), and Joshi et al. (2005)

focusing on nanoelectrochemical sensors using zirconia nanoparticles as selective sorbents, disposable carbon nanotube modified screen-printed nanobiosensors, porous membrane-protected carbon nanotube microsolid-phase extraction, rejection of aromatic pesticides with nanofiltration membranes, and disposable nanobiosensors based on carbon nanotubes modified thick film strip electrodes, respectively.

There was a similar trend for the hottest papers published in the 2010s. For example, the hottest paper with 131 citations was related to graphene-coated solid-phase microextraction fibers (Chen et al., 2010). Wu et al. (2011), Xie et al. (2010), Wang et al. (2011), Aragay et al. (2012), and Liu et al. (2012) were the other hottest top papers relating to graphene-based magnetic nanocomposites, gold nanoparticle modified glassy carbon electrodes, gold nanoparticle-graphene nanosheet hybrids, nanomaterials in general, and gold nanoparticles, respectively.

2 Nanopesticides

2.1 The Most Cited Papers in Nanopesticides—Overview

The field of nanopesticides has been one of the most dynamic research areas in recent years with 25 citation classics. These citation classics were located and key emerging issues from these papers were presented under two main headings in the decreasing order of the number of citations (Table 19.1).

Lin Y.H. was the most prolific author with five papers. The other most prolific authors were Wang J. and Du D. with four and three papers, respectively. Chen W., Joshi K.A., Kiso Y., Kitao T., Liu G.D., Mulchandani A., Nishimura K., Van Der Bruggen B., Vandecasteele C., and Wang Z. published two papers each. In total, 99 authors contributed to these 25 citation classics in this field. Thus, the average number of authors per paper was nearly four.

China was the most prolific country with 10 papers, closely followed by the United States with eight papers. Belgium, Germany, Japan, Poland, and South Korea published two papers each. On the other hand, Croatia, England, India, Singapore, and Spain had one paper each. In total, 12 countries contributed to these 25 citation classics in this field. The average number of papers per country was nearly 0.5.

Central China Normal University and New Mexico State University were the most prolific individual institutions with three papers each. These were followed by Arizona State University, the Toyohashi University of Technology, and the University of

Table 19.1 Citation Classics in Nanopesticides

No.	Paper Reference	Year	Document	Affiliation	Country	Number of Authors	M/F	Journal	Subject Area	Topic	Total Number of Citations WS
1	Liu & Lin	06	A	Pacific NW Natl. Lab.	United States	2	M	Anal. Chem.	Chem. Anal.	Carbon nanotube biosensors	260
2	Liu & Lin	06	A	Pacific NW Natl. Lab.	United States	2	M	Anal. Chem.	Chem. Anal.	Electrochemical sensors	223
3	Lin et al.	04	A	Pacific NW Natl. Lab., New Mexico State Univ.	United States	3	M	Electroanalysis	Chem. Anal., Electrochem.	Carbon nanotube biosensors	161
4	Basheer et al.	06	A	Natl Univ. Singapore, Pune Univ.	India, Singapore	5	M	Anal. Chem.	Chem. Anal.	Carbon nanotube microsolid-phase extraction	153
5	Kiso et al.	01	A	Toyohashi Univ. Technol.	Japan	4	M	J. Membr. Sci.	Eng. Chem., Polym. Sci.	Nanofiltration membranes	140
6	Joshi et al.	05	A	Univ. Calif Riverside, New Mexico State Univ.	United States	6	M	Electroanalysis	Chem. Anal., Electrochem.	Carbon nanotube biosensors	137
7	Chen et al.	10	A	Xiamen Univ. +1	China, S. Korea	8	F	Anal. Chim. Acta	Chem. Anal.	Graphene-coated solid-phase microextraction fiber	131

(Continued)

Table 19.1 Citation Classics in Nanopesticides (*cont.*)

No.	Paper Reference	Year	Document	Affiliation	Country	Number of Authors	M/F	Journal	Subject Area	Topic	Total Number of Citations WS
8	Deo et al.	05	A	New Mexico State Univ., Ernst Moritz Arndt Univ. Greifswald +2	United States, Poland, Germany	9	M	Anal. Chim. Acta	Chem. Anal.	Carbon nanotube biosensors	128
9	Kiso et al.	00	A	Toyohashi Univ. Technol.	Japan	4	M	J. Membr. Sci.	Eng. Chem., Polym. Sci.	Nanofiltration membranes	123
10	Wu et al.	11	A	Agr. Univ. Hebei	China	5		J. Chromatogr. A	Bioch. Res. Meth., Chem. Anal.	Graphene-based magnetic nanocomposites	120
11	Xie et al.	10	A	W Anhui Univ., Chinese Acad. Sci.	China	5	M	Anal. Chem.	Chem. Anal.	Gold nanoparticle modified glassy carbon electrode	118
12	Wang et al.	11	A	Tsinghua Univ., Pacific NW Natl. Lab. +1	China, United States	9	F	J. Mater. Chem.	Chem. Phys., Mats. Sci. Mult.	Gold nanoparticles-graphene nanosheet hybrids	110
13	Van der Bruggen et al.	98	A	Katholieke Univ. Leuven	Belgium	5	M	Desalination	Eng. Chem., Water Res.	Nanofiltration	110
14	Van der Bruggen et al.	01	A	Katholieke Univ. Leuven	Belgium	5	M	Desalination	Eng. Chem., Water Res.	Nanofiltration	108
15	Wang et al.	07	A	Wuhan Univ., Univ. Bristol	China, England	5	F	J. Colloid Interface Sci.	Chem. Phys.	Oil-in-water nanoemulsions	99

16	Du et al.	07	A	Cent China Normal Univ. +1	China	4	F	Biosens. Bioelectron.	Biophy., Ciot. Appl. Microb., Chem. Anal., Electrochem., Nanosci. Nanotech.	Gold nanoparticles embedded in sol–gel film	99
17	Yoon et al.	07	A	Arizona State Univ. +3	S. Korea, United States	5	M	Desalination	Eng. Chem., Water Res.	Nanofiltration and ultrafiltration membranes	99
18	Jiang et al.	08	A	Zhejiang Univ., Univ. Arkansas	China, United States	7	M	Biosens. Bioelectron.	Biophy., Ciot. Appl. Microb., Chem. Anal., Electrochem., Nanosci. Nanotech.	Immunosensors	98
19	Aragay et al.	12	R	Catalan Inst. Nanotechnol. +1	Spain	3	F	Chem. Rev.	Chem. Mult.	Nanomaterials for sensing	95
20	Liu et al.	12	A	Chinese Acad. Sci. +1	China	6	M	Anal. Chem.	Chem. Anal.	Gold nanoparticles	94
21	Kosutic et al.	05	A	Univ. Zagreb	Croatia	4	M	Sep. Purif. Technol.	Eng. Chem.	Nanofiltration membranes	94
22	Viswanathan et al.	09	A	Polish Acad. Sci.	Poland	3	M	Biosens. Bioelectron.	Biophy., Ciot. Appl. Microb., Chem. Anal., Electrochem., Nanosci. Nanotech.	Electrochemical biosensor	93
23	Berg et al.	97	A	Univ. Duisburg	Germany	3	M	Desalination	Eng. Chem., Water Res.	Nanofiltration	92

(Continued)

Table 19.1 Citation Classics in Nanopesticides (*cont.*)

No.	Paper Reference	Year	Document	Affiliation	Country	Number of Authors	M/F	Journal	Subject Area	Topic	Total Number of Citations WS
24	Du et al.	08	A	Cent China Normal Univ. +1	China	6	F	Biosens. Bioelectron.	Biophy., Ciot. Appl. Microb., Chem. Anal., Electrochem., Nanosci. Nanotech.	Multiwalled carbon nanotubes	89
25	Sun Wang	10	A	Shandong Univ. Technol.	China	2	F	Biosens. Bioelectron.	Biophy., Ciot. Appl. Microb., Chem. Anal., Electrochem., Nanosci. Nanotech.	Acetylcholinesterase biosensors	86

A, Article; R, review; M, male; F, female.

California–Riverside with two papers each. In total, 24 individual institutions contributed to these citation classics.

On the other hand, at the national or regional basis, the most prolific institutions were the Pacific Northwest National Laboratory and the United States Department of Energy, with five papers each. These are followed by the Chinese Academy of Sciences and the University of California system with two papers each. In total, 17 such institutions contributed to these citation classics.

The most prolific publication year was 2005, when four papers were published. This was followed by 2007 and 2010 with three papers each. There were two papers published in each of the years 2001, 2006, 2008, 2011, and 2012. In 1997, 1998, 2000, 2004, and 2009, one paper was published in each year. Thus, it is significant to note that these citation classics have been relatively recent.

The most prolific journal was *Analytical Chemistry* with five papers, closely followed by *Biosensors Bioelectronics* with four papers. *Desalination* and the *Journal of Membrane Science* published three papers each, while *Analytica Chimica Acta* and *Electroanalysis* had two papers each. Additionally, five journals published one paper each. In total, 12 journals published these citation classics. Thus, the average number of papers per journal was nearly two.

The most prolific subject category was Chemistry Analytical with 14 papers, nearly half of the total papers. This was followed by Electrochemistry and Engineering Chemical, with seven papers each. Additionally, Biophysics, Biotechnology Applied Microbiology, and Nanoscience Nanotechnology had four papers each. In total, 12 subject categories had these citation classics. Thus, the average number of papers per category was nearly two.

The citation impact of these classical papers was significant with 123 citations per paper and an H-index of 25. The number of citations ranged from 86 to 260 for the Web of Science database.

There was a significant gender deficit among these papers, as there were only 7 out of 24 papers with a female first author out.

Only two of these classical papers were reviews in this field, while 23 of them were articles.

These classical papers were grouped under three major headings: general studies on the use of nanomaterials and processes on pesticides including the nanoextraction of pesticides (general studies—nanoextraction), nanosensors for the detection of pesticides (nanosensors), and nanofiltration of pesticides (nanofiltration).

In the following part, brief information on the most cited papers will be provided under these major topical headings.

2.2 The Most Cited Papers in Nanopesticides—Nanobiosensors

Liu and Lin (2006) discuss nanobiosensors based on self-assembling AChE on carbon nanotubes (CNTs) in a paper originating from the United States with 260 citations. AChE is immobilized on the negatively charged CNT surface by alternatively assembling a cationic poly(diallyldimethylammonium chloride) (PDDA) layer and an AChE layer. The electrocatalytic activity of CNT leads to a greatly improved electrochemical detection of the enzymatically generated thiocholine product. The developed PDDA/AChE/PDDA/CNT/GC nanobiosensor integrated into a flow injection system was used to monitor organophosphate pesticides and nerve agents, such as paraoxon. Under the optimal conditions, the biosensor was used to measure as low as 0.4 pM paraoxon with a 6-min inhibition time. The biosensor had excellent operational lifetime stability with no decrease in the activity of enzymes for more than 20 repeated measurements over a 1-week period.

Liu and Lin (2005) discuss electrochemical nanosensors using zirconia (ZrO_2) nanoparticles as selective sorbents in a paper originating from the United States with 223 citations. Zirconia nanoparticles were electrodynamically deposited onto the polycrystalline gold electrode by cyclic voltammetry. Nitroaromatic organophosphates strongly bind to the ZrO_2 nanoparticle surface. The authors find that the stripping voltammetric response is highly linear over the 5–100 ng/mL (ppb) methyl parathion range examined, with a detection limit of 3 ng/mL and good precision. The detection limit was improved to 1 ng/mL by using 10-min adsorption time.

Lin and Lu (2004) discuss carbon nanotube modified screen-printed nanobiosensors in a paper originating from the United States with 161 citations. They find that these nanobiosensors using acetycholinesterase (AChE)/choline oxidase (CHO) enzymes provided a high sensitivity, large linear range, and low detection limits for the analysis of organophosphate compounds. The authors reason that this is due to the catalytic activity of carbon nanotube to promote the redox reaction of hydrogen peroxide produced during AChE/CHO enzymatic reactions with their substrate, as well as the large surface area of carbon nanotube materials.

Joshi et al. (2005) discuss nanobiosensors based on carbon nanotubes modified thick filmstrip electrodes in a paper originating from the United States with 1337 citations. They find that the large surface area and electrocatalytic activity of carbon nanotubes lowered the overpotential for thiocholine oxidation to

200 mV without the use of mediating redox species and enzyme immobilization by physical adsorption. The biosensor detected as low as 0.5 nM (0.145 ppb) of the model organophosphate nerve agent paraoxon with good precision, electrode-to-electrode reproducibility, and stability.

Deo et al. (2005) discuss carbon nanotube (CNT)/organophosphorus hydrolase (OPH) electrochemical nanobiosensors in a paper originating from Germany, Poland, and the United States with 128 citations. A bilayer approach with the OPH layer atop of the CNT film was used for preparing the CNT/OPH biosensor. They find that the CNT layer leads to a greatly improved anodic detection of the enzymatically generated p-nitrophenol product, including higher sensitivity and stability. Under the optimal conditions, the biosensor measured as low as 0.15 muM paraoxon and 0.8 muM methyl parathion with sensitivities of 25 and 6 nA/muLM, respectively.

Xie et al. (2010) discuss electropolymerized poly(p-aminothiophenol) (PATP) membranes on a gold nanoparticle (AuNP) modified glassy carbon (gc) electrodes in a paper originating from China with 118 citations. They find that the cyclic voltammetric response of the imprinted PATP-AuN-P-gc sensor to pesticide is about 3.2-fold as compared with the imprinted PATP-Au sensor, and the detection limit for pesticide is about two orders of magnitude lower than that by the imprinted PATP-Au sensor. An excellent electrochemical selectivity for CPF over other pesticides was also achieved. The authors assert that the combination of surface molecular self-assembly with electropolymerized molecular imprinting on a larger surface area of an AuNP-modified electrode produces a high ratio of imprinted sites and, thus, provides an ultrasensitive electrochemical detection of organophosphate pesticide.

Wang et al. (2011) discuss the self-assembly of AChE on a gold nanoparticles (AuNPs)–graphene nanosheet (cr-Gs) hybrid in a paper originating from China and the United States with 110 citations. An enzyme nanoassembly (AChE/AuNPs/cr-Gs) was prepared by self-assembling AChE on Au NP/cr-Gs nanohybrid. An electrochemical sensor based on AChE/Au NPs/cr-Gs was further developed for ultrasensitive detection of organophosphate pesticide. The authors find that the developed approach provides a promising strategy to improve the sensitivity and enzyme activity of electrochemical biosensors.

Du et al. (2007) discuss gold nanoparticles (AuNPs) with AChE on silica sol–gel (SiSG) film in a paper originating from China with 99 citations. The large quantities of hydroxyl groups in the sol–gel composite provided a biocompatible microenvironment around the enzyme molecule and stabilized its biological activity to a large extent. The immobilized AChE could catalyze the hydrolysis of acetylthiocholine chloride (ATCI) to form thiocholine. AuNPs catalyzed the electrooxidation of thiocholine, thus increasing detection sensitivity. The authors find that the inhibition of monocrotophos was proportional to its concentration ranging from 0.001 to 1 μg/mL and 2 to 15 μg/mL. The detection limit was 0.6 ng/mL at a 10% inhibition.

Jiang et al. (2008) discuss immunonanosensors in a paper originating from China and the United States with 98 citations. They present an overview of various transduction systems, such as electrochemical, optical, piezoelectric, and nanomechanics methods, used in the design and fabrication of immunosensors for pesticide detection. The authors then evaluate the techniques of regeneration, signal amplification, miniaturization, and antibodies for the development and applications of these immunosensors.

Aragay et al. (2012) discuss nanomaterials for sensing and destroying pesticides in general in a review paper originating from Spain with 95 citations.

Liu et al. (2012) discuss the rhodamine B-covered gold nanoparticle (RB-AuNP)-based assays in a paper originating from China with 94 citations. They note that the detection mechanism is based on the fact that these pesticides can inhibit the activity of AChE, thus preventing the generation of thiocholine. This assay allows detection of pesticides in real samples such as agricultural products and river water. The results in detecting pesticide residues collected from food samples via this method are consistent with those from high-performance liquid chromatography (HPLC).

Viswanathan et al. (2009) discuss nanobiosensors based on AChE with carbon nanotubes (CNTs) in a paper originating from Poland with 93 citations. The self-assembled monolayers (SAMs) of single-walled carbon nanotubes (SWCNT) wrapped by thiol-terminated single strand oligonucleotide (ssDNA) on gold were utilized to prepare nano size polyaniline matrix for AChE enzyme immobilization. The key step of this biosensor was an AChE-acetylcholine enzymatic reaction, which causes the small changes of local pH in the vicinity of an electrode surface. The authors find that the dynamic range for the determination of methyl parathion and chlorpyrifos was between 1.0×10^{-11} and 1.0×10^{-6} M with good reproducibility and stability, while the detection limit of the biosensor for both pesticides was 1×10^{-12} M.

Sun and Wang (2010) discuss AChE nanobiosensors based on a Prussian blue (PB)-modified electrode modifying glassy carbon electrode (GCE) in a paper originating from China with 86 citations. The authors find that the chitosan membrane as carrier can absorb a large amount of enzyme, and PB has a significant synergistic effect toward enzymatic catalysis. As a result of these two important enhancement factors, the proposed biosensor exhibited extreme sensitivity to OP pesticides compared to the other kinds of AChE biosensor. The authors further find that under optimum conditions, the inhibition rates of these pesticides were proportional to their concentrations while the detection limits were 2.5 ng L^{-1} for dichlorvos, 15 ng L^{-1} for omethoate, 5 ng L^{-1} for trichlorfon, and 10 ng L^{-1} for phoxim.

2.3 The Most Cited Papers in Nanopesticides—Nanofiltration

Kiso et al. (2001) discuss the rejection of a number of aromatic pesticides with nanofiltration (NF) membranes in a paper originating from Japan with 140 citations. They find that the highest desalting membrane rejected all pesticides at > 92.4%, except tricyclazole. Although the other membranes showed lower rejections, some pesticides were rejected at very high rates by all membranes. The authors reason that all the pesticides are adsorbed on the membranes and adsorption properties were controlled by both hydrophobicity and the molecular shape of the solute. They conclude that steric hindrance is an important factor for solute permeation even in the case of hydrophobic pesticides.

Kiso et al. (2000) discuss rejection of a number of nonphenylic pesticides with nanofiltration membranes in a paper originating from Japan with 123 citations. They find that the membrane with the highest desalting degree rejected all pesticides except dichlorvos at more than 96.7% while the other membranes showed a rather less effective property, and that chlorpyrifos was rejected at a very high rate by all membranes. They further find that the rejection was influenced mainly by hydrophobicity and all pesticides adsorbed on the membranes, and that the adsorption was controlled by hydrophobicity of the pesticide.

Van der Bruggen et al. (1998) discuss nanofiltration of pesticides from ground waters for four pesticides and four membranes in a paper originating from Belgium with 110 citations. They find that NF-70 is a suitable membrane for the removal of pesticides. They argue that the size of the molecule is the most important parameter, and may be represented by molecular weight or more accurately by a molecular diameter calculated from the molecular structure. They further find that a higher dipole moment results in a lower retention while the matrix of the groundwater caused an increase of the pesticide retention, resulting in a decrease of the water flux through the membrane.

Van der Bruggen et al. (2001) discuss nanofiltration of four pesticides with four membranes in a paper originating from Belgium with 108 citations. They find that pesticide rejections are satisfactory and that hardness is also very efficiently removed, whereas only a small fraction of nitrate is removed for most membranes, except for NF70. The authors then discuss the economics of nanofiltration. Price calculations at different pressures resulted in an optimal pressure of 8 bar. They argue that the final price for treatment of groundwater is realistic, suggesting that nanofiltration is a valuable option for groundwater treatment.

Yoon et al. (2007) discuss nanofiltration of endocrine disrupting compounds (EDCs) and pharmaceuticals and personal care products (EDC/PPCPs) from various drinking water sources in a paper originating from the United States and South Korea with 99 citations. They find a general separation trend due to hydrophobic adsorption as a function of octanol–water partition coefficient between hydrophobic compounds and the porous hydrophobic membrane during membrane filtration. They further find that both hydrophobic adsorption and size exclusion mechanisms are dominant to retain EDC/PPCP for the NF membrane, while the UF membrane retained typically hydrophobic EDC/PPCPs due mainly to hydrophobic adsorption.

Kosutic et al. (2005) discuss the nanofiltration of pesticides and arsenic from drinking water in a paper originating from Croatia with 94 citations. They find that the rejection of the sodium dibasic arsenate as well as the arsenate anion from the natural groundwater by the nanofiltration membranes are satisfactorily high, and one of the nanofiltration membranes exhibits superior permeation rate values. The authors reason that the prevailing mechanism of ion retention by negatively charged nanotiltration membranes is the charge exclusion. The size exclusion mechanism is also important but not sufficient for the uncharged organic molecules rejection while the membrane material and the membrane pore size distribution (PSD) also influence the uncharged organic molecules rejection.

Berg et al. (1997) discuss the nanofiltration of pesticides in a paper originating from Germany with 92 citations. They find that the rejection of uncharged trace organics is mainly influenced by steric hindrances while the high rejection of polar trace organics can be explained by electrostatic interactions with the charged membrane surface. As the dissociation of polar organics and the surface charge of the membrane depend on pH value, the authors further find that rejection increases with increased pH. At neutral pH values, which are normal in the drinking water treatment, a nearly complete rejection of polar organics was observed.

2.4 The Most-Cited Papers in Nanopesticides—Other Studies Including Nanoextraction

Basheer et al. (2006) discuss multiwalled carbon nanotube (MWCNT) microsolid-phase extraction (mu-SPE) in a paper originating from India and Singapore with 153 citations. A 6-mg sample of MWCNTs was packed inside a sheet of porous polypropylene membrane. The mu-SPE device, which was wetted with dichloromethane, was then placed in a stirred sewage sludge sample solution to extract organophosporous pesticides. The authors find that the π–π electrostatic interaction with the analytes and the large surface area of MWCNTs facilitated the adsorption of analytes, with good selectivity and reproducibility. The method showed good linearity, repeatability of the extractions, and low limits of detection.

Chen et al. (2010) discuss graphene (G)-coated solid-phase microextraction (SPME) fibers through extraction of six pyrethroid pesticides in a paper originating from China and South Korea with 131 citations. They find that although the thickness of G-coated fiber was only 6–8 μm, its extraction efficiencies were higher than those of two commercial fibers. They attribute this high extraction efficiency to the huge delocalized π-electron system of G, which shows strong π-stacking interaction with pyrethroid pesticide. The method developed was successfully applied to three pond water samples, and the recoveries were 83–110% with a spike of 1 μg L^{-1}.

Wu et al. (2011) discuss graphene-based magnetic nanocomposites as an effective adsorbent in a paper originating from China with 120 citations. They find that this nanocomposite showed great adsorptive ability toward the analytes. The method takes advantage of both nanoparticle adsorption and magnetic phase separation from the sample solution. Under optimum conditions, the enrichment factors of the method for analytes were in the range from 474 to 868. Compared with the dispersive liquid–liquid microextraction and the ultrasound assisted–surfactant enhanced emulsification microextraction, the authors assert that much higher enrichment factors and sensitivities were achieved with this method.

Wang et al. (2007) discuss oil-in-water (O/W) nanoemulsions in system water/poly(oxyethylene) nonionic surfactant/methyl decanoate in a paper originating from England and China with 99 citations. They find that bluish transparent nanoemulsions were formed only when the concentrate was located in the bicontinuous microemulsion (BC) or oil-in-water microemulsion (Wm) region. They note that both the phase behavior and the composition of the concentrate are important factors in nanoemulsion formation.

Du et al. (2008) discuss multiwalled carbon nanotubes (MWCNTs) as a new sorbent for solid-phase extraction (SPE) of organophosphate (OP) pesticides. They find that a combination of SPE with square-wave voltammetric (SWV) analysis resulted in a fast, sensitive, and selective electrochemical method for determination of OP pesticide using methyl parathion (MP) as a representative. Due to the strong affinity of MWCNT for the phosphoric group, the authors reason that nitroaromatic OP compounds can strongly bind to the MWCNT surface. The macroporosity and heterogeneity of MWCNT allow the extraction of a large amount of MP in less than 5 min.

3 Conclusions

The field of nanopesticides has emerged as a distinct research area in recent years, building on the underlying research areas of nanomaterials and nanoprocesses and pesticides in general. Thus, this new research field shows strong signs of interdisciplinarity booming in the 2010s.

The sensing of pesticides through the use of nanobiosensors (nanobiosensing), extraction of pesticides through the use of a number of nanomaterials and processes (nanoextraction), and the nanofiltration of pesticides using nanomembranes and a number of nanoprocesses (nanofiltration) emerged as the key research subfields.

These citation classics deal with important health and nutrition-related research issues with strong public policy implications since the exposure to pesticides has adverse effects on human and animal health as evidenced in studies on pesticides in general.

The citation classics presented in this paper were helpful in highlighting important papers influencing the development of the research field as well as in determining the key research areas in this field.

Further research is recommended for detailed studies including scientometric studies and citation classic studies in combination with corresponding studies in the underlying research fields with a special emphasis on nanobiosensing, nanofiltration, and nanoextraction of pesticides to minimize the adverse effects of pesticides on both human and animal health.

References

Anastassiades, M., Lehotay, S.J., Stajnbaher, D., Schenck, F.J., 2003. Fast and easy multiresidue method employing acetonitrile extraction/partitioning and "dispersive solid-phase extraction" for the determination of pesticide residues in produce. J. AOAC Int. 86 (2), 412–431.

Aragay, G., Pino, F., Merkoci, A., 2012. Nanomaterials for sensing and destroying pesticides. Chem. Rev. 112 (10), 5317–5338.

Atwater, H.A., Polman, A., 2010. Plasmonics for improved photovoltaic devices. Nat. Mater. 9 (3), 205–213.

Bae, S., Kim, H., Lee, Y., Xu, X.F., Park, J.S., Zheng, Y., et al., 2010. Roll-to-roll production of 30-inch graphene films for transparent electrodes. Nat. Nanotechnol. 5 (8), 574–578.

Baltussen, A., Kindler, C.H., 2004a. Citation classics in anesthetic journals. Anesth. Analg. 98, 443–451.

Baltussen, A., Kindler, C.H., 2004b. Citation classics in critical care medicine. Intensive Care Med. 30, 902–910.

Basheer, C., Ainedhary, A.A., Rao, B.S.M., Valliyaveettil, S., Lee, H.K., 2006. Development and application of porous membrane-protected carbon nanotube micro-solid-phase extraction combined with gas chromatography/ mass spectrometry. Anal. Chem. 78 (8), 2853–2858.

Berg, P., Hagmeyer, G., Gimbel, R., 1997. Removal of pesticides and other micropollutants by nanofiltration. Desalination 113 (2–3), 205–208.

Betarbet, R., Sherer, T.B., MacKenzie, G., Garcia-Osuna, M., Panov, A.V., Greenamyre, J.T., 2000. Chronic systemic pesticide exposure reproduces features of Parkinson's disease. Nat. Neurosci. 3 (12), 1301–1306.

Chen, J.M., Zou, J., Zeng, J.B., Song, X.H., Ji, J.J., Wang, Y.R., et al., 2010. Preparation and evaluation of graphene-coated solid-phase microextraction fiber. Anal. Chim. Acta 678 (1), 44–49.

Chiou, C.T., Malcolm, R.L., Brinton, T.I., Kile, D.E., 1986. Water solubility enhancement of some organic pollutants and pesticides by dissolved humic and fulvic-acids. Environ. Sci. Technol. 20 (5), 502–508.

Deo, R.P., Wang, J., Block, I., Mulchandani, A., Joshi, K.A., Trojanowicz, M., et al., 2005. Determination of organophosphate pesticides at a carbon nanotube/ organophosphorus hydrolase electrochemical biosensor. Anal. Chim. Acta 530 (2), 185–189.

Dreyer, D.R., Park, S., Bielawski, C.W., Ruoff, R.S., 2010. The chemistry of graphene oxide. Chem. Soc. Rev. 39 (1), 228–240.

Du, D., Chen, S., Cai, J., Zhang, A., 2007. Immobilization of acetylcholinesterase on gold nanoparticles embedded in sol–gel film for amperometric detection of organophosphorous insecticide. Biosens. Bioelectron. 23 (1), 130–134.

Du, D., Wang, M.H., Zhang, J.M., Cai, H., Tu, H.Y., Zhang, A.D., 2008. Application of multiwalled carbon nanotubes for solid-phase extraction of organophosphate pesticide. Electrochem. Commun. 10 (1), 85–89.

Dubin, D., Hafner, A.W., Arndt, K.A., 1993. Citation-classics in clinical dermatological journals: Citation analysis, biomedical journals, and landmark articles 1945–1990. Arch. Dermatol. 129, 1121–1129.

Gehanno, J.F., Takahashi, K., Darmoni, S., Weber, J., 2007. Citation classics in occupational medicine journals. Scand. J. Work Environ. Health 33, 245–251.

Geim, A.K., Novoselov, K.S., 2007. The rise of graphene. Nat. Mater. 6 (3), 183–191.

Henry, M., Beguin, M., Requier, F., Rollin, O., P. Odoux, J.F., et al., 2012. A common pesticide decreases foraging success and survival in honey bees. Science 336 (6079), 348–350.

Hullmann, A., Meyer, M., 2003. Publications and patents in nanotechnology—an overview of previous studies and the state of the art. Scientometrics 58 (3), 507–527.

Iijima, S., 1991. Helical microtubules of graphitic carbon. Nature 354 (6348), 56–58.

Isman, M.B., 2006. Botanical insecticides, deterrents, and repellents in modern agriculture and an increasingly regulated world. Ann. Rev. Entomol. 51, 45–66.

Jiang, X.S., Li, D.Y., Xu, X., Ying, Y.B., Li, Y.B., Ye, Z.Z., et al., 2008. Immunosensors for detection of pesticide residues. Biosens. Bioelectron. 23 (11), 1577–1587.

Joshi, K.A., Tang, J., Haddon, R., Wang, J., Chen, W., Mulchandani, A., 2005. A disposable biosensor for organophosphorus nerve agents based on carbon nanotubes modified thick film strip electrode. Electroanalysis 17 (1), 54–58.

Kiso, Y., Nishimura, Y., Kitao, T., Nishimura, K., 2000. Rejection properties of non-phenylic pesticides with nanofiltration membranes. J. Membr. Sci. 171 (2), 229–237.

Kiso, Y., Sugiura, Y., Kitao, T., K. Nishimura, K., 2001. Effects of hydrophobicity and molecular size on rejection of aromatic pesticides with nanofiltration membranes. J. Membr. Sci. 192 (1–2), 1–10.

Konur, O., 2000. Creating enforceable civil rights for disabled students in higher education: an institutional theory perspective. Disabil. Soc. 15, 1041–1063.

Konur, O., 2002a. Assessment of disabled students in higher education: current public policy issues. Assess. Eval. Higher Educ. 27, 131–152.

Konur, O., 2002b. Access to employment by disabled people in the UK: Is the Disability Discrimination Act working? Int. J. Discrimin. Law 5, 247–279.

Konur, O., 2002c. Access to Nursing Education by disabled students: rights and duties of Nursing programs. Nurse Educ. Today 22, 364–374.

Konur, O., 2006a. Participation of children with dyslexia in compulsory education: current public policy issues. Dyslexia 12, 51–67.

Konur, O., 2006b. Teaching disabled students in Higher Education. Teach. Higher Educ. 11, 351–363.

Konur, O., 2007a. A judicial outcome analysis of the Disability Discrimination Act: a windfall for the employers? Disabil. Soc. 22, 187–204.

Konur, O., 2007b. Computer-assisted teaching and assessment of disabled students in Higher Education: the interface between academic standards and disability rights. J. Comput. Assist. Learn. 23, 207–219.

Konur, O., 2011. The scientometric evaluation of the research on the algae and bio-energy. Appl. Energy 88, 3532–3540.

Konur, O., 2012a. 100 citation classics in Energy and Fuels. Energy Educ. Sci. Technol. Part A 30 (si 1), 319–332.

Konur, O., 2012b. What have we learned from the citation classics in Energy and Fuels: a mixed study. Energy Educ. Sci. Technol. Part A 30 (si 1), 255–268.

Konur, O., 2012c. The gradual improvement of disability rights for the disabled tenants in the UK: the promising road is still ahead. Soc. Polit. Econ. Cult. Res. 4, 71–112.

Konur, O., 2012d. The policies and practices for the academic assessment of blind students in higher education and professions. Energy Educ. Sci. Technol. Part B 4 (si 1), 240–244.

Konur, O., 2012e. Prof. Dr. Ayhan Demirbas' scientometric biography. Energy Educ. Sci. Technol. Part A 28, 727–738.

Konur, O., 2012f. The evaluation of the research on the biofuels: a scientometric approach. Energy Educ. Sci. Technol. Part A 28, 903–916.

Konur, O., 2012g. The evaluation of the research on the biodiesel: a scientometric approach. Energy Educ. Sci. Technol. Part A 28, 1003–1014.

Konur, O., 2012h. The evaluation of the research on the bioethanol: a scientometric approach. Energy Educ. Sci. Technol. Part A 28, 1051–1064.

Konur, O., 2012i. The evaluation of the research on the microbial fuel cells: a scientometric approach. Energy Educ. Sci. Technol. Part A 29, 309–322.
Konur, O., 2012j. The evaluation of the research on the biohydrogen: a scientometric approach. Energy Educ. Sci. Technol. Part A 29, 323–338.
Konur, O., 2012k. The evaluation of the biogas research: a scientometric approach. Energy Educ. Sci. Technol. Part A 29, 1277–1292.
Konur, O., 2012l. The scientometric evaluation of the research on the production of bio-energy from biomass. Biomass Bioenerg. 47, 504–515.
Konur, O., 2012m. The evaluation of the global energy and fuels research: a scientometric approach. Energy Educ. Sci. Technol. Part A 30, 613–628.
Konur, O., 2012n. The evaluation of the biorefinery research: a scientometric approach. Energy Educ. Sci. Technol. Part A 30 (si 1), 347–358.
Konur, O., 2012o. The evaluation of the bio-oil research: a scientometric approach. Energy Educ. Sci. Technol. Part A 30 (si 1), 379–392.
Konur, O., 2013. What have we learned from the research on the International Financial Reporting Standards (IFRS)? A mixed study. Energy Educ. Sci. Technol. Part D 5, 29–40.
Konur, O., 2014. The periodical research on the experiences of the college students with ADHD: a mixed study. Int. J. Res. Teacher Educ. 5, 12–33.
Konur, O., 2015a. Algal biosorption of heavy metals from wastes. In: Kim, S.K., Lee, C.G. (Eds.), Marine Bioenergy: Trends and Developments. CRC Press, Boca Raton, Florida, pp. 597–626.
Konur, O., 2015b. Algal economics and optimization. In: Kim, S.K., Lee, C.G. (Eds.), Marine Bioenergy: Trends and Developments. CRC Press, Boca Raton, Florida, pp. 691–716.
Konur, O., 2015c. Algal high-value consumer products. In: Kim, S.K., Lee, C.G. (Eds.), Marine Bioenergy: Trends and Developments. CRC Press, Boca Raton, Florida, pp. 653–682.
Konur, O., 2015d. Algal photobioreactors. In: Kim, S.K., Lee, C.G. (Eds.), Marine Bioenergy: Trends and Developments. CRC Press, Boca Raton, Florida, pp. 81–108.
Konur, O., 2015e. Algal photosynthesis, biosorption, biotechnology, and biofuels. In: Kim, .S.K. (Ed.), Springer Handbook of Marine Biotechnology. Springer, Berlin, Heidelberg, Germany, pp. 1131–1161.
Konur, O., 2015f. Current state of research on algal biodiesel. In: Kim, S.K., Lee, C.G. (Eds.), Marine Bioenergy: Trends and Developments. CRC Press, Boca Raton, Florida, pp. 487–512.
Konur, O., 2015g. Current state of research on algal bioelectricity and algal microbial fuel cells. In: Kim, S.K., Lee, C.G. (Eds.), Marine Bioenergy: Trends and Developments. CRC Press, Boca Raton, Florida, pp. 527–556.
Konur, O., 2015h. Current state of research on algal bioethanol. In: Kim, S.K., Lee, C.G. (Eds.), Marine Bioenergy: Trends and Developments. CRC Press, Boca Raton, Florida, pp. 217–244.
Konur, O., 2015i. Current state of research on algal biohydrogen. In: Kim, S.K., Lee, C.G. (Eds.), Marine Bioenergy: Trends and Developments. CRC Press, Boca Raton, Florida, pp. 393–422.
Konur, O., 2015j. Current state of research on algal biomethane. In: Kim, S.K., Lee, C.G. (Eds.), Marine Bioenergy: Trends and Developments. CRC Press, Boca Raton, Florida, pp. 273–302.
Konur, O., 2015k. Current state of research on algal biomethanol. In: Kim, S.K., Lee, C.G. (Eds.), Marine Bioenergy: Trends and Developments. CRC Press, Boca Raton, Florida, pp. 327–370.
Konur, O., 2015l. The scientometric study of the global energy research. In: Prasad, R., Sivakumar, S., Sharma, U.C. (Eds.), Energy Science and Technology. V.1. Opportunities and Challenges. Studium Press LLC, Houston, TX, pp. 475–489.

Konur, O., 2015m. The review of citation classics on the global energy research. In: Prasad, R., Sivakumar, S., Sharma, U.C. (Eds.), Energy Science and Technology. V.1. Opportunities and Challenges. Studium Press LLC, Houston, TX, pp. 490–526.

Konur, O., 2016a. Scientometric overview regarding antimicrobial nanobiomaterials. In: Grumezescu, A.M. (Ed.), Applications of Nanobiomaterials. Volume VI: Nanobiomaterials in Antimicrobial Therapy. Elsevier, Amsterdam.

Konur, O., 2016b. Scientometric overview regarding surface chemistry of nanobiomaterials. In: Grumezescu, A.M. (Ed.), Applications of Nanobiomaterials. Volume 3: Surface Chemistry of Nanobiomaterials. Elsevier, Amsterdam, pp. 463–486.

Konur, O., 2016c. Scientometric overview regarding nanobiomaterials in dentistry. In: Grumezescu, A.M. (Ed.), Applications of Nanobiomaterials. Volume 11: Nanobiomaterials in Dentistry. Elsevier, Amsterdam.

Konur, O., 2016d. The scientometric overview in nanobiodrugs. In: Grumezescu, A. (Ed.), Nanoarchitectonics for Smart Delivery and Drug Targeting. Elsevier, Amsterdam.

Konur, O., 2016e. The scientometric overview in cancer targeting. In: Grumezescu, A. (Ed.), Nanoarchitectonics for Smart Delivery and Drug Targeting. Elsevier, Amsterdam.

Konur, O., 2016f. Scientometric overview regarding water nanopurification. In: Grumezescu, A. (Ed.), Nanotechnology in Food Industry: Water Purification. Academic Press, Elsevier.

Konur, O., 2016g. The hot papers in the surface engineering of nanobiomaterials. In: Grumezescu, A. (Ed.), Therapeutic Nanostructures. Volume 1: General Approach. Elsevier, Amsterdam.

Konur, O., 2016h. The recent citation classics in antimicrobial nanobiomaterials. In: Grumezescu, A. (Ed.), Therapeutic Nanostructures. Volume 3: Antimicrobials. Elsevier, Amsterdam.

Konur, O., 2016i. Glycoscience: the current state of the research. In: Kim, S.K. (Ed.), Marine Glycobiology: Principles and Applications, Part 1. Introduction to Marine Glycobiology. CRC Press, Boca Raton, Florida.

Konur, O., 2016j. Algal Omics: the current state of the research. In: Kim, S.K. (Ed.), Marine Omics: Principles and Applications. Part 1. Introduction to Marine Omics. CRC Press, Boca Raton, Florida.

Konur, O., 2016k. The citation classics in algal enzymes. In: Kim, S.K. (Ed.), AFNR: Marine Enzymes Biotechnology: Production and Industrial Applications. Part II - Marine Organisms Producing Enzymes. Elsevier, Amsterdam.

Konur, O., 2016l. Scientometric overview in food nanopreservation. In: Grumezescu, A.M. (Ed.), Nanotechnology in the Agro-Food Industry: Food Preservation. Elsevier, Amsterdam.

Kosutic, K., Furac, L., Sipos, L., Kunst, B., 2005. Removal of arsenic and pesticides from drinking water by nanofiltration membranes. Sep. Purif. Technol. 42 (2), 137–144.

Kroto, H.W., Heath, J.R., Obrien, S.C., Curl, R.F., Smalley, R.E., 1985. C_{60}: Buckminsterfullerene. Nature 318 (6042), 162–163.

Lehotay, S.J., Son, K.A., Kwon, H., Koesukwiwat, U., Fu, W.S., Mastovska, K., et al., 2010. Comparison of QuEChERS sample preparation methods for the analysis of pesticide residues in fruits and vegetables. J. Chromatogr. A 1217 (16), 2548–2560.

Lin, Y.H., Lu, F., Wang, J., 2004. Disposable carbon nanotube modified screen-printed biosensor for amperometric detection of organophosphorus pesticides and nerve agents. Electroanalysis 16 (1–2), 145–149.

Liu, G.D., Lin, Y.H., 2005. Electrochemical sensor for organophosphate pesticides and nerve agents using zirconia nanoparticles as selective sorbents. Anal. Chem. 77 (18), 5894–5901.
Liu, G.D., Lin, Y.H., 2006. Biosensor based on self-assembling acetylcholinesterase on carbon nanotubes for flow injection/amperometric detection of organophosphate pesticides and nerve agents. Anal. Chem. 78 (3), 835–843.
Liu, D.B., Chen, W.W., Wei, J.H., Li, X.B., Wang, Z., Jiang, X.Y., 2012. A highly sensitive, dual-readout assay based on gold nanoparticles for organophosphorus and carbamate pesticides. Anal. Chem. 84 (9), 4185–4191.
Mullin, C.A., Frazier, M., Frazier, J.L., Ashcraft, S., Simonds, R., vanEngelsdorp, D., et al., 2010. High levels of miticides and agrochemicals in North American apiaries: implications for honey bee health. PLoS One 5 (3).
North, D., 1994. Economic-performance through time. Am. Econ. Rev. 84, 359–368.
Novoselov, K.S., Geim, A.K., Morozov, S.V., Jiang, D., Zhang, Y., Dubonos, S.V., et al., 2004. Electric field effect in atomically thin carbon films. Science 306 (5696), 666–669.
Oregan, B., Gratzel, M., 1991. A low-cost, high-efficiency solar-cell based on dye-sensitized colloidal TiO_2 films. Nature 353 (6346), 737–740.
Paladugu, R., Chein, M.S., Gardezi, S., Wise, L., 2002. One hundred citation classics in general surgical journals. World J. Surg. 26, 1099–1105.
Porter, A.L., Youtie, J., Shapira, P., Schoeneck, D.J., 2008. Refining search terms for nanotechnology. J. Nanopart. Res. 10 (5), 715–728.
Radisavljevic, B., Radenovic, A., Brivio, J., Giacometti, V., Kis, A., 2011. Single-layer MoS_2 transistors. Nat. Nanotechnol. 6 (3), 147–150.
Rafols, I., Meyer, M., 2010. Diversity and network coherence as indicators of interdisciplinarity: case studies in bionanoscience. Scientometrics 82 (2), 263–287.
Rezaee, M., Assadi, Y., Hosseinia, M.R.M., Aghaee, E., Ahmadi, F., Berijani, S., 2006. Determination of organic compounds in water using dispersive liquid–liquid microextraction. J. Chromatogr. A 1116 (1–2), 1–9.
Schummer, J., 2004. Multidisciplinarity, interdisciplinarity, and patterns of research collaboration in nanoscience and nanotechnology. Scientometrics 59 (3), 425–465.
Sinha, B., 2012. Global biopesticide research trends: a bibliometric assessment. Indian J. Agric. Sci. 82 (2), 95–101.
Sun, X., Wang, X.Y., 2010. Acetylcholinesterase biosensor based on Prussian blue-modified electrode for detecting organophosphorous pesticides. Biosens. Bioelectron. 25 (12), 2611–2614.
Tanner, C.M., Kamel, F., Ross, G.W., Hoppin, J.A., Goldman, S.M., Korell, M., et al., 2011. Rotenone, paraquat, and Parkinson's Disease. Environ. Health Perspect. 119 (6), 866–872.
Van der Bruggen, B., Schaep, J., Maes, W., Wilms, D., Vandecasteele, C., 1998. Nanofiltration as a treatment method for the removal of pesticides from ground waters. Desalination 117 (1–3), 139–147.
Van der Bruggen, B., Everaert, K., Wilms, D., Vandecasteele, C., 2001. Application of nanofiltration for removal of pesticides, nitrate and hardness from ground water: Rejection properties and economic evaluation. J. Membr. Sci. 193 (2), 239–248.
Viswanathan, S., Radecka, H., Radecki, J., 2009. Electrochemical biosensor for pesticides based on acetylcholinesterase immobilized on polyaniline deposited on vertically assembled carbon nanotubes wrapped with ssDNA. Biosens. Bioelectron. 24 (9), 2772–2777.
Wang, L.J., Li, X.F., Zhang, G.Y., Dong, J.F., Eastoe, J., 2007. Oil-in-water nanoemulsions for pesticide formulations. J. Colloid Interface Sci. 314 (1), 230–235.

Wang, Y., Zhang, S., Du, D., Shao, Y.Y., Li, Z.H., Wang, J., et al., 2011. Self assembly of acetylcholinesterase on a gold nanoparticles-graphene nanosheet hybrid for organophosphate pesticide detection using polyelectrolyte as a linker. J. Mater. Chem. 21 (14), 5319–5325.

Whitehorn, P.R., O'Connor, S., Wackers, F.L., Goulson, D., 2012. Neonicotinoid pesticide reduces bumble bee colony growth and queen production. Science 36 (6079), 351–352.

Wrigley, N., Matthews, S., 1986. Citation-classics and citation levels in geography. Area 18, 185–194.

Wu, Q.H., Zhao, G.Y., Feng, C., Wang, C., Wang, Z., 2011. Preparation of a graphene-based magnetic nanocomposite for the extraction of carbamate pesticides from environmental water samples. J. Chromatogr. A 1218 (44), 7936–7942.

Xie, C.G., Li, H.F., Li, S.Q., Wu, J., Zhang, Z.P., 2010. Surface molecular self-assembly for organophosphate pesticide imprinting in electropolymerized poly(p-aminothiophenol) membranes on a gold nanoparticle modified glassy carbon electrode. Anal. Chem. 82 (1), 241–249.

Yella, A., Lee, H.W., Tsao, H.N., Yi, C.Y., Chandiran, A.K., Nazeeruddin, M.K., et al., 2011. Porphyrin-sensitized solar cells with Cobalt (II/III)-based redox electrolyte exceed 12 percent efficiency. Science 334 (6056), 629–634.

Yoon, Y., Westerhoff, P., Snyder, S.A., Wert, E.C., J. Yoon, J., 2007. Removal of endocrine disrupting compounds and pharmaceuticals by nanofiltration and ultrafiltration membranes. Desalination 202 (1–3), 16–23.

INDEX